Vitamins and Elements

		Vitamin A (µg)[b,c]	Vitamin C (mg)	Vitamin D (µg)[d,e]	Vitamin E (mg)[f,g,h]	Vitamin K (µg)	Thiamin (mg)	Riboflavin (mg)	Niacin (mg)[h,i]	Vitamin B6 (mg)	Folate (µg)[h,j]
RDA or AI[1]											
Age 51-70	Male	**900**	**90**	10*	**15**	120*	**1.2**	**1.3**	**16**	**1.7**	**400**
	Female	**700**	**75**	10*	**15**	90*	**1.1**	**1.1**	**14**	**1.5**	**400**
Age 70+	Male	**900**	**90**	15*	**15**	120*	**1.2**	**1.3**	**16**	**1.7**	**400**
	Female	**700**	**75**	15*	**15**	90*	**1.1**	**1.1**	**14**	**1.5**	**400**
Tolerable Upper Intake Levels[a]											
Age 51-70	Male	3000	2000	50	1000	ND	ND	ND	35	100	1000
	Female	3000	2000	50	1000	ND	ND	ND	35	100	1000
Age 70+	Male	3000	2000	50	1000	ND	ND	ND	35	100	1000
	Female	3000	2000	50	1000	ND	ND	ND	35	100	1000

		Vitamin B12 (µg)[k]	Pantothenic Acid (mg)	Biotin (µg)	Choline (mg)[l]	Boron (mg)	Calcium (mg)	Chromium (µg)	Copper (µg)	Fluoride (mg)	Iodine (µg)
RDA or AI[1]											
Age 51-70	Male	**2.4**	5*	30*	550*	ND	1200*	30*	**900**	4*	**150**
	Female	**2.4**	5*	30*	425*	ND	1200*	20*	**900**	3*	**150**
Age 70+	Male	**2.4**	5*	30*	550*	ND	1200*	30*	**900**	4*	**150**
	Female	**2.4**	5*	30*	425*	ND	1200*	20*	**900**	3*	**150**
Tolerable Upper Intake Levels[a]											
Age 51-70	Male	ND	ND	ND	3500	20	2500	ND	10000	10	1100
	Female	ND	ND	ND	3500	20	2500	ND	10000	10	1100
Age 70+	Male	ND	ND	ND	3500	20	2500	ND	10000	10	1100
	Female	ND	ND	ND	3500	20	2500	ND	10000	10	1100

[1] Recommended Dietary Allowances (RDAs) are in **bold type** and Adequate Intakes (AIs) are in ordinary type followed by an asterisk (*).

ND - Indicates values not determined.

Footnotes

[a] UL = The maximum level of daily nutrient intake that is likely to pose no risk of adverse effects. Unless otherwise specified, the UL represents total intake from food, water, and supplements. Due to lack of suitable data, ULs could not be established for vitamin K, thiamin, riboflavin, vitamin B12, pantothenic acid, biotin, or carotenoids. In the absence of ULs, extra caution may be warranted in consuming levels above recommended intakes.

[b] As retinol activity equivalents (RAEs). 1 RAE = 1 µg retinol, 12 µg β-carotene, or 24 µg β-cryptoxanthin. To calculate RAEs from the REs of provitamin A carotenoids in foods, divide the REs by 2. For preformed vitamin A in foods or supplements and for provitamin A carotenoids in supplements, 1 RE = 1 RAE.

[c] ULs - As preformed vitamin A only.

[d] cholecalciferol. 1 µg cholecalciferol = 40 IU vitamin D.

[e] In the absence of adequate exposure to sunlight.

[f] as α-tocopherol. α-Tocopherol includes RRR-α-tocopherol, the only form of α-tocopherol that occurs naturally in foods, and the 2R-stereoisomeric forms of α-tocopherol (RRR-, RSR-, RRS-, and RSS-α-tocopherol) that occur in fortified foods and supplements. It does not include the 2S-stereoisomeric forms of α-tocopherol (SRR-, SSR-, SRS-, SSS-α-tocopherol), also found in fortified foods and supplements.

[g] ULs - as α-tocopherol; applies to any form of supplemental α-tocopherol.

[h] The ULs for vitamin E, niacin, and folate apply to synthetic forms obtained from supplements, fortified foods, or a combination of the two.

[i] As niacin equivalents (NE). 1 mg of niacin = 60 mg of tryptophan: 0-6 months = preformed niacin (not NE).

[j] As dietary folate equivalents (DFE). 1 DFE = 1 µg food folate = 0.6 µg of folic acid from fortified food or as a supplement consumed with food = 0.5 µg of a supplement taken on an empty stomach.

[k] Because 10 to 30 percent of older people may malabsorb food-bound B12, it is advisable for those older than 50 years to meet their RDA mainly by consuming foods fortified with B12 or a supplement containing B12.

[l] Although AIs have been set for choline, there are few data to assess whether a dietary supply of choline is needed at all stages of the life cycle, and it may be that the choline requirement can be met by endogenous synthesis at some of these stages.

[m] The ULs for magnesium represent intake from a pharmacological agent only and do not include intake from food and water.

[n] Although vanadium in food has not been shown to cause adverse effects in humans, there is no justification for adding vanadium to food and vanadium supplements should be used with caution. The UL is based on adverse effects in laboratory animals and this data could be used to set a UL for adults but not children and adolescents.

The values for this table were excerpted from the Institute of Medicine Food and Nutrition Board. *Dietary Reference Intakes: The Essential Guide to Nutrient Requirements.* Washington, DC: National Academy Press, 2006. The table was compiled by and is reprinted with permission of the National Resource Center on Nutrition and Aging at Florida International University.

National Resource Center on Nutrition and Aging, Florida International University, Revised 3/19/04

Nutrition *for the* Older Adult

Melissa Bernstein, PhD, RD, LD
Assistant Professor
Rosalind Franklin University of Medicine and Science

Ann Schmidt Luggen, PhD, GNP
Professor Emeritus
Northern Kentucky University

JONES AND BARTLETT PUBLISHERS
Sudbury, Massachusetts
BOSTON   TORONTO   LONDON   SINGAPORE

World Headquarters
Jones and Bartlett Publishers
40 Tall Pine Drive
Sudbury, MA 01776
978-443-5000
info@jbpub.com
www.jbpub.com

Jones and Bartlett Publishers
Canada
6339 Ormindale Way
Mississauga, Ontario L5V 1J2
Canada

Jones and Bartlett Publishers
International
Barb House, Barb Mews
London W6 7PA
United Kingdom

Jones and Bartlett's books and products are available through most bookstores and online booksellers. To contact Jones and Bartlett Publishers directly, call 800-832-0034, fax 978-443-8000, or visit our website, www.jbpub.com.

Substantial discounts on bulk quantities of Jones and Bartlett's publications are available to corporations, professional associations, and other qualified organizations. For details and specific discount information, contact the special sales department at Jones and Bartlett via the above contact information or send an email to specialsales@jbpub.com.

The authors, editor, and publisher have made every effort to provide accurate information. However, they are not responsible for errors, omissions, or for any outcomes related to the use of the contents of this book and take no responsibility for the use of the products and procedures described. Treatments and side effects described in this book may not be applicable to all people; likewise, some people may require a dose or experience a side effect that is not described herein. Drugs and medical devices are discussed that may have limited availability controlled by the Food and Drug Administration (FDA) for use only in a research study or clinical trial. Research, clinical practice, and government regulations often change the accepted standard in this field. When consideration is being given to use of any drug in the clinical setting, the health care provider or reader is responsible for determining FDA status of the drug, reading the package insert, and reviewing prescribing information for the most up-to-date recommendations on dose, precautions, and contraindications, and determining the appropriate usage for the product. This is especially important in the case of drugs that are new or seldom used.

Production Credits
Acquisitions Editor: Shoshanna Goldberg
Editorial Assistant: Kyle Hoover
Production Director: Amy Rose
Production Assistant: Julia Waugaman
Associate Marketing Manager: Jody Sullivan
V.P., Manufacturing and Inventory Control: Therese Connell
Composition: Publishers' Design and Production Services, Inc.
Cover and Title Page Design: Scott Moden
Photo Research and Permissions Manager: Kimberly Potvin
Assistant Photo Researcher: Bridget Kane
Cover and Title Page Image: © Pierdelune/ShutterStock, Inc.
Printing and Binding: Malloy Incorporated
Cover Printing: Malloy Incorporated

Library of Congress Cataloging-in-Publication Data
Bernstein, Melissa.
    Nutrition for the older adult / by Melissa Bernstein and Ann Schmidt Luggen.
        p. ; cm.
    Includes bibliographical references and index.
    ISBN 978-0-7637-3624-8 (pbk.)
    1. Older people—Nutrition. 2. Diet therapy for older people. 3. Older people—Nutrition.
I. Luggen, Ann Schmidt. II. Title.
    [DNLM: 1. Nutritional Physiological Phenomena. 2. Aged.   WT 115 B531n 2010]
    TX361.A3B47 2010
    613.2084'6—dc22
                                                        2009011050
6048

Printed in the United States of America
13 12 11 10 09   10 9 8 7 6 5 4 3 2 1

To the memory of my father, Stephen Allen, who continues to be a source of inspiration to me.

—Melissa Bernstein

This work is dedicated to my loving husband, Michael, who has been so supportive of all my books.

—Ann Schmidt Luggen

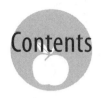

Contents

Preface

With the number of older adults on the rise, we are pleased to bring you *Nutrition for the Older Adult*, a book that fills a much needed role in the textbook market. Given the depth and breadth of the information available and the continually expanding, exciting research in the area of nutrition, this book serves as an introduction to the subject. It is our ambition to educate students and those working with older adults so that we can share the common goal of providing the highest quality nutritional care to promote healthy, successful aging for all adults.

This book serves as an introduction to older adult nutrition for both undergraduate nutrition students and graduate students seeking a broader nutrition knowledge for working with older adults. The book can also be utilized by health professionals who are active with older adults and interested in learning more about nutritional connections with the diseases and disorders common in this population.

The format of the book is basic and contains succinct chapters written by experts in the fields of nutrition and clinical health science. Each chapter is written so that it stands alone; however, it is best viewed in the context of the broader whole. To bring nutrition alive to the reader, we discuss actual patients and nutritional disorders that are seen in community and clinical settings throughout the text. The book is as current as possible in terms of the research and guidelines that the health care environment has available.

The basic fundamentals of nutrition as they apply to older adults are discussed so that students who are new to nutri-tion will be well grounded in this knowledge. The book contains essential nutrition information as a background for use by nutritionists who work in the many areas where older adults are seen. This book also has a chapter that discusses changes that commonly occur naturally with aging so that it is understood that disease is not a natural consequence of growing old. Further, the diseases that often occur in older adults are presented as well as nutritional elements that may contribute to the problems or are part of the treatment. To provide students with a comprehensive knowledge when working with this population, we have also included chapters on nutritional assessment and exercise, as well as nutrition services, health promotion, and cultural diversity. Many chapters include case studies, questions, and activities that will guide classroom discussion and independent study to reinforce learning. For current updates and more information as well as TestBanks and PowerPoints available for instructor access, please visit our textbook Web site at http://nutrition.jbpub.com/olderadults. Also on this Web site are numerous student resources, including a glossary, flashcards, crossword puzzles, and nutrition resources, including a BMI calculator, links to nutrition journals, healthy recipes, and nutrition science animations.

Finally, dear reader, student, and faculty, we are confident that this text will provide an improved learning base for you so that you may provide quality care to those older adults with whom we work and love.

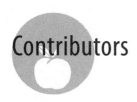

Contributors

Jill H. Arnold, PharmD
Clinical Pharmacy Specialist
Bath VAMC

Julie L. Baron, PharmD
Clinical Pharmacy Specialist–Primary Care
Kaiser Permanente, Ohio

Odilia I. Bermudez, PhD, MPH, LDN
Assistant Professor
Tufts University School of Medicine
Department of Public Health and Family Medicine

Bonnie L. Callen, RN, PhD, CPHCNS-BC
Assistant Professor
University of Tennessee
College of Nursing

Karen Chapman-Novakoski, RD, LDN, PhD
Professor, Nutrition
College of Agricultural, Consumer & Environmental
    Sciences
College of Medicine; Extension Specialist, Nutrition
University of Illinois, Urbana-Champaign
Editor-in-Chief, Journal of Nutrition Education and
    Behavior

Maria A. Fiatarone Singh, MD, FRACP
John Sutton Chair of Exercise and Sport Science
Discipline of Exercise, Health and Performance
Faculty of Health Sciences
Professor of Medicine
Faculty of Medicine
University of Sydney

Barbara Kamp, MS, RD

Timothy J. Legg, PhD, GNP-BC, CHES
Assistant Professor
College of Health Sciences
TUI University

Jacqueline Marcus, MS, RD, LD, FADA
Dietician, Nutritionist
Wellness.com®

Mary B. Neiheisel, BSN, MSN, EDD, CNS, APRN-FNP,
    FAANP
Professor of Nursing and Pfizer/Ardoin Endowed Professor
University of Louisiana at Lafayette
Nurse Practitioner
Faith House, Inc.

Susan Saffel-Shrier, MS, RD, CD, Certified Gerontologist
Associate Professor
Department of Family and Preventive Medicine
University of Utah School of Medicine

William S. Schwab III, MD, PhD, AGSF
Chief of Geriatrics, Ohio Permanente Medical Group

Joseph R. Sharkey, PhD, MPH, RD
Associate Professor, Social and Behavioral Health
Director, Texas Healthy Aging Research Network
Director, Program for Research in Nutrition and Health
    Disparities
School of Rural Public Health
Texas A&M Health Science Center

Kathy J. Shattler, MS, RD
Nutri-Care Consulting

Ardith L. Sudduth, PhD, GNP, FNP-BC
Assistant Professor
College of Nursing and Allied Health Profession
University of Louisiana at Lafayette
The Hamilton Medical Group Endowed Professorship in
    Nursing
Distinguished Professor University of Louisiana 2008

Colleen Tsarnas, MS, RD, CNSD, LDN
Clinical Dietitian
Thomas Jefferson University Hospital

CHAPTER 1

Introduction and Demographics of Aging

Melissa Bernstein, PhD, RD, LD and
Ann Schmidt Luggen, PhD, GNP

CHAPTER OBJECTIVES   Upon completion of this chapter, the reader will be able to:

1. Identify nutrition-related challenges facing the aging population
2. Identify nutritional recommendations for older adults based on the Dietary Guidelines for Americans and Healthy People 2010
3. Describe the modernization of the Older Americans Act in the area of health promotion for older adults
4. Describe the factors that affect the nutritional status of various ethnic groups
5. Discuss the preparation of the health care workforce to deliver services to older adults

KEY TERMS AND CONCEPTS

Administration on Aging (AoA)

Healthy People 2010

Modified MyPyramid for Older Adults

Old age

Eating is one of life's greatest pleasures; therefore, food is much more than a vehicle for promoting and protecting health. Unlike many disease factors, such as genetics, gender, and age, diet is a risk factor that can be changed positively (or negatively) to reduce (or increase) the risk of disease. Nutritional health throughout a lifetime influences how a person will age; in turn, the process of aging affects nutrition (**Figure 1-1**). Older adults are an extremely heterogeneous group and arrive at **old age** with dramatically different nutritional as well as health and social requirements. The challenges in meeting these requirements are as different as the older adults themselves. In addition, the population of older adults is rapidly growing in its ethnic and racial

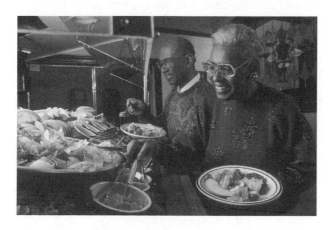

old age Often defined as ages nearing the average human lifespan. Although organizations providing services to older adults define their own age criteria, most people still think of old age as those adults ages 65 and older. Some organizations' minimum age requirements are:

- The Older Americans Act (OAA): 60 years
- USDA programs: 60 years
- DRIs: 51 to 70 years and 70+ years.
- Medicare: 65 years
- Social Security: 67 years
- AARP: 51 years

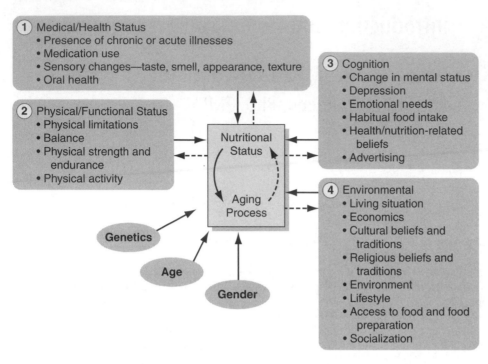

FIGURE 1-1 Factors That Influence Aging and Quality of Life

Source: Adapted from American Dietetic Association. Position paper of the American Dietetic Association: Nutrition across the spectrum of aging. *J Am Diet Assoc.* 2005; 105(4): 616–633.

diversity. This trend will continue in the United States as minority populations continue to increase. It is of utmost importance that older adults of all groups adopt healthy lifestyle practices and dietary habits to reduce the burden of chronic disease and maximize quality of life and healthy aging.

The population of older adults in the United States is growing and changing rapidly as the baby boomers enter their later years and become more entrenched within the older generation, with the "oldest old" becoming the most rapidly growing group. According to a report by the **Administration on Aging (AoA)** of the Department of Health and Human Services, the population aged 65 and older increased 11.2% or 3.8 million since 1997 to 37.9 million in 2007 and are ex-

Administration on Aging The Administration on Aging (AoA) is one of the nation's largest providers of home- and community-based care for older adults and their caregivers. It awards annual grants to state governments to support programs mandated by Congress in the Older Americans Act. The six core services funded by the AoA are: supportive services, nutrition services, preventive health services, the National Family Caregiver Support Program (NFCSP), services that protect the rights of vulnerable older adults, and services for Native Americans.

pected to increase to 55 million in 2020 (a 36% increase for that decade). By 2030, there will be approximately 72 million older persons, almost twice that in 2007 (**Figure 1-2**). Specifically, adults aged 65 and older represented 12.6% of the population in 2007, but are expected to grow to 19% of the population by 2030. In addition, the AoA projects that the population aged 85 and older will increase from 5.5 million in 2007 to 5.7 million in 2010, and then to 6.6 million in 2020, a 15% increase for that decade (**Figure 1-3**).

This emerging cohort of older adults aged 45 to 64 is better educated, better positioned financially, and more nutrition conscious than previous generations. **Table 1-1** provides U.S. Census characteristics from 2006 for adults aged 65 years and older. As people age, their ability to independently shop for, prepare, and eat an adequate diet decreases. In addition, older adults are living longer, with those 85 years and older at increased risk of being hospitalized or institutionalized and having or developing severe undernutrition. Therefore, nutrition is vitally important to maintaining a high quality of life and preventing chronic health problems.

In rural areas, the elderly population has increased, because older people are relocating to rural areas following retirement and those who have spent their lives in these

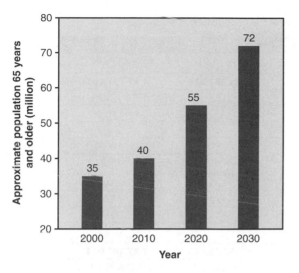

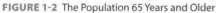

FIGURE 1-2 The Population 65 Years and Older

Source: Data from Department of Health and Human Services, Administration on Aging, Projected Future Growth of the Older Population. Available at http://www.aoa.gov/AoARoot/Aging_Statistics/future_growth/future_growth.aspx#age. Accessed May 6, 2009.

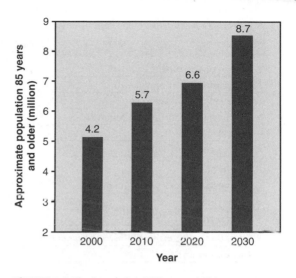

FIGURE 1-3 The Population 85 Years and Older

Source: Data from Department of Health and Human Services, Administration on Aging, Projected Future Growth of the Older Population. Available at http://www.aoa.gov/AoARoot/Aging_Statistics/future_growth/future_growth.aspx#age. Accessed May 6, 2009.

TABLE 1-1 Characteristics of the Population Aged 65 Years and Older in the United States

Subject	Total Population	65 Years and Older
Total population	**299,398,485**	**37,191,004**
Sex and Age		
Male	49.2%	42.0%
Female	50.8%	58.0%
Median age (years)	36.4	74.8
Race and Hispanic or Latino Origin		
One race	98.0%	99.3%
White	73.9%	85.1%
Black or African American	12.4%	8.3%
American Indian and Alaska Native	0.8%	0.5%
Asian	4.4%	3.2%
Native Hawaiian and other Pacific Islander	0.1%	0.1%
Some other race	6.3%	2.1%
Two or more races	2.0%	0.7%
Hispanic or Latino origin (of any race)	14.8%	6.3%
White alone, not Hispanic or Latino	66.2%	81.1%
Marital Status		
Population 15 years and older	**238,585,682**	**37,191,004**
Now married, except separated	50.4%	53.2%
Widowed	6.4%	31.7%
Divorced	10.5%	9.3%
Separated	2.3%	1.2%
Never married	30.5%	4.6%

(continues)

TABLE 1-1 Characteristics of the Population Aged 65 Years and Older in the United States (Cont.)

Subject	Total Population	65 Years and Older
Educational Attainment		
Population 25 years and older	**195,932,824**	**37,191,004**
Less than high school graduate	15.9%	27.2%
High school graduate (includes equivalency)	30.2%	34.5%
Some college or associate degree	26.9%	19.6%
Bachelor's degree or higher	27.0%	18.7%
Disability Status		
Civilian population 5 years and older	**273,835,465**	**35,570,460**
With any disability	15.1%	41.0%
No disability	84.9%	59.0%
Place of Birth, Citizenship Status, and Year of Entry		
Total population	**299,398,485**	**37,191,004**
Native	261,850,696	32,863,975
Foreign born	37,547,789	4,327,029
Entered 2000 or later	25.3%	6.5%
Entered 1990 to 1999	30.5%	13.0%
Entered before 1990	44.1%	80.6%
Naturalized U.S. citizen	42.0%	72.8%
Not a U.S. citizen	58.0%	27.2%
Language Spoken at Home and Ability to Speak English		
Population 5 years and older	**279,012,712**	**37,191,004**
English only	80.3%	86.1%
Language other than English	19.7%	13.9%
Speak English less than "very well"	8.7%	8.1%
Employment Status		
Civilian population 16 years and older	**233,254,741**	**37,191,004**
In labor force	64.8%	14.5%
Employed	60.7%	13.9%
Unemployed	4.2%	0.5%
Percent of civilian labor force	6.4%	3.7%
Not in labor force	35.2%	85.5%
Income in the Past 12 Months (in 2006 inflation-adjusted dollars)		
Households	**111,617,402**	**22,719,664**
With earnings	80.3%	32.9%
Mean earnings (dollars)	66,733	40,044
With Social Security income	26.8%	93.0%
Mean Social Security income (dollars)	13,877	14,936
With Supplemental Security Income	4.0%	5.7%
Mean Supplemental Security Income (dollars)	7,388	6,885
With cash public assistance income	2.4%	1.5%
Mean cash public assistance income (dollars)	3,139	3,246
With retirement income	17.4%	49.8%
Mean retirement income (dollars)	19,141	18,616
With Food Stamp benefits	8.1%	5.6%

(continues)

TABLE 1-1 Characteristics of the Population Aged 65 Years and Older in the United States (Cont.)

Subject	Total Population	65 Years and Older
Poverty Status in the Past 12 Months		
Population for whom poverty status is determined	**291,531,091**	**35,570,460**
Below 100 percent of the poverty level	13.3%	9.9%
100 to 149 percent of the poverty level	8.9%	12.0%
At or above 150 percent of the poverty level	77.8%	78.1%

Source: U.S. Census Bureau. American Community Survey. 2006. Available at: http://www.census.gov/acs/www/index.html. Accessed May 12, 2008.

areas are choosing to remain in their own homes. Approximately 20% of older adults in the United States live in rural areas. Older adults living in rural areas are more likely to suffer from poor health, have lower incomes, and have less education compared to their urban counterparts. Additionally, unhealthy behaviors, such as tobacco use, that damage health occur with greater frequency in rural populations. High alcohol consumption is another unhealthy behavior that is more prevalent in rural areas, especially among non-Hispanic Whites, Hispanics, and American Indians. Obesity is also a problem in these areas.

Demographics

Over 2.4 million persons celebrated their 65th birthday in 2007. In that year, nearly 1.8 million died. Older adults comprised 12.6% of the U.S. population in 2008, meaning that one in every eight Americans is over the age of 65. By 2030, older adults will make up 19.3% of the population. Conservative estimates predict that the number of adults 65 and older will grow from 35 million in 2000 to 40 million in 2010. The number of old-old (85+) will grow even more—from 4 million in 2000 to 5.7 million in 2010 (a 36% increase), then to 6.6 million (a 15% increase for that decade) in 2020.

Older women outnumber older men 21.9 million to 16 million. In rural areas, women constitute 53% of the rural population aged 60 to 64 and 63% of the rural population aged 85 and older. These statistics underscore the importance of ensuring adequate nutritional intake for all older adults as an essential factor for maintaining functional independence and for preventing malnutrition and related complications, such as increased susceptibility to illness, impaired immune function, and prolonged hospital stay.

Older adults often find it difficult to meet their nutritional needs because they have increased requirements for some nutrients and a decreased energy requirement. Numerous barriers to food intake complicate the task of maximizing nutrition in older adults (**Figure 1-4**). Multiple chronic and acute illnesses, changes in absorption and digestion, polyp-

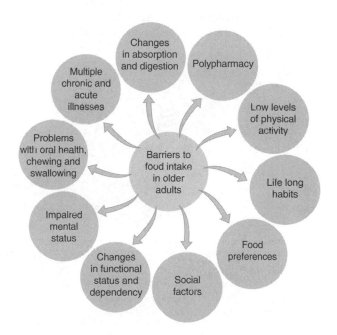

FIGURE 1-4 Barriers to Food Intake in Older Adults

harmacy, low levels of physical activity, lifelong habits and food preferences, social factors, changes in functional status and dependency, impaired mental status, and problems with oral health, chewing, and swallowing have all been shown to influence the eating habits and nutritional status of both institutionalized and noninstitutionalized older adults. Age-related complications that could potentially interfere with food intake emphasize the need for multiple food choices to maximize nutritional intake.

Dietary Guidance

Meeting the nutritional needs of older adults can be difficult because of the many age-related changes that interfere with optimal food intake. Emphasizing a nutritionally

Modified MyPyramid for Older Adults A modification of the MyPyramid educational tool that translates the principles of the 2005 Dietary Guidelines for Americans and other nutritional standards to help consumers age 70 and older in making healthier food and physical activity choices.

adequate and nutrient-dense diet is essential to promoting health and preventing nutrition-related complications that could contribute to increased functional dependency and frailty. Aging and age-related problems can impose significant barriers to achieving a healthy diet as defined by the Dietary Guidelines, which have been established for healthy Americans. With its focus on health promotion and risk reduction, the Dietary Guidelines currently forms the basis of federal food, nutri-

tion education, and information programs. The "well" older adults may benefit from the same dietary recommendations as those provided for the general adult population; however, the appropriateness of and ability to adhere to these recommendations may decrease as an individual becomes increasingly functionally dependent and frail.

Although the recommendations of the Dietary Guidelines for Americans and the USDA food pyramid, known as MyPyramid, are designed for all Americans over the age of 2 years, some modifications of MyPyramid are appropriate for those older than the age of 70 to optimize their nutrient intake, as shown in **Figure 1-5**. While maintaining MyPyramid's emphasis on vegetables and fruits, the **Modified MyPyramid for Older Adults** addresses the unique dietary needs of adults over 70 by emphasizing nutrient-dense food

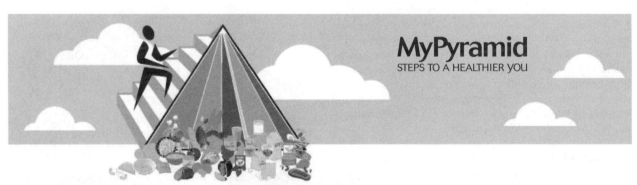

Based on the information you provided, this is your daily recommended amount from each food group.

GRAINS 5 ounces	VEGETABLES 2 cups	FRUITS 1 1/2 cups	MILK 3 cups	MEAT & BEANS 5 ounces
Make half your grains whole	**Vary your veggies**	**Focus on fruits**	**Get your calcium-rich foods**	**Go lean with protein**
Aim for at least **3 ounces** of whole grains a day	Aim for these amounts **each week:** **Dark green veggies** = 2 cups **Orange veggies** = 1 1/2 cups **Dry beans & peas** = 2 1/2 cups **Starchy veggies** = 2 1/2 cups **Other veggies** = 5 1/2 cups	Eat a variety of fruit Go easy on fruit juices	Go low-fat or fat-free when you choose milk, yogurt, or cheese	Choose low-fat or lean meats and poultry Vary your protein routine— choose more fish, beans, peas, nuts, and seeds

Find your balance between food and physical activity

Be physically active for at least **30 minutes** most days of the week.

Know your limits on fats, sugars, and sodium

Your allowance for oils is **5 teaspoons a day.**

Limit extras—solid fats and sugars—to **130 calories a day.**

Your results are based on a 1600 calorie pattern.   Name: _____

This calorie level is only an estimate of your needs. Monitor your body weight to see if you need to adjust your calorie intake.

FIGURE 1-5 MyPyramid for an Older Woman

Source: Courtesy of U.S. Department of Agriculture [www.mypyramid.gov]

Modified MyPyramid for Older Adults

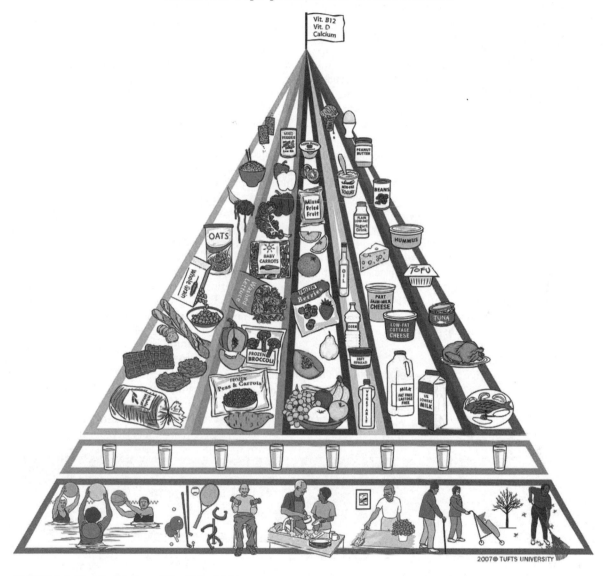

FIGURE 1-6 Modified MyPyramid for Older Adults

Source: Copyright 2007 Tufts University. Reprinted with permission from Lichenstein AH, Rasmussen H, Yu WW, Epstein SR, Russel RM. Modified MyPyramid for Older Adults. *J Nutr.* 2008; 138:78–82.

choices and the importance of fluid balance (**Figure 1-6**). The Modified MyPyramid for Older Adults also provides additional guidance about forms of foods that could best meet the unique needs of older adults and stresses the importance of regular physical activity.

The Modified MyPyramid for Older Adults emphasizes the importance of choosing adequate amounts of fiber-rich foods, focusing on whole-grain products and whole fruits and vegetables rather than their highly refined and processed forms. Food choices that are easier to prepare, that have a longer shelf life, and that minimize waste are important when a person has limited income, lives alone, or has health problems. Therefore, the Modified MyPyramid for Older Adults includes icons depicting packaged fruits and vegetables in addition to fresh examples. Fresh, frozen, canned, and dried fruits and vegetables are excellent sources of many nutrients as well as fiber. Examples include bags of frozen precut vegetables that can be resealed or single servings of canned fruit. In addition, by having a row of glasses as its foundation, the Modified MyPyramid for Older Adults emphasizes the importance of fluid consumption for older adults.

Although current food guidelines continue to emphasize that the majority, if not all, of the nutrients an older adult consumes should come from food rather than supplements, the flag at the top of the Modified MyPyramid for Older Adults is there to serve as a reminder that some people find it difficult to get adequate amounts of some nutrients from food alone, especially when calorie needs are reduced (**Box 1-1**). Therefore, older adults may need certain supplemental nutrients, such as calcium, vitamin D, and vitamin B12, the needs for which increase with age. Physiologic changes related to age and their impact on nutritional intake, nutrition requirements, and health status are discussed in detail in Chapter 2.

Healthy People 2010

The Healthy People initiative (Healthy People 1990, 2000, and now 2010) began in 1979 in the U.S. Department of Health and Human Services. Over the years, the initiative's goals and objectives have changed in order to serve as the basis for development of state and community planning.

The first major goal of the newest initiative, **Healthy People 2010**, is to increase the years and quality of healthy life. This goal was developed in response to the rapidly aging population. During the 20th century, Americans gained 30 years of life expectancy. In 1900, life expectancy was 47 years for white men and 49 years for white women. Now, those older than age 85 constitute the fastest-growing age group in the United States, leading to the focus on quality of life.

The initiative's second major goal is to eliminate racial and ethnic disparities in health care. This goal was initiated because of the rapidly increasing diversity of the U.S. population and the need to address this in the nation's health care system. Many of these disparities are seen in the older population. Although Americans enjoy better health today because of major medical and basic scientific advances in the care of many diseases, such as cancer, hypertension, heart disease, and diabetes, high-quality care is not available to all. For example, African American women are 40% more likely to die from heart disease than White women. American Indians suffer rates of diabetes that are three times the national average. No older racial or ethnic group is doing very well when it comes to immunizations for influenza or pneumococcus.

Healthy People 2010 has ten Leading Health Indicators that serve as a mechanism for monitoring national progress in meeting goals and objectives. Five of the ten indicators focus on lifestyle: tobacco use, obesity and overweight, physical activity, substance (alcohol) abuse, and responsible sexual behavior (**Box 1-2**). Most of these are applicable to the older adult and are addressed in this book.

BOX 1-1 Changes in Aging That Affect Nutrient Needs

Change in Body Composition or Physiologic Function	Impact on Nutrient Requirements
Decreased muscle mass	Decreased need for energy
Decreased bone density	Increased need for calcium and vitamin D
Decreased immune function	Increased need for vitamin B6, vitamin E, and zinc
Increased gastric pH	Increased need for vitamin B6, folic acid, calcium, iron, and zinc
Decreased skin capacity for cholecalciferol synthesis	Increased need for vitamin D
Increased wintertime parathyroid hormone production	Increased need for vitamin D
Decreased calcium bioavailability	Increased need for calcium and vitamin D
Decreased efficiency in metabolic use of vitamin B6	Increased need for vitamin B6
Increased oxidative stress	Increased need for beta-carotene, vitamin C, and vitamin E
Increased levels of homocysteine	Increased need for folate, vitamin B12, and vitamin B6
Decreased vitamin absorption	Increased need for food choices with high nutrient density
Decreased gastric motility	Increased need for fiber and water

Source: Data from Blumberg J. Nutritional needs of seniors. *J Am Coll Nutr.* 1997;16(6):517–523.

BOX 1-2 First Five Leading Health Indicators for Healthy People 2010

1. **Tobacco use.** This is the leading cause of preventable death in the United States. More than 3,000 young people become new smokers every day. Half will die prematurely from a tobacco-related illness.

2. **Obesity and overweight.** This problem results mainly from poor nutrition and physical inactivity. It has reached epidemic proportions in adults, especially African Americans, Hispanic women, and children. Type 2 diabetes (adult-onset diabetes) is now occurring in children. The American diet consists of fats and sugars and is deficient in vegetables, grains, and fruits. The prescription is to eat at least five servings of vegetables and fruits each day.

3. **Physical inactivity.** This is the second leading cause of preventable deaths in the United States when coupled with dietary factors, resulting in 300,000 deaths every year. The prescription is moderate physical activity at least five days every week for 30 minutes per day.

4. **Alcohol and other substance abuses.** This is a major health problem. The leading drug of choice among adolescents is alcohol. Alcohol abuse is a hidden problem in older adults. The prescription is to avoid toxins, including alcohol and illicit drugs.

5. **Sexual behaviors.** Protect oneself and others from sexually transmitted diseases. Relationships should not begin with sex, but with mutual respect, commitment, communication, and understanding.

Source: U.S. Department of Health and Human Services. *Healthy People 2010: Understanding and Improving Health.* 2nd ed. Washington, DC: U.S. Government Printing Office; November 2000.

The remaining five Leading Health Indicators are mental health, injury and violence, environmental quality, immunization, and access to health care (**Box 1-3**). Many older people die from influenza and pneumonia because of lack of immunization. The final category, access to health care, is an important problem in older adults. Nearly 43 million Americans are uninsured and less likely to receive regular or quality health care, especially minority older adults. Further, most of our health care dollars are spent managing disease (90%), and many of these dollars are spent in the last stages (months to weeks) of life. Too little is spent on disease prevention (<2%), which is a new and vital focus.

Administration on Aging

In an effort to promote health and eliminate health disparities among older persons and, in particular, older minority adults, the AoA is encouraging the national Aging Network to participate in the Healthy People 2010 initiative by using it as a planning and evaluation tool for programs and services. The AoA targets health disparities in three areas: diabetes, cardiovascular disease, and adult immunization.

In 2007, the Assistant Secretary on Aging of the AoA, Josefina Carbonell, presented testimony to the U.S. Senate in which she discussed the modernization of the Older Americans Act in the area of health promotion for older adults at risk for disability and chronic disease. The AoA is working with senior centers and faith centers to begin evidence-based prevention programs that have proven effective in reducing the risk of disease, injury, and disability in older adults. Often these are simple tools and techniques that older adults can use to self-manage their chronic problems, such as reducing the risk of falling, improving nutrition, and enhancing physical and mental health. The goal is to take it nationwide. The AoA has set ambitious performance targets in terms of programs, efficiency measurement, and outcomes. The AoA has increased the number of older adults served per million dollars of funding over the past five years by 22%. The detailed discussion in the following section highlights some of the specific nutritional concerns of various minority and ethnic groups.

Older Minority Groups

Minority groups are projected to increase from 5.7 million in 2000 (16.3% of the older population) to 8 million in 2010 (20.1%) and then to 12.9 million in 2020 (23.6%).

Hispanic Americans

In 2007, the percentage of minority older adults reached 19.3%. Currently, older adults of Hispanic origin represent 7.1% of minorities, but this is expected to increase to more than 17.5% by 2050. By 2028, Hispanic older adults are projected to be the largest racial/ethnic minority group of older Americans. Most Hispanic Americans (72%) live in four states: California, Florida, New York, and Texas.

This population group is less educated than other groups of older Americans: 42.2% have completed high school,

BOX 1-3 Second Five Leading Health Indicators for Healthy People 2010

1. **Mental health.** Our knowledge and understanding of mental health has evolved significantly over the past 25 years. One in five Americans suffers from a mental disorder each year. Because of shame or stigma, less than one-half seek care. The goals are to ease access to mental health care, erase the stigma associated with mental illness, and broaden awareness that many mental problems come from physical causes resulting from changes in chemical secretions in the brain, rendering them treatable by the health care provider.

2. **Injury and violence.** Vehicle crashes, suicides, and homicides are serious public health problems. They are often associated with substance abuse.

3. **Environmental quality.** About 25% of preventable illness worldwide is attributable to toxins in air, water, and soil. African Americans and Hispanics make up 25% of the population but constitute 40% of those who live near dangerous toxin sites. This puts them at greater risk for asthma, lead poisoning, and other illnesses.

4. **Immunization.** Rates of immunization for adults and older adults are poor, even among the majority population. The rates for children are good, having expanded markedly in recent years. African Americans and Hispanics have great need to improve in this area.

5. **Access to health care.** Nearly 43 million Americans were uninsured in 2000. Members of minority groups are most likely to be uninsured or underinsured. They are less likely to obtain quality care management. Related issues are socioeconomic status, education, income, and housing. Minorities are underrepresented in the health care professions, and it is important that culturally competent health care providers become available.

Source: U.S. Department of Health and Human Services. *Healthy People 2010: Understanding and Improving Health.* 2nd ed. Washington, DC: U.S. Government Printing Office; November 2000.

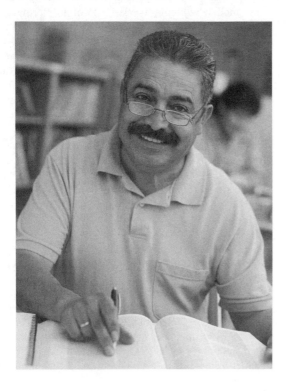

compared with 76% of the total population of older Americans. Further, 8% of older Hispanic adults have completed college, compared with 19% of all older Americans. Poverty is an important problem for Hispanic older adults: the poverty rate is 17%, more than twice that of the total older American population (7.4%).

In 2007, 39% of noninstitutionalized older adults reported very good to excellent health. Racial and ethnic groups are less likely to rate their health care this high. In all populations, these percentages decline with increasing age. Nearly 21% of all older adults have been diagnosed with diabetes; however, the rate of diabetes among older Black adults is much higher (24.5%) than that for non-Hispanic Whites (21.9%), (**Box 1-4**). As recently as 2004, only 34% of older Hispanics had obtained a pneumococcal vaccination, compared with 69% of non-Hispanic Whites and 39% of non-Hispanic Blacks. Twice the number of older adult Hispanic persons required assistance for personal care, compared with 5.6% of non-Hispanic Whites and 8.6% of non-Hispanic Blacks.

Most older Hispanics report that they have access to medical care. In 2000, 6.7% said that they did not have access to medical care. Another 6.5% reported delays in access to care because of the cost of care; furthermore,

▶ BOX 1-4 Prevalence of Chronic Conditions Among Adults Aged 65 and Older by Race/Ethnicity (2002–2003)

High blood pressure		Any cancer	
Black, non-Hispanic	68.4%	White, non-Hispanic	22.7%
White, non-Hispanic	49.7%	Black, non-Hispanic	11.2%
Hispanic	45%	Hispanic	8.8%
Arthritis		**Diabetes**	
Black, non-Hispanic	53.4%	Black, non-Hispanic	24.5%
White, non-Hispanic	48.6%	White, non-Hispanic	14.9%
Hispanic	42.6%	Hispanic	21.9%
Coronary heart disease		**Stroke**	
White, non-Hispanic	21.9%	Black, non-Hispanic	9.6%
Black, non-Hispanic	17.4%	White, non-Hispanic	8.6%
Hispanic	14.3%	Hispanic	8.0%

Source: CDC, National Center for Health Statistics. National Health Interview Survey, 2006. An Introduction to the Health of Older Americans, p. 4.

20.7% reported that they were dissatisfied with the quality of health care received. This is not very different from the total older adult population.

African Americans

Older African Americans comprise 8.2% of the minority older adult population. **Table 1-2** shows the history of population growth of this racial/ethnic group. By 2050, 12% of older Americans will be African American. African Americans live predominantly in eight U.S. states: New York, California, Florida, Texas, Georgia, Illinois, North Carolina, and Virginia.

Educational attainment among African Americans has increased significantly over the past 40 years. Approximately 55.1% of older African Americans have finished high school; in 1970, only 9% had attained this level of education. Today, 10.7% of older African Americans have a bachelor's degree or higher. The poverty rate for African American older adults is 23.2%. This is more than twice the percentage for the total U.S. older population, which is 9.7%.

Positive evaluations of good health diminish with continued aging. Among African Americans, fewer than 23.7% were likely to report good to excellent health compared to older Whites.

African Americans are living longer than in the past. Since 1960, life expectancy for African American men has increased 1.9 years and it has increased 2.9 years for African American women. At age 65, African American men have a life expectancy of 14.6 years (to 79.6 years of age); women have 18.0 years more (to 83 years of age). These data are similar to those for all older American men and women.

The most common chronic illness affecting older African Americans is hypertension (68%), followed by arthritis (53%), heart disease of all types (25%), diabetes (25%), sinusitis (15%), and cancer (11%). These rates are similar for all older Americans, with the exception of hypertension, which is lower in the general population—51%. Diabetes is 16% lower in the general population of older adults, whereas heart disease (31%) and cancer (21%) are both higher in other racial/ethnic groups than in African American older adults.

A large majority of older African American adults state that they have access to health care (96%). However, 17% report that they or their family members have been unable to obtain care or were delayed in receiving necessary medical care. Seventy-three percent of older African American adults do not have supplemental private health insurance,

TABLE 1-2 History of Growth of the Older African American Population

Year	Number (in millions)
1980	2.1
2000	2.8
2020	5.2
2040	8.9

Source: Administration on Aging. A statistical profile of Black older Americans aged 65+. June 2006. Available at: http://www.aoa.gov/PRESS/prodsmats/fact/pdf/Facts-on-Black-Elderly2008.doc. Accessed February 18, 2009.

relying solely on Medicare. Of all U.S. older adults, 37% lack private health insurance.

Native Americans

There is little information on American Indians and Alaska Natives, especially of the older population and those living in rural-frontier/urban areas. This is thought to be because of the expense of accessing small populations located in isolated areas or because the sample size is often too small for statistical analysis in national studies. However, this population is projected to increase 167% between 2000 to 2010.

The U.S. government recognizes 562 American Indian/ Alaska Native tribes. The Indian Health Service (IHS) budget provides funds for health care; these funds are often managed by the tribe, but they may also be managed through the IHS. Care is provided through more than 500 hospitals and clinics on or near reservations and through specialty services off the reservations.

Nearly half of Native Americans have private insurance coverage (49%). The IHS requires that patients exhaust all possible sources of medical funding prior to payment, so that IHS is the provider of last resort. Many Native Americans/Alaska Natives may be eligible for Medicare.

According to a survey conducted from 1988 to 1994, older Native Americans have a high prevalence of arthritis, congestive heart failure, stroke, asthma, prostate cancer, hypertension, and diabetes compared with the general population aged 55 and older. Their functional limitations are lower than the general population.

Older women in this group have a significantly higher prevalence of diabetes, hypertension, cancers (not including breast, colorectal, and lung), cataracts, asthma, and arthritis and have moderately severe to severe functional limitations. As these women continue to age, the prevalence of arthritis, heart failure, hypertension, stroke, colorectal cancer, and cataracts increase. Men have an increased prevalence of prostate cancer with increasing age.

Stroke is a common cause of death in Native Americans. This is related to hypertension, diabetes, and heart disease. Native American women are more likely to be obese and are less likely to exercise, which contributes to these diseases.

As Native Americans age, certain chronic problems, such as asthma and diabetes, diminish in prevalence. People in the younger old age groups are more likely to have asthma (171%) and diabetes (154%) compared with those 85 and older. Among impoverished Native Americans, there is increasing severity of functional limitation, diabetes, stroke, and arthritis.

Life expectancy for American Indians is 71.1 years—lower than that for the U.S. population (76.9 years). However, this varies by regional area. For example, the life expectancy in the California Indian Health Service Area is 76.3 years.

Native Americans face barriers to primary, secondary, and tertiary health care. In rural and frontier communities, this lack of access causes problems. Fifty-one percent of Native American older adults live in frontier areas, 28% live in rural areas, and 21% live in urban areas. Increasing access to health care is a critical step toward eliminating racial and ethnic health disparities. Further, lower health status correlates with lower socioeconomic status. Poverty is a vulnerability of Native American older adults.

Targeted interventions are being developed and implemented to improve the health of American Indian and Alaska Native older adults. **Table 1-3** lists specific policy recommendations.

Asian Americans and Pacific Islanders

Approximately 4.3% (10.9 million) of older Americans are Asian Americans or Pacific Islanders (AAPIs). These groups are frequently categorized as Asian Americans and as Hawaiian and other Pacific Islanders. Asian Americans may be from the Philippines, Korea, Vietnam, China, Pakistan, India, Cambodia, Laos, Thailand, or Japan.

The Asian population in the United States is increasing, growing by 3% between 2004 and 2005. This population group is expected to increase 213% between 2000 and 2010. Of the 421,000 Asian Americans in the United States, 239,000 are immigrants. Most of this population is quite young, with a median age of 32.2 years. Most Asians live in Hawaii; 42% of all people in Hawaii are Asian. Other areas with high Asian populations are San Francisco (18.4%), Los Angeles (10.4%), Sacramento (9%), San Diego (8.9%), Seattle (7.9%), and New York (6.8%).

AAPIs comprise 32 different ethnic groups and speak 500 distinct languages and dialects. They comprise approx-

TABLE 1-3 Policy Recommendations for Native Americans

1. Increase disease prevention efforts, including health promotion and wellness programs.
2. Increase chronic disease management programs to prevent comorbidity and increase access to services.
3. Increase availability of home- and community-based long-term care services in rural areas.
4. Increase availability of health care services and homes that are equipped with necessary plumbing and sanitation along with handicap accessibility to those Native elders living in rural reservation areas.
5. Increase access to educational opportunities that would result in increased income for future generations of Native elders.

Source: Center for Rural Health. *Prevalence of Chronic Disease Among American Indian and Alaska Native Elders.* University of North Dakota School of Medicine and Health Sciences; October 2005. Reprinted with permission.

imately 4% of the total U.S. population and are projected to reach 11% by 2070. Most AAPIs have large families. The population growth of AAPIs exceeds any other racial/ethnic group; thus, the average age of the U.S. population will decrease in the future.

In 1998, AAPIs had the highest median household income of any racial group; their current median income is slightly less than (sometimes quoted as more than) that of non-Hispanic Whites. More members of an Asian family work compared with other racial/ethnic groups. However, their income is bipolar; this group has both the highest incomes of any racial/ethnic group and the lowest incomes, especially among new immigrants. A high proportion of AAPIs own their own homes and complete college.

AAPIs have the longest life expectancy (80.3 years) among the different racial groups in the United States, according to 1992 data. Some of the common diseases of this group are liver cancer, viral hepatitis, liver cirrhosis, nasopharyngeal cancer, stomach cancer, and tuberculosis. Difficulty with language is a barrier to health care access, especially for the poor and newly immigrated. Further, there is a lack of culturally competent health care professionals in the U.S. health care system. Given the unmet needs for health care, AAPIs may use traditional medicine, including acupuncture, herbal medicine, and massage. Lead poisoning is occasionally reported as occurring from folk remedies.

The population of Native Hawaiian and other Pacific Islanders (NHPIs) rose by 1.5%, or 15,000, between 2004 and 2005. The median age of this group is 28.2 years. Adults aged 65 to 74 constitute 7% of the population, and those aged 75 and older about 8%. Most NHPIs live in Hawaii; only 1% live in all other states. However, 25% of the NHPI population is Caucasian; 22% are native Hawaiian. NHPIs originate from any of 22 islands and speak as many as 1,000 languages. Most NHPIs (53%) live above the poverty level. Just 5% are uninsured, and 3% live at the poverty level.

The cuisine of NHPIs varies from culture to culture and is a blend of native foods and Japanese, Asian, American, and European foods. Food plays a central role in the cultures. The usual number of meals each day is three. Starchy foods are the foundation of the traditional diet.

The traditional diet of NHPIs has become Americanized. Many NHPIs now eat fast foods and highly processed items such as white flour, white sugar, canned meat and fish, butter, margarine, mayonnaise, candy, cookies, carbonated drinks, and sweetened cereals. Rice has become a staple, displacing yams and taro.

The prevalence of chronic problems among NHPIs is somewhat different from other ethnic groups. The most common chronic condition is elevated cholesterol (15–17%) (not usually singled out in other demographics), followed closely by hypertension. Next in frequency are arthritis,

asthma, and diabetes. The prevalence of diabetes in this group is twice as high as projected for the Healthy People 2010 goal. It is highest among Native Hawaiians compared with Whites and other ethnic groups on the islands. Cancer occurs in less than 4% of the NHPI population. However, 49.5% of Hawaii's adult population is categorized as overweight or obese based on body mass index. Nearly 56% of older adults are overweight or obese in the 65-to-74-year age category. Thirty-six percent of those 75 and older are overweight or obese. However, nearly 70% of other adult Hawaiians are overweight or obese, making this a major problem in this population.

NHPIs with more education and higher income have better access to health care. Access to ongoing care is high and exceeds the Healthy People 2010 expectations. However, the number of insured is diminishing, according to recent statistics evaluating the Healthy People initiative.

In terms of disease prevention, the number of Native Hawaiians receiving a fecal blood occult test for colorectal cancer has diminished over recent years, as has the number of those receiving a colonoscopy after age 50. The percentage of women in this population who had mammograms declined from 80% in 2001 to 70% in 2002. The percentage of elderly Hawaiians who have been immunized against influenza is much lower than the Healthy People 2010 goal of 90% and has been diminishing since 1990, down to 73.5% in 2002. Pneumococcal immunization is low (59.5%). Those Hawaiians who are the least educated participate in the least amount of leisure time physical activity. More men meet the Healthy People 2010 physical activity goal than do women.

Caucasian Americans (Non-Hispanic Whites)
Compared to other racial/ethnic groups, the non-Hispanic White population has the highest median age (40.0 years). For Hispanics, it is 26.9 years; for Alaska Natives, 29.2 years; Asians, 34.1 years; and African Americans, 30.8 years.

The proportion of people 65 and older is highest among non-Hispanic Whites—15% compared with 12% of the total U.S. population. These older adults can expect to live longer than ever before. Although life expectancy varies by race, the difference decreases with age. In 2001, the life expectancy at birth was 5.5 years greater for Whites than for African Americans. At age 65, a White adult can expect to live an average of nearly two years longer than an African American adult. Interestingly, among those who survive to age 85, life expectancy is higher for African Americans than for Whites.

Health and Well-Being
Almost half of men and women aged 65 and older report very good or excellent health. However, as people age, self-reported health diminishes: 34% of older adults aged 75 to

84 report very good or excellent health, whereas only 28% of those aged 85 and older report this. These data vary by race. Forty percent of Whites aged 65 years and older report very good or excellent health, whereas only 25% of African Americans report the same.

Chronic diseases are very common among older adults of all races. Actual prevalence of chronic conditions supports racial differences in self-reported health (Box 1-4). White Americans have a lower incidence of hypertension (49.7%) compared with African Americans (68.4%) and Hispanic Americans (45%). Diabetes is another chronic illness that occurs less commonly in Whites: only 14.9% of White older adults have diabetes, compared with 21.9% of older Hispanic Americans and 24.5% of older African Americans. However, older Whites have higher cancer rates than older Hispanic Americans: 22.7% versus 8.8%.

Overall, health and well-being are influenced by numerous interrelated factors accumulated over a lifetime. Nutrition is proving to be a major determinant in successful aging. Eighty-five percent of noninstitutionalized older adults have one or more chronic health condition that could be improved with proper nutrition, and up to half may have clinical evidence of various forms of malnutrition. The most common conditions in older adults in 2004 and 2005 were hypertension (48%), diagnosed arthritis (47%), all types of heart disease (29%), cancer (20%), diabetes (16%), and sinusitis (14%) (**Box 1-5**). Many of these diseases limit activity and diminish quality of life. Figure 1-7 highlights the dietary and non-dietary risk factors for common diseases in older adults.

Food choice and dietary intake are multifactorial and are influenced by physiologic, behavioral, social, environmental, and psychological factors. These factors are compounded in older adults by functional and health factors that also contribute to food intake (**Figure 1-8**).

Consumption of a poor-quality diet can result in inadequate intake of energy and essential nutrients, resulting in malnutrition and worsening of health status (**Figure 1-9**). Malnourished older adults are more prone to infections and diseases, their injuries take longer to heal, surgery is riskier, and their hospital stays are longer and more expensive.

The Health Care Workforce

Is the health care workforce ready for the graying of America? It is widely believed that universities and schools are not well prepared for fulfilling the upcoming need for health professionals who are qualified to manage the numbers of older adults who will be entering the health care system. In 2012, nearly 10,000 Americans will turn 65 years of age *every day*. The number of those aged 65 and older who are eligible for Medicare will double to 70 million by 2030. The number of people aged 85 and older will increase *five times*, to nearly 19 million, by midcentury. **Figures 1-10** and **1-11** illustrate the geographic distribution and percentages of the total population who are 65 years and older and 85 years and older, respectively.

Older adults use more health care services than any other age group. Although this group currently comprises only 13% of the population, it uses half of all physician visits and half of all hospital stays. The average adult aged 75 has three chronic health problems and uses five prescription drugs. These issues and the changes of aging constitute a challenge for those who are unprepared to care for adults of this age group.

The number of health care professionals prepared in geriatrics is small. Of a total of 650,000 practicing physicians, fewer than 9,000 have a specialty in geriatrics. This means that there are 2.5 geriatricians for every 10,000 older adults. The number of geriatricians is expected to fall to 6,000 in the near future. Fewer than 3% of medical students currently take elective geriatric courses.

Of the approximately 200,000 practicing pharmacists, only 720 have geriatric certification. A survey of nursing baccalaureate programs showed that only 23% require a single course in geriatrics, although most require a course in nutrition. Less than 0.5% of nurses have advanced certification in geriatrics as geriatric nurse practitioners. Among social workers, less than 5% have identified themselves as practicing in geriatrics. In nutrition, the numbers are much better. Nutritionists and dieticians have long practiced in long-term care settings and hospitals in which the management of older adults is common.

Despite the low numbers of qualified health care professionals, the largest training gap in any medical educational field is in geriatrics. Only 0.5% of geriatricians are edu-

---

BOX 1-5 Chronic Diseases That Are the Leading Causes of Death Among U.S. Adults Aged 65 and Older (2002)

Heart disease

Cancer

Stroke

Chronic lower respiratory diseases

Influenza and pneumonia

Alzheimer's disease

Diabetes

All other causes

Source: CDC, National Center for Health Statistics. National Health Interview Survey, 2006. An Introduction to the Health of Older Americans, p. 4.

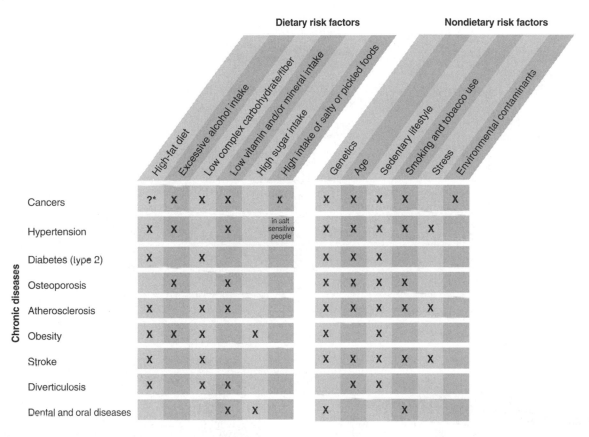

FIGURE 1-7 Risk Factors for Disease in Older Adults

*The Nurses' Health Study, a large prospective study, found no evidence linking higher total fat intake with increased risk of breast cancer. These results call into question theories that link dietary fat to other cancers.

cators. Sixty percent of nursing schools have no geriatrics faculty at all.

One trend in family medicine is to make geriatrics a curricular requirement. Currently, 92% of family medicine residency programs have this requirement. Medical schools are beginning to establish departments or divisions of geriatric medicine within internal medicine or family medicine divisions. Unfortunately, the Medicare system discourages young physicians from entering geriatrics because of the very poor reimbursement rates (which continue to drop) for the care of older adults. Medicare payments are set lower than those of commercial insurers. For example, whereas the charge for a basic checkup at the office is $55, commercial insurers pay $45 and Medicare pays $35. These differences continue based on the type of visit.

The American Medical Association (AMA) states that of the physicians it has surveyed, 45% plan to stop seeing

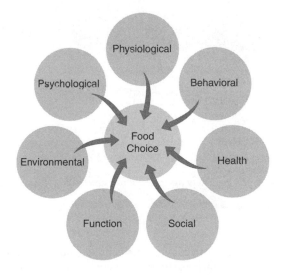

FIGURE 1-8 Classification of Factors That Affect Food Choice in Older Adults

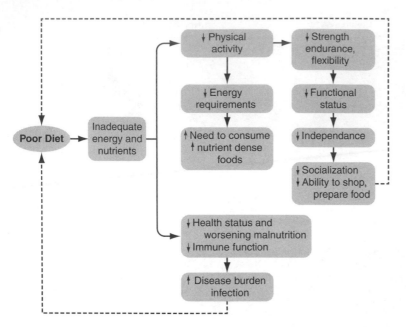

FIGURE 1-9 Poor Diet Affects the Older Adult

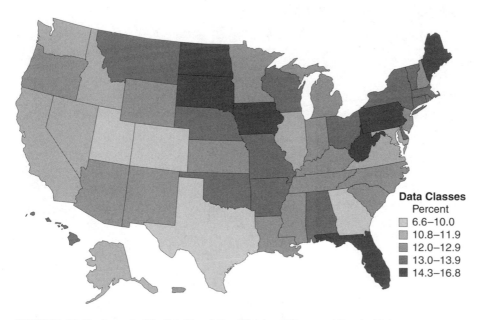

FIGURE 1-10 The Percent of the Total Population Who Are 65 Years and Over by State

Source: U.S. Census Bureau, 2006 American Community Survey.

Medicare patients because reimbursement continues to lag behind the cost to practice. Other professional groups, such as the American Geriatrics Society and the American Academy of Family Physicians, echo this concern. This is a sad state given the demographic imperative. One small light is the number of private and public organizations working diligently to fund geriatric training and education and research to provide the essential care needed for older Americans.

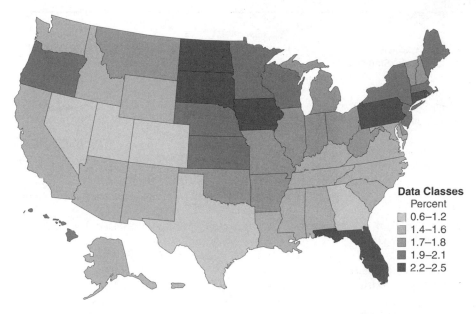

FIGURE 1-11 The Percent of the Total Population Who Are 85 Years and Over by State

Source: U.S. Census Bureau, 2006 American Community Survey.

Data Classes
Percent
- 0.6–1.2
- 1.4–1.6
- 1.7–1.8
- 1.9–2.1
- 2.2–2.5

Conclusion

Older adults are particularly vulnerable to compromised nutrient intake because of declines in food intake and the decreasing energy needs that accompany aging. Therefore, a high-quality, nutritionally adequate diet becomes more critical. However, multiple chronic and acute illnesses, multiple medications, impaired health, low levels of physical activity, poor dentition, impaired mental status, depression, an inability to self-feed, and anorexia have all been shown to influence the eating habits and nutritional status of older adults. As shown in Figure 1-1, these factors alone or in combination may contribute to dietary inadequacies and lead to the consumption of a low-quality diet, thereby worsening many of the conditions. This limits an individual's ability to remain independent and can lead to other complications such as increased medical burden, polypharmacy, and reduced socialization and physical activity. Maintenance of health, independence, and functional status is related to an individual's ability to shop, cook, and eat independently, which is directly related to food intake and nutritional status. Ultimately, the goals for nutrition intervention in the older population should be to maintain health and quality of life throughout the continuum of the aging process. Specific attention should be given to address the individuality of each older adult, including cultural and ethnic considerations with regard to nutritional requirements, food preferences, and disease prevalence to promote overall healthy aging.

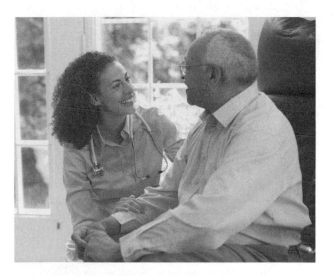

Activities Related to This Chapter

1. List nutrition-related challenges facing the aging population based on the classifications of factors that affect food choices for older adults. List two to three specific examples for each group. As you go through the text, you can add to each list.

REFERENCES

Administration on Aging. A profile of older Americans: 2005. Available at: http://www.aoa.gov/PROF/Statistics/profile/2005/2.asp. Accessed January 12, 2007.

Administration on Aging. A profile of older Americans: 2007. Available at: http://www.aoa.gov/prof/Statistics/profile/2007/profiles2007.aspx. Accessed February 18, 2009.

Administration on Aging. A statistical profile of Black older Americans aged 65 + . June 2006. Available at: http://www.aoa.gov/press/prodsmats/fact/pdf/Facts-on-Black-Elderly.pdf.

Administration on Aging. A statistical profile of Hispanic older Americans aged 65 + . September 2005. Available at: http://www.aoa.gov/press/prodsmats/fact/pdf/Facts-on-Hispanic-Elderly.pdf.

American Dietetic Association. Position paper of the American Dietetic Association: Nutrition across the spectrum of aging. *J Am Diet Assoc.* 2005;105(4):616–633.

American Dietetic Association. Position of the American Dietetic Association: Nutrition, aging, and the continuum of care. *J Am Dietetic Assoc.* 1996;96:1048–1052.

Ausman LM, Russell RM. *Nutrition in the Elderly*. Philadelphia: Lea & Febiger; 1994.

Center for Rural Health. *Prevalence of Chronic Disease Among American Indian and Alaska Native Elders*. University of North Dakota School of Medicine and Health Sciences; October 2005.

Centers for Disease Control and Prevention. National health and nutrition examination survey III. 1988–1994. Available at: http://www.cdc.gov/nchs/products/elec_prods/subject/nhanes3.htm. Accessed February 18, 2009.

Centers for Disease Control and Prevention. National health interview survey (NHIS). 2004. Available at: http://www.cdc.gov/nchs/about/major/nhis/quest_data_related_1997_forward.htm. Accessed February 18, 2009.

Centers for Disease Control and Prevention. *The State of Aging and Health in America 2004*. 2005. Available at: http://www.cdc.gov/aging/pdf/State_of_Aging_and_Health_in_America_2004.pdf. Accessed February 18, 2009.

Chen T, Hsu C-C. Asian Americans. In: Encyclopedia of Public Health. Available at: http://www.answers.com/topic/asian-american. Accessed January 15, 2007.

Chernoff R. *Geriatric Nutrition: The Health Professional's Handbook*. Sudbury, MA: Jones & Bartlett; 2006.

Chernoff R. Meeting the nutritional needs of the elderly in the institutional setting. *Nutr Rev.* 1994;52:132–136.

Federal Interagency Forum on Aging-Related Statistics. *Older Americans 2004: Key Indicators of Well-Being*. Hyattsville, MD: National Center for Health Statistics; 2004. Available at: http//www.agingstats.gov/chartbook2004/healthstatus.html. Accessed February 7, 2005.

Free Health Encyclopedia. Health care careers. 2007. Available at: http://www.faqs.org/health/Healthy-Living-V2/Health-Care-Careers.html. Accessed March 1, 2007.

Goodwin JS. Social, psychological and physical factors affecting the nutrient status of elderly subjects: separating cause and effect. *Am J Clin Nutr.* 1989;50:1201–1209.

Grey-Donald K. The frail elderly. *J Am Dietetic Assoc.* 1995;95:538–540.

Hawaii Department of Health. Tracking Hawaii's progress toward Healthy People 2010. 2006. Available at: http://www.brfsshi@mail.health.state.hi.us. Accessed January 17, 2007.

Hawaii Department of Health. *Vital Statistics Report: 2006*. 2006. Available at: http://www.hawaii.gov/health/statistics/vital-statistics/vr_06/index.html. Accessed January 17, 2007.

Hawaii Department of Health, Office of Health Status Monitoring. Hawaii health survey, 2005. 2005. Available at: http://hawaii.gov/health/statistics/hhs/hhs_05/index.html. Accessed February 18, 2009.

Kumanyika S. Improving our diet, still a long way to go. *N Engl J Med.* 1996;335:738–739.

Lichtenstein AH, Rasmussen H, Yu WW, Epstein SR, Russell RM. Modified MyPyramid for older adults. *J Nutr.* 2008;138:78–82.

LoCicero J III, et al. Cross-cutting issues. In: American Geriatrics Society, eds. *New Frontiers in Geriatrics Research: An Agenda for Surgical and Related Medical Specialties* (Chapter 13). 2006. Available at: http://www.frycomm.com/ags/rasp/chapter.asp?ch = 13. Accessed March 28, 2006.

Nutrition and Well-Being A to Z. Diet of Pacific Islander Americans. 2006. Available at: http://www.faqs.org/nutrition/Ome-Pop/Pacific-Islander-Americans-Diet-of.html. Accessed January 16, 2007.

Office on Women's Health. The health of minority women. 2003. Available at: http://www.4women.gov/owh/pub/minority/index.htm. Accessed January 16, 2007.

Satcher D. Healthy People 2010. In: Encyclopedia of Public Health. Available at: http://www.answers.com/topic/health-people-2010.

Stefanacci RG. Medicare part D: reimbursement politics. *Clin Geriatr.* 2007;15(2):1070–1389.

Stevenson K. 1900–2000: Changes in life expectancy in the United States. March 23, 2006. Available at: http://www.elderweb.com/home/node/2838. Accessed February 18, 2009.

U.S. Census Bureau. Nation's population one-third minority. May 10, 2006. Available at: http://www.census.gov/Press-Release/www/releases/archives/population/006808.html. Accessed January 16, 2007.

U.S. Census Bureau. Population profile of the United States: dynamic version. Available at: http://www.census.gov/population/www/pop-profile/profiledynamic.html. Accessed February 18, 2009.

U.S. Congress, Senate Special Committee on Aging. Testimony of J. Carbonell, Assistant Secretary of Aging, Administration on Aging. February 15, 2007.

U.S. Department of Health and Human Services and U.S. Department of Agriculture. *Dietary Guidelines for Americans, 2005*. Washington, DC: Department of Health and Human Services; 2005.

Physiologic Changes with Aging

Ann Schmidt Luggen, PhD, GNP

. . . .

CHAPTER OBJECTIVES   Upon completion of this chapter, the reader will be able to:

1. Describe the physical changes in each system that are related to the aging process
2. List the functional changes of aging
3. Discuss the changes in each body system with regard to aging and how they affect the body's function

KEY TERMS AND CONCEPTS

Actinic keratoses

Anorexia

Collagen

Cytokines

Dysphagia

Hypogeusia

Lentigines

Melanocytes

Olfactory

Pruritus

Sarcopenia

Seborrheic keratoses

Sensorineural hearing loss

Sicca

Telangiectasias

. . . .

General Changes with Aging

The average lifespan has been increasing, particularly due to decreases in childhood mortality. The maximum lifespan is thought to be about 125 years in women, slightly less in men. This has changed little, and death is usually related to heredity, lifestyle, and environmental toxins.

Age changes are most evident after the age of 85. These changes often involve a functional decline and decline in response to stress.

Physical decline does not equate to functional decline. In older adults who do not exercise strenuously on a frequent basis, the need for oxygen can be met with about half the usual cardiac output. However, when there are demands on the body—for example, an acute illness—the significance of physical decline becomes evident, because at advanced age few or no reserves are available. Body functions may decline with chronic or acute conditions or mental illness, such as Alzheimer's disease. However, with proper nutrition, care, and physical and mental exercise, good function can continue with advancing age.

With increasing age, the amount of tissue in the body decreases. By age 80, the decline is about 50%. There is also a predictable decrease in lean body mass, mainly skeletal muscle, which occurs even with a good diet. This decrease

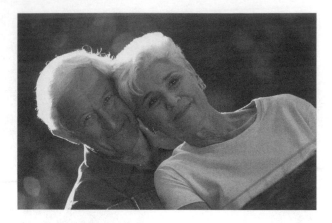

collagen Main content of connective tissue and much of the whole body protein content.

pruritus Itchy skin.

melanocytes Cells in the skin that produce and contain the pigment melanin.

lentigines Harmless flat sunspots seen on the sun-exposed skin of older adults. Freckles.

seborrheic keratoses Benign proliferation of basal cells producing smooth or warty lesions. Very common in older adults; who usually have multiple lesions on the chest, back, and face. Lesions are brown, tan, waxy, or flesh colored. They may be very small (mm) to large (several cm).

telangiectasias Fine, irregular red lines on the skin that are produced by capillary dilatation. Often seen on the cheeks and nose of older adults with rosacea.

actinic keratoses Premalignant lesions that appear in areas of skin exposed to sunlight. Most common in adults after long exposure to ultraviolet light; especially common in those with fair complexion, blue eyes, and light hair. Rare in people with dark skin.

may be caused by a lack of regular exercise. The loss of muscle makes the older adult more susceptible to falls and chronic illness.

Skin, Hair, and Nails

As a person ages, the skin becomes less elastic and there is a loss of **collagen** and adipose tissue, which manifests as wrinkling. The amount of wrinkling depends on the skin's exposure to the sun, which enhances this effect. Because of thinning of the skin and loss of collagen fibers, the skin is more susceptible to tears. If the skin becomes injured, healing is slowed because of decreased immunologic responsiveness. These functional changes lessen the skin's ability to provide mechanical protection, sensory perception, thermoregulation, and vitamin D production.

Beginning in early adulthood, the glands that provide lubrication diminish production by about 23% each decade, so that skin becomes much dryer. Dryness, also known as *xerosis*, is often accompanied by **pruritus** (itching).

Production of sweat by the sweat glands slows with age. This decrease in sweating makes it more difficult for the older adult to cope with temperature changes.

The thinned skin has diminished turgor; that is, when the skin is pinched, it remains pinched for some seconds. This does not occur in younger adults unless they are very dehydrated. Skin turgor is used as a means of assessing hydration; however, it can be poor even in well-hydrated older adults.

Although **melanocytes**, which give the skin color, diminish with aging, hyperpigmentation occurs in areas of the skin exposed to the sun. Other terms for this phenomenon include *liver spots*, *age spots*, and **lentigines**. Lentigines are commonly found on the hands, wrists, and face.

The capillaries in the skin become more fragile with advancing age. This means that bruising or merely brushing against a hard object may cause bleeding. Some sensation is lost to light touch.

Many different skin lesions are seen with aging. Most are benign. Blue venous lakes or small bluish blood vessels may pop up on the lip, especially in sun-exposed areas or in smokers. **Seborrheic keratoses** are very common and can look small and innocent or large and abnormal, although they are usually benign. They occur on sun-exposed areas of the skin, often on the face, neck, back, and arms.

The older person might also have **telangiectasias**, small dilated blood vessels that often occur on the face and arms. As with seborrheic keratoses, these are worse in areas that are exposed to the sun.

Actinic keratoses are a type of premalignant skin lesion. The lesions are scaly and reddish and may bleed easily. They occur in sun-exposed areas. Although they are not caused by age-related changes to the skin, they occur with increasing frequency with age.

Hair grays or whitens in about 50% of adults by age 50 as a result of an age-related loss of melanocytes. Hair growth also slows. Hair loss, caused by an age-related loss of hair follicles, occurs in both men and women, but more so with men. Hair loss occurs not only on the head, but also in the axillae and pubic areas. Following menopause, loss of hair from the head is often not very pronounced in women. Diffuse hair loss in both sexes may be caused by iron deficiency, hypothyroidism, chronic renal failure, and undernutrition. In men, new hair growth occurs in the ears and nose. Eyebrows take on a bushy appearance. Due to the loss of estrogen production following menopause, women may begin to grow hair in new places, most notably on the chin.

Nails thicken with aging, becoming brittle and hard. Nail growth slows, and longitudinal lines appear. The nails are dry. They become very susceptible to fungal infections, especially in the feet. It is uncommon in very old age not to have these infections.

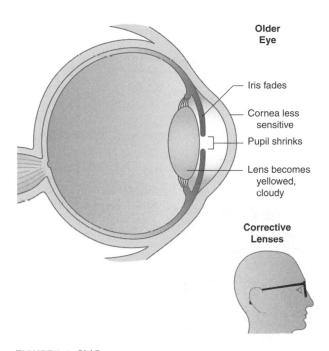

Older
Eye

— Iris fades

— Cornea less
sensitive

— Pupil shrinks

— Lens becomes
yellowed,
cloudy

Corrective
Lenses

FIGURE 2-1 Old Eye

Source: National Institutes of Health, 2008.

Eyes and Vision

Changes in vision begin early in the aging process, especially in the lens of the eye. Over time, these changes create loss of function in terms of reading, driving, increased susceptibility to accidents, and decreased quality of life unless adequately managed (**Figure 2-1**).

With age, the skin becomes darkened in the area of the eye orbits due to a loss of periorbital fat. This loss of periorbital fat also causes enophthalmos, sinking of the eyeball into the eye orbit. Crow's feet (wrinkles) appear at the lateral corners of the eyes. Laxity of the skin around the eye can cause ectropion, in which the eyelid everts, thus exposing the eye to drying and infection. Entropion, or inversion of the eyelid with the lashes inverted inward toward the eye, causes the eyelashes to brush against the cornea, causing pain and potential infection.

The sclerae may be white or yellowish, with yellow deposits of fat. Fat deposits (xanthomas) may also be seen around the outside of the eye and may be associated with high blood lipid levels.

With age, the lens of the eye becomes less transparent, decreasing the amount of light that reaches the retina. A 60-year-old person's retina receives only a fraction of the light that a 20-year-old's receives. With time, the lens becomes cloudy. It becomes yellowish and is a cataract. Sun exposure increases the risk of cataracts, as does exposure to cigarette smoke.

The pupils decrease in size as a person ages. The pupils do not dilate as effectively, which can impair a person's night vision and make it more difficult to adapt to poor lighting. With age, the eyes do not constrict in bright light as fast as they once did, causing increased sensitivity to bright light. Thus, driving in the dark or through a tunnel or entering a movie theater or unlighted room can increase the risk for accidents. Appropriate lighting is very important for the continuing safety of the older adult.

Tear production slows with aging. This results in dry eyes (**sicca**), which can be very irritating. Dry eyes are predisposed to conjunctivitis (red eye) caused by viruses or bacteria. Conjunctivitis can be painful, purulent and infectious.

Arcus senilis is a thin line or grayish band around the upper part of the eye. It is very common in those aged 65 and older; it may be innocent or it may indicate elevated cholesterol levels.

The retina of the eye contains the macula, an area of the retina with the highest visual acuity. This area degenerates in many older adults so that central vision is lost but peripheral vision is maintained. Risk factors for this debilitating visual disorder, called macular degeneration, include smoking, hypertension, and diabetes. Some loss of peripheral vision is normal as is the ability to judge depth. Other common alterations of the eye with aging are myopia (nearsightedness) and hyperopia (farsightedness). These can usually be managed well with ophthalmologic consultation and glasses or laser therapy; however, 20/20 vision is often not possible in the very old. If these conditions are not treated, the older adult can become isolated from his or her usual world and confusion can ensue. Another normal phenomenon is diminished clarity of color, especially blues and pastels. Many older adults have "floaters" which are tiny specks or "cobwebs" that appear to float across the eye. They are especially noticeable in bright light or outdoors.

Ears and Hearing

The earlobes become elongated with age (**Figure 2-2**). Cerumen (earwax) production diminishes, but cerumen continues to accumulate in the ear canal, which can cause impaction that requires special cleaning. Cerumen buildup can cause conductive hearing loss, which can be prevented with diligent attention to the cleaning task. Other causes of conductive hearing loss include the thickening of the tympanic membrane in the middle ear and the presence of foreign bodies in the ear. Hearing loss causes the older adult to become isolated from communication, often resulting in irritability.

sicca Condition of having dry eyes and/or dry mouth.

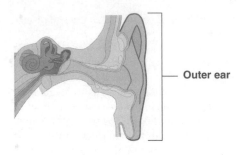

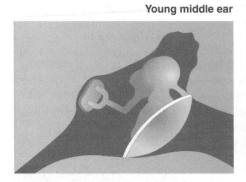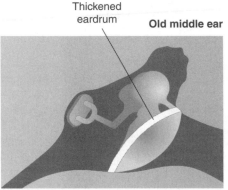

FIGURE 2-2 Young Versus Old Ear

Source: National Institutes of Health, 2008.

Presbycusis (**sensorineural hearing loss**) is the diminished ability to hear high-frequency sounds; it is common in older adults and increases with aging. When people speak louder so that older adults can "hear better," it becomes even more difficult for them to hear. When there is background noise, such as in a crowded room, there is diminished ability to distinguish sounds. Many sounds become unintelligible, for example, *f*, *th*, *ch*, and *sh*. The key to enhancing communication is to speak in lower tones. However, many older adults have both types of hearing loss—conductive and sensorineural—and should be referred to an audiologist.

Nose and Mouth

The tip of the nose elongates with aging. This causes the cartilage to separate, which widens and lengthens the nose. Vasomotor rhinitis (runny nose) is common in older adults, as is allergic (atopic) rhinitis and sinusitis.

Smell (**olfactory** sensation) diminishes steadily after age 60, becoming significantly impaired by age 80. The older adult may be unable to smell the pleasurable aroma of favorite foods being cooked or served on the dinner plate. Olfactory sensation can be tested by having the individual close his or her eyes, placing an odor (e.g., nutmeg, alcohol, perfume) beneath a nostril, and asking the person to identify the smell.

Olfactory sensation is closely related to taste, but taste declines more gradually than smell. Flavors need to be highly concentrated in order to be tasted. With the loss of taste and smell, the appearance and consistency of foods become more important.

The number of papillae on the tongue decreases with age, by about 50% by age 50. This results in a decrease in taste sensation known as **hypogeusia**. (The loss of the ability to taste is called *ageusia*.) The anterior taste buds, which are sensitive to sweet and salt, are lost before those on the posterior aspect of the tongue, which predominantly taste bitter and sour. This results in foods tasting bitter and sour rather than sweet or salty. This is known as *parageusia*, a perversion of taste. This means that foods that the older adult once enjoyed may have an unpleasant taste.

The sensation of thirst is absent in many older adults. Adequate fluid intake for older adults is 30 mL of water per kilogram of body weight per day or 1 mL of water per ingested kilocalorie. Fluid requirements are higher in those with fever or those who are undergoing diuretic therapy, as

sensorineural hearing loss Unknown cause of hearing loss; however, it is related to nerve damage. More common in older adults.

olfactory Sense of smell; one of the chemosensory functions that often declines with aging. Also negatively affected by smoking, sinusitis, respiratory disorders, dental infections, and poor oral hygiene.

hypogeusia Reduced ability to taste; ageusia is total loss of taste.

BOX 2-1   Typical Reports of Swallowing Problems

"I cough and choke a lot."

"Mashed potatoes stick in my throat."

"She pockets food in the side of her mouth."

"One side of his mouth droops."

"He drools a lot."

dysphagia Difficulty swallowing. It may result from a neurological disorder that impairs esophageal motility or a mechanical obstruction of the esophagus.

well as in other situations. The older adult does not respond to serum osmolarity, so dehydration may go undetected.

Common changes in the mouth with aging are dry mouth (xerostomia), swallowing problems (**dysphagia**), taste problems, gum problems (periodontal disease), and dental caries (tooth decay). Dry mouth is caused by diminished saliva production. Saliva is essential, because it has antibacterial, antifungal, and cleansing properties. It also facilitates swallowing. Dryness can be assessed by looking at the tongue and mucous membranes. Swallowing problems (dysphagia) can be caused by illness, such as stroke, or by neurologic changes that occur with advancing age. Swallowing can be assessed by watching the older adult drink water and eat foods of differing quality and thickness. Reports from the patient that may indicate dysphagia are noted in **Box 2-1**.

Periodontal disease and loss of teeth are common. States where complete tooth loss are highest are Kentucky, Tennessee, and Oklahoma. It is important to check the area beneath the dentures to watch for areas of irritation, ulcerations, or lesions.

Lungs and Thorax

Lung function diminishes gradually after age 20, eventually leaving the older adult without great respiratory reserve. The size of the airways in older adults is diminished, and the alveolar sacs—the site of air exchange—become shallow. The costovertebral joints and costal cartilage, which allow movement of the ribs, become calcified. Kyphoscoliosis, a change in the shape of the spinal column, occurs in many older adults to some degree and begins at about age 55. These changes result in increasing weakness of the respiratory muscles and reduced compliance. The intercostal muscles atrophy and reduce diaphragm strength by about 25%. These changes do not affect function in a meaningful way unless the older adult is compromised by an infection such as pneumonia. The cough reflex is diminished also.

The loss of elastin and collagen that occurs in the skin also occurs in the lungs, beginning at about age 30. Lung mucous membranes become progressively dry, also. This decreases the ability of the lungs to expand and recoil with

respiration. When this occurs, accessory muscle use in the thorax or neck may be seen. These changes mean that older adults are less able to expire all of the air inhaled with inspiration. The result is that more air stays in the lung at expiration, so that residual lung volume is higher in older adults. Maximum breathing capacity diminishes with each decade of life. In addition, the loss of resilience and loss of skeletal muscle in the chest contribute to the development of a barrel chest in many older adults.

Cellular immunity declines with age. Older adults previously exposed to tuberculosis (TB) may experience reactivation of TB infection. Frail older adults who are malnourished are at great risk for pulmonary infections, including pneumonia, bronchitis, and tuberculosis. They are also at risk for aspiration pneumonias.

Heart

A discussion of cardiac changes related to aging is complicated, because heart disease is the most common cause of death in older adults in our society. Some of the strictly age-related changes that occur are listed in **Box 2-2**. With age,

BOX 2-2   Age-Related Changes of the Heart

Heart muscle cells (myocytes)	Loss with aging
	Hypertrophy (increase in size with aging)
Left heart ventricle	Becomes stiffer
Left ventricle wall	Thickens
Filling of the left ventricle	Decreases
Heart rate	Slight decrease
Maximum heart rate	Diminishes
Cardiac output	Unchanged; slight decrease in women
Maximum cardiac output	Decreases
Vasodilation related to exercise	Decreases
Ability of heart to secrete sodium	Decreases

Source: Adapted from American Geriatric Society (AGS). *Geriatric Review Syllabus.* 6th ed. New York: American Geriatric Society; 2006; McCance K and Huether S. *Pathophysiology.* 5th ed. Philadelphia: Elsevier Mosby; 2006.

the amount of fibrotic tissue in the heart increases and the amount of elastic tissue decreases. This change means that the older heart is less able to expand and contract, and it may become stiff and noncompliant. The maximum pumping rate and the heart's ability to extract oxygen from the blood both diminish with progressive aging.

Some tissues calcify and stiffen. For example, the aortic and mitral valves are commonly affected by calcification and stiffening. This causes a new heart sound, a murmur, to occur. A murmur is especially problematic if the older adult has heart failure, the most common cause of hospital admissions in older adults.

Older adults commonly experience arrhythmias of the heart with aging. These are caused by deposition of lipofuscin, amyloid, collagen, and fats in the pacemaker part of the heart over time. The arrhythmias may manifest as a fast heart rate, an irregular heart rate, or a very slow heart rate. All of these cause decompensation of the heart, which affects most areas of the body.

Blood pressure increases with age due to stiffening of the aorta and nearby arteries and loss of elasticity of the blood vessels. High blood pressure can cause cardiovascular events, dementia, and even death. A most common change with aging is isolated systolic hypertension, a blood pressure of more than 140mmHg with a diastolic blood pressure of less than 90. This is caused by arterial wall thickening and stiffness resulting in decreased compliance, left ventrical hypertrophy, and sclerosis of the atrial and mitral valves. This can result in decreased peripheral pulses with cold extremities, risk of arrhythmias, and postural hypotension.

Older adults often suffer from hypotension when they stand up after sitting, lying down, or eating a meal. Postural hypotension is often caused by drugs used to treat hypertension or from age-related diminished sensitivity of the body's baroreceptors. Hypotension is a major cause of falls in older adults.

Understanding of the changes that occur within the intima, or lining of arteries, has increased in recent years. Within the intima, there is an age-related cross-linking of collagen, an increase in the amount of collagen, and changes in elastin. Aging also affects the vessels' extracellular matrix, inflammatory molecules, endothelial cell function, and reactive oxygen species (**Figure 2-3**). The changes shown in Figure 2-3 can occur at different times and to different extents in older adults. Even among those at risk genetically, exercise, good nutrition, and drug therapy can slow the aging of the blood vessels and delay or prevent cardiovascular diseases.

Cardiac changes in older people vary in terms of changes at rest versus changes with exercise. Regular exercise can slow the rate of decline of the heart. Decreases in cardiac function are much smaller in the older adult who exercises

on a regular basis. It is essential to assess the older adult's fitness level and tolerance for exercise.

Abdomen

Age-related changes in the gastrointestinal (GI) system begin in middle age. In addition to changes in taste, smell, saliva secretion, and dental health, discussed previously, many other changes occur in the GI tract. There is a decrease in the muscles of mastication and thirst perception. In the esophagus, motility diminishes, which can affect swallowing. The lower esophageal sphincter at the stomach relaxes, allowing stomach contents to enter the esophagus more frequently. Reflux is not a normal part of aging, but it occurs in a large percentage of older adults.

Gastric motility is also diminished with delayed emptying. Secretion of bicarbonate and gastric mucus, the protective mucosa, is diminished, decreasing the ability of the gastric mucosa to resist damage. The stomach's antral cells atrophy, resulting in diminished secretion of hydrochloric acid and intrinsic factor. These, as well as other physiologic changes, could lead to potential alterations in the digestion and absorption of numerous nutrients, such as protein, vitamin B12, vitamin D, folic acid, and calcium.

The abdominal muscles in older adults are often weak, increasing the risk of hernias. The amount of subcutaneous abdominal fat increases, normally in many healthy older adults. However, a longitudinal study has indicated that a large waist circumference is related to high mortality when controlled for in those older adults with a high body mass index. A low BMI (less than 19) is also implicated in high mortality rates.

The intestinal villi atrophy, which can result in lactose intolerance in those who may never have had this problem. Lactose intolerance commonly occurs for the first time in advanced age. Intestinal absorption, motility, and blood flow diminish with age, somewhat impairing nutrient absorption. The following nutrients are absorbed more slowly: proteins, fats, minerals (e.g., iron and calcium) and vitamins, and carbohydrates, especially lactose. Thus, the dietary requirement for calcium is higher for older adults.

The motility or movement of digestion (peristalsis) is slowed in older people. Among the many causes is a loss of muscle tone. Decreased motility increases the incidence of constipation because it increases the transit time of stools. In addition, this slowing causes more water to be reabsorbed by the intestines, thus increasing the hardness of the stool. Lack of dietary fiber increases the problem of constipation, as does lack of exercise and insufficient fluids.

Pancreatic function diminishes with age. However, enough function remains to digest normal amounts of dietary fat—up to 100 g/day. Fecal fat is excreted at 120 to 130 g/day.

The liver becomes smaller in size and weight with increasing age. Cell numbers and the ability to regenerate

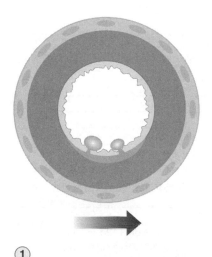
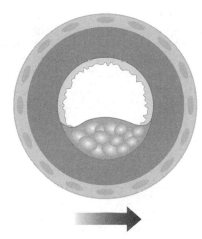
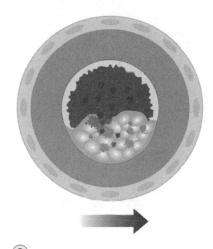

① Inflammation is a key factor in the development of atherosclerosis. As LDL cholesterol accumulates in the arterial wall, it undergoes chemical changes and signals to endothelial cells to latch onto white blood cells circulating in the blood.

② These immune cells penetrate the intima and trigger an inflammatory response, devouring LDLs, to become fat-laden "foam cells", and form a fatty streak, the earliest stage of atherosclerotic plaque.

③ The plaque continues to grow and forms a fibrous cap. Substances released by foam cells can eventually destabilize the cap, allowing it to rupture, causing a blood clot which can block blood flow and trigger a heart attack.

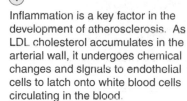

FIGURE 2-3 Intimal Changes in Coronary Arteries

Source: National Institute on Aging/National Institutes of Health.

diminish. Liver function, however, remains near normal. The liver's blood flow decreases with age, which can influence the efficiency of drugs metabolized by the liver.

Additional age-related changes in the GI tract are provided in **Table 2-1**.

Kidneys

Many age-related changes occur in the kidneys. The kidneys of a 90-year-old are smaller and weigh 20% to 30% less than those of a 30-year-old. The membranes in the glomeruli and tubules thicken, and the tubules diminish in length and volume. In the kidneys of a 90-year-old, 30% to 40% of the glomeruli are gone and nearly 40% of the remaining glomeruli are sclerosed. Blood flow, glomerular filtration rate (with a 10% decrease per decade after age 30), and diminished drug clearance occurs. These changes occur throughout the lifespan (**Figure 2-4**).

With aging, nephrons become fewer in number (see kidney terms in **Box 2-3**) and renal blood flow decreases. These changes accelerate between the ages of 40 to 80, so that by old age the kidneys' glomerular filtration is often diminished by nearly 50%. Glomerular capillaries atrophy and may even disappear. Supplying arteries become tortuous and may contribute to ischemia.

Kidney function often diminishes about 1% per year after age 40. However, a longitudinal study found that although two-thirds of older adults had deterioration in their glomerular filtration rates (GFR), one-third did not. Loss of function is not inevitable but would be unusual.

The ability of the kidneys to excrete concentrated urine diminishes significantly over time, and the specific gravity of the urine may be below normal and less concentrated. The older person usually excretes lower levels of glucose, acid, and potassium. Hyperkalemia becomes more common as a result of diminished secretion by the tubules. Reabsorption of sodium, bicarbonate, and glucose is diminished. Changes of fluid balance and pH are not responded to as quickly, and the older person may become hyper- or hypovolemic. Acute deficits of fluid may cause renal insufficiency.

The serum creatinine level often increases without negative consequences. The blood urea nitrogen (BUN) level may increase dramatically. Electrolytes and fluids are excreted more often during the night, in contrast to younger adults, who excrete more during the daytime hours.

The kidney demonstrates a decline in renal activation and diminished intestinal absorption of calcium. Older adults require more vitamin D to compensate for the loss of

TABLE 2-1 Age-Related Changes in the Gastrointestinal Tract

Area	Change	Implications	Contributors
Oropharynx	Decr. neuromuscular coordination; loss of tooth supports, dentin	Choking, dysphagia, aspiration	Stroke, other neuromuscular problems
	Decr. taste buds	Loss of appetite	Alcohol
	Decr. taste sensation	Impaired taste	Old-old age
	Decr. olfactory sensation		
	Loss of teeth	Impaired chewing	Poor care
	Sarcopenia	Decr. chewing	Decr. exercise; malnutrition
Esophagus	Decr. motility	Indigestion, GERD	Obesity, DM, hiatal hernia, medications, cancer, peppermints, stroke, PD
	Decr. LES function	Slow emptying	
		Incr. acid injury—PUD	
Stomach	Decr. acid response	Mucosa unprotected	Tobacco, alcohol, DM, heart failure, herbals, NSAIDs, medications, *Helicobacter pylori*
	Decr. blood flow	Incr. injury—PUD	
	Slow emptying		Early satiety
	Decr. motility, volume		
Small intestine	Relaxed villi	Decr. absorption of most nutrients	Vascular disease
	Atrophy of muscle fibers		
	Decr. mucosal surface		
Gallbladder	Decr. contractility	Cholelithiasis	Obesity, multiparity
	Incr. cholecystokinin levels	Decr. appetite	
Liver	Decr. size, blood flow, perfusion, and fibrosis	Decr. effectiveness of function	Alcohol, herbs
	Decr. regeneration	Decr. metabolism of medications	
Pancreas	Decr. endocrine function	DM risk	DM
Colon	Decr. mucus production, elasticity, and perception of distention	Constipation, loss of urge	DM, dementia
Rectum/anus	Decr. resting pressure	Fecal incontinence	Dementia, neurologic disease

Decr., decreased; GERD, gastroesophageal reflux disease; DM, diabetes mellitus; PD, Parkinson disease; LES, lower esophageal sphincter; Incr., increased; PUD, peptic ulcer disease; NSAIDs, nonsteroidal anti-inflammatory drugs.

Source: Mayhew M, Edmunds M, Wendel V. *Gerentological Nurse Practitioner Review Manual.* Washington, DC: American Nurses Credentialing Center; 2001. Miller CA. *Nursing for Wellness in Older Adults.* 4th ed. Philadelphia: Lippincott; 2004; Huether S. Structure and function of the digestive system. In: McCance K, Huether S, eds. *Pathophysiology.* 4th ed. St. Louis: Mosby; 2002:1231–1337; American Geriatric Society. *Geriatrics Review Syllabus.* 6th ed. New York: American Geriatric Society; 2006.

this function. If there have been urinary tract problems in the past, this loss of function may be accentuated.

With aging, there is reduced elasticity of the bladder. Muscle tone and capacity are diminished and the older adult has frequency of urination. Post-void residual is often found and nocturnal urine production increases. Urinary incontinence is common in older adults. Changes in bladder structure and function may contribute to these symptoms. Changes in neurotransmission influence the micturition response and may lead to an overactive bladder. **Box 2-4** lists

some additional changes. **Figure 2-5** depicts the structure of the urinary tract.

In men, urinary tract obstruction is common and most often caused by benign prostatic hyperplasia (BPH). Symptoms include urinary frequency, urinary retention with overflow incontinence, urinary tract infections, difficulty starting the stream of urine, nocturia (increased urination at night), and ejaculation problems. BPH occurs with sufficient frequency to consider it an age-related issue. Eighty percent of men will develop this condition by age 80. At

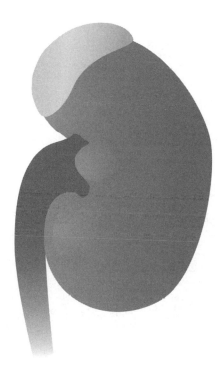

FIGURE 2-4 Kidney

Sources: Data from McCance K, Huether S. *Pathophysiology*. 5th ed. Philadelphia: Elsevier Mosby; 2006; Crowley I.V. *Human Disease*. 6th ed. Sudbury, MA: Jones & Bartlett; 2004.

BOX 2-3 Kidney Terms and Definitions

Nephron	Functional unit of the kidney, contains a glomerulus and a renal tubule. Filters plasma and reabsorbs and secretes substances from the various parts of the nephron. Its main function is to form a filtrate of protein-free plasma.
Glomerulus	Capillaries supplied by an afferent arteriole and combined into an efferent arteriole; supplies the renal tubule.
Renal tubules	Long tubes (4 cm) that join the glomerulus (proximal end) with the collecting tubule (distal end). The renal tubule has three parts: the proximal convoluted tubule, the loop of Henle, and the distal convoluted tubule. The tubules selectively reabsorb water, minerals, and other materials that need to be conserved. They excrete unwanted substances to be eliminated.
Reabsorption	Sodium chloride (NaCl), glucose, potassium ions (K^+), amino acids, bicarbonate (HCO_3), phosphate (PO_4), urea, protein, water
Secretion	Hydrogen ions (H^+), foreign substances, organic anions and cations, urea, K^+, ammonia (NH_3), some drugs

birth, the prostate is the size of a pea and grows slowly until puberty, at which point it grows rapidly until the 30s. At 40 to 45 years of age, BPH begins and continues until death. The cause of BPH is unclear, but it is thought to be related to levels and ratios of androgens, estrogens, growth-stimulatory factors, and growth-inhibitory factors. Medication, urinary catheters, and surgery are useful for management.

Breasts and Genitalia

In older women, a loss of elastin and subcutaneous fat and an increase in fibrosis causes pendulous breasts, reducing breast size and fullness. Breast mass decreases due to loss of estrogen following menopause and a decrease in the number of mammary ducts. The nipples of the breast may retract; the areola becomes smaller and may nearly disappear. The breasts often flatten and sag (**Figure 2-6**). The risk for breast cancer in older women is high.

Beginning at menopause, which occurs, on average, at age 50, the ovaries, uterus, and cervix atrophy. The ovaries no longer release eggs, and menstrual periods stop. The ovaries continue to produce small amounts of estrogen and testosterone. Pituitary hormones diminish.

The vagina becomes thin, dry, and loses elasticity. Lubrication, which becomes watery, is diminished. The vagina narrows and shortens, and there is a loss of rugae. This is known as atrophic vaginitis. In addition, the vagina becomes pale because of diminished vascularity. The result of these changes is decreased sexual functioning because of pain (dyspareunia) and diminished pleasure unless measures are taken to promote lubrication.

Common problems as a result of these changes are vaginal prolapse, bladder prolapse, and uterine prolapse. These changes can cause stress incontinence (leakage of urine). Some women experience hot flashes due to hormonal changes. Vaginal yeast infections become more common because changes in hormones affect the microorganisms in the vagina.

Some women take hormone replacement therapy (HRT) to reduce menopausal symptoms. HRT may heighten the risk of breast cancer, but it does help prevent the osteoporosis that occurs with diminished estrogen levels. **Figure 2-7** depicts changes in the female reproductive system with aging.

⬤ BOX 2-4 Age-Related Changes That Predispose to Urinary Incontinence

Change	Potential Problem
Atrophic vaginitis/urethritis	Diminished urethral mucosal seal
Benign prostatic hyperplasia	Outlet obstruction, frequency, urgency
Inability to postpone urination	Frequency, urgency, nocturia
Increase in urine concentration during sleep hours	Nocturia
Diminished detrusor contractility	Diminished urine flow, hesitancy
Decrease in bladder capacity	Frequency, urgency, nocturia
Detrusor overactivity	Frequency, urgency, nocturia
Increase in residual urine after voiding	Frequency, nocturia

Sources: Adapted from American Geriatric Society (AGS). *Geriatric Review Syllabus.* 6th ed. New York: American Geriatric Society; 2006; Tabloski, P. *Gerontological Nursing.* Upper Saddle River, NJ: Prentice Hall; 2006.

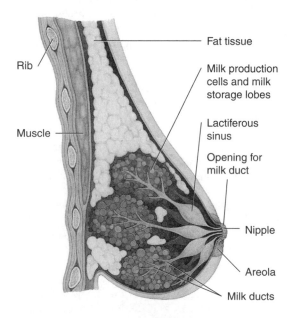

FIGURE 2-5 Urinary Tract System

Source: National Institutes of Health, 2007.

In men, testosterone production declines with age, and sperm counts diminish to nearly 50% of those of younger men. Less seminal fluid is produced. Libido, muscle strength, energy, and well-being all decrease. Men also face an increased risk of osteoporosis. These changes are much more gradual than the menopausal changes in older women and result from changes in the testes. **Figure 2-8** illustrates the reproductive systems of young and older adult males.

Musculoskeletal Changes

All older adults experience age-related changes in gait and posture. Coordination is affected by changes in the muscles and joints and movement becomes slower.

Bone mass and bone density diminish beginning between the ages of 40 to 50. In women, these losses occur more quickly following menopause. The bone becomes more brittle with age and less strong. Bone remodeling takes longer to complete, and the rate of mineralization slows. This predisposes older men and women to fractures, often as a result of minimal trauma, especially in the proximal end of the long bones and in the spine.

With advancing age, articular cartilage has a slowed response to growth factors, becomes brittle, and accumulates calcium pyrophosphate. This can cause synovitis (inflam-

FIGURE 2-6 Anatomy of Female Breast

Younger female reproductive system

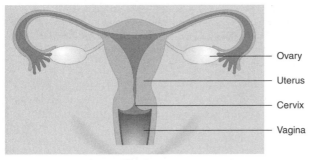

Older female reproductive system

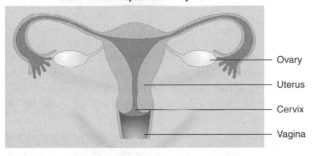

FIGURE 2-7 Comparison of Younger and Older Female Reproductive Systems

Source: National Library of Medicine/National Institutes of Health, 2008.

mation) in the lining of a joint where the calcium pyrophosphate settles.

The intervertebral discs in the spine become thinner and drier with advancing age. This decreases the amount of space between the intervertebral discs, resulting in a decrease in height. In addition, the arch of the foot becomes less pronounced, further contributing to loss of height. The older adult can lose 2 to 4 inches of his or her maximum adult height.

The vertebrae lose minerals, causing the bones to become thinner. The spinal column becomes curved and compressed.

Figure 2-9 compares a young spine with an older woman's spine. Osteoporosis is common in the adult of advanced age.

The connective tissue in the ligaments and tendons loses its tensile strength, elasticity, and regenerative capacity over time. The tendons and ligaments stiffen, decreasing joint flexibility. The connective tissue can be easily damaged, ruptured, or torn.

Muscle mass decreases with age, beginning at about age 30. As much as 30% to 40% of muscle mass and strength may be lost between the ages of 30 and 90. Muscle bulk is lost due to both a reduction in the number and size of muscle fibers. The muscles atrophy and degenerate, and the proportion of adipose tissue to muscle increases. Handgrip strength diminishes, making routine activities, such as opening a jar, difficult. The heart muscle is less able to propel large quantities of blood quickly, and older adults tire more quickly and take longer to recover from exercise. **Table 2-2** summarizes changes in muscle mass over time.

Younger male reproductive system

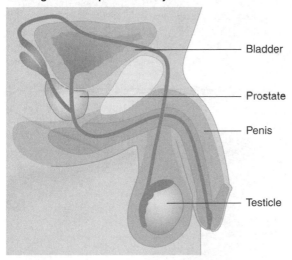

Older male reproductive system

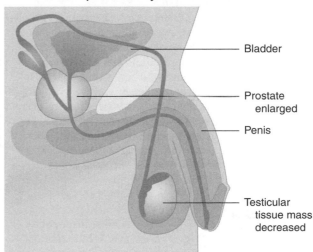

FIGURE 2-8 Comparison of Younger and Older Male Reproductive Systems

Source: National Library of Medicine/National Institutes of Health, 2008.

a)   b)

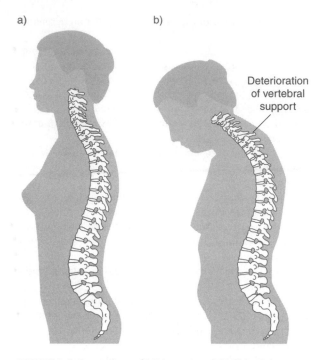

Deterioration
of vertebral
support

FIGURE 2-9 Comparison of (a) Younger and (b) Older Spine

Source: National Library of Medicine/National Institutes of Health, 2008.

TABLE 2-2 Changes in Muscle Mass with Aging

Age Group	Body Weight Muscle (%)	Adipose Tissue (%)	Bone (%)
Young adults	30	20	10
Older adults (75+)	15	40	8

Source: Data from *Merck Manual of Geriatrics*, Aging and the musculoskeletal system (Ch. 48, Sec. 7), May, 2005.

Neurologic Changes

Structural changes occur in the brain with aging. The brain and spinal cord lose neurons. The brain atrophies, with most of the decrease in size and weight occurring in the frontal hemispheres. There is fibrosis and thickening of the meninges. The gyri narrow and the sulci widen, increasing the size of the subarachnoid space. **Figure 2-11** depicts the anatomy of the brain.

Strength training can reduce **sarcopenia** (muscle wasting and lost of strength), and most older adults can continue to function well. However, fewer than 10% of Americans participate in regular exercise, and the most sedentary group is those adults older than 50.

With advancing age, movement slows because it takes longer for the muscles to respond and osteoarthritis (OA) can limit movement and decrease range of motion. The gait becomes slower and shorter. There is less arm swinging, and the gait becomes less steady. These changes increase the risk of injury due to lack of balance.

Osteoarthritis-related symptoms increase with age and can occur in any bone in the body. Pain in the neck may be cervical OA and can result in diminished range of motion of the neck and pain down the arms, shoulders, and upper back. Pain in the midspine is thoracic OA. Osteoarthritis in the lower spine (lumbar and sacral OA) may present as pain in the buttocks or down the legs. These changes are not as visible as those in the hands, knees, and ankles. Hip and knee OA are very common with increasing age and are worsened by overweight and obesity (**Figure 2-10**).

sarcopenia Age-associated loss of muscle mass, associated with muscle weakness, functional limitations, and disability, as well as impairments in cardiovascular capacity and metabolic health.

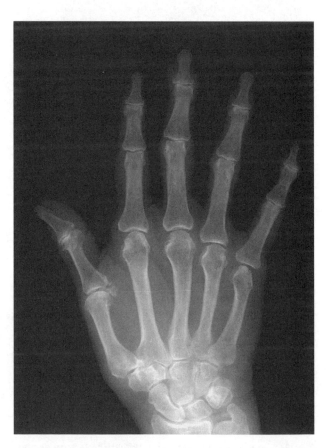

FIGURE 2-10 X-Ray Showing Osteoarthritis in the Hand of an Older Adult

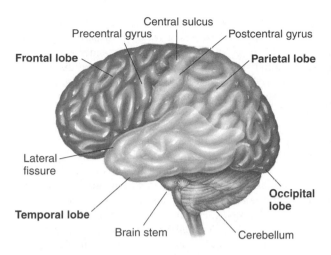

Central sulcus
Precentral gyrus   Postcentral gyrus
Frontal lobe   **Parietal lobe**

Lateral
fissure

**Occipital
lobe**

Temporal lobe

Brain stem   Cerebellum

FIGURE 2-11 Anatomy of the Brain

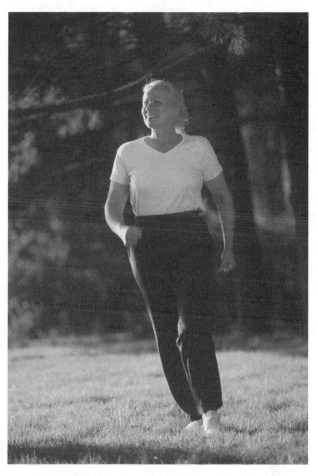

Cognitive function may decline with aging. Those abilities that commonly decline include selective attention, the ability to name objects, verbal fluency, complex visuospatial skills, and logical analysis. Most of these age-related losses of cognitive function are mild. Self-reported memory loss by older adults is usually caused by depression rather than cognitive impairment due to dementia. Dealing with the depression may improve cognitive function. Often families are much less concerned about the memory loss than is the older adult, who fears dementia.

Distant memories are more accessible to the older adult than recent ones. The ability to acquire, store, and retrieve newer memories is reduced. Older adults are able to learn as well as younger adults; however, it takes more time. Intelligence is stable with aging. Much intellectual function is maintained with continued intellectual activity. Playing card games such as bridge, doing puzzles (especially crossword), reading, learning a new skill such as playing a musical instrument, and continuing social interactions will all help maintain function.

Personality also seems to be stable with aging. A pleasant, easygoing younger adult will be a pleasant older adult. An irritable, angry young adult will probably be the same when older. There are many theories of personality in aging, but no single theory has been proven.

Fewer neurotransmitters are produced and those that are produced are conducted more slowly. Neuronal cell death and dysfunction occur. These changes translate into slower movements, slower responses, and slower reflexes. In addition, it might take the older adult longer to make decisions.

It is easier for the older adult to move large muscle groups than to move smaller groups for fine movements. Older adults are susceptible to tremors not associated with a dis-

ease entity; this is known as benign senile or benign essential tremor. This type of tremor is more noticeable when the older adult is stressed or tired.

The autonomic nervous system (ANS) becomes less efficient with age. Because of this, the older adult is less able to recover from a stressful event, such as surgery, than when young. The diminished functioning of the ANS also renders the older adult more susceptible to orthostatic hypotension (dizziness when standing up from a sitting or supine position). The older adult is also subject to hypo- and hyperthermia.

Age-related changes of the ANS include diminished light-touch sensation, diminished vibratory sense (especially in the lower extremities), less brisk deep tendon reflexes, and diminished ability for upward gaze and sometimes downward gaze. The Achilles tendon reflex is often absent. The older adult is at an increased risk of falling due to postural instability. Recovery from walking on an unstable surface is slowed.

The very old are at risk for neurologic abnormalities such as delirium. Almost any acute health problem—for example, fever—can cause a sudden deficit in oxygenation in the brain, which manifests as delirium.

Sleep and Aging

Many older adults have difficulty with sleep. About 50% of older adults complain of sleep difficulties. They take a longer time to fall asleep and have difficulty staying asleep, awakening frequently during the night. **Box 2-5** describes the stages of sleep.

In older adults, total sleep time is diminished. The older adult becomes sleepy much earlier in the evening than a younger adult and awakens much earlier in the morning. This is thought to be caused by an alteration of the body's circadian rhythm. *Sleep efficiency* is diminished; that is, more time is spent in bed, but less time is spent in productive sleep. Sleep efficiency is about 95% in younger adults and but is less than 80% in older adults. Although experts disagree as to which changes in sleep occur normally with aging, most agree that the net effect of age-related changes in non-REM (non–rapid-eye movement) sleep is that less time is spent in the deep, physical restorative stages of sleep. Stages 3 and 4 of non-REM sleep are probably better preserved in older women than in older men.

REM sleep appears to be important for mental and psychological restoration, because being deprived of REM sleep causes irritability and diminished concentration. REM sleep may be constant in older adults, but the amount of it may be diminished as a result of overall reduced night sleep time, with the result of irritability and loss of concentration. In addition, older adults are less able to tolerate sleep deprivation than younger adults.

Sleep changes associated with aging occur earlier in men than women (by about 10 years). Age-related changes in other body systems may contribute to sleep problems.

Drugs, arthritis, depression, bereavement, social isolation, dementia, thyroid diseases, Parkinson disease, and osteoporotic fractures may all affect sleep in older adults. One study found that the frequency of respiratory disturbances increased dramatically with age. Only 5% of subjects younger than 50 years old had a respiratory index of more than 15 incidents per hour. More than 50% of adults older than 65 years had more than 15 respiratory disturbances (often sleep apnea) per hour of sleep. It has been suggested that this phenomenon is normal in the older adult.

Measures to promote sleep include moderate exercise in the afternoon and avoidance of stimulants such as caffeine, colas, and teas, or medications that have a stimulant. A light bedtime snack, especially warm milk, can be helpful in promoting sleep. The older adult should try to go to bed at the same time every night and avoid naps during the day. If a person cannot attain sleep after about 20 minutes, he or she should get out of bed and do some quiet activity such as reading or listening to music. Many older adults believe that having a drink of alcohol helps with sleep. It does make one sleepy; however, alcohol increases awakenings later during the night.

Mental Health

Maintaining mental acuity by participating in activities that stimulate the mind and body helps a person to retain normal functioning and a healthy lifestyle. Severe mental decline is not inevitable. The aged brain can maintain the ability to make new connections, absorb new information, and acquire new skills.

Physical disorders can affect psychological disorders or precipitate latent ones. More than 25% of older adults have impaired hearing. Sensory deprivation can cause symptoms of delusion. The frail older adult with depression and psychosis may be unable to correctly take drugs to treat his or her physical illnesses. Older adults living in the community setting often have the same degree of physical disability as do those in nursing homes. However, social supports such as family members, church, and others are more available in the community setting.

Vague physical decline does not always indicate physical aging or the progression of underlying illness. In one study of depressed adults older than 60, physical complaints were reported by more than 60% of respondents. The nature and rate of physical decline in a depressed older adult may reflect his or her will to live or die.

Although aging may affect cognition, memory, intelligence, personality, and behavior, many changes in mental health are difficult to attribute to aging. A decline may be due to treatable illnesses, such as depression, hypothyroidism, or vitamin B12 deficiency. The prevalence of psychiatric disorders is 15% to 25% among those 65 and older who live in the community. It is 27% to 55% among those who

---

▶ BOX 2-5 Stages of Non-REM Sleep (Sleep Needed for Physical Recuperation)

Stage I	Light sleep	Easily arousable
Stage II	Deeper sleep	Easily aroused
Stage III	Deeper	Difficult to arouse
Stage IV	Deepest	All body functions reduced; restorative sleep

REM sleep (dream sleep) is psychologically restorative sleep.

are hospitalized. Psychiatric disorders are a primary or secondary diagnosis in 70%, 80%, or 94% of those in a nursing home, depending on the particular study. Dementia is a brain disorder affecting 10% of adults aged 65 and older and 25% or more of those aged 85 and older.

Nutritional Aspects of Aging

Considerable changes in body composition occur with aging, making standardized comparisons with younger adults impossible. The body's water content, lean mass, and bone mass all diminish with age. Fat mass increases, and there are usually greater abdominal fat stores. All of these changes affect nutrition in aging.

In general, older adults have a diminished basal metabolic rate, which reflects the loss of muscle mass. The basal metabolic rate is the principal determinant of total energy expenditure. **Box 2-6** shows a method of determining a person's basal energy expenditure and needs.

Many of the physiologic changes of aging place older adults at risk for malnutrition. In general, food intake is diminished in aged individuals. About 16% of older persons living in the community consume fewer than 1,000 kcal/day, which is insufficient for adequate nutrition. Those older adults who are underweight in middle age are at greater risk of death than those who are overweight. However, this may be changing as more adults, especially those in their 60s and 70s, are obese.

Older adults seem to feel full with less food. This may be due to a decrease in the natural opioid dynorphin, which affects the feeding drive. Further, the satiety effect of cholecystokinin is increased. A number of **cytokines** (e.g., interleukin-2) cause a decrease in food intake. Many elders have increased cytokine levels, which contributes to **anorexia**. Stresses such as surgery increase the cytokine levels. High levels of cytokines inhibit production of albumin; the albumin present in the body moves to the extracellular spaces. Even minor stressors can cause this situation.

Leptin, a protein hormone produced by fat cells, decreases food intake and increases energy metabolism. Leptin is related to prolonged postprandial satiety. Postmenopausal women with high leptin levels have a tendency to eat less than women who have low leptin levels. In women older than 70, leptin levels diminish with the decline in body fat that occurs at this age. In older men, leptin levels increase despite the decline in body fat because of declining testosterone production.

Some drugs commonly taken by older adults contribute to undernutrition, such as those used to treat hypertension (e.g., diuretics and digoxin), hypothyroidism (thyroxine), respiratory conditions (e.g., theophylline), and cancer (e.g., cisplatin). Halting the use of some psychotropic drugs that cause weight gain (anti-anxiety and antipsychotic medications) can cause weight loss, as can consumption of alcohol.

● BOX 2-6 Prediction of Basal Energy Expenditure and Need

Predictive Equations for Basal Energy Expenditure (BEE)

Men: $66.5 + (13.75 \times kg) + (5.003 \times cm) - (6.775 \times age)$

Women: $655.1 + (9.563 \times kg) + (1.850 \times cm) - (4.676 \times age)$

Source: Adapted from Cornell University. Medical calculators: basal energy expenditure—Harris-Benedict equation. October 2000. Available at: http://www-users.med.cornell.edu/~spon/picu/calc/beecalc.htm.

Vitamin D

Older people have an increased requirement for vitamin D because of their diminished capacity to produce the vitamin, absorb it intestinally, and activate it renally (**Figure 2-12**). Vitamin D is essential to skeletal health, muscle strength, and protection against heart disease and cancers. Because it is found in so few foods, older adults may not consume adequate amounts of it in the diet. Indeed, vitamin D deficiency is highly prevalent in the United States and worldwide, affecting as many as one-third to one-half of otherwise healthy middle-aged and older adults. The precursor to vitamin D, 7-dehydrocholesterol, is 75% less productive in older age compared with younger adults. Vitamin D deficiency may be related to diminished exposure to sunlight and poor intake of dietary products.

The skin is only 40% as efficient in the synthesis of vitamin D in older years as in youth. Even older adults living in Florida have insufficient vitamin D, and in the winter months vitamin D levels can be as much as 40% below recommended levels. Dark-skinned people may require as much as six times the amount of ultraviolet radiation as light-skinned people in order to stimulate the production of vitamin D. Further, the kidney is less responsive in converting the inactive form of vitamin D to the active hormonal form (1,25-dihydroxy vitamin D) in advanced age. This vitamin is essential for the body's absorption of calcium.

Vitamin D is considered to be both a vitamin and a hormone. It is not a true

cytokines Low-molecular-weight proteins or glycoproteins. Function as chemical signals between cells. They play an important role in inflammation and in the acquired immune response.

anorexia Loss of interest in eating.

North of 42 degrees latitude, sunlight is too weak to synthesize vitamin D from late October through early March. The same effect occurs during the winter in the southern hemisphere south of 42 degrees latitude

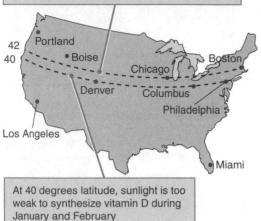

At 40 degrees latitude, sunlight is too weak to synthesize vitamin D during January and February

FIGURE 2-12 Mapping Vitamin D Synthesis

Source: Insel P, Turner RE, Ross D. *Nutrition.* 3rd ed. Sudbury, MA: Jones & Bartlett; 2007, p. 405. Reproduced with permission.

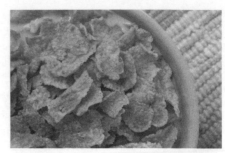

VITAMIN D

Daily Value = 400 IU

Exceptionally good sources		
Cod liver oil	1 Tbsp	1,360 IU
Salmon, canned, solids + bones	55 g (2 oz)	420 IU
Sardines, canned, solids + bones	55 g (2 oz)	150 IU
Milk, 1% milkfat	240 ml (1 cup)	129 IU
Milk, nonfat	240 ml (1 cup)	103 IU
Milk, whole, 3.25% milkfat	240 ml (1 cup)	99 IU
Fortified, ready-to-eat cereals	30 g	40–50 IU

High: 20% DV or more

FIGURE 2-13 Food Sources of Vitamin D

Source: U.S. Department of Agriculture, Agricultural Research Service. USDA National Nutrient Database for Standard Reference, Release 18. 2005. http://www.ars.usda.gov/nutrientdata.

vitamin, because it is synthesized in the skin in the presence of sunlight. It exists in dietary sources such as fish oils, fatty fish, egg yolk, fortified milk, and other fortified foods (**Figure 2-13**). In 1997, Dietary Reference Intakes (DRIs) were developed for vitamin D intake (**Table 2-3**). However, since that time it has been found that vitamin D deficiency is widespread worldwide.

Experts believe that previously recommended levels of vitamin D are insufficient, especially for older adults, and particularly for those who are frail and have multiple comorbidities. It has been suggested that vitamin D supplements (cholecalciferol) of 400 to 800 IU/day are associated with decreases in mortality. These supplements are inexpensive and safe for most older adults.

Calcium

The requirement for calcium increases at menopause. Adequate calcium intake is a key component of any bone-protective therapeutic program. Calcium also has beneficial effects on nonskeletal disorders, including hypertension, colorectal cancer, and obesity. To receive the nutritional benefits of calcium, adequate vitamin D is required. The target for postmenopausal women is 1,200 mg of calcium, which can be obtained through diet by consuming three cups of dairy products daily or from diet and supplements. Nonfat milk is the most nutrient-dense source because of

its high calcium content and low fat and calorie content. **Figure 2-14** illustrates the functions of calcium.

The body normally absorbs 25% to 75% of dietary calcium depending on a person's age, the presence of adequate vitamin D, the body's need for calcium, and calcium intake. The older adult usually absorbs only 25% when absorption is lowest.

Absorption of calcium is inversely related to calcium intake. An increase in dietary calcium diminishes absorption. A decrease in dietary calcium causes an increase in absorption. Without vitamin D, calcium absorption can drop to less than 10% of the dietary source of calcium. Some foods, such as phytates (e.g., nuts, seeds, and grains) and oxalates, *decrease* absorption of calcium. In addition, supplements containing high levels of phosphorus and magnesium can also decrease calcium absorption. The Adequate Intake (AI) level for calcium in older adults is 1,200 mg/day. Rich sources of calcium include tofu (calcium processed); yogurt; nonfat milk; sesame seeds; Swiss, mozzarella, and cheddar cheeses; and canned sardines.

Vitamin K

Vitamin K is the blood-clotting vitamin. Many older adults do not get sufficient amounts of vitamin K, despite the fact that they are consuming more of it than younger adults. The body only needs small amounts of vitamin K. The vitamin may be essential in the prevention of bone loss, fractures, arteriosclerosis, and osteoarthritis. The low levels of

TABLE 2-3 Dietary Reference Intakes for Vitamin D Established in 1997

Age (yrs)	Adequate Intake	Upper-Limit Intake (mcg/day)
Children (1–8)	5 mcg (200 IU)	25
Males (9–50)	5 mcg	50
Men (51–70)	10 mcg (400 IU)	50
Men (71+)	15 mcg (600 IU)	50
Females (9–50)	5 mcg	50
Women (51–70)	10 mcg (same as for older men)	50
Women (71+)	15 mcg (same as for older men)	50

Source: Adapted from Standing Committee on the Scientific Evaluation of Dietary References Intake. *Dietary Reference Intakes: Calcium, Phosphorus, Magnesium, Vitamin D, and Fluoride.* National Academy Press: Washington, DC; 1997.

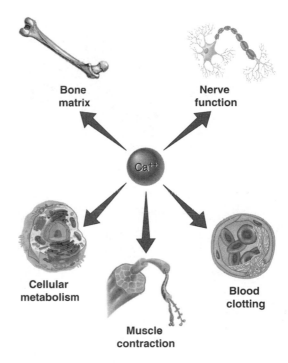

FIGURE 2-14 Functions of Calcium

Source: Insel P, Turner RE, Ross D. *Nutrition.* 3rd ed. Sudbury, MA: Jones & Bartlett; 2007, p. 477. Reproduced with permission.

estrogen that occur in menopause change the way vitamin K is metabolized in women.

Older adults with fat-malabsorption syndromes, such as celiac, sprue, ulcerative colitis, and Crohn's disease, can become deficient in vitamin K. Prolonged use of antibiotics may cause a vitamin K deficiency because the drugs destroy intestinal bacteria that produce the vitamin. Vitamin K status is assessed prior to surgery because patients often are given antibiotics with surgery. Large doses of vitamin A and E counteract the absorption and action of vitamin K. Vitamin E promotes bleeding. **Figure 2-15** shows food sources of vitamin K.

Changes in Laboratory Values with Aging

Laboratories do not provide a different "normal range" for older adults. However, many age-related differences are reflected in the laboratory values of older adults. **Box 2-7** shows changes that occur in these values with aging that must be taken into consideration when assessing whether a value is normal or abnormal. One of the best ways to determine what is normal is continuity of care; that is, following a patient over time, determining the patient's normal values, and then reviewing laboratory results every few years for changes to abnormal values or maintenance of normal values for that individual.

Vitamin B12, an essential water-soluble vitamin, is found in a wide variety of foods, including fish, meats, and dairy products. It can be stored in the body for several years, so unless the diet is poor, it is uncommon to be deficient in this vitamin. However, many older adults have slightly low blood levels of B12. It may be that older adults are unable to use the vitamin. Those who cannot absorb the vitamin in the intestinal tract and vegetarians who consume it in

insufficient amounts will be deficient. Because only *slightly low* levels of vitamin B12 (without anemia) can cause severe problems, it is important to watch this laboratory level on a regular basis. This is also true with thyroid levels, because hypothyroidism is common in older adults.

Drugs commonly used by older adults in the treatment of chronic health problems may spuriously alter laboratory test results. These drugs include penicillin G, levodopa, morphine, nalidixic acid, and isoniazid, which may lead to false-positive urine glucose test results. Vitamin C supplements can also alter laboratory test results. No vitamin supplements should be taken in excess, and patients should be warned that "*more is not better.*"

A low serum albumin level in a healthy person is usually a result of diet. However, low levels can also indicate serious disease when accompanied by undernutrition.

Blood glucose levels increase with aging, but usually remain within the nondiabetic range. Lack of exercise, obesity, and some drugs may affect glucose tolerance more than aging. The renal threshold for glucose does decrease with aging. Glucose may be found in the urine of older patients even when the blood glucose level is less than 200 mg/dL.

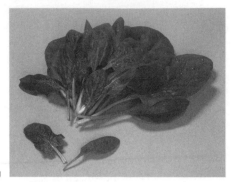

VITAMIN K

Daily Value = 80 μg

Exceptionally good sources

Kale, cooked	85 g (~1/2 cup)	694 μg
Spinach, raw	85 g (~3 cups)	410 μg
Turnip greens, raw	85 g (~3 cups)	213 μg
Broccoli, cooked	85 g (~1/2 cup)	120 μg
Romaine lettuce, raw	85 g (~1 1/2 cups)	87 μg
Cabbage, raw	85 g (~1 1/4 cups)	51 μg
Asparagus, cooked	85 g (~1/2 cup)	43 μg
Okra, cooked	85 g (~1/2 cup)	34 μg
Black-eyed peas, cooked	90 g (~1/2 cup)	33 μg
Blackberries, raw	140 g (~1 cup)	28 μg
Soybean oil	1 Tbsp.	27 μg
Blueberries, raw	140 g (~3/4 cup)	27 μg
Green beans, cooked	85 g (~2/3 cup)	14 μg
Cauliflower, raw	85 g (~3/4 cup)	13.6 μg
Artichokes, cooked	85 g (~1/2 cup)	13 μg
Tomato, green, raw	85 g (1 small)	8.6 μg

High: 20% DV or more

Good: 10–19% DV

FIGURE 2-15 Food Sources of Vitamin K

Source: U.S. Department of Agriculture, Agricultural Research Service. USDA National Nutrient Database for Standard Reference, Release 18. 2005. http://www.ars.usda.gov/nutrientdata.

◗ BOX 2-7   Changes in Laboratory Values with Aging

Increase in Value	Decrease in Value
Uric acid	Vitamin B6
Triglycerides	Vitamin B12
Prostate-specific antigen (PSA)	Vitamin C
Postprandial glucose	Phosphorus
Ferritin	Calcium
Cholesterol	Creatinine kinase
Alkaline phosphatase	Thiamine
Copper	Estrogen
Serum cholesterol	Growth hormone
Glucose, postprandial serum	Serum iron
Parathyroid hormone	Selenium
	Zinc
	Testosterone
	Plasma vitamin E
	Triiodothyronine (T3)

Source: Adapted from *Merck Manual of Geriatrics* [online]. Laboratory values. 2000. Available at: http://www.merck.com/mkgr/mmg/appndxs/app1.jsp. Accessed April 23, 2008.

The erythrocyte sedimentation rate (ESR) is not affected by aging, but it is often higher in the older adult. This is a result of the number of chronic health problems of an inflammatory nature that occur in older people, each of which may raise the ESR. Some of these conditions include rheumatoid arthritis, cancer, temporal arteritis, and infection. If the ESR is elevated, it should be rechecked and evaluated further if the cause is not known.

The prostate-specific antigen (PSA) level increases with age. It may increase even with benign conditions. An increase of the PSA of more than 5% to 8% in a year may be quite significant, requiring follow-up with ultrasound and perhaps a biopsy to eliminate the possibility of false-positive tests.

Protein-to-creatinine ratios in urine are used to estimate the magnitude of proteinuria, which increases with old age. Ratios above 3.0 indicate massive proteinuria; ratios below 2.0 indicate insignificant proteinuria.

Creatinine clearance decreases with age, but the serum creatinine level remains stable because older adults lose muscle mass over time. When serum creatine is measured,

it might appear that renal function is good; however, practitioners should use the Cockcroft-Gault formula to better estimate renal function, especially before prescribing drugs. This formula is as follows:

$$\text{Creatinine clearance (mL/min)} = \frac{(140 - \text{age in years}) \times \text{body weight in kilograms}}{72 \times \text{serum creatinine level (mg/dL)}}$$

In women, the calculated value is multiplied by 0.85.

Conclusion: Quality of Life

Quality of life is often described on both objective and subjective dimensions. Most older adults assess their quality of life (QOL) positively based on their social contacts, level of independence, health, material goods, and social comparisons. Adaptation and resilience may play a part in the maintenance of good QOL. Two major factors that have to be considered with QOL in old age are dementia and

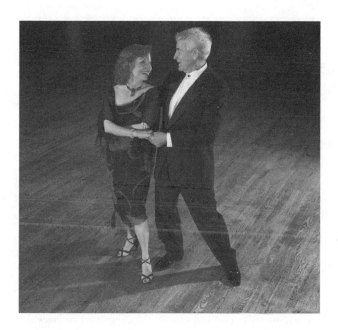

depression. However, with all other influences controlled, aging in and of itself does not influence QOL negatively. A long period of good QOL is possible. The maintenance and improvement of QOL should be included among the goals of clinical management.

Activities and Questions Related to This Chapter

1. What are the clinical consequences of slowed digestion in the elderly patient?
2. How does one estimate renal function of older adults?
3. State what a socially managed mealtime is and why it is important.
4. Describe the vitamin and mineral changes in aging, how they affect the older adult, and how dietary management can help.
5. List the changes that occur in laboratory values in older adults compared with younger adults.

REFERENCES

A.D.A.M. Medical Encyclopedia [online]. Aging changes in the bones—muscles—joints. August 22, 2006. Available at: http://www.nlm.nih.gov/medlineplus/ency/article/004015.htm. Accessed April 21, 2008.

A.D.A.M. Medical Encyclopedia [online]. Aging changes in sleep. August 22, 2006. Available at: http://www.nlm.nih.gov/medlineplus/ency/article/004018.htm. Accessed April 21, 2008.

A.D.A.M. Medical Encyclopedia [online]. Aging changes in the female reproductive system. August 19, 2006. Available at: http://www.nlm.nih.gov/medlineplus/ency/article/004016.htm. Accessed April 21, 2008.

A.D.A.M. Medical Encyclopedia [online]. Aging changes in the male reproductive system. September 26, 2006. Available at: http://www.nlm.nih.gov/medlineplus/ency/article/004017.htm. Accessed April 21, 2008.

American Academy of Orthopaedic Surgeons. Effects of aging. July 2007. Available at: http://orthoinfo.aaos.org/topic.cfm?topic = A00191. Accessed April 20, 2008.

American Academy of Sleep Medicine (AASM). New study in the journal SLEEP finds that respiratory disturbances during sleep increase significantly with age, even in healthy individuals. 2008. Available at: http://www.aasmnet.org/Articles.aspx?id = 724. Accessed February 3, 2009.

American Geriatric Society. *Geriatric Review Syllabus*. 6th ed. New York: American Geriatric Society; 2006.

Area Agency on Aging. What is normal aging? n.d. Available at: http://www.agingcarefl.org/aging/normalAging. Accessed February 3, 2009.

Booth S. Vitamin K status in the elderly. *Curr Opin Clin Nutr Metabol Care*. 2007;10(1):20–23.

Centers for Disease Control and Prevention. National oral health surveillance system. n.d. Available at: http://apps.nccd.cdc.gov/nohss/ListV.asp?akev = 8&DataSet = 2. Accessed February 3, 2009.

Cherniack EP, Levis S, Troen BR. Hypovitaminosis D: a stealthy epidemic that requires treatment. *Geriatrics*. 2008;63(4):24–30.

Di Francesco V, Zamboni M, Zoico E, Mazzali G, Dioli A, Omizzolo F, et al. Unbalanced serum leptin and ghrelin dynamics prolong postprandial satiety and inhibit hunger in healthy elderly: another reason for the "anorexia of aging." *Am J Nutr*. 2006;83(5):1149–1152.

Gallo JJ, Fulmer T, Paveza GJ, Reichel W. *Handbook of Geriatric Assessment*. 4th ed. Sudbury, MA: Jones & Bartlett; 2006.

Giese K. Do your patients have a vitamin D deficiency? *Clin Advisor*. Apr 2007;70–75.

Insel P, Turner RE, Ross D. *Nutrition*. 3rd ed. Sudbury, MA: Jones & Bartlett; 2007.

Janssen I, Katzmarzyk P, Ross R. Body mass index is inversely related to mortality in older people after adjustment for waist circumference. *J Am Geriatr Soc*. 2006;53(12):2112–2118.

Jockers BS. Vitamin D sufficiency: an approach to disease prevention. *Am J Nurse Pract*. 2007;11(10):43–48.

McCance K, Huether S. *Pathophysiology*. 5th ed. Philadelphia: Elsevier Mosby; 2006.

Merck Manual: Home Edition [online]. Undernutrition: disorders of nutrition and metabolism. August 2007. Available at: http://www.merck.com/mmhe/sec12/ch153/ch153a.html. Accessed April 23, 2008.

Merck Manual of Geriatrics. 3rd ed. Whitehouse Station, NJ: Merck Research Laboratories; 2000.

Merck Manual of Geriatrics [online]. Age-associated changes in cardiac function. In: Aging and the cardiovascular system. 2000. Available at: http://www.merck.com/mkgr/tables/83t2.jsp. Accessed March 23, 2006.

Merck Manual of Geriatrics [online]. Age-related changes in ocular function. May 2005. Available at: http://www.merck.com/mkgr/mmg/sec15/ch126/ch126b.jsp. Accessed March 27, 2009.

Merck Manual of Geriatrics [online]. Aging and the gastrointestinal tract. May 2005. Available at: http://www.merck.com/mkgr/mmg/sec13/ch102/ch102a.jsp. Accessed March 27, 2009.

Merck Manual of Geriatrics [online]. Aging and the lungs. April 2006. Available at: http://www.merck.com/mkgr/mmg/sec10/ch75/ch75a.jsp. Accessed March 27, 2009.

Merck Manual of Geriatrics [online]. Aging and the musculoskeletal system. May 2005. Available at: http://www.merck.com/mkgr/mmg/sec7/ch48/ch48a.jsp. Accessed March 27, 2009.

Merck Manual of Geriatrics [online]. Aging and the skin. March 2006. Available at: http://www.merck.com/mkgr/mmg/sec15/ch122/ch122b.jsp. Accessed February 8, 2007.

Merck Manual of Geriatrics [online]. Biology of aging. June 2006. Available at: http://www.merck.com/mkgr/mmg/sec1/ch1/ch1a.jsp. Accessed March 27, 2009.

Merck Manual of Geriatrics [online]. Effects of psychologic dysfunction on physical health. 2000. Available at: http://www.merck.com/mkgr/mmg/sec4/ch32/ch32d.jsp. Accessed March 23, 2006.

Merck Manual of Geriatrics [online]. Laboratory values. 2000. Available at: http://www.merck.com/mkgr/mmg/appndxs/app1.jsp. Accessed April 23, 2008.

Merck Manual of Geriatrics [online]. Sleep disorders. March 2006. Available at: http://www.merck.com/mkgr/mmg/sec6/ch47/ch47a.jsp. Accessed March 27, 2009.

National Institute on Aging. AgePage: Aging and your eyes. n.d. Available at: http://www.nia.nih.gov/HealthInformation/Publications/eyes.htm. Accessed February 3, 2009.

National Institute on Aging. Baltimore longitudinal study on aging. n.d. Available at: http:// www.nia.nih.gov/NK/rdonlyres/F1B25F15-BB89-4A73-842A-SE7A2A2F69C2/0/BLSA_FNL_110708FINa1dPDF.pdf. Accessed February 2, 2009.

National Institute on Aging. Blood vessels and aging: the rest of the journey. 2006. Available at: http://www.nia.nih.gov/HealthInformation/Publications/AgingHeartsandArteries/chapter04.htm. Accessed February 4, 2007.

National Institute on Aging. Subgoal 2: Maintain and enhance brain function, cognition, and other behaviors. 2008. Available at: http://www.nia.nih.gov/About NIA/StrategicPlan/ResearchGoalB/Subgoal2.htm. Accessed April 21, 2008.

Netuveli G, Blane D. Quality of life in older ages. *Br Med Bull.* 2008;85(1):113–126.

North American Menopause Society. Updated position statement for calcium intake in postmenopausal women. *Menopause* 2006;13:859–862.

O'Neill PA. *Caring for the Older Adult.* New York: Saunders; 2002.

Perez-Lopez FR. Review article: vitamin D acquisition and breast cancer risk. *Reprod Sci.* 2009;16(1):7–19.

Pilz S, Marz W, Wellnitz B, Seelhorst U, Fahrietner-Pammer A, Dimai H, et al. Association of vitamin D deficiency with heart failure and sudden cardiac death in a large cross-sectional study of patients referred for coronary angiography. *J Clin Endocrinol Metab.* 2008;93(10):3927–3935.

Russell R, Mason J. Future health needs: nutrition and aging. 1999. Available at: http://www.cyberounds.com/conferences/nutrition/conferences/0999/conference.html. Accessed September 1, 2000.

Science Daily. Vitamin D deficiency study raises new questions about disease and supplements. January 27, 2008. Available at: http://www.sciencedaily.com/releases/2008/01/080125223302.htm. Accessed April 23, 2008.

Smith CM, Cotter VT. Practice protocol: age-related changes in health. 2008. Hartford Institute for Geriatric Nursing. Available at: http://www.consultgerirn.org/topics/normal_aging_changes/want_to_know_more. Accessed February 3, 2009.

Tabloski P. *Gerontological Nursing.* Upper Saddle River, NJ: Prentice Hall; 2006.

Weber J, Kelley J. *Health Assessment in Nursing.* 2nd ed. Baltimore: Lippincott; 2003.

Zembrzuski CD. *Clinical Companion for Assessment of the Older Adult.* Albany, NY: Delmar Thomson Learning; 2001.

Macronutrient Requirements for Older Adults

Melissa Bernstein, PhD, RD, LD

· ·

CHAPTER OBJECTIVES   Upon completion of this chapter, the reader will be able to:

1. Describe the different dietary recommendations for older adults
2. Discuss the changes in energy needs that occur with advancing age
3. List the nutritional and lifestyle factors that contribute to nutrition recommendations in older adults
4. Identify food sources of carbohydrates, fats, and proteins that can help older adults meet nutrition recommendations
5. Understand how age-related changes in metabolism and health affect requirements for carbohydrates, fats, proteins, and fluids

KEY TERMS AND CONCEPTS

Biological value	MyPyramid
Dietary fiber	Nitrogen balance
Dietary Guidelines for Americans 2005	Nonviscous fiber
Dietary Reference Intakes (DRIs)	Sarcopenia
Discretionary calories	Viscous fiber
Essential fatty acids	

· ·

Older adults require specialized nutrition services aimed at maintaining independence and health. The older population is a heterogeneous group with diverse needs and available resources. With advancing age, there is a general loss of body weight and lean body mass and an increase in the proportion of body fat. In addition, body water is reduced and bone density decreases. These age-related changes in body composition influence nutrient metabolism and requirements. The nutritional status and needs of older people are multifactorial and are related to age-associated biological changes, as well as to socioeconomic changes. The decreased food intake, sedentary lifestyle, and reduced energy expenditure commonly seen in this population place older adults at risk for malnutrition, especially protein and micronutrient deficiencies. Persistent, chronic conditions impose difficulty on older adults in carrying out their activities of daily living and may result in an increased requirement for some nutrients because of changes in absorptive and metabolic capacity.

Nutrient Recommendations

Dietary Reference Intakes

The Food and Nutrition Board of the Institute of Medicine publishes the dietary reference values for intake of nutrients

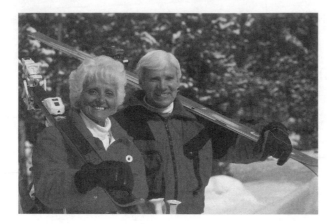

by Americans. **Dietary Reference Intakes (DRIs)** serve as reference values of nutrients to form the basis for planning and assessing the diets of healthy people. The DRIs replace the 1989 Recommended Daily Allowances. The 2005 DRIs are quantitative estimates of nutrient intakes for healthy individuals. Recommendations for nutrient values for energy, carbohydrate, fiber, fat, fatty acids, cholesterol, protein, and amino acids, as well as the scientific basis for them, can be found in *Dietary Reference Intakes for Energy, Carbohydrate, Fiber, Fat, Fatty Acids, Cholesterol, Protein, and Amino Acids (Macronutrients) 2005.*

The Dietary Reference Intake table on the inside cover of this textbook presents the DRI values for men and women aged 51 to 70 and 70 and older. The values include the Recommended Dietary Allowances (RDAs), Adequate Intakes (AIs), and Tolerable Upper Limits (ULs). See **Box 3-1** for definitions of these and related terms.

Table 3-1 reviews the uses of DRIs in dietary assessment and planning for individuals as well as groups. It is important to realize that these recommendations are based on the DRIs for healthy adults and that additional interpretation may be necessary when applying them to older adults, who have multiple medical conditions. Although specific ULs are not set for macronutrients, the absence of a definitive value does not signify that people can tolerate long-term intakes of these substances at high levels. Chronic excessive intake can produce adverse effects; therefore, caution should be exercised when consuming levels significantly above those typically found in food-based diets. This is especially a concern for older adults who may have either long-term monotonous diets contributing to high intake or reduced physiologic ability to metab-

Dietary Reference Intakes (DRIs) A framework of dietary standards that includes Estimated Average Requirement (EAR), Recommended Dietary Allowance (RDA), Adequate Intake (AI), and Tolerable Upper Intake Level (UL).

▶ BOX 3-1 Dietary Reference Intakes: Summary of Terminology

Dietary Reference Intakes: A set of recommendations for healthy people in the United States and Canada used for planning and assessing diets of individuals and groups.

1. *Recommended Dietary Allowances (RDAs)* are nutrient intake goals for individuals for which there is *significant scientific agreement* to the average daily nutrient intake level to meet the needs of 97% of healthy people of a specific age category and gender.

2. *Adequate Intakes (AIs)* are nutrient intake goals for which there is *supportive scientific agreement* to the average daily nutrient intake level to meet the needs of 97% of healthy people of a specific age category and gender.

3. *Tolerable Upper Limit (UL)* is the highest average daily nutrient intake level that is unlikely to pose harm or risk of toxicity to almost all healthy individuals of a specific age category and gender. Intakes above this level increase the risk of toxicity and illness.

4. *Estimated Average Requirement (EAR)* is the level used in nutrition research and policy. EAR is the average daily intake of nutrient estimated to meet the requirement of half of the healthy individuals of a specific age category and gender. EAR serves as the basis for the RDA values.

5. *Acceptable Macronutrient Distribution Ranges (AMDRs)* are values for carbohydrates, fats, and proteins which are expressed as a percentage of total calorie intake. AMDRs are the amounts sufficient to provide adequate calories, nutrients, and health benefits while reducing the risk of chronic diseases.

6. *Daily Values (DVs)* are the nutrient standards used on food labels. DVs are intended to serve as a guide to allow consumers to compare the nutrition composition of foods.

Source: Adapted from Institute of Medicine, Food and Nutrition Board. *Dietary Reference Intakes for Energy, Carbohydrate, Fiber, Fat, Fatty Acids, Cholesterol, Protein and Amino Acids (Macronutrients).* Washington, DC: National Academies Press; 2005.

TABLE 3-1 Uses of Dietary Reference Intakes for Healthy Adults

Type of Use	Value	Individual	Group
Assessment	EAR	Examine the probability that usual intake is inadequate.	Estimate the prevalence of inadequate intake within a group.
	EER	Examine the probability that usual energy intake is inadequate.	Estimate the prevalence of inadequate intakes within a group.
	RDA	If usual intake is at or above this level, then there is a low probability of inadequacy.	Should not be used to assess intakes of groups.
	AI	If usual intake is at or above this level, then there is a low probability of inadequacy.	Mean usual intakes at or above this level will imply a low prevalence of inadequate intakes.
	UL	Usual intakes above this level will place the individual at risk of adverse effects from excessive nutrient intake.	Estimate the percentage of the population at potential risk for adverse effects from excess nutrient intake.
Planning	RDA	Goal intake.	NA
	EAR	NA	Plan an intake distribution with a low prevalence of inadequate intakes.
	EER	NA	Plan an energy distribution with a low prevalence of inadequate intakes.
	AI	Goal intake.	Plan mean intakes.
	UL	An upper guide to limit intake; chronic intake higher than this amount may increase risk of adverse outcomes.	Plan intake distributions with a low prevalence of risk for adverse outcomes.

EAR, Estimated Average Requirement; EER, Estimated Energy Requirement; RDA, Recommended Dietary Allowance; AI, Adequate Intake; UL, Tolerable Upper Intake Level; NA, not applicable.

Source: Adapted from Institute of Medicine, Food and Nutrition Board. *Dietary Reference Intakes for Energy, Carbohydrate, Fiber, Fat, Fatty Acids, Cholesterol, Protein and Amino Acids (Macronutrients).* Washington, DC: National Academies Press; 2005.

olize and eliminate nutrients, therefore increasing the risk of harmful effects.

Energy Needs

Energy is required to sustain the body's functions. This includes involuntary functions, such as respiration and circulation, as well as physical work. Energy is supplied to the body through the consumption of dietary carbohydrates, proteins, fats, and alcohols. An individual's energy balance depends on his or her energy intake and energy expenditure. Energy output can be divided into three main components: resting energy expenditure (REE), physical activity (PA), and the thermic effect of food (TEF), as shown in **Figure 3-1**. The most variable component is physical activity. Dietary intake studies have shown that energy intake declines with advancing age. Measurement of energy consumption can be used as a guide when assessing energy needs if the individual's weight is stable. It is important to consider that, in general, dietary studies tend to underestimate caloric intake.

For a weight-stable individual, his or her energy requirement is the energy intake from food that equals energy expenditure. The Estimated Energy Requirement (EER) is defined as the dietary energy intake that is predicted to maintain energy balance in a healthy adult. The EER is specific to age, gender, weight, height, and activity level. Prediction equations to calculate the EER for normal-weight individuals were developed from data on total daily energy expenditure, as measured by the doubly labeled water technique. The EERs for healthy adults over the age of 19 with active lifestyles are 3,067 calories per day for men (minus 10 calories per day for each additional year over 19) and 2,403 for women (minus 7 calories per day for each additional year). RDA and UL are not provided for energy, because energy intakes above the EER or above an individual's energy requirement would be expected to result in undesirable weight gain.

Although commonly used for adults, prediction equations, such as the Mifflin St Joer and the Harris-Benedict equations, may overestimate needs and should be used cau-

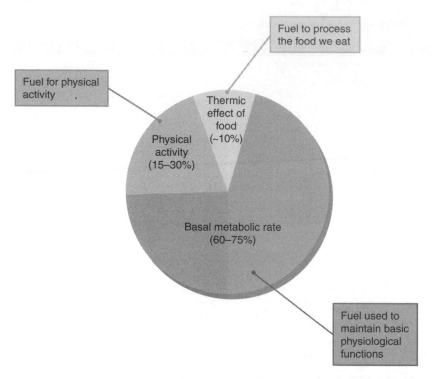

FIGURE 3-1 Major Components of Energy Expenditure: Thermic Effect of Food (TEF), Basal Metabolic Rate (BMR), and Physical Activity (PA)

tiously to estimate energy requirements in older adults. A comparison of dietary intake estimated caloric needs and the basal energy expenditure estimated from prediction equations should serve as a guideline for caloric requirements. Approaches to measuring caloric requirements such as indirect calorimetry, doubly labeled water, and total body potassium may produce more reliable results; however, they are not widely available. Regardless of the method used to estimate the energy needs of older adults, careful attention to dietary intake to meet nutrient requirements as well as regular monitoring for changes in body weight must be implemented to ensure adequate nutritional health.

The decline in energy requirement with age can be attributed to decreased basal metabolic rate (BMR), decreased TEF, and decreased physical activity. The cause of the reduction in BMR that occurs with advancing age is multifactorial and includes changes in body composition, primarily a reduction in lean mass, which is metabolically active tissue, thus

MyPyramid An educational tool that translates the principles of the 2005 Dietary Guidelines for Americans and other nutritional standards to help consumers in making healthier food and physical activity choices.

contributing to the reduction in BMR. In addition, declines in energy expenditures that are related to reduced physical activity (increased sedentary behavior) contribute to lower caloric requirements.

Decreased energy expenditure causes a unique problem for many older individuals. In general, older adults require less energy to maintain their weight, but their nutrient needs stay the same, and in some cases increase. Meeting nutrient intake recommendations while staying within energy needs is fundamental to current dietary guidance. Older adults who do not reduce their caloric intake to balance this decreased energy expenditure may become overweight. This possibility emphasizes the need for older individuals to choose nutrient-dense foods. In applying the **MyPyramid** program, this means maintaining an appropriate discretionary calorie allowance after choosing the suggested amounts of high-nutrient foods from each group. The **Dietary Guidelines for Americans 2005** recommends consuming a variety of foods within and among the basic food groups while staying within energy needs. Choosing a variety of nutrient-dense foods from all food groups is associated with better nutritional status and should be an important goal for older individuals.

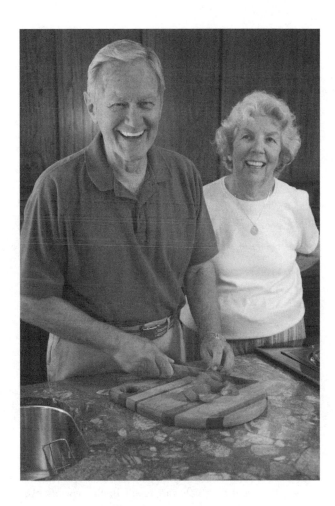

Carbohydrate Recommendations

A growing body of evidence has shown that macronutrients, particularly fats and carbohydrates, play a role in the risk for chronic disease. For health promotion and disease prevention, the majority of dietary carbohydrates should come from complex, unrefined carbohydrates such as grains, vegetables, legumes, and fruit. The Acceptable Macronutrient Distribution Range (AMDR) for a nutrient is the range of intake that is associated with reduced risk of chronic disease while providing essential nutrient intake. Consumption of a nutrient in excess of the AMDR increases the risk for chronic disease. The DRI committee of the Institute of Medicine recommends that carbohydrates should ideally provide 45% to 65% of daily calories. This range allows for adequate intake of all essential nutrients while minimizing the risk for coronary heart disease, obesity, and diabetes. Additionally, the 2005 Dietary Guidelines for Americans recommend "choosing carbohydrates wisely for good health"; specifically, choosing fiber-rich foods and increasing intake of fruits, vegetables, whole grains, and nonfat or low-fat milk products to obtain the recommended amounts of carbohydrates and moderating the intake of processed grains and refined sugars. These guidelines apply to all healthy adults, including those older individuals who are not in need of a medically prescribed diet.

An Estimated Average Requirement (EAR) for carbohydrate is established based on the average amount of glucose utilized by the brain and is set at 100 g/day for both men and women aged 50 and older. The RDA for carbohydrate is set for men and women aged 51 and older at 130 g/day; however, most Americans exceed these amounts. By utilizing the AMDR, professionals can quickly calculate a healthy range of carbohydrates for their older clients based on energy requirements.

Older adults, as well as other individuals who need to monitor their caloric intake and their **discretionary calories** according to the recommendations made in the Dietary Guidelines and MyPyramid, should also be careful not to eat too many simple sugars. These carbohydrates are low in nutrient content and can contribute

Body weight generally increases up to the sixth decade of life. Then, deteriorating health in combination with sedentary lifestyle and the resulting loss in lean mass (termed **sarcopenia**) contribute to increased frailty and result in increased dependence. This often then results in a vicious cycle of illness-increased disability and functional dependence. Loss of additional bone muscle mass leads to reduced flexibility and decreased independence.

Dietary Carbohydrates

Carbohydrates, sugars, starches, and fibers found in grains, fruits, vegetables, and milk products are an important part of a healthy diet. In most diets, carbohydrates are the major energy source. Carbohydrates supply important fuel for most body functions. Sugars and starches from carbohydrates provide energy to all the cells in the body, including the brain and nervous system. Foods contain different types of carbohydrates, such as complex carbohydrates (starches and fiber) and simple carbohydrates (sugars).

Dietary Guidelines for Americans 2005 Foundation of federal nutrition policy; they are developed by the U.S. Department of Agriculture (USDA) and the Department of Health and Human Services (DHHS). These science-based guidelines are intended to reduce the number of Americans who develop chronic diseases such as hypertension, diabetes, cardiovascular disease, obesity, and alcoholism.

sarcopenia Age-associated loss of muscle mass, associated with muscle weakness, functional limitations, and disability, as well as impairments in cardiovascular capacity and metabolic health.

discretionary calories Extra calories above the minimum required to meet essential nutrient needs.

to excess calories and inadequate intake of essential nutrients. Although the AMDR for added sugar is not more than 25% of total daily calories, currently there is no suggested daily intake of sugar, thus emphasizing that carbohydrate requirements should be met with nutritious whole grains, fruits, and vegetables. Essential micronutrients are low in foods and beverages that are the major sources of added sugars. Therefore, lowering intake of sugars and sweets helps to ensure sufficient intake of nutrients without ingesting excess empty calories. Despite the MyPyramid recommendations for people to "make half the grains whole," which is designed to help reduce the risk of coronary heart disease, provide dietary fiber, and maintain adequate bowel function, women aged 31 to 50 only consume 13% of their grains as whole grains. For individuals, especially older adults who need to maximize their nutrient intake while keeping energy intake at a level for weight maintenance, complex carbohydrates are a better choice. Given that the RDA for carbohydrates for men and women aged 50 and older is 130 g/day, this translates to an allowance of only 260 calories from refined carbohydrates, which can easily be exceeded without careful food planning.

Dietary Fiber

Fibers are the structural components in plant-based foods. **Dietary fiber** is a term used to describe carbohydrates from plants that are not digestible by the human gastrointestinal system. *Functional fibers* are those that have been shown to have beneficial physiologic effects in humans. *Total fiber* is the sum of dietary fiber and functional fibers. Fiber plays a beneficial role in numerous medical conditions that affect many older people. Consumption of high-fiber-containing foods is recommended by the American Diabetes Association for the management of diabetes mellitus, as well as by the American Heart Association to reduce the risk of cardiovascular disease and the National Cancer Institute to reduce the risk of various types of cancer.

Both nonviscous and viscous fibers are important for the health of older adults. By slowing glucose absorption, **nonviscous fiber** reduces postprandial blood glucose concentrations and therefore has been shown to be beneficial for the management of diabetes mellitus. Foods with high amounts of insoluble fiber, such as

dietary fiber Plant carbohydrates that are not digestible by the gastrointestinal tract.

nonviscous fiber Dietary fibers that are insoluble in water; include cellulose, lignins, resistant starches, and many hemicelluloses.

viscous fiber Dietary fibers that are fermentable and are soluble in water to form a gel-like consistency; include gums and mucilages, pectins, psyllium, and some hemicelluloses.

▶ BOX 3-2 Fiber Sources and Functions

Type	Food Sources	Functions in Body
Soluble viscous fiber	Barley, oats (oat bran), bran, rye, fruits, legumes, vegetables	• Lowers blood cholesterol • Slows glucose absorption • Bulks stool by holding moisture • Increases satiety by slowing upper gastrointestinal (GI) tract transit
Insoluble nonviscous fiber	Fruits, legumes, seeds, vegetables, wheat bran, brown rice, whole grains	• Increases speed of transit of fecal mass through lower GI tract, which alleviates constipation • Increases "bulk" to diet, increasing feelings of fullness

wheat bran, whole-grain breads and cereals, and vegetables, increase fecal bulk and decrease transit time in the colon. This helps to reduce the incidence of constipation and formation of diverticula, conditions common in older adults. Fiber delays gastric emptying of ingested foods into the small intestine, which can result in the sensation of fullness and therefore be helpful for weight management.

Fiber also interferes with the absorption of dietary fats and cholesterol, which may result in lower blood cholesterol concentrations, reducing the risk of cardiovascular disease. **Viscous fibers,** such as gums and pectins, decrease the rate of cholesterol and triglyceride absorption in the small intestine by binding with intestinal contents. Oat bran and high-fiber foods, such as cereals, starchy vegetables, and beans, have been shown to lower serum lipid levels, providing protection against heart disease. **Box 3-2** outlines the types of fibers, their main sources, and their primary functions in the body.

The Dietary Guidelines for Americans and My Pyramid recommend choosing fiber-rich foods for a health-promoting diet. Recommendations range from 25 to 35 g/day, with the AI for total fiber set at 30 g/day and 21 g/day for men and women, respectively, over the age of 51 (based on 14 g fiber per 1,000 kcal). Data from national studies for mean nutrient intake by older adults show that fiber consumption is 14.0 and 14.4 grams daily for women aged 71 and older and women between 50 and 70 years, respectively, and 17.5 and 18.5 grams daily for men aged 71 and older and men between 51 and 70, respectively. Other national surveys support these findings that fiber intake is consistently lower than the recommended levels in adults of all ages.

Choosing a variety of fiber-rich foods from fresh fruits, vegetables, legumes, whole grains, and breakfast cereals is the best way to increase fiber consumption. To meet carbohydrate recommendations, older individuals should choose fewer processed foods and select more natural and whole-grain products. For example, selecting whole-grain bread instead of a more refined product, such as white bread, is a healthier choice, because the former contains more nutrients and fiber. In addition, fruits and vegetables provide a high-carbohydrate energy source while also contributing a significant amount of nutrients and fiber.

Care should be taken, however, when planning the diet of *frail* older adults with regard to foods high in dietary fiber. These foods increase the feeling of satiety and therefore may cause overall food intake to decrease, thereby limiting intake of necessary nutrients from food sources and contributing to difficulties in maintaining an appropriate body weight. When choosing a diet high in fiber, it is also important to ensure adequate water intake to prevent fecal impaction.

Water Balance and Recommended Intakes

Water is an essential nutrient, and it requires special consideration with regards to the older adult. Water provides the environment for almost all of the body's activities; it is required for many metabolic reactions; and it supplies a medium for transport of materials, nutrients, and wastes throughout the body. The body actively maintains fluid balance to support these vital body functions by balancing intake with output. With advancing age, both sides of this equation are challenged. The body attempts to adjust imbalances promptly; however, in older adults this adjustment is impaired as a result of declines in thirst and reduced renal function.

Water Intake

Water constitutes approximately 45% to 50% of an older adult's body weight. This is 10% to 15% less than a younger adult, due to the losses in lean body mass seen with advancing age. Water makes up about three-fourths of the weight of lean tissue and less than one-fourth of the weight of fat; therefore, body composition influences total body water. Because of age-related changes in body composition (older people have a smaller proportion of lean body mass), the proportion of body water is smaller in older adults.

Thirst and renal function are the main controllers of water and electrolyte balance. Endocrine changes, hemodynamic factors, environmental factors, medication use, and

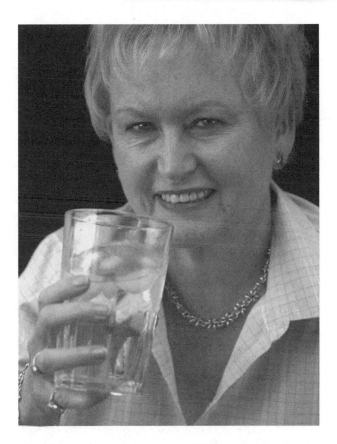

voluntary restriction can all independently or cumulatively contribute to reduced fluid intake. All of these factors make older adults more prone to problems with fluid balance and disruptions in homeostasis. Water imbalance is more likely during times of metabolic stress, such as illness or hospitalization, as well as in extreme weather conditions.

Numerous mechanisms that stimulate thirst, and therefore the desire to drink, are reduced in the older adult. Thirst, which is stimulated by increased plasma osmolality, is the major signal for a person to drink. As individuals age, the thirst sensation is delayed and reduced compared with that of a younger person. Reduced thirst in the older adult can also be attributed to medication use. Polypharmacy and combinations of medications with numerous side effects, such as mouth distaste, nausea, and anorexia, can also contribute to reduced fluid intake.

Declines in mental status, cognitive abilities, and depression can lead to dehydration as a result of forgetfulness or deliberate fluid restriction. Older adults may also voluntarily restrict fluid intake in an attempt to manage incontinence. Attempts to minimize trips to the restroom may be another motivator for older adults who are functionally impaired.

Fluid Output

Normal physiologic losses of fluid occur through the skin, lungs, kidneys, and gastrointestinal tract. In addition, alterations in factors such as cardiac output and blood pressure can contribute to age-related impairments in water conservation and sodium balance. The aged kidney has a decreased urinary-concentrating ability, leading to reduced ability to conserve water. Additionally, medications such as diuretics and laxatives can increase water output.

Older adults also have decreased sweating and thermoregulatory responses. Therefore, environmental conditions such as extreme heat and humidity, which increase fluid loss, are especially problematic for older adults. The increased fluid lost in hot, humid weather, combined with a reduced ability to sweat and cool body temperature, places an older adult at exceptionally high risk for dehydration and heat-related illness.

Dehydration

Normally, water intake equals water output. Dehydration results from imbalances in this equation when body water output exceeds water input. Dehydration is the most common fluid and electrolyte disturbance in older adults, and severe imbalances in body water can be life threatening.

Inadequate fluid intake, as well as reduced total body water with age, places older adults at increased risk for dehydration. Numerous physiologic, medical, environmental, and lifestyle factors associated with aging can interfere with fluid homeostasis and contribute to dehydration. Illness, fever, diarrhea, vomiting, infection, dementia, chronic renal disease, diabetes mellitus, and use of diuretics and laxatives all increase the risk of dehydration and may contribute to a chronic dehydrated state in many older adults. **Table 3-2** outlines signs and symptoms of dehydration in older adults.

Inadequate fluid intake can lead to rapid dehydration in older adults. Potential complications include hypotension, constipation, nausea, vomiting, mucosal dryness, decreased urinary output, elevated body temperature, and mental confusion, many of which can worsen dehydration. Some medications commonly used by older adults may contribute to dehydration or require adequate body water for proper metabolism, emphasizing the need for adequate fluid consumption. Dehydration is associated with increased morbidity and mortality; therefore, prevention is ideal.

Water Recommendations

Older adults generally do not consume adequate fluids. It has been well documented that institutionalized older adults do not consume enough fluids and are therefore at increased risk of dehydration.

Total water intake is defined as drinking water, water in beverages, and water that is part of food. The AI for *total* water is set at 2.7 and 3.7 liters daily for women and men,

TABLE 3-2 Signs and Symptoms of Dehydration in Older Adults

Clinical Symptoms
Thirst
Change in mental status, including increased combativeness or confusion
Dry mouth, cracked lips
Diarrhea or constipation
Fever
Hypotension or postural hypertension
Tachycardia (>100 beats per minute)
Recent rapid weight loss
Oliguria and/or dark urine
Sunken or dry eyes
Urinary tract infection
Vomiting
High ratio of blood urea nitrogen (BUN) to creatinine
High urinary specific gravity
High plasma sodium
Health-Related Indicators
Needs help drinking from a cup or glass
Drinks fewer than six cups of liquids daily
Trouble swallowing liquids
Confusion
Headaches and dizziness
Lethargy
Muscle weakness
Falls frequently
Change in abilities to perform activities of daily living
Chronic diuretic or laxative use
Polypharmacy

Older individuals with one or more of the symptoms listed may be at risk for dehydration.

Source: Niedert KC, Dorner B. *Nutrition Care of the Older Adult: A Handbook for Dietetics Professionals Working Throughout the Continuum of Care.* 2nd ed. Chicago: American Dietetic Association; 2004.

respectively, aged 51 and older. This amount is intended to prevent the deleterious, primarily acute, effects of dehydration, which include metabolic and functional abnormalities. In addition to using the AI as a guideline for daily fluid recommendations, **Box 3-3** shows clinical formulas for estimating daily fluid requirements that are commonly used for normal older adults.

Fluid intake should be adequate to compensate for normal physiologic losses through the kidney, the respiratory and gastrointestinal systems, and the skin. Additional fluid will be needed to compensate for losses associated with illness, such as those arising from fever, vomiting, and

BOX 3-3   Methods for Estimating Daily Fluid Requirements in Older Adults

Using Age

Ages 55–65:   30 mL/kg/day (min 1,500 mL/day)

Ages >65:   25 mL/kg/day (min 1,500 mL/day)

Using Caloric Intake

1 mL per kilocalorie consumed

Using Body Weight

100 mL/kg for the first 10 kg of (actual) body weight

+50 mL/kg for the next 10 kg of (actual) body weight

+15 mL/kg for the remaining body weight

Sources: Adapted from Niedert KC, Dorner B. *Nutrition Care of the Older Adult: A Handbook for Dietetics Professionals Working Throughout the Continuum of Care.* 2nd ed. Chicago: American Dietetic Association; 2004; Chernoff R. *Geriatric Nutrition: The Health Professional's Handbook.* 3rd ed. Sudbury, MA: Jones & Bartlett; 2006; Chidester JC, Spangler AA. Fluid intake in the institutionalized elderly. *J Am Dietetic Assoc.* 1997;97:23–28.

diarrhea. Numerous factors, including physiologic, environmental, and social ones, interact to affect the fluid requirements of older adults. In addition, many medications, both prescription and over the counter, can influence fluid requirements and hydration status or have side effects that interfere with fluid intake, such as nausea, confusion, or alterations in gastrointestinal status.

Daily fluid intake can come from food and beverages. Individuals who require nutrition support and interventions can meet their fluid requirements through enteral or parenteral feedings. As discussed in Chapter 1, eight 8-ounce glasses of fluids are presented near the base of the Modified MyPyramid for Older Adults, which emphasizes the importance of adequate fluid intake for older adults. This amount would provide almost 2 liters of water daily toward total water needs. Examples of good choices to meet recommendations for fluid intake include beverages such as water, fruit or vegetable juice, and nonfat or low-fat milk, as well as low-sodium soups. Alcohol and caffeinated beverages should not count toward water intake. Meeting the recommendations for fluid intake is more challenging in older adults because of the decline in the thirst mechanism reminding them to drink.

Fats

Fats are lipids found in foods or in the body. They are composed mostly of triglycerides and small amounts of phospholipids and sterols. Triglycerides provide the body with a valuable source of energy. Fats from foods also carry fat-soluble vitamins (A, D, E, and K), fat-soluble phytochemicals (carotenoids), and **essential fatty acids** (linoleic acid and linolenic acid). In addition to being an essential energy reserve, stored fat acts as an insulator, keeping the body warm and protecting internal organs from damage. Fatty acids are used to make hormonal regulators. Phospholipids are sterols that contribute to cellular structure. Cholesterol, a sterol, is used to make hormones, vitamin D, and bile.

Fat is an essential source of energy for the body. Dietary fat provides more than twice the calories per gram than either protein or carbohydrates, making it a concentrated source of energy. The AMDR for fats is 20% to 35% of total calories for men and women aged 50 and older. The upper end of this AMDR is based on decreasing the risk of chronic disease as well as ensuring an adequate intake of other nutrients. The lower end of the AMDR is based on elevated plasma triglycerides and lowered concentrations of high density lipoprotein (HDL) cholesterol levels seen in very low-fat diets.

By keeping fat and carbohydrate intake within the recommended ranges, the risk for heart disease, obesity, and diabetes can be kept to a minimum. However, fat provides a valuable source of concentrated energy for frail older individuals who may be struggling to consume enough calories to maintain an appropriate body weight. Limiting fat too far can lead to weight loss and nutrient deficiencies.

Older adults should be careful to choose dietary fats in similar distributions to those recommended for younger adults. Saturated fat should be limited to no more than 8% to 10% of total calories, polyunsaturated fats approximately 10%, and monounsaturated fats 10% to 15%. These recommendations also include a minimum of 10% of total energy derived from fats to ensure adequate energy and essential fatty acid intake.

Essential Fatty Acids

Foods high in dietary fat provide a necessary source of the essential fatty acids linoleic acid and linolenic acid. Linoleic acid (*n*-6), an omega-6 fatty acid, is an essential structural component of cell membranes. It is also involved in cell signaling processes and is a precursor for eicosanoids. The AI for linoleic acid for men aged 50 and older is 14 g/day, and for women aged 50 and older it is 11 g/day. Nuts, seeds, and vegetable oils, such as corn, soybean, safflower, and sesame, are good sources of linoleic acid.

Linolenic acid (*n*-3), an omega-3 fatty acid, is required for neurologic growth and development. It also is a precursor for the production of the eicosanoids eicosa-

essential fatty acids Fatty acids that the body needs but cannot synthesize and must obtain from diet.

pentaenoic acid (EPA) and docosahexaenoic acid (DHA). Canola, soybean, and flax seed oils, nuts and seeds, and soybeans and fatty fish are all good dietary sources of linolenic acid. The AIs for men and women older than 50 are 1.6 g/day and 1.1 g/day, respectively. Deficiency of linoleic and linolenic acids leads to reduced production of arachidonic acid, EPA, and DHA.

The AMDR for n-6 linoleic acid is 5% to 10% of daily calories. The AMDR for n-3 alpha-linolenic acid is 0.6% to 1.2% of daily calories. These amounts are based on long-term studies that have demonstrated beneficial health effects from this level of consumption. Although no UL is defined for these nutrients, higher amounts may lead to increased lipid peroxidation, free-radical formation, and compromised immunity, as well as the possibility of additional adverse effects from higher amounts of polyunsaturated fatty acids.

The AI and AMDR for polyunsaturated fatty acids are established to maintain the appropriate balance between linoleic and alpha-linolenic fatty acids. A ratio of 6:1 is recommended for omega-6 fatty acids to omega-3 fatty acids for essential brain functioning and for the management of cardiovascular disease, arthritis, and cancer.

Heart Disease

Lifestyle changes such as reduction of dietary fat and cholesterol in addition to exercise may contribute to weight loss and a reduction in cardiovascular disease risk factors in older adults. Elevated total cholesterol levels remain a risk factor for death from coronary artery disease in older adults and are associated with a similar pattern of death from coronary heart disease as seen in younger adults. In addition, HDL cholesterol levels below 35 mg/dL predict heart disease mortality and occurrence of new events in individuals older than age 70. Reduction of dietary fat will reduce overall caloric intake and contribute to weight loss and the avoidance of obesity in older adults.

The Adult Treatment Panel III (ATP III) guidelines of the National Cholesterol Education Program (NCEP) serve as the standard for treatment of high blood cholesterol. Numerous observational studies and clinical trials support cholesterol-lowering approaches (diet, exercise, and medications) to reduce coronary heart disease. However, there is less evidence concerning these approaches in older populations, and it is important to consider that management may be different for free-living versus institutionalized (well versus frail) older adults. The NCEP recommendations include limiting dietary saturated fat to 8% to 10% of total calories, with approximately 10% of calories from polyunsaturated fats and the rest of total fat intake from monounsaturated fats; dietary cholesterol intake should be limited to less than 300 mg/day for all adults while consuming a nutritionally adequate diet. The 2005 DRIs for additional

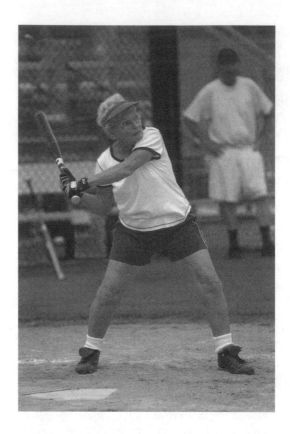

nutrients recommend that dietary cholesterol, trans-fatty acids, and saturated fatty acids be kept as low as possible, while consuming a nutritionally adequate diet.

For older adults with the aforementioned barriers to a healthy diet, these recommendations may be difficult to achieve. It is necessary to recommend dietary changes that incorporate low-fat dairy products, lean meats, dried beans, and adequate soluble fiber that limit trans-fatty acids. Management of weight appears to be a significant factor in the health status and cardiovascular health of older individuals. For overweight adults, goals to achieve and maintain a healthy body weight should be established with a nutrition professional. Dietary restrictions should be liberalized for people who cannot maintain appropriate body weight in order to ensure adequate calorie, protein, and nutrient intake.

Proteins

Proteins form the major structural components of all cells in the body. Proteins, along with amino acids (the dietary components of proteins), have a number of metabolic functions, including acting as enzymes, membrane carriers, and hormones. The nine essential (or indispensable) amino acids must be obtained from dietary sources, because they cannot be made by the body or they cannot be made in sufficient amounts to support physiologic needs. Nonessential (or dispensable) amino acids are those that can be made by the body under normal physiologic conditions.

Physiologic Aging and Protein Requirements

Advancing age is associated with changes in appetite, food intake, and physical activity, which can all influence protein and amino acid metabolism and are critical risk factors for malnutrition. As people age, there is a reduction in total body protein that accompanies changes in body composition. Decreases in the amount of skeletal muscle, along with physiologic changes, contribute to sarcopenia. Increased frailty, skin fragility, impaired wound healing, overall reduction in reserve capacity, and impaired immune function are all consequences of reduced body proteins. The reduction in lean mass, along with other physiologic changes resulting in loss of protein, is a manifestation of the age-related loss in total body protein.

The requirements for dietary protein for older adults is a topic of vigorous debate. Limited information is available to establish evidence-based dietary protein recommendations for older adults. The current RDA for men and women is set at 56g/d for males and 46g/d for female or 0.80g/kg body weight/day of protein based on **nitrogen balance** studies.

The potential exists for influence of metabolic adaptations on dietary requirements. Free-living healthy adults have been shown to accommodate to low protein intake. However, with age, both protein intake and efficiency of utilization appear to decrease.

While there is currently no consensus on actual dietary protein needs, evidence suggests that the RDA for protein may not be adequate to meet the metabolic and physiologic needs even as a minimum level for older adults. Moderate increases in protein intake above 0.80g/protein/day may contribute to enhanced muscle protein metabolism as well as provide a mechanism for reducing progressive muscle loss that commonly accompanies aging. Reduced whole-body protein turnover means that older adults require more protein per kilogram body weight than younger adults. Data from a review of nitrogen balance studies to evaluate the relevance of the recommended protein intake, indicate that a protein intake of 1.0-1.3g/d/d is required to maintain nitrogen balance in healthy older persons. This higher protein requirement may be explained by lower energy intake, impaired insulin action, and a decrease in the efficacy of protein utilization.

Although older adults may adapt to lower dietary protein intake, this is not physiological desirable and attempts should be made to attenuate the resulting consequences. Exercise, specifically resistance training, will result in an increase in muscle size and results in a decrease in nitrogen excretion thus lowering dietary protein needs. Increased dietary protein intakes up to 1.6g.kg.d should adequately and safely meet the needs of older adults with normal renal function, and may enhance hypertrophic response to resistance training provided energy needs are met. Higher levels of dietary protein may be needed to meet additional demands of physiologic stress. **Table 3-3** summarizes the DRI values for carbohydrates, proteins, fats, and water.

> **nitrogen balance** Nitrogen intake minus the sum of all sources of nitrogen excretion.

Dietary Protein

Data from NHANES suggests there is a trend towards decreased protein intake with advancing age. Obtaining

TABLE 3-3 Summary Table: Dietary Recommended Intakes (DRIs) for Carbohydrate, Fiber, Fat, Protein, and Water for Adults Aged 51 Years and Older

Nutrient	Value	Recommendation
Carbohydrates	AMDR	45–65% total daily calories
	DRI	130 g/day
	EAR	100 g/day
Fiber	AI: Men	30 g/day
	AI: Women	21 g/day
Fat	AMDR	20–35% total daily calories
n-6 PUFA (linoleic acid)	AMDR	5–10% total daily calories
	AI: Men	14 g/day
	AI: Women	11 g/day
n-3 PUFA (alpha-linolenic acid)	AMDR	0.6–1.2% total daily calories
	AI: Men	1.6 g/day
	AI: Women	1.1 g/day
Protein	AMDR	10–35% total daily calories
	RDA	0.8 g/kg/day
	EAR	0.66 g/kg/day
	RDA: Men	56 g/day
	RDA: Women	46 g/day
Water	AI: Men	3.7 L/day
	AI: Women	2.7 L/day

AMDR, Acceptable Macronutrient Distribution Range; EAR, Estimated Average Requirement; AI, Adequate Intake; PUFA; polyunsaturated fatty acid; RDA, Recommended Dietary Allowance.

Source: Adapted from Institute of Medicine, Food and Nutrition Board. *Dietary Reference Intakes for Energy, Carbohydrate, Fiber, Fat, Fatty Acids, Cholesterol, Protein and Amino Acids (Macronutrients).* Washington, DC: National Academies Press; 2005.

biological value (BV) Extent to which the protein in a food can be incorporated by the body. Expressed as the percentage of the absorbed dietary nitrogen retained by the body.

adequate high-quality dietary protein intake may be challenging for older adults, many of whom have reduced appetite, functional and social limitations, and economic hardship. Inadequate protein consumption likely contributes to an acceleration of sarcopenia and related morbidities. In addition, protein undernutrition aggravates diseases and conditions commonly observed in older adults, resulting in increased susceptibility to disease and poor clinical outcomes.

To meet the RDA for protein as well as the AMDR of 10% to 35% of total daily calories, proteins with a high **biological value**—such as those from animal sources, which provide high-quality proteins and essential amino acids, along with iron, vitamin B12, and other vital nutrients—should be regularly included in the diet of older adults. Higher protein intake may compensate for the decrease in availability of muscle amino acids and spare muscle mass.

In addition, a recent cohort study entitled the Health ABC Study found significantly less lean body mass loss over 3 years in subjects in the highest quintile of protein intake. Sedentary older adults are at risk for low protein intake because of their low energy requirements. Increased dietary amino acid density becomes more important for this population, as well as increased physical activity and higher food intakes to reduce the extent of any deficiency. To ensure adequate protein intake, older adults may benefit from an even distribution of protein throughout the day. Some experts are now recommending that older adults consume 25-30g of high-quality protein with each meal to stimulate muscle protein synthesis. Encouraging increased dietary protein intake with protein-rich foods has numerous advantages over supplementation with protein and amino acid products including cost, accessibility, socialization and dietary variety.

Greater dietary variety in older institutionalized adults is associated with better nutritional status, whereas community-dwelling older adults who have a low body mass index and consume a limited variety of micronutrient-dense foods were determined to be at nutritional risk, with only 65.4% consuming the RDA for protein.

Frailty exacerbates age-related changes in protein metabolism by inducing an increase in muscle protein catabolism and a decrease in muscle mass. A protein-enriched diet in frail older women has been found to increase endogenous protein balance and positive nitrogen balance in less than 2 weeks. If sustained over a long enough time to result in lean tissue accretion, increased protein intakes and nitrogen retention could convey desirable health benefits.

Conclusion

For older adults, achievement of macronutrient recommendations requires consideration of numerous factors, which can change with alterations in heath and social status. Older adults should be encouraged to consume a nutrient-dense diet and strive to maintain a healthy body weight and physically active lifestyle. Reduction of fat, saturated fat, and trans fats, as well as simple sugars, can help to lower calorie intake and reduce the risk of developing chronic conditions. Meeting fluid and fiber needs may be an increasing challenge depending on health status; however, they are important considerations for maintaining optimal health in persons of any age. Encouraging regular physical activity improves functional status and allows for higher energy consumption, thereby providing an important vehicle for meeting nutritional requirements.

Activities and Questions Related to This Chapter

1. Explain how age affects the nutritional requirements for energy, carbohydrate, fiber, fat, protein, and water.
2. Using www.mypyramid.gov, develop a dietary plan for an older woman or an older man. Suggest how this plan might need to be altered given a chronic medical condition such as diabetes, heart disease, or Alzheimer's disease. What recommendations would you make to ensure dietary adequacy?
3. How does reduced lean body mass affect the energy and macronutrient needs of older adults? What suggestions would you make to help ensure that nutrient needs are met?

REFERENCES

Ballesteros MN, Cabrera RM, Saucedo MS, et al. Dietary fiber and lifestyle influence serum lipids in free living adult men. *J Am Coll Nutr.* 2001;20(6):649–655.

Beers MH, Berkow R. *The Merck Manual of Geriatrics.* 3rd ed. Whitehouse Station, NJ: Merck Research Laboratories; 2000.

Bernstein MA, Tucker KL, Ryan ND, et al. Higher dietary variety is associated with better nutritional status in frail elderly people. *J Am Diet Assoc.* 2002;102(8):1096–1104.

Black AE, Prentice AM, Goldberg GR, et al. Measurements of total energy expenditure provide insights into the validity of dietary measurements of energy intake. *J Am Diet Assoc.* 1993;93:572–579.

Blanc S, Schoeller DA, Bauer D, et al. Energy requirements in the eighth decade of life. *Am J Clin Nutr.* 2004;79(2):303–310.

Campbell WW, Trappe TA, Wolfe RR, Evans WJ. The recommended dietary allowance for protein may not be adequate for older people to maintain skeletal muscle. *J Gerontol A Biol Sci Med Sci.* 2001;56(6):M373–M380.

Centers for Disease Control and Prevention. Trends in intake of energy and macronutrients—United States, 1971–2000. *MMWR.* 2004;53(4):80–82.

Chernoff R. Protein and older adults. *J Am Coll Nutr.* 2004;23(6 suppl):627s–630s.

Chernoff R. Thirst and fluid requirements in the elderly. *Nutr Rev.* 1994;52:132–136.

Chevalier S, Gougeon R, Nayar K, Morais JA. Frailty amplifies the effects of aging on protein metabolism: the role of protein intake. *Am J Clin Nutr.* 2003;78(3):422–429.

Corti MC, Guralnik JM, Salive ME, et al. Clarifying the direct relation between total cholesterol levels and death from coronary heart disease in older persons. *Ann Intern Med.* 1997;126:753–760.

Corti MC, Guralnik JM, Salive ME, et al. HDL cholesterol predicts coronary heart disease mortality in older persons. *JAMA.* 1995;274:539–544.

Dietary Guidelines Advisory Committee. *The Report of the Dietary Guidelines Advisory Committee on* Dietary Guidelines for Americans, 2005: *Executive Summary.* Washington, DC: U.S. Department of Health and Human Services; 2004. Available at: http://www.health.gov/dietaryguidelines/dga2005/report/HTML/A_ExecSummary.htm.

Evans WJ. Protein nutrition, exercise and aging. *J Am Coll Nutr.* 2004;23(6 suppl):601s–609s.

Fox AA, Thompson JL, Butterfield GE, et al. Effects of diet and exercise on common cardiovascular disease risk factors in moderately obese older women. *Am J Clin Nutr.* 1996;63:225–233.

Frankenfield D, Roth-Yousey L, Compher C. Comparison of prediction equations for resting metabolic rate in healthy, non-obese individuals: a systematic review. *J Am Diet Assoc.* 2005;105(5):775–789.

Fulgoni VL. Current protein intake in America: Analysis of the National Health and Nutrition Examination Survey, 2003–2004. *Am J Clin Nutr.* 2008;87(suppl):154s–1557s.

Harris J, Benedict F. *A Biometric Study of Basal Metabolism in Man.* Washington, DC: Carnegie Institution; 1919:40–44. Publication 279.

Harris TB, Savaga PJ, Tell GS, et al. Carrying the burden of cardiovascular risk in old age: associations of weight and weight change with prevalent cardiovascular disease, risk factors, and health status in the Cardiovascular Health Study. *Am J Clin Nutr.* 1997;66:837–844.

Houston DK, Nicklas BJ, Ding J, et. al. Dietary protein intake is associated with lean mass change in older, community-dwelling adults: the Health, Aging, and Body Composition (Health ABC Study). *Am J Clin Nutr.* 2008;87(1):150–155.

Institute of Medicine, Food and Nutrition Board. *Dietary Reference Intakes for Energy, Carbohydrate, Fiber, Fat, Fatty Acids, Cholesterol, Protein and Amino Acids (Macronutrients).* Washington, DC: National Academies Press; 2005.

Institute of Medicine, Food and Nutrition Board. *Dietary Reference Intakes for Water, Potassium, Sodium, Chloride, and Sulfate.* Washington, DC: National Academies Press; 2004.

Johnson RK. What are people really eating and why does it matter? *Nutr Today.* 2000;35:40–45.

Kleiner SM. Water: an essential but overlooked nutrient. *J Am Diet Assoc.* 1999;99(2):200–206.

Lichtenstein AH, Rasmussen H, Yu WW, et al. Modified MyPyramid for older adults. *J Nutr.* 2008;138:98–82.

Lucas M, Heiss CJ. Protein needs of older adults engaged in resistance training: a review. *J Aging Phys Act.* 2005;13(2):223–236.

Marshall TA, Stumbo PJ, Warren JJ, Xie XJ. Inadequate nutrient intakes are common and are associated with low diet variety in rural, community-dwelling elderly. *J Nutr.* 2001;131:2192–2196.

McGrandy RB, Barrows CH, Spanias A, et al. Nutrient intakes and energy expenditure in men of different ages. *J Gerontol.* 1966;21:581–587.

Meydani M. Nutrition interventions in aging and age-associated disease. *Ann NY Acad Sci.* 2001;928:226–235.

Mifflin MD, St. Jeor ST, Hill LA, et al. A new predictive equation for resting energy expenditure in healthy individuals. *Am J Clin Nutr.* 1990; 51:241–247.

Millward DJ. Macronutrient intakes as determinants of dietary protein and amino acid adequacy. *J Nutr.* 2004;134(6 suppl):1569s–1574s.

Morais JA, Chevalier S, Gougeon R. Protein turnover and requirements in the healthy and frail elderly. *J Nutr Health Aging.* 2006;10(4):272–283.

National Cholesterol Education Program. Second report of the Expert Panel on Detection, Evaluation, and Treatment of High Blood Cholesterol in Adults. *Circulation.* 1994;89:1333–1432.

National Institutes of Health. *Third Report of the National Cholesterol Education Program Expert Panel on Detection, Education, Evaluation, and Treatment of High Blood Cholesterol in Adults (Adult Treatment Panel III).* Bethesda, MD: National Institutes of Health; 2001.

Paddon Jones D, Rasmussen BB. Dietary protein recommendations and the prevention of sarcopenia. *Curr Opin Clin Nutr Metab Care.* 2009;12(1):86–90.

Paddon-Jones D, Short KR, Campbell WW, et al. Role of dietary protein in the sarcopenia of aging. *Am J Clin Nutr.* 2008; 87(suppl):1562S–1566S.

Perier C, Triuleyre P, Terrat C, et al. Energy and nutrient intake of elderly hospitalized patients in a steady metabolic status versus catabolic status. *J Nutr Health Aging.* 2004;8(6):518–520.

Roberts SB. Energy requirements for older individuals. *Eur J Clin Nutr.* 1996;50(suppl):S112–S118.

Roberts SB, Hajduk CL, Howarth NC, et al. Dietary variety predicts low body mass index and inadequate macro and micronutrient intake in community-dwelling older adults. *J Gerontol A Biol Sci Med Sci.* 2005;60(6):613–621.

Roubenoff R, Hughes, VA, Dallal, GE, et al. The effect of gender and body composition method on the apparent decline in lean mass–adjusted resting metabolic rate with age. *J Gerontol Med Sci.* 2000;55A(12):M757–M760.

Simopoulos AP. Omega-6/omega-3 essential fatty acid ratio: the scientific evidence. *World Rev Nutr Dietetics.* 2003;92:1–22.

U.S. Department of Agriculture. MyPyramid.gov. Available at: http://www.mypyramid.gov.

U.S. Department of Agriculture. MyPyramid.gov. Grain recommendations compared to consumption. Available at: http://www.MyPyramid.gov/downloads/MyPyramid%20 Peer%20to%20Peer.ppt#358,27.

U.S. Department of Health and Human Services and U.S. Department of Agriculture. *Dietary Guidelines for Americans 2005.* 6th ed. Washington, DC: U.S. Department of Health and Human Services; 2005.

Wakimoto P, Block G. Dietary intake, dietary patterns and changes with age: an epidemiological perspective. *J Gerontol.* 2001;56A(special issue II):65–90.

Weinberg AD, Minaker KL. Dehydration: evaluation and management in older adults. *JAMA.* 1995;274:1552–1556.

Wolfe RR. Protein summit: Consensus areas and future research. *Am J Clin Nutr.* 2008;87(suppl):1582s–1583s.

Vitamin Status and Requirements of the Older Adult

Susan Saffel-Shrier, MS, RD, CD

· ·

CHAPTER OBJECTIVES   Upon completion of this chapter, the reader will be able to:

1. Identify the key features of vitamins and their alterations in metabolism and health effects in older adults
2. Outline the requirements and key features that influence the requirements of vitamins in older adults
3. Describe the role of individual vitamins in health promotion and disease prevention
4. List the roles of vitamins in the prevention of chronic conditions and diseases that affect older adults
5. Suggest appropriate recommendations and dietary modifications to ensure adequate intake of vitamin-rich foods

KEY TERMS AND CONCEPTS

Antioxidant

Carotenoids

Coenzymes

Fortification

Homocysteine

Oxidative stress

Provitamin

Tocopherols

· ·

Interest in vitamin nutrition in older adults has increased in recent years because in most Western countries the 60+ age group constitutes the fastest-growing population demographic. In the past, research on vitamin nutrition focused on prevention of deficiency diseases. In recent years, important new discoveries have been made in how vitamins play a role in the prevention and modulation of chronic disease. This is of special interest to the aging population, because lifelong nutrition plays a role in healthy aging. Although many adults are living longer and more healthfully, for many the aging process represents a continued decline in health and well-being. The goal of nutritional therapy in the aging population thus is not only one of disease management, but also of health protection, so that individuals not only live long, but also enjoy good health.

It is important to remember that the aging population is an extremely heterogeneous group. Recommended intakes of vitamins and minerals for older adults are listed in the tables on the inside cover of this book. These recommendations attempt to take into consideration the variability among older adults by offering recommendations for those aged 51 to 70 and for those aged 70 and older for many nutrients. Adequate intake of these essential nutrients becomes increasingly important with advancing age, but attainment of these goals becomes an increasing challenge. Declines in functional, medical, and mental status all play an interconnected role in the attainment of adequate nutrition. This chapter discusses selected vitamins and aspects of their metabolism in relation to the aging process and chronic diseases. This chapter discusses both fat-soluble

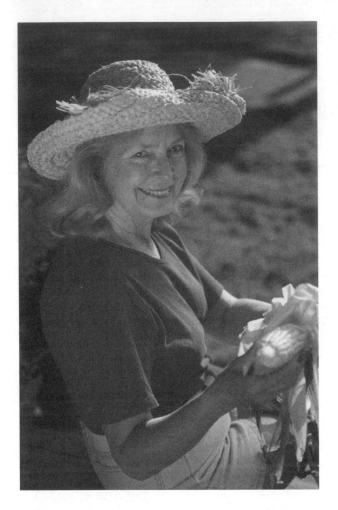

retinoic acid. Provitamin A forms are classified as **carotenoids**, of which over 700 have been identified. The principal dietary carotenoids are alpha-carotene, beta-carotene, beta-cryptoxanthin lycopene, lutein, and zeaxanthin. Of the carotenoids with provitamin A activity, food composition data are available for three: alpha-carotene, beta-carotene, and beta-cryptoxanthin.

Function

Preformed vitamin A plays a role in maintaining vision and in systemic functions such as cellular differentiation, growth, bone development, reproduction, and immunity. In a reversible process, retinol can be converted to retinal. Retinal can be converted to retinoic acid, which is an irreversible process.

Vitamin A is most well known for its role in vision, particularly night vision. Vitamin A as cis-retinal is needed to form rhodopsin found in the rod cells of the retina. Systemically, vitamin A in the hormonal form, retinoic acid, is needed for epithelial cell growth; it also affects gene expression. Vitamin A is required in the functioning of osteoblasts and osteoclasts of bone. Vitamin A's role in immunity involves T-lymphocyte function and antibody response to viral, parasitic, and bacterial infections.

Provitamin A carotenoids have **antioxidant** properties and have been implicated in the prevention of various cancers, age-related macular degeneration, dementia, cardiovascular disease, and arthritis. As antioxidants, carotenoids reduce the potential oxidative damage of lipid peroxidation, membrane disruption, and cellular DNA damage.

Absorption

Retinols and carotenoids are fat soluble and require micellar formation to be absorbed. Retinol absorption is estimated to be 70% to 90% from dietary sources, whereas beta-carotene absorption is estimated to be between 20% and 50%. Carotenoid lycopene bioavailability is impaired in persons 60 years and older. There appears to be no age difference in the bioavailability of beta- and alpha-carotene or lutein. Older adults, when given both preformed vitamin A and carotenoids, have been found to have increased absorption and a decreased clearance of retinyl esters from the blood.

Metabolism

In recent years, the role of carotenoids in disease risk has received a great deal of attention. Collectively, carotenoids function as antioxidants, but in some instances they have been shown to inhibit cell proliferation or delay cell cycle progression, or both. Like other antioxidants, carotenoids provide protection against oxidative reactions that produce free radicals resulting in tissue damage and increased risk of age-related diseases. Carotenoids have been found in three antioxidant levels: protection against oxidative reactions,

vitamins (those associated with lipid absorption and transportation as well as the presence of bile salts) and water-soluble vitamins. The water-soluble vitamins discussed in this chapter are classified as B-complex vitamins and, in part, have a hematopoietic function.

Vitamin A

Vitamin Forms and Precursors

The term *vitamin A* refers to both the preformed and **provitamin** forms. Preformed vitamin A forms are the retinols: retinol, retinal, and

provitamin Inactive forms of vitamins that the body can convert into active usable forms. Also referred to as vitamin precursors.

carotenoids A group of yellow, orange, and red pigments found in plants. Many of these compounds are precursors of vitamin A.

antioxidant A substance that combines with or otherwise neutralizes a free radical, thus preventing oxidative damage to cells and tissues.

scavenging free radicals, and repair of damaged molecules. The following list highlights the major dietary carotenoids:

- *Beta-carotene:* Epidemiologic and intervention studies have indicated a role of beta-carotene in heart disease, dementia, and cancer. Beta-carotene antioxidant activity includes scavenging free radicals and inhibiting lipid peroxidation as well as decreasing damage to DNA. It has also been shown to modulate carcinogenesis; this may be, in part, due to its ability to be converted to the provitamins that regulate gene expression. Another possible mechanism is through the increase of detoxifying enzymes. However, intervention trials have not shown a protective effect of B-carotene supplementation on health or cancer prevention.
- *Lutein and zeaxanthin:* Lutein and zeaxanthin are found in the macula of the eye and filter out phototoxic light. This protective effect is thought to be due to the scavenging of free radicals. Both have been indicated in protecting against age-related macular degeneration and cataracts, common conditions that affect many older adults.
- *Lycopene:* Lycopene has been associated with decreased risk of cardiovascular disease and lung and prostate cancer. The scavenging effects of lycopene are superior to those of beta-carotene. As an antioxidant, lycopene has shown a protective effect against oxidative DNA damage in Alzheimer's disease. The anticancer effect of lycopene is related to its antioxidant properties and inhibition of cell proliferation.
- *Beta-cryptoxanthin:* Both lung and colon cancer risk are reduced by beta-cryptoxanthin, as is the risk of arthritis. Beta-cryptoxanthin has an antioxidant effect and influences gene expression as a precursor to provitamin A.

Although observational studies have shown a strong association of carotenoids with decreased disease risk, intervention studies have been inconclusive. This inconclusiveness demands strict evaluation of the scientific process and an understanding of the metabolism of carotenoids. Currently, there is a lack of understanding of the synergistic relationships among antioxidants. This is most evident when positive effects are seen when whole foods are studied in disease-risk reduction but not when single nutrients are manipulated. Other scientific challenges include determining the appropriate time to assess the nutrient over the lifespan, recommended intakes, and duration of particular intakes.

Food Sources

Preformed vitamin A is found in foods of animal origin such as egg yolks, butter, milk (fortified), liver, and fish liver oils. Carotenoids are the red, yellow, and orange pigments found in plants. **Box 4-1** lists prominent food sources of the carotenoids.

▶ BOX 4-1 Food Sources of Carotenoids

Alpha-carotene: Pumpkin, carrots, winter squash, tangerines

Beta-carotene: Carrots, spinach, kale, cantaloupe, apricots

Lutein and zeaxanthin: Turnips, collard and mustard greens, spinach, kale, broccoli, kiwi, honeydew melon

Lycopene: Tomatoes, pink grapefruit, watermelon

Beta-cryptoxanthin: Papaya, mango, peaches, oranges, bell peppers, corn, watermelon

---

Recommendations

Vitamin A is currently being measured in Retinol Activity Equivalents (RAEs). One RAE is equal to 1 mcg retinol, 12 mcg of dietary beta-carotene, and 21 mcg of other carotenoids. The Institute of Medicine's Food and Nutrition Board set its recommendation for vitamin A at 900 mcg for men and 700 mcg for women. The National Cancer Institute recommends five to nine servings of fruits and vegetables per day, with the most benefit seen from nine servings per day.

Deficiencies

Although numerous studies have found a low dietary intake of vitamin A among older adults, serum retinol blood levels remain normal. As discussed earlier, this is thought to be due to increased absorption or clearance, or both. When considering carotenoid deficiencies, the factor of age-related **oxidative stress** needs to be addressed, as well as the role of suboptimal intakes and blood levels. Aging in and of itself results in increased oxidative stress, and this increases with most chronic diseases.

In these situations when demand for antioxidants is high, suboptimal blood levels may occur, which, in turn, could affect disease severity or progression of the aging process. In particular, a low plasma lycopene level has been shown to be associated with increased dependency among older women. Nutritional intervention studies have been shown to increase plasma levels of carotenoids.

oxidative stress Condition caused by an imbalance between the body's level of prooxidants (free radicals, reactive oxygen, and reactive nitrogen species) and its antioxidant capabilities, resulting in tissue damage, accelerated aging, impaired immune function, and degenerative diseases. Increased oxidative stress has many causes, including factors related to nutrition, illness, and the environment.

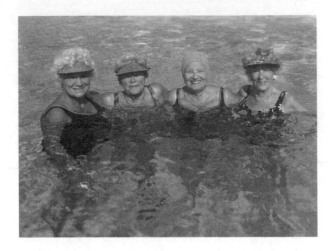

Toxicity

The Tolerable Upper Intake Level (UL) for vitamin A is 3,000 IU/day as set by the Institute of Medicine's Food and Nutrition Board. Persons with high alcohol consumption, liver disease, hyperlipidemia, or severe malnutrition may be susceptible to adverse effects of excessive preformed vitamin A. High intakes of preformed vitamin A have been shown to increase the risk of osteoporosis and hip fractures. Symptoms of toxicity include nausea and vomiting, headache, dizziness, blurred vision, and mental disturbances. High-dose supplements of beta-carotene have been shown to increase lung cancer.

Vitamin D

Forms

Vitamin D is acquired from dietary sources and through the skin's conversion of ultraviolet rays from sunlight. The dietary precursors of vitamin D include cholecalciferol and ergocalciferol. The precursor found in skin, 7-dehydrocholesterol, is converted to cholecalciferol when exposed to sunlight (ultraviolet B, or UVB). Cholecalciferol is further converted to 25-hydroxycholecalciferol—25(OH)D—in the liver and is also considered a precursor. The active form of vitamin D is 1,25-dihydroxycholecalciferol—1,25(OH)D—and is produced in the kidney via the hydroxylation of 25(OH)D. The 1,25(OH)D form has hormonal activity.

Functions and Metabolism

Vitamin D has a well-established function in bone metabolism and calcium homeostasis. In more recent years, additional physiologic functions have been identified. Vitamin D sometimes functions like a steroid hormone by activation of signal transduction pathways.

- *Bone health and osteoporosis:* Vitamin D coupled with parathyroid hormone (PTH) plays a significant role in bone health and prevention of osteoporosis. PTH is re-

sponsible for maintaining normal serum calcium levels. When serum calcium levels decline, PTH stimulates the production of 1,25(OH)D, which, in turn, acts on the calcium homeostasis target tissues: intestine, bone, and kidney. Serum calcium levels are increased as a result of the increased absorption of calcium in the intestine, the reabsorption of calcium in the kidneys, and the resorption of calcium from bone. If inadequate vitamin D is present, PTH rises, resulting in increased bone resorption. This can lead to the development of osteoporosis.

- *Muscle and falls:* Vitamin D has a direct effect on skeletal muscle formation via the vitamin D receptor (VDR), which promotes protein synthesis. Both ATP and creatine phosphate production are stimulated by vitamin D and are required for muscle contraction. VDRs are also required for intracellular regulation. When vitamin D levels drop and PTH levels rise, there is an increase in protein catabolism, a reduction in muscle fibers, and a reduction in ATP and oxygen uptake by the mitochondria. As muscle strength declines, balance becomes poor and the propensity to fall increases. It is estimated that in both institutionalized and ambulatory individuals, adequate vitamin D reduces fall risk by more than 20%.

- *Cancer:* Vitamin D exerts a protective effect against certain cancers by increasing the production of 1,25(OH)D. In cancers, vitamin D regulates cell cycles and cell differentiation and increases apoptosis of malignant cells. Cancer risk has been shown to decrease with increased UVB light and subsequent vitamin D synthesis.

- *Cardiovascular disease:* Development of atherosclerosis has been linked to a chronic inflammatory process and the production of cytokines. Suppression of cytokines has been demonstrated by 1,25(OH)D, and the VDR has been identified in heart muscle. Observational studies have shown an inverse relationship between myocardial infarction and vitamin D serum levels.

- *Diabetes mellitus:* Vitamin D plays a role in blood glucose levels and insulin secretion and action. As vitamin D status declines, fasting blood glucose levels have been shown to rise.

Absorption

Because it is a fat-soluble vitamin, vitamin D is absorbed from micellar formation through passive diffusion into the intestinal wall. The absorption rate of dietary vitamin D is approximately 50% and occurs in the duodenum and distal small intestine.

Recommendations

Vitamin D status is typically determined by measuring plasma 25(OH)D levels. The biologically active form is not measured because of tight metabolic regulation, whereas 25(OH)D is not regulated. There is no current consensus on normal 25(OH)D levels. There is, however, a consensus that the normal range should be determined based on normal PTH levels. The Institute of Medicine has determined that a 25(OH)D level of greater than 50 nmol/L is required to maintain normal PTH levels. Others have recommended levels of 75 to 80 nmol/L.

In addition to sunlight exposure, the Institute of Medicine has set vitamin D requirements at 10 mcg (400 IU) for men and women aged 51 to 70 years and 15 mcg (600 IU) for men and women older than 70 years. Current research has established a need for a minimum of 1,000 IU/day. Vitamin D supplementation, providing between 400–1000 IU daily is often recommended for older adults with poor milk intake or limited sunlight exposure.

Food Sources

The main source of dietary vitamin D is milk. Studies have shown that vitamin D intake is below two-thirds of the Recommended Dietary Allowance (RDA) in up to 75% of the older population. Additional food sources include fatty fish, fish oil, and egg yolks, along with fortified margarines, milk, and cereals. Although increased **fortification** of food could assist in addressing the deficiencies seen in the older population, there are concerns regarding the safety of such food for children.

Deficiency

Vitamin D insufficiency or deficiency is common in the older population due to reduced dietary intake and skin synthesis and decreased renal production and resistance of 1,25(OH) D. It is estimated that 50% of nursing home residents and 57% of hospitalized patients have vitamin D deficiencies or insufficiencies. In addition to decreased dietary intake of vitamin D, older persons experience a fourfold decrease in capacity to produce vitamin D from sunlight exposure, as well as resistance to 1,25(OH)D calcium absorption. Both vitamin D deficiency and insufficiency can result in osteomalacia, osteoporosis, and elevated PTH. Vitamin D insufficiency is defined as the lowest threshold value that prevents elevated PTH level, bone turnover, and bone mineral loss.

Toxicity

The UL set by the Institute of Medicine is 2,000 IU/day (50 mcg/day). The main adverse effects are hypercalcemia and enhanced bone resorption. Short-term high doses of 4,000 to 10,000 IU have been shown to not produce toxicities. Adverse effects have been shown when serum levels of 25(OH)D are 200 nmol/L, which corresponds to a daily intake of 40,000 IU.

Vitamin E

Forms and Other Names

There are eight naturally occurring forms of vitamin E. Natural vitamin E is a mixture of **tocopherols** and tocot-

rienols. However, only alpha-tocopherol in the RRR-alpha form is maintained in human plasma. Vitamin E in fortified foods and supplements is available in different forms. It can be found as a mixture of tocopherols and tocotrienols, natural alpha-tocopherol, synthetic alpha-tocopherol, or a mixture of synthetic esters. Esterification produces a more stable product, thus protecting the vitamin from oxidation. Esterified vitamin E is the form most often used in food supplements and cosmetic products.

Functions

Vitamin E functions primarily as a chain-breaking antioxidant that prevents lipid peroxidation. In fact, vitamin E is considered one of the most effective natural hydrophobic scavengers of free radicals. The tocopherols have similar antioxidant potential, but the higher levels of alpha-tocopherol in the plasma and at the hepatic level result in alpha-tocopherol being considered the most biologically active form. Recently, an alternative function of vitamin E has been proposed. Vitamin E appears to be involved in cellular signaling, interference with enzymatic activity, apoptosis, and gene modulation.

Absorption

Vitamin E is absorbed with other dietary lipids in the proximal part of the intestine. All forms of vitamin E are absorbed equally well. The overall absorption efficiency of vitamin E is thought to be low in humans, 20% to 50%, and is inversely related to intake. That is, the higher the intake, the less that is absorbed. Absorption of pharmacologic doses (200 mg) is less than 10%. In healthy persons, plasma levels of alpha-tocopherol cannot increase more than two to three times the intake, and in some healthy persons only minimal increases are seen. Therefore, it appears that there is significant variation in absorption responses. In addition, both natural and synthetic vitamin E are efficiently absorbed, but synthetic vitamin E plasma levels are not maintained, as compared with natural vitamin E. This does not change with age.

After absorption, vitamin E is secreted within the chylomicrons and is transported through the lymph system. Vitamin E is hydrolyzed and released to the peripheral tissues or transported to the liver. In the liver, vitamin E is incorporated into very low density lipoproteins (VLDLs) and redistributed to peripheral tissues in low-density lipoproteins (LDLs) or high-density lipoproteins (HDLs). It is mainly alpha-tocopherol that is recognized by the hepatic alpha-tocopherol transfer protein

fortification The addition of vitamins or minerals to a food that were not originally present in the food.

tocopherols Chemical name for vitamin E. There are four tocopherols: alpha, beta, gamma, and delta. Only alpha-tocopherol is active in the body.

(TPP). TPP mediates this salvage pathway, which is essential in maintaining adequate levels of alpha-tocopherol.

Metabolism

Two hypotheses currently exist concerning the mode of action of vitamin E in numerous disease states that affect older adults, such as certain cancers, heart disease, chronic inflammatory response, dementia, respiratory infections, and age-related eye disease. These two hypotheses are the oxidative theory and the injury response theory. Both theories consider oxidation a key factor in the progression of disease.

Oxidative Theory

In the oxidative theory, lipid peroxidation is the initial event. Lipid peroxidation occurs when normal metabolism generates potentially damaging free radicals, such as reactive oxygen, which in turn react with the unsaturated fatty acids in the cell membrane, resulting in oxidative cellular damage. Therefore, it is the role of vitamin E to scavenge the free radicals so as to maintain cell membrane integrity. Vitamin E inhibits lipid peroxidation by accepting the unstable free radicals. The resulting vitamin E–free radical can be once again reduced to the unoxidized form via vitamin C.

Injury Response Theory

Although the function of vitamin E as an antioxidant has been well recognized, specific nonantioxidant effects of vitamin E have been more recently acknowledged. This theory has been identified in the etiology of atherosclerosis and taste and smell disorders. In the injury response theory, vitamin E inhibits or interferes with enzymatic activity through cell signaling and results in reduced inflammatory responses. Such enzymes include cyclooxygenase-2 (COX-2), which plays a role in prostaglandin production, cytokines, and interleukins. Vitamin E has been shown to prevent the induction of apoptosis after lipid peroxidation.

Recommendations

The current Institute of Medicine recommendation for vitamin E is based on the alpha-tocopherol form, which is considered the most biologically active. The Daily Recommended Intake (DRI) for men and women in both the 51-to-70-year and the 70-plus brackets is 15 mg daily. The older population has been found to have inadequate intakes of vitamin E compared with persons younger than 60 years. However, higher dietary variety appears to improve vitamin E intake.

Food Sources

The natural forms of vitamin E are synthesized only by plants. Excellent food sources are vegetable oils, nuts, seeds, whole grains, and dark green leafy vegetables. The U.S. population consumes mainly gamma-tocopherol, but this form does not have significant biological activity.

Deficiencies

Overt deficiencies are rare and result from genetic abnormalities, fat malabsorption syndromes, and protein energy malnutrition. Subclinical deficiencies of vitamin E and their implication in chronic diseases were discussed previously.

Toxicity

The UL for vitamin E established by the Food and Nutrition Board of the Institute of Medicine is 1,000 mg/day; adverse effects include hemorrhagic toxicity from vitamin E–containing supplements.

An increase in prothrombin time and bleeding has been observed with co-administration of vitamin E and warfarin. Vitamin E can prolong prothrombin time by inhibiting vitamin K–dependent carboxylase.

Other adverse effects of vitamin E supplementation, including fatigue, weakness, and emotional disturbances have been observed at levels of 800 IU/day. Nausea and gastric distress have been reported at intake levels of 2,000 to 2,500 IU/day. At levels of 3,200 IU/day of vitamin E, diarrhea and cramps have been reported.

Vitamin K

Forms

The three biologically active groups of vitamin K are phylloquinones (K1), menaquinones (K2), and menadione (K3). Phylloquinones are naturally occurring in plants, and menaquinone is synthesized by bacteria. Menadione is the synthetic form of vitamin K.

Functions

Vitamin K has two major functions:

- *Blood clotting:* Vitamin K is involved in the blood-clotting process as cofactors in enzymes in the synthesis of 4 of the 13 blood-clotting factors. The four vitamin K–dependent factors are II (prothrombin), VII, IX, and X.
- *Bone formation:* Vitamin K is required in the synthesis of osteocalcin, a bone matrix protein. Osteocalcin is considered a marker of bone formation. Vitamin K has also been shown to reduce urinary calcium excretion.

Absorption

The absorption of phylloquinone, a fat-soluble vitamin, is enhanced by the presence of bile salts and pancreatic juice. Phylloquinone is absorbed in the jejunum of the small intestine through a saturable, energy-dependent process. Dietary vitamin K absorption varies between 40% and 80%. Menaquinones and menadione are absorbed in the distal small intestine and colon by passive diffusion.

Metabolism

The role of vitamin K in bone metabolism and its possible protective role against osteoporosis is of significant interest in the study of nutrition and aging. Observational studies have reported association of vitamin K intake and serum levels and the risk of low bone mineral density and hip fractures. Osteocalcin levels have also been found to be low in older persons with low serum vitamin K levels.

Recommendations

The DRI for vitamin K is 120 mcg for men in both older age groups and 90 mcg for women in both older age groups. These levels have been challenged by research demonstrating that 90 mcg in older women is inadequate to support maximal osteocalcin synthesis; an intake of 1,000 mcg has been recommended for optimal osteocalcin levels. Typical dietary intake for the older adult is estimated between 130 and 150 mcg/day.

Food Sources

Food sources of vitamin K include green leafy vegetables, collards, spinach, broccoli, brussels sprouts, cabbage, plant oils, and margarine. Although not sufficient to meet daily needs, anaerobic bacteria found in the lower gastrointestinal tract produce menaquinones, providing a source of vitamin K for humans.

Deficiency

Dietary intake studies have found adequate intake among the older population. The emerging evidence of the role of vitamin K in bone health requires further study before revisions of the current recommendations can be made. The drug coumarin may place the older person at risk of bone fracture through possible reduced production of osteocalcin.

Toxicities

The Institute of Medicine has reported no adverse effects associated with dietary or supplementary vitamin K. There is currently no UL.

Table 4-1 summarizes fat-soluble and water-soluble vitamins along with their functions, food sources, deficiency and toxicity symptoms, and special considerations for older adults.

The B-Complex Vitamins: Vitamin B12, Vitamin B6, and Folate

The vitamins B12, B6, and folate have distinct metabolic interactions and are of particular interest in the older population. These metabolic interactions, along with the aging process, place the older person at risk for a cascade of nutritional health concerns and disorders. Therefore, these nutrients are discussed as a composite so as to assist in fully understanding their nutritional implications.

Forms

The term *vitamin B12* includes a group of corrinoids that contain a cobalt-centered corrin nucleus having the biological activity of cyanocobalamin. Vitamin B12 is water soluble. *Vitamin B6* is also water soluble and includes three forms: pyridoxine, pyridoxal, and pyridoxamine. *Folate* is a generic term that includes numerous forms of this vitamin. Food folates are polyglutamate derivatives. Folic acid, the form used in fortified food products and vitamin supplements, is a pteroylmonoglutamic acid.

Functions

Collectively, vitamin B12, vitamin B6, and folate function as **coenzymes** involved in one-carbon metabolism. Vitamin B12 is a cofactor for two enzymes, methionine synthase and l-methylmalonyl-CoA. These enzymes are essential for blood formation and neurologic function; inadequate concentrations result in elevated **homocysteine** and methylmalonic acid levels, the implications of which are discussed later in this chapter. Vitamin B6 in a phosphorylated form is a coenzyme in over 100 enzymes involved in amino acid metabolism. Most notably, vitamin B6 is a coenzyme in heme synthesis and the transfer of sulfur from homocysteine to cysteine. Folate functions as part of coenzymes in numerous reactions that require the transfer of single-carbon units in amino acid metabolism. These folate coenzymes are involved in DNA synthesis, purine synthesis, and interconversion of amino acids, particularly homocysteine to methionine. Homocysteine is a common denominator in the functioning of these vitamins and is the focus of discussion in the metabolism section.

Absorption

Vitamins B12, B6, and folate have uniquely different methods of absorption and are discussed individually.

Vitamin B12 Absorption

Normal aging changes of the gut along with common disorders of older adults have significant negative influences on the absorption of vitamin B12. **Figure 4-1** shows the complex absorptive process of vitamin B12. Changes in the gastrointestinal tract that commonly accompany aging are discussed in detail in Chapter 7.

coenzymes Organic compounds, often B-vitamin derivatives that combine with an inactive enzyme to form an active one. Coenzymes associate closely with these enzymes, allowing them to catalyze certain metabolic reactions in a cell.

homocysteine An amino acid precursor of cysteine and a risk factor for heart disease.

TABLE 4-1 Summary Table of Vitamins

Vitamin	Function	Food Sources	Deficiency	Toxicity	Special Considerations
Vitamin A	Vision, cellular differentiation, bone development, immunity, antioxidant	Preform: Egg yolks, fish liver oils, milk Carotenoids: Dark red, green, and yellow vegetables	Aging & chronic disease-related oxidative stress	UL: 3,000 IU/day Symptoms: Nausea, vomiting, headache, mental changes	Increased absorption of retinol with age
Vitamin D	Bone health, cancer, cardiovascular disease, diabetes mellitus	Milk, fatty fish, egg yolks, fortified foods	Osteoporosis, bone fractures, muscle weakness, cancer, diabetes	UL: 2,000 IU/day Symptoms: Hypercalcemia-related anorexia, nausea, diarrhea	Increased dietary dependency with age
Vitamin C	Antioxidant, connective tissue, hormone, neurotransmitter synthesis	Citrus fruits, strawberries, cantaloupe, tomatoes, peppers	Aging & chronic disease-related oxidative stress	UL: 2,000 mg/day Symptoms: Diarrhea, kidney stones	Possible decreased absorption with age
Vitamin E	Antioxidant in age-related eye disease, cancer, inflammation, dementia, heart disease	Vegetable oils, nuts, seeds, whole grains, dark green leafy vegetables	Aging & chronic disease-related oxidative stress	UL: 1,000 mg/day Symptoms: Increased bleeding	Caution regarding supplementation when using anticoagulants
Vitamin K	Blood clotting, bone formation	Dark green leafy vegetables	Osteoporosis	NA	Encourage adequate vegetable intake
Vitamin B12	Coenzyme, RBC formation, neurologic	Animal products, fortified foods	Anemia, cognitive decline	NA	Poor absorption with age
Folate	Coenzyme, RBC formation	Green leafy vegetables, orange juice, fortified foods	Anemia, dementia	UL: 1,000 mcg Masks vitamin B12 deficiency	Fortification has improved folate status
Vitamin B6	Coenzyme, RBC formation, and neurotransmitter synthesis	Animal protein, spinach, bananas	Anemia, dementia	UL: 100 mg/day Symptom: Sensory neuropathy	High metabolic turnover with age

Normal aging changes include a decrease in gastric acid (hypochlorhydria or achlorhydria). Other factors include atrophic gastritis with accompanying small bowel bacterial overgrowth, gastric surgery, and certain drugs. It is estimated that 10% to 30% of older adults have atrophic gastritis. When bacterial overgrowth is present, the bacteria utilize vitamin B12 for their own metabolism. Older adults without atrophic gastritis have midrange blood levels of vitamin B12, whereas older adults with atrophic gastritis have the lowest blood levels.

Prior to absorption, vitamin B12 must be cleaved from the protein food to which it is bound. This requires the presence of hydrochloric acid and pepsin. After the cleav-age, the free vitamin binds to the R factor protein and the complex is transported to the small intestine, where the R protein is released. It is in the small bowel that vitamin B12 binds with intrinsic factor; absorption occurs in the ileum. When vitamin B12 is unable to be digested from its protein-bound food, malabsorption occurs, resulting in the main cause of vitamin B12 deficiency in older adults.

Vitamin B6 Absorption

The absorption of vitamin B6 does not appear to be affected by age. Absorption occurs through passive diffusion, and high doses are easily absorbed.

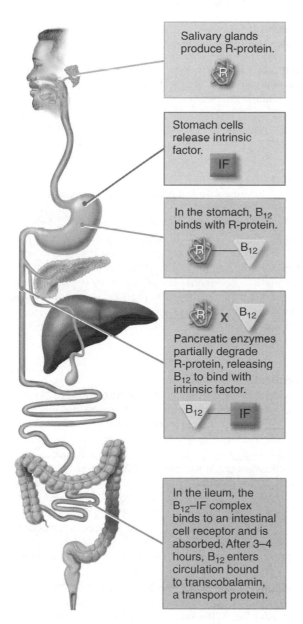

Salivary glands produce R-protein.

Stomach cells release intrinsic factor.

IF

In the stomach, B_{12} binds with R-protein.

R — B_{12}

R X B_{12}

Pancreatic enzymes partially degrade R-protein, releasing B_{12} to bind with intrinsic factor.

B_{12} — IF

In the ileum, the B_{12}–IF complex binds to an intestinal cell receptor and is absorbed. After 3–4 hours, B_{12} enters circulation bound to transcobalamin, a transport protein.

FIGURE 4-1 Absorption of Vitamin B12
Source: Insel P, Turner RE, Ross D. *Nutrition.* 3rd ed. Sudbury, MA: Jones & Bartlett; 2007, p. 44. Reproduced with permission.

Folate Absorption

Food folates are hydrolyzed to monoglutamate forms prior to absorption. Food folate, as well as supplemental folate, is absorbed via a nonsaturable mechanism involving passive diffusion in the proximal small intestine. It is unclear whether an aging change in folate digestion and/or absorption exists.

Metabolism

As illustrated in **Figure 4-2**, one of the important combined roles of vitamins B12, B6, and folate is their function as coenzymes in the metabolism of one-carbon units and homocysteine. Homocysteine is a nonessential sulfur-containing amino acid produced in the metabolism of methionine or transsulfuration of cysteine.

Elevated serum homocysteine (hyperhomocysteinemia) is an independent risk factor for vascular diseases of the coronary, cerebral, and peripheral vessels. Therefore, it plays an important role in atherosclerosis, cognitive disorders, diabetes mellitus, and inflammatory bowel disease through oxidative stress, proinflammatory, and immune responses. Homocysteine has also been suggested to play a role in osteoporosis, bone fractures, certain cancers, systemic lupus erythematosus, multiple sclerosis, and rheumatoid arthritis. Vitamins B12, B6, and folate status are the main determinants of homocysteine blood levels. The third National Health and Nutrition Examination Survey (NHANES III) found that approximately 14% of older persons had elevated homocysteine levels.

Homocysteine is metabolized via two pathways. The methionine synthase pathway requires both vitamin B12 and folate; the cystathionine pathway requires vitamin B6. In the remethylation of homocysteine, cyanocobalamin acts as a cofactor for methionine synthase, which catalyzes the conversion of homocysteine to methionine using the folate metabolite 5-methytetrahydrofolic acid as the methyl donor. The cystathionine pathway requires pyridoxine (vitamin B6) as a cofactor in the metabolism of homocysteine to cysteine. It is thought that there is a higher metabolic turnover of vitamin B6 in the older adult. Finally, vitamin B12 is solely involved as a coenzyme in the conversion of methylmalonyl-CoA to succinyl-CoA, a metabolite of the Kreb cycle. When there is inadequate vitamin B12, the production of methylmalonic acid increases. Therefore, methylmalonic acid is considered a highly specific measure of vitamin B12 status.

Recommendations

The DRI for vitamin B12 for men and women in the 51-to-70-year age group and the 70-plus age group is 2.4 mcg/day. The vitamin B6 DRI is 1.7 mg/day for men and 1.5 mg/day for women in both age groups. The folate DRI is 400 mcg for all sex and age groups.

Food Sources

Vitamin B12 is mainly found in animal sources and foods fortified with vitamin B12, such as cereals and grain products. Vitamin B6 is found in a variety of foods, such as fortified cereals, fish, meats, bananas, beans, peanut butter, and many vegetables. The best sources of dietary folate are liver, leafy greens, fortified grain products, and citrus fruits.

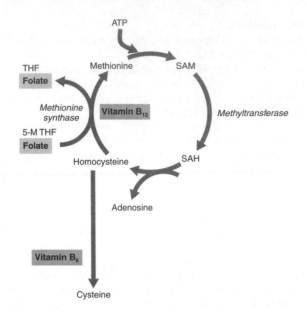

FIGURE 4-2 Folate, Vitamin B12, and Vitamin B6 Metabolism. SAM=S-adenosyl-methionine; SAH=S-adenosyl-homocysteine; 5-M THF=5-methyl tetrahydrofolate; THF=tetrahydrofolate

Deficiency

Folate Deficiency

The prevalence of a folate deficiency in the older population is approximately 30%, with neuropsychiatric older adults having a much higher prevalence of deficiency—80%. Post-menopausal women on the National Cholesterol Education Program Step II diet were found to have inadequate intake of folic acid. Fortification of grains, while primarily intended to lower incidence of neural tube defects should prove beneficial in raising serum folate levels of older adults.

The FDA mandated the fortification of grains with folic acid in 1998 at a level of 140 mcg per 100 g of cereal grain. After fortification, the prevalence of high serum folate levels rose from 7% to 38%. Because there has been some evidence to suggest that fortification can mask a vitamin B12 deficiency, there has been concern about older adults as an at-risk population. It has been recommended that vitamin B12 status be regularly monitored in the older population.

Vitamin B12 Deficiency

Deficiencies in vitamin B12 are primarily caused by malabsorption. However, dietary intake of vitamin B12-rich foods may be inadequate in older adults and should be assessed. The NHANES data has shown a small but significant increase in serum vitamin B12 levels. It has been suggested that vitamin supplements and fortified foods are the best sources of vitamin B12 in the older population. In addition, postmenopausal women on a low-fat vegan diet had inadequate vitamin B12 intakes.

Vitamin B6 Deficiency

Conservatively, 10% of the older population is defined as being vitamin B6 deficient based on blood vitamin levels. The DRI for B6 has been set higher in the older age groups than younger adults because of the higher metabolic turnover, and thus higher requirement, in the former.

Toxicity

High intakes of folate (median intake 742 mcg/day) have been associated with a faster rate of cognitive decline in community-dwelling older adults. The Institute of Medicine recommends that folic acid intake from food and supplements not exceed 1,000 mcg daily in healthy older adults, because larger amounts can mask the neurologic damage of a vitamin B12 deficiency. The UL as set by the Institute of Medicine for vitamin B6 is 100 mg/day. Sensory neuropathy has occurred from high intakes of vitamin B6. There is no UL set for vitamin B12, and no adverse effects noted by the Institute of Medicine.

Vitamin C

Vitamin C is a water-soluble vitamin with a variety of functions. It is an antioxidant and plays a role in connective tissue, hormone, and neurotransmitter synthesis. As an antioxidant, vitamin C is a potential preventive agent against cognitive impairment. Vitamin C functions synergistically with other antioxidants, particularly vitamin E, and may require the presence of other antioxidants to be most effective. Vitamin C supplementation in combination with other antioxidants may have a role in preventing dementia.

High fruit and vegetable intakes have been associated with lower incidences of cardiovascular disease, age-related macular degeneration, and cancer. Vitamin C, found mainly in fruits and vegetables, has been indicated to be one of many antioxidants that lowers the risk of these diseases. Vitamin C supplementation may reduce the incidence of coronary heart disease; however, additional research is required in this area.

In general, caloric intake declines with age and can reflect a reduced intake of vitamin C. Vitamin C tissue and plasma levels decline with age and more so in men than in women. Vitamin C is absorbed via an active transport mechanism, and older adults may have a reduced absorption. This reduced absorption has led to the suggestion that older adults may require as much as twice the requirement of younger adults. The current DRI for vitamin C is 90 mg/day for men and 75 mg/day for women over age 50. High supplemental doses of vitamin C can lead to diarrhea and renal stone formation. Smokers have a higher requirement

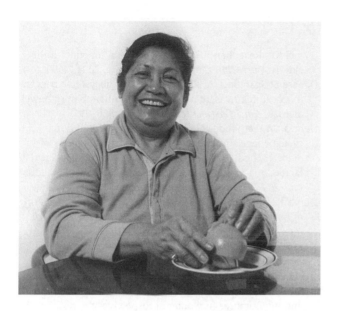

for vitamin C. Current recommendations are for adequate (five to nine) servings of fruits and vegetables per day.

Other B Vitamins

The B vitamins thiamin, niacin, riboflavin, biotin, and pantothenic acid are all involved in the release of energy from the energy-yielding nutrients: carbohydrates, proteins, and fats. Little evidence suggests changes in the metabolism of these vitamins occurs with aging. National data have found that these nutrients are adequately consumed among older adults. However, multiple nutrient deficiencies can be seen with poor dietary intake or as a result of chronic medication use. Deficiencies have also been found to occur when

factors such as social isolation, food insecurity, low socioeconomic status, chronic disease, and limited functionality are present, and generally accompany an underlying malnutrition.

Conclusion

The physiologic changes of aging and how they relate to nutritional needs is a topic of current research; much more knowledge is needed to fully understand the nutritional needs of the older adult. Maintaining adequate dietary intake is essential in preserving health and independence, along with controlling health care costs. Supplementation should be considered when dietary intake is inadequate.

Activities Related to This Chapter

1. Interview a friend or relative to find out his or her food likes and dislikes. Plan a menu that meets the DRIs for that person while still meeting his or her personal preferences.
2. Conduct a diet interview of an older person in your neighborhood. Using reliable diet analysis software, determine whether this person's nutrient intake meets the DRI recommendations. For which nutrients does this person meet the recommendations? For which nutrients is this person above or below the recommendations? What suggestions can you make to improve this person's overall diet quality?
3. List the vitamins most likely to be found deficient in an older adult. Offer food suggestions and preparation methods to improve intake of these nutrients.
4. List all the vitamins and describe how age affects the requirement for each.

REFERENCES

Adunsky A, Arinzon Z, Krasniznsky I, et al. Plasma homocysteine levels and cognitive status in long-term stay geriatric patients: a cross sectional study. *Arch Gerontol Geriatr*. 2005;40:129–138.

Alpha-Tocopherol Beta-Carotene Cancer Prevention Study Group. The effects of vitamin E and beta-carotene on the incidence of lung cancer and other cancers in male smokers. *N Engl J Med*. 1994;330:1029–1035.

Araki A, Hosoi T, Orimo H, Ito H. Association of plasma homocysteine with serum interleukin-6 and C-peptide levels in patients with type 2 diabetes. *Metabolism*. 2005;54(6):809–814.

Bailey LB, Gregory JF. Folate metabolism and requirements. *J Nutr*. 1999;129:779–782.

Baker H, Jaslow SP, Frank O. Severe impairment of dietary folate utilization in the elderly. *J Am Geriatr Soc*. 1978;26(5):218–221.

Binkley NC, Krueger DC, Engelke JA, et al. Vitamin K supplementation reduces serum concentrations of under-gamma-carboxylated osteocalcin in healthy young and elderly adults. *Am J Clin Nutr*. 2000;72:1523–1528.

Bischoff-Ferrari HA, Willett WC, Wong JB, et al. Fracture prevention with vitamin D supplementation: a meta-analysis of randomized controlled trials. *JAMA*. 2005;293(18):2257–2264.

Booth SL, Broe KE, Peterson JW, et al. Association between vitamin K biochemical measures and bone mineral density in men and women. *J Clin Endocrinol Metab*. 2002;89:4904–4909.

Bottiglieri T, Diaz-Arrasitia R. Hyperhomocysteinemia and cognitive function: more than just a causal link? *Am J Clin Nutr*. 2005;82:493–494.

Broekmans WMR, Klöpping-Ketelaars IAA, Schuurman CRW, et al. Fruits and vegetables increase plasma carotenoids and vitamins and decrease homocysteine in humans. *J Nutr*. 2000;130:1578–1583.

Brubacher D, Moser U, Jordan P. Vitamin C concentrations in plasma as a function of intake: a meta-analysis. *Int J Vitamin Nutr Res*. 2000;70:226–237.

Cardinault N, Tyssandier V, Grolier P, et al. Comparison of the postprandial chylomicron carotenoid responses in young and older subjects. *Eur J Nutr*. 2003;42(6):315–323.

Chernoff R. Micronutrient requirements in older women. *Am J Clin Nutr*. 2005;81(5):1240S–1245S.

Cherubini A, Martin A, Andres-Lacueva C, et al. Vitamin E levels, cognitive impairment and dementia in older persons: the InCHIANTI study. *Neurobiol Aging*. 2005;26:987–994.

Costa EM, Blau HM, Fledman D. 1,25-hydroxyvitamin D3 receptors and hormonal responses in cloned human skeletal muscle cells. *Endocrinology*. 1986;119:2214–2220.

D'Anci KE, Rosenberg IH. Folate and brain function in the elderly. *Curr Opin Clin Nutr Metab Care*. 2004;7:659–664.

Danese S, Sgambato A, Papa A, et al. Homocysteine triggers mucosal microvascular activation in inflammatory bowel disease. *Am J Gastroenterol*. 2005;100:886–895.

DeLuis DA, Fernandez N, Arranz ML, et al. Total homocysteine levels relation with chronic complications of diabetes, body composition and other cardiovascular risk factors in a population of patients with diabetes mellitus type 2. *J Diabetes Complications*. 2005;19(1):42–46.

Durga J, van Tits LJH, Schouten EG, et al. Effect of lowering of homocysteine levels on inflammatory markers. *Arch Intern Med*. 2005;165:1388–1394.

Englehart MJ, Geerlings MI, Ruitemeberg A. Dietary intake of antioxidants and risk of Alzheimer disease. *JAMA*. 2002;287(24):3223–3229.

Feskanich D, Wever P, Willett WC, et al. Vitamin K intake and hip fractures in women: prospective study. *Am J Clin Nutr*. 1999;82:719–724.

Garcia A, Zanibbi K. Homocysteine and cognitive function in elderly people. *CMAJ*. 2004;171(8):897–904.

Garland CF, Garland RC, Gorham ED. The role of vitamin D in cancer prevention. *Am J Public Health*. 2006;96:252–261.

Genkinger JM, Platz EA, Hoffman EA, et al. Fruit, vegetable, and antioxidant intake and all cause, cancer and cardiovascular disease mortality in a community dwelling population in Washington County, Maryland. *Am J Epidemiol*. 2004;106:1223–1233.

Giovannucci ERE, Liu Y, Stampfer MJ, Willett WC. A prospective study of tomato products, lycopene, and prostate cancer risk. *J Natl Cancer Inst*. 2002;94:391–398.

Gori AM, Corsi AM, Fedi F, et al. A proinflammatory state is associated with hyperhomocysteinemia in the elderly. *Am J Clin Nutr*. 2005;82:335–341.

Grant WB. Ecologic studies of solar UV-B radiation and cancer mortality. *Recent Results Cancer Res*. 2003;164:371–377.

Gray SH, Hanlon JT, Landerman LR, et al. Is antioxidant use protective of cognitive function in the community dwelling elderly? *Am J Geriatr Pharmacotherapy*. 2003;1(1):3–10.

Greenspan SL, Resnick NM, Parker A. Vitamin D supplementation in older women. *J Gerontol Med Sci*. 2005;60A:754–759.

Groff JL, Gropper SS, Hunt SM. *Advanced Nutrition and Human Metabolism*. 2nd ed. Minneapolis/St. Paul: West Publishing; 1995.

Gross MD, Snowdon DA. Plasma antioxidant concentrations in a population of elderly women: findings from the nun study. *Nutr Res*. 1996;16(11–12):1881–1890.

Heaney RP. Vitamin D: how much do we need and how much is too much? *Osteoporosis Int*. 2000;11:553–555.

Heber D, Lu QY. Overview of mechanisms of action of lycopene. *Exp Biol Med*. 2002;227(10):920–930.

Holick MF. Sunlight and vitamin D for bone health and prevention of autoimmune diseases, cancers and cardiovascular disease. *Am J Clin Nutr*. 2004;80(suppl):1678–1688S.

Holick MF. Vitamin D deficiency. *N Engl J Med*. 2007;357:266–281.

Institute of Medicine. Dietary reference intakes: vitamins. 2004. Available at: http://www.iom.edu/DBFile.asp?id=7296. Accessed December 2007.

Institute of Medicine, Food and Nutrition Board. *Dietary Reference Intakes for Vitamin C, Vitamin E, Selenium and Carotenoids*. Washington DC: National Academies Press; 2000.

Institute of Medicine, Food and Nutrition Board. Vitamin D. In: *Dietary Reference Intakes for Calcium, Phosphorus, Magnesium, Vitamin D and Fluoride*. Washington, DC: National Academies Press; 1999.

Institute of Medicine, Food and Nutrition Board. Vitamin D. In: *Dietary Reference Intakes for Thiamin, Riboflavin, Niacin, Vitamin B6, Folate, Vitamin B12, Pantothenic Acid, Biotin and Choline*. Washington, DC: National Academies Press; 1998.

Kado DM, Bucur A, Selhub J, et al. Homocysteine levels and decline in physical function: MacArthur studies of successful aging. *Am J Med*. 2002;113:537–542.

Kanai T, Takagi T, Masuhiro K, et al. Serum vitamin K level and bone mineral density in post-menopausal women. *Int J Gynaecol Obstet*. 1997;56:25–30.

Karas M, Amir H, Fishman D, et al. Lycopene interferes with cell cycle progression and insulin-like growth factor I signaling in mammary cancer cells. *Nutr Cancer*. 2000;36(1):101–110.

Knekt P, Ritz J, Pereira MA, et al. Antioxidant vitamins and coronary heart disease risk: a pooled analysis of 9 cohorts. *Am J Clin Nutr*. 2004;80:1508–1520.

Krazinski SD, Russell RM, Otradovec CL, et al. Relationship of vitamin A and E intake to fasting plasma retinol, retinol binding protein, retinyl esters, carotene, alpha-tocopherol and cholesterol among elderly people and young adults: increased plasma retinyl esters among vitamin A supplement users. *Am J Clin Nutr*. 1989;49:112–120.

Lamberti P, Zoccolella S, Armenise E, et al. Hyperhomocysteinemia in L-dopa treated Parkinson's disease patients: effect of cobalamin and folate administration. *Eur J Neurol*. 2005;12(5):365–368.

Lewerin C, Matousek M, Steen G, et al. Significant correlations of plasma homocysteine and serum methylmalonic acid with movement and cognitive performance in elderly subjects but no improvement from short term

vitamin therapy: a placebo-controlled randomized study. *Am J Clin Nutr*. 2005;81(5):1155–1162.

Mecocci P, Polidori MC, Troiano L, et al. Plasma antioxidants and longevity: a study on healthy centenarians. *Free Radic Biol Med*. 2000;28:1243–1248.

Meydani SN, Ham SN, Hamer DH. Vitamin E and respiratory infection in the elderly. *Ann NY Acad Sci*. 2004;1031:214–222.

Morris MC, Evans DA, Bienias JL, et al. Dietary folate and vitamin B12 intake and cognitive decline among community dwelling older persons. *Arch Neurol*. 2005;62:641–645.

Morris MC, Evans DA, Tangney CC, et al. Relation of tocopherol forms to incident Alzheimer disease and to cognitive change. *Am J Clin Nutr*. 2005;1:508–514.

Mosekilde L. Vitamin D and the elderly. *Clin Endocrinol*. 2005;62:265–281.

Munteanu A, Zingg JM, Azzi A. Anti-atherosclerotic effects of vitamin E: myth or reality? *J Cell Mol Med*. 2004;18(1):59–76.

Nieves JW. Osteoporosis: the role of micronutrients. *Am J Clin Nutr*. 2005;8(suppl):1232S–1296S.

Nelson JL, Bernstein PS, Schmidt MC, et al. Dietary modification and moderate antioxidant supplementation differentially affect serum carotenoids, antioxidant levels and markers of oxidative stress in older humans. *Nutrition*. 2003;133:3117–3123.

Omenn GS, Goodman GE, Thornquist MD, et al. Effects of a combination of beta-carotene and vitamin A on lung cancer and cardiovascular disease. *N Eng J Med*. 1996;334:1150–1155.

Pattanaungkul S, Riggs BL, Yergey AL, et al. Relationship of intestinal calcium absorption to 1,25-dihydroxyvitamin D levels in young vs elderly women: evidence for age related intestinal resistance to 1,25-(OH)2 action. *J Clin Endocrinol Metab*. 2000;85:4023–4027.

Peeters AC, van der Molen EF, Blom HJ, den Heijer M. The effect of homocysteine reduction by B-vitamin supplementation on markers of endothelial dysfunction. *Thromb Haemost*. 2004;92(5):1086–1091.

Pfeifer M, Begerow B, Minne HW. Vitamin D and muscle function. *Osteoporosis Int*. 2002;13:187–194.

Pfeiffer CM, Caudill SP, Gunter EW, et al. Analysis of factors influencing the comparison of homocysteine values between the third National Health and Nutrition Examination Survey (NHANES) and NHANES 1999. *J Nutr*. 2000;130:2850–2854.

Polidori MC, Cherubini A, Senin U, Mecocci P. Peripheral non-enzymatic antioxidant changes with human aging: a selective status report. *Biogerontology*. 2001;2(2):99–104.

Pufulete M, Al-Ghnaniem R, Khushal A, et al. Effect of folic acid supplementation on genomic DNA methylation in patients with colorectal adenoma. *Gut*. 2005;54:648–653.

Rao AV, Balachandran B. Role of oxidative stress anti-oxidants in neurodegenerative disease. *Nutr Neurosci.* 2003;5(5):291–309.

Rao AV, Rao LG. Carotenoids and human health. *Pharmacol Res.* 2007;55:207–216.

Ricciarelli R, Zinngg JM, Azzi A. Vitamin E: protective role of a Janus molecule. *FASEB.* 2001;15:2314–2325.

Russell RM. The aging process as a modifier of metabolism. *Am J Clin Nutr.* 2000;72(suppl):529S–530S.

Russell RM. The vitamin A spectrum: from deficiency to toxicity. *Am J Clin Nutr.* 2000;71(4):878–884.

Sato Y, Honda Y, Iwamoto J, et al. Effect of folate and meco-balamin on hip fracture patients with strokes. *JAMA.* 2005;293:1082–1088.

Scraggs R, Khaw KT, Murphy S. Effect of winter oral vitamin D3 supplementation on cardiovascular risk factors in elderly adults. *Eur J Clin Nutr.* 1995;49:640–646.

Seddon JM. Multivitamin multimineral supplements and eye disease: age related macular degeneration and cataracts. *Am J Clin Nutr.* 2007;85(suppl):30S–37S.

Selhub J, Jacques PF, Wilson PW, et al. Vitamin status and intake as primary determinants of homocysteinemia in an elderly population. *JAMA.* 1993;270(22):2693–2697.

Staehelin H. Micronutrients and Alzheimer's disease. *Proc Nutr Soc.* 2005;64:565–570.

Szule P, Chapuy MC, Meunier PJ, Delmas PD. Serum undercarboxylated osteocalcin is a marker of the risk of hip fracture: a three year follow-up study. *Bone.* 1996;18:487–498.

Takami M, Nakatsuda K, Naka H, et al. Vitamin K2 (me-naquinone 4) reduces serum undercarboxylated osteo-calcin level as early as two weeks in elderly women with established osteoporosis. *J Bone Mineral Metab.* 2003;21:161–165.

Tucker KL, Qiao N, Scott T, et al. High homocysteine and low B vitamins predict cognitive decline in aging men: VA Normative Aging Study. *Am J Clin Nutr.* 2005;82:627–635.

Turner-McGrievy GM, Barnard ND, Scialli AR, Lanou AJ. Effects of a low-fat vegan diet and a Step II diet on macro and micronutrient intakes in overweight postmenopausal women. *Nutrition.* 2004;20(9)738–746.

Vieth R, Chan PC, MacFarlene GD. Efficacy and safety of vitamin D3 intake exceeding the lowest observed effect level. *Am J Clin Nutr.* 2001;73:288–294.

Visioli F, Hagen TM. Nutritional strategies for healthy cardiovascular aging: focus on micronutrients. *Pharmacol Res.* 2007;55:199–206.

Vogel S, Contois JH, Tucker KL, et al. Plasma retinol and plasma and lipoprotein tocopherol and carotenoid con-centrations in healthy elderly participants of the Framing-ham Heart Study. *Am J Clin Nutr.* 1997;66:950–958.

Weaver CM, Fleet JC. Vitamin D requirements: current and future. *Am J Clin Nutr.* 2004;80(suppl):1735S–1739S.

Willcox JK, Ash SL, Catignaini GL. Antioxidants and prevention of chronic disease. *Crit Rev Food Sci Nutr.* 2004;44:275–295.

Wolters M, Strohle A, Hahn A. Cobalamin: a critical vitamin in the elderly. *Preventive Med.* 2004;39:1256–1266.

Zandi P, Anthony JC, Khachaturian AS, et al. Reduced risk of Alzheimer disease in users of antioxidant vitamin supplements. *Arch Neurol.* 2004;61:82–81.

Zittermann A, Schleithoff SS, Tenderrich G, et al. Low vita-min D status: a contributing factor in the pathogenesis of congestive heart failure. *J Am Coll Cardiol.* 2003;41:105–112.

Mineral Requirements of the Older Adult

Karen Chapman-Novakoski, RD, LDN, PhD

CHAPTER OBJECTIVES   Upon completion of this chapter, the reader will be able to:

1. Describe the functions of minerals and special considerations for their requirements in aging
2. Identify minerals whose requirement is more or less for older adults
3. Recognize areas where the usual mineral intake of the older adult may need improvement to achieve recommended levels of intake for health

KEY TERMS AND CONCEPTS

Electrolytes

Major minerals

Osteoporosis

Renal disease

Trace minerals

Minerals comprise only about 4% of body weight and, although inorganic, are essential to tissues, fluid balance, metabolic function, and organ systems. As a group, they are involved in both regulatory processes and structural functions.

The **major minerals** include calcium, phosphorus, magnesium, sodium, chloride, and potassium. These minerals are at times referred to as **electrolytes**, meaning that they can have a negative or positive charge, thus conducting electricity. In the body, these anions (negatively charged) and cations (positively charged) are important for the action potentials of cells, nerve conduction, and muscle excitation. The anions include chloride and phosphorus and when combined with oxygen molecules to become phosphate. The cations include calcium, magnesium, sodium, and potassium.

These charged minerals are balanced within cells (intracellular) and outside of cells (extracellular). Maintaining this balance is part of metabolism and is important in body water and blood volume regulation, blood pH, nerve conduction, and muscle contraction. In a healthy person, the normal range of electrolytes in the blood is kept fairly constant and is usually fairly narrow. Only in trauma or disease states do electrolytes rise above or fall below the normal range.

The **trace minerals** are so called because only very small amounts are needed on a daily basis. Recommended intakes have been established for most minerals, with the exception of chloride, aluminum, and nickel. The recommended intakes are expressed as Dietary Reference Intakes (DRIs): the Recommended Dietary Allowance (RDA)

trace minerals Minerals present in the body and required in the diet in relatively small amounts compared with major minerals. Also known as microminerals

major minerals A major mineral is required in the diet and is present in the body in large amounts compared with trace minerals.

electrolytes Substances that dissolve into charged particles (ions) when dissolved in water or other solvents and thus are capable of conducting an electrical current. The terms electrolyte and ion are often used interchangeably.

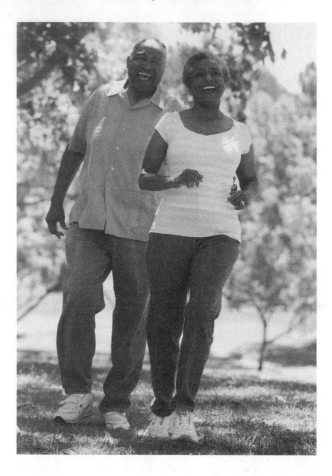

and Adequate Intake (AI) levels. In addition, for many of the micronutrients Tolerable Upper Intake Level values (ULs) have also been established.

Although requirements for different minerals vary, the body's mineral balance (homeostasis) is usually achieved through regulation of how much of a nutrient is absorbed in the intestine and how much is excreted in the urine. The appropriate amount of a mineral is important, because too little may lead to deficiency symptoms and too much may be toxic, both situations possibly leading to deleterious health consequences. A more subtle issue is the optimal amount for aging. For example, several minerals, such as zinc, copper, manganese, and selenium, have antioxidant properties. Antioxidants can prevent damage by free radicals. The relationship between free radical damage and the aging process continues to be investigated.

The amounts of minerals in a particular food often vary depending on the soil a plant is grown in or the feed an animal consumes. For trace minerals, the content in foods may even vary with the cooking utensils used. However, minerals are inorganic and cannot be destroyed with cooking or processing. The DRI values for minerals for older adults can be found on the inside cover of this textbook.

The Major Minerals

Calcium

Calcium's primary role is in maintaining the structure of bone. Inorganic components such as calcium phosphate crystals and salts constitute approximately 65% of bone dry weight. Calcium in the blood and extracellular fluid has a role in vasodilation and vasocontraction, muscle contraction, blood clotting, and nerve transmission.

Absorption and Metabolism

Calcium is absorbed through two mechanisms: (1) a saturable, regulated route that is dependent on vitamin D and (2) a nonsaturable mechanism that is not tightly regulated. The vitamin D–regulated system occurs primarily in the duodenum and proximal jejunum of the small intestine. Vitamin D increases calcium uptake at the intestinal brush border by stimulating production of a calcium-binding protein. The passive vitamin D–independent system occurs along the length of the intestine. Usually only 10% to 30% of calcium is absorbed, although absorption can be influenced by a number of factors. Fortunately, a greater need for calcium stimulates greater absorption. Calcium is best absorbed in an acid medium, as occurs in the proximal duodenum. Calcium within a meal is better absorbed than when taken alone, possibly because of the increased acid production stimulated by food. **Box 5-1** lists factors that influence the absorption of calcium.

Factors that have been investigated for having a negative effect on calcium absorption include fiber, oxalic acid, phytic acid, caffeine, fat, and phosphorus. The effect of fiber on intestinal absorption of calcium is quite variable and may in fact enhance calcium absorption, depending on the type of fiber. Oxalic acid and phytic acid often are associated with fiber. As with fiber, their effect on calcium absorption is highly variable. Caffeine and fat have been shown to have negligible effects on calcium absorption. Although phosphorus, especially in the form of soft drinks, is often believed to have a negative effect on calcium absorption, phosphorus-intake studies have failed to support this opinion.

Calcium balance may be influenced by factors that affect the renal handling of calcium. Both high protein and high sodium intake increase urinary loss of calcium. A high sodium intake increases urinary sodium loss, and with it an obligatory increase in urinary calcium. Thus, it is recommended to keep sodium intake within a moderate range and to consume adequate amounts of calcium. Low-protein *and* high-protein diets have been shown to have a negative effect on bone health. The negative effects of either extreme are more pronounced with inadequate calcium intake than with adequate intake.

Caffeine has been shown *not* to have a significant effect on calcium excretion. Inadequate calcium intake combined with caffeine can have a negative impact on bone health,

BOX 5-1   Factors That Influence Calcium Absorption in Older Adults

Overall nutritional status

Vitamin D status

Calcium status

Gut pH

Presence of other food in the intestine

Dietary fiber

Oxalic acid

Phytic acid

Caffeine

Dietary fat

Phosphorus

Renal function

Dietary protein

Medication use

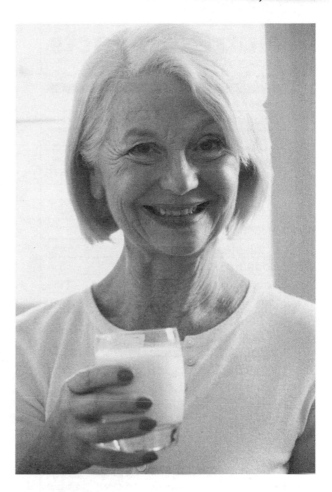

such as in cases where caffeine-containing beverages replace milk in the diet.

Calcium balance is affected by calcium intake. If intake should change from adequate to inadequate, a higher percentage of calcium would be absorbed to compensate for poor intake. In general, this adaptive mechanism is not great enough to compensate for poor intake completely. The degree of compensation declines with age.

Ingested calcium is normally excreted in feces and urine in approximately equal amounts. However, fecal calcium is a more reliable measure of calcium intake, because urinary excretion will decrease during growth and with decreases in the kidney's glomerular filtration, which is often seen in advanced age.

Calcium in the blood is maintained within a narrow range. If calcium in the blood begins to fall, levels are returned to normal by a combination of an increase in intestinal absorption, an increase in renal reabsorption, and an increase in calcium release from bone.

Recommendations

The AI for men and women aged 51 and older is 1,200 mg calcium per day. This is 200 mg higher than recommended during the preceding two decades. Although milk is one of the best sources of calcium, with 300 mg of calcium per 8 ounces, to achieve this intake would require four 8-ounce servings each day. Therefore, for many older adults to meet the recommended intake level, supplements may be re-

quired for those whose diets are not sufficient in calcium because of food preferences, medical conditions, or personal beliefs.

Typical Intakes of Older Adults

Poor calcium intake was found in the National Health and Nutrition Examination Survey III (NHANES III) for men and women older than 60 years. Mean intakes for men were 735 mg/day for nonsupplement users and 900 mg/day for supplement users when diet and supplemental intake were considered. Even so, 60% of the men who used supplements had total calcium intakes below the AI. Whereas mean intakes for women who used supplements were similar to that of men, nonsupplement users had a mean intake of 580 mg/day.

Food Sources

Most dietary calcium is obtained from dairy products, although more grain-based foods and fruit juices are being fortified with calcium. Dark green leafy vegetables, shellfish, and tofu set with calcium are good sources of calcium,

Nutrition Facts

Serving Size 1 Bar (85g)
Servings Per Container 4

Amount Per Serving

Calories 170   Calories from Fat 50

	% Daily Value *
Total Fat 6g	**9%**
Saturated Fat 4g	**19%**
Trans Fat 0g	
Polyunsaturated Fat 0.5g	
Monounsaturated Fat 1g	
Cholesterol 13mg	**4%**
Sodium 83mg	**3%**
Total Carbohydrate 33g	**11%**
Dietary Fiber 4g	**16%**
Sugar 25g	
Protein 3g	

Vitamin A 110%	•	Vitamin C 2%
Calcium 10%	•	Iron 3%

*Percent Daily Values are based on a 2,000 calorie diet.
Your daily values may be higher or lower depending on
your calorie needs.

		Calories	2,000	2,500
Total Fat	Less than		65g	80g
Sat Fat	Less than		20g	25g
Cholesterol	Less than		300mg	300mg
Sodium	Less than		2,400mg	2,400mg
Total Carbohydrate			300g	375g
Dietary Fiber			25g	30g

Calories per gram:
Fat 9   •   Carbohydrate 4   •   Protein 4

although they are not usually consumed on a daily basis. The amount of calcium in a food product can be found on the Nutrition Facts label as a percentage. The percentage is multiplied by 1,000 mg calcium. For instance, if the Nutrition Facts label reads calcium 40%, then the food contains 400 mg of calcium (0.40 × 1,000).

Deficiency and Toxicity

Chronic poor intake results in **osteoporosis**, a condition of reduced bone mass and increased bone fragility. The other functions of calcium are maintained even with chronic poor intake at the ex-

osteoporosis Bone disease characterized by a decrease in bone mineral density and the appearance of small holes in bones due to loss of minerals.

pense of the calcium stored in bone. Osteoporosis primarily affects older adults. Postmenopausal women are especially susceptible to osteoporosis because of the loss of estrogen, which has a positive influence on bone turnover.

The UL is set at 2,500 mg of calcium. For most healthy people, a dietary intake of calcium above this level is probably safe, more so than intake from supplements over this level. However, those with kidney disease, those taking certain diuretics, and those having low intake of other minerals may be more susceptible to the toxic effects of high levels of calcium intake. The possible adverse effects at levels of intake above the UL include kidney stones, kidney damage, and alteration in the absorption or metabolism of other minerals.

Special Considerations

A deficiency in vitamin D can lead to poor calcium absorption. The active absorption of calcium in the intestine is dependent on vitamin D. In bone, osteoclasts are stimulated by vitamin D. In both instances, the net desired effect is to increase calcium availability.

Lactose intolerance may result in an avoidance of dairy products. Lactose is usually tolerated if small amounts of dairy products are consumed. If it is preferable to avoid dairy products, many foods are good or excellent sources of calcium, including many fortified foods and beverages. The enzyme lactase may be consumed as capsules or purchased already added to milk. Lactase activity may vary, however, and all products may not produce consistent results.

Serum calcium is maintained in a narrow range. A hormone, parathyroid hormone (PTH), is sensitive to changes in serum calcium, increasing when serum calcium levels begin to fall. Increased PTH enhances calcium reabsorption in the kidneys as well as calcium release from bone. With normal kidney function, increased PTH will also stimulate renal activation of vitamin D so that calcium intestinal absorption is increased. This mechanism may not function as efficiently in older adults because of a decrease in kidney function and an increase in PTH levels.

Phosphorus

Most of the phosphorus in an adult's body is in bone as hydroxyapatite. However, phosphorus also occurs as phospholipids in most cell membranes and it is a component of nucleic acids. Phosphorus has an important role in metabolism as an acid-base buffer, in enzymatic reactions, and in energy transfer.

Absorption and Metabolism

Adults absorb from 55% to 70% of the phosphorus they consume. Most phosphorus is absorbed by a passive diffusion across the intestinal mucosa. Some is also absorbed by an active transport dependent on vitamin D. Phosphorus absorption is not reduced by dietary components, but can be reduced by aluminum-containing antacids or medications and by pharmacologic doses of calcium carbonate.

The kidneys are the main regulators of phosphorus retention. However, hormones exert their influence on the kidneys so that phosphorus is either reabsorbed or excreted. The hormones involved with calcium homeostasis, vitamin D and PTH, are also involved in phosphorus homeostasis, in addition to insulin, growth hormone, and steroid hormones. In kidney diseases, both body and blood phosphorus increase.

Recommendations

The RDA for phosphorus for men and women older than 51 years is the same as for all adults: 700 mg/day.

Typical Intakes of Older Adults

Phosphorus intakes for older adults have been estimated by What We Eat in America, NHANES 2005–2006. Women aged 50–59 are reported to have an intake of 1134 mg/day, and those aged 60–69 years have an intake of 1061 mg/day. Women aged 70 or older have an intake of approximately 993 mg/day. Men ages 50–59, 60–69, and 70 and older have intakes of 1152 mg/day, 1434 mg/day, and 1234 mg/day, respectively.

Food Sources

Phosphorus is found in nearly all foods. Good sources include meat, milk products, eggs, grains, and legumes. Soft drinks are also high in phosphorus.

Deficiency and Toxicity

Phosphorus is found in so many foods that phosphorus deficiency is known only to occur with starvation. Refeeding a severely malnourished person very quickly parenterally without providing adequate phosphorus has been noted to produce a hypophosphatemia that can be life threatening. Severe hypophosphatemia can also occur with poor phosphorus intake during refeeding following alcoholic binges or diabetic ketoacidosis. Very high intake of aluminum-containing antacids can also cause hypophosphatemia.

Toxicity due to high phosphorus intake is not known to occur in persons with healthy kidney function. High phosphorus intake has not been shown to be the cause of negative calcium balance or bone resorption. At one time, there was concern that the phosphorus in carbonated beverages had a negative effect on bone health. However, the effect appears to be due to the substitution of high-calcium beverages with carbonated beverages rather than a direct effect of the phosphorus.

Special Considerations

In persons with severe **renal disease**, high phosphorus intake can lead to calcification of soft tissue. The UL for adults up to age 70 is 4.0 g/day. For those older than 70, the upper limit is reduced to 3.0 g/day because of the increased prevalence of impaired renal function.

Magnesium

Approximately half of the body's magnesium is found in bone. Magnesium is a cofactor for hundreds of enzyme reactions, and as such is involved in energy metabolism, protein and fatty acid synthesis, and glucose metabolism. Magnesium is required for adequate purine and pyrimidine reserves that are needed for DNA and RNA synthesis. Muscle contraction requires magnesium. Through its interaction with sodium, potassium, and calcium, magnesium is important for maintaining cellular ionic balance.

Absorption and Metabolism

Intestinal magnesium absorption is proportional to the amount ingested and occurs through both passive and active mechanisms. Absorption occurs throughout the intestinal tract, but appears to be greatest in the distal jejunum and ileum. The kidneys control the urinary excretion of magnesium, with output being low when magnesium intake is low and higher when magnesium balance is positive. As with other minerals, the normal serum magnesium concentration (1.8–2.3 mg/dL) does not reflect skeletal magnesium.

Recommendations

The RDA for men aged 51 or older is 420 mg magnesium per day, and for women of a similar age it is 320 mg/day. These recommendations are the same as those for adults during the preceding two decades, but slightly more than the 400 and 300 mg recommended for men and women, respectively, aged 19 through 30 years.

Typical Intakes of Older Adults

The mean intake of magnesium for adults is approximately 300 mg. However, magnesium intake varies with caloric intake. A nationwide study reported the magnesium intake of older men as approximately 300 mg; that of older women was close to 200 mg. Because older adults generally consume fewer calories than younger adults, magnesium intake is also usually lower. Several studies have reported low magnesium intake in the older population. Reports of institutionalized older adults indicate that their magnesium intake is lower than their free-living counterparts.

Magnesium metabolism may be changed in the older adult with decreased intestinal absorption and increased urinary excretion. Bone magnesium may also decrease with aging.

Food Sources

Magnesium is found in many foods, but the amount of magnesium found in any particular food varies greatly.

renal disease Disease of the kidneys.

Green leafy vegetables, fruits, grains, and nuts provide almost half of the average American intake of magnesium. One-third of the usual intake is provided by milk, meat, and eggs. Shellfish can also be a good source of magnesium.

Deficiency and Toxicity

Magnesium deficiency rarely occurs except as secondary to a medical condition or disease. However, excessive alcohol intake can lead to magnesium deficiency through increased urinary losses. Many medications also increase urinary losses of magnesium, the most common being thiazide and loop diuretics used to treat hypertension and congestive heart failure. Magnesium deficiency has been associated with hypertension, cardiac diseases, and diabetes.

High amounts of dietary magnesium have not been found to have toxic effects. However, supplemental magnesium in high doses will cause diarrhea.

Hypermagnesemia occurs only with renal disease when large amounts of magnesium have been consumed, usually as a supplement or antacid. Hypermagnesemia in such cases can result in neurologic and cardiac symptoms. The UL for everyone older than 8 years is 350 mg of supplemental magnesium.

Special Considerations

Those with impaired renal function are at greater risk of magnesium toxicity. However, there are medical conditions for which prescribed supplemental magnesium exceeding the UL is beneficial with medical supervision. Some medications may increase magnesium excretion and require a higher magnesium intake to achieve optimal magnesium levels.

Sodium

Sodium is the main extracellular cation and is required in the maintenance of extracellular fluid volume and plasma volume. Sodium is also important for membrane potential and active transport of nutrients.

Absorption and Metabolism

Most ingested sodium is absorbed in the small intestine. A narrow range of sodium in the blood is maintained through hormones and their effect on the kidneys. With moderate to high sodium intake, most sodium is excreted in the urine, with much smaller amounts retained. Although sodium can also be lost through the skin with sweating, sodium homeostasis is largely controlled by the kidneys under the influences of the renin–angiotensin hormonal system.

Recommendations

The AI for men and women aged 51 to 70 years is 1,300 mg of sodium per day. This is lower than recommended for younger adults due to the high prevalence of hypertension with age and changes in the metabolism of sodium. For men and women older than 70, the AI is set at 1,200 mg. The lower AI for those older than 70 is based on an overall reduced caloric intake. The AI does not apply to competitive athletes or workers exposed to extreme heat.

The Dietary Guidelines for Americans advises adults to consume less than 2,300 mg of sodium each day, and older adults to consume no more than 1,500 mg/day. This recommendation is more liberal than the RDA but remains much lower than usual intake.

Typical Intakes of Older Adults

Usual intake of sodium for men aged 51 to 70 is 3,800 mg/day, and for men older than 70 it is 3,200 mg/day. Usual intake for women aged 51 to 70 is 2,600 mg, and for women older than 70 it is 2,400 mg/day.

Food Sources

Most sodium is ingested as sodium chloride, or salt. Salt is 40% sodium and 60% chloride. Sodium may also be added to foods for either flavor or preservation. Common additives include monosodium glutamate, sodium carbonate, sodium benzoate, and sodium bicarbonate. High-sodium foods include processed meats such as ham, bacon, or luncheon meats; snack foods with visible salt such as chips; canned soups; cheese; smoked or canned fish; and salted nuts. The milligrams of sodium in a food product can be found on the Nutrition Facts label. The percent Daily Value is based on a 2,000-calorie diet, but is 2,400 mg of sodium regardless of calorie level.

Deficiency and Toxicity

High sodium intake is associated with hypertension, a condition found in at least half of older adults. The UL for sodium is 2.3 g/day (2,300 mg). The ability to excrete sodium is reduced in older adults, who are more sensitive to sodium intake with respect to their blood pressure.

Low blood sodium, hyponatremia, usually occurs as a result of medications or a medical condition. Hyponatremia is a common complication of thiazide diuretic medications.

Special Considerations

Salt sensitivity refers to the response of blood pressure to an acute change in salt intake. Those whose blood pressure falls with an acute decrease in salt intake are categorized as "salt sensitive." About half of those with hypertension and about one-fourth of those without hypertension are salt sensitive. However, the percentage of those who are salt sensitive increases with age. In addition, the kidneys' ability to excrete sodium declines with age. Carefully reading labels to watch for added and unnecessary sodium is an effective way for older adults to limit their sodium intake. **Table 5-1** lists common label terms for sodium.

Chloride

Chloride is an important anion in extracellular fluid and therefore is important in maintaining fluid and electrolyte balance. Together, sodium and chloride are the main determinants of extracellular volume. Chloride is also important in digestion as part of the hydrochloric acid secreted in the stomach.

Absorption and Metabolism

Most ingested chloride is absorbed in the intestine and excreted in the urine. As is true of sodium, chloride homeo-stasis is largely controlled by the kidneys under the influences of the renin–angiotensin hormonal system.

Recommendations

The AI for chloride is 2.0 g/day for men and women aged 51 to 70 years. As with sodium, this recommendation is lower than for younger adults. For those older than 70, the AI is set at 1.8 g/day. Chloride recommendations are based on an equimolar ratio with sodium.

Food Sources

The primary source of dietary chloride is sodium chloride, commonly known as salt. Therefore, salted foods that are high in sodium are also high in chloride, such as salted snack foods or crackers, salted nuts, and processed foods with added salt.

Deficiency and Toxicity

Deficiency symptoms of chloride do not occur in healthy adults. Adverse effects of high chloride intake reflect a high salt intake and are more attributable to the sodium ingested than to the chloride.

Special Considerations

Excess vomiting can lead to chloride loss because of the hydrochloric acid content of the stomach. Diuretics can increase urinary losses of water, sodium, and chloride.

Potassium

Potassium is the main intracellular cation, with very small amounts of potassium located in the extracellular compartments. A pump at the cell membrane works to move potassium into cells and sodium out of cells. The difference between the amount of potassium inside and outside the cell creates a voltage difference that is important in maintaining the resting membrane potential of the cell. Potassium has a role in cardiac function, neural transmission, muscular contraction, vascular tone, acid-base metabolism, and glucose metabolism.

TABLE 5-1 Label Terms for Sodium

Term on Label	Definition	Food Examples
Sodium-free	Less than 5 mg sodium per serving	Fresh fruits and vegetables; pasta
Very low sodium	35 mg or less sodium per serving	Very low sodium canned tuna
Low sodium	140 mg or less per serving	Low-sodium soups, broths, and bouillons; low-sodium peanut butter; low-sodium canned salmon; low-sodium cheese; low-sodium catsup, baking powder, and sauces
Reduced or less sodium	At least 25% less sodium than the regular food product	Reduced-sodium bacon; reduced-sodium canned vegetables; lower-sodium soy sauce
No salt added, or unsalted		Unsalted margarine or butter; canned vegetables with no added salt; unsalted crackers, nuts, pretzels, potato chips, and popcorn

Absorption and Metabolism

Most potassium is absorbed in the small intestine. The kidneys are responsible for potassium retention or excretion and maintain potassium balance through a wide range of potassium intake. As with the other major minerals, serum potassium levels do not reflect body potassium status.

A large amount of the body's potassium is in the muscles because of potassium's key role in membrane polarization, which is needed for neural stimulation of muscle and muscle contraction.

Recommendations

The AI for men and women older than 50 is 4.7 g/day. This recommendation is the same for all adults older than 19 and is in agreement with the Dietary Guidelines for Americans.

Typical Intakes of Older Adults

Mean intake of potassium for men aged 51 to 70 is 3,300 mg/day, and for men older than 70 is 2,900 mg/day. Mean intake of potassium for women aged 51 to 70 is 2,500 mg/day and for women older than 70 is 2,400 mg/day.

Food Sources

Fruits and vegetables are high in potassium. Meat and dairy products are also fairly high in potassium. Tea and coffee are also sources of potassium, but water is usually low in potassium. Potassium may be added to foods as a preservative, such as potassium bicarbonate.

Deficiency and Toxicity

Potassium deficiency rarely occurs because of poor intake. Most often hypokalemia (low blood potassium) results because of increased potassium excretion, usually as a result of medications such as diuretics.

Low potassium intake is linked to a higher prevalence of hypertension. A diet higher in fruits and vegetables as a source of potassium has been shown to reduce blood pressure.

Toxicity has not been found with high dietary potassium intake in healthy adults; therefore, there is currently no UL for healthy adults. Hyperkalemia (high blood potassium) occurs with kidney disease because the diseased kidneys are unable to excrete potassium.

Special Considerations

Increased losses of potassium can occur with exercise and heat exposure as a result of increased potassium losses through sweat. Certain types of diuretics used in the treatment of hypertension and heart failure can substantially increase potassium losses. A lower tolerance of potassium is found with renal insufficiency.

Table 5-2 summarizes the discussion of the major minerals.

TABLE 5-2 Summary Table for the Major Minerals

Name	Main Functions	Food Sources	Toxicity	Deficiency	Special Considerations of Older Adults
Calcium	Bone and teeth; nerve conduction; blood clotting; muscle contraction; cellular ionic balance	Dairy products, fortified foods	Kidney stones; calcification of soft tissue	Osteoporosis	Osteoporosis is most prevalent in older adults.
Phosphorus	Bone and teeth; energy transfer; enzymatic reactions; cellular ionic balance	Dairy products, meat, grains, soft drinks	Rare	Rare	—
Magnesium	Bone and teeth; muscle contraction; energy metabolism; coenzyme; cellular ionic balance	Green leafy vegetables; fruits, grains, and nuts; milk, meat, and eggs	Rare; low intakes associated with hypertension	Diarrhea	Deficiency can occur with diuretics.
Sodium	Cellular ionic balance; extracellular fluid volume, plasma volume; membrane potential; active transport of nutrients	Salt, processed foods	Rare	Associated with hypertension	May need to limit intake.
Potassium	Cellular ionic balance; membrane potential; muscle contraction	Fruits and vegetables; meat and dairy products; tea, coffee	Low intakes associated with hypertension		Diuretics may increase losses.
Chloride	Cellular ionic balance; membrane potential; gastric hydrochloric acid	Salt	Rare	Rare	—

The Trace Minerals

Iron

Red blood cells transport hemoglobin, a protein that contains iron in the center of four heme protein subunits. Each heme subunit has the polypeptide globin attached. Iron is essential for oxygen transport through hemoglobin, moving oxygen from the lungs to tissues without becoming oxidized itself.

Myoglobin also contains iron, but is found exclusively in muscle. Like hemoglobin, the primary function of myoglobin is to transport oxygen. Whereas hemoglobin transports oxygen through the bloodstream throughout the body, myoglobin only transports oxygen within the muscles. Because muscles contract frequently, myoglobin releases oxygen to meet the demand.

Cytochromes are also heme-containing compounds that are necessary for cellular respiration and metabolism. Cytochromes are found in the mitochondria of cells. It is in the mitochondria through the iron-containing cytochromes that energy metabolism occurs. These heme enzymes are important to prevent lipid oxidation within the body.

Enzymes containing nonheme iron are also important to energy metabolism, although they are present in smaller quantities. In addition, iron also has a central role in immune function.

Absorption and Metabolism

Iron is absorbed in the duodenum of the small intestine. Because iron is recycled within the body, with little iron being excreted, only a small amount of dietary iron is normally absorbed. Iron absorption is inversely related to body stores, so that absorption is higher when body stores are low. Absorption may also be increased when red blood cell production is increased, as may occur after blood loss. If blood loss has been excessive or is continuous, such as is found with chronic blood loss from the colon in some medical conditions, then increased iron absorption may not be adequate to meet the body's needs. **Box 5-2** lists factors that influence iron absorption.

> **BOX 5-2 Factors That Influence Iron Absorption**
>
> Body stores
> Red blood cell production
> Food source
> Dietary intake
> Vitamin C

Absorption of nonheme iron from cereals or plants is enhanced if meat or a source of vitamin C is eaten at the same time. Iron absorption may be decreased by dietary fiber. Although it has been believed that iron and zinc compete for intestinal transport, there is evidence that zinc does not inhibit iron absorption.

Iron is stored as ferritin in the lining of the intestine and in the plasma and as hemosiderin in the liver. However, most of the body's iron is present in the hemoglobin in red blood cells (**Figure 5-1**). Most of the iron in red blood cells is recycled and used again after the red blood cell dies. The iron from the dead red blood cell is transported in the plasma bound to the protein transferrin. The iron in transferrin is transported to the bone marrow for the synthesis of new hemoglobin for new red blood cells. Transferrin usually does not carry all of the iron that it is capable of transporting. This is referred to as iron-binding capacity,

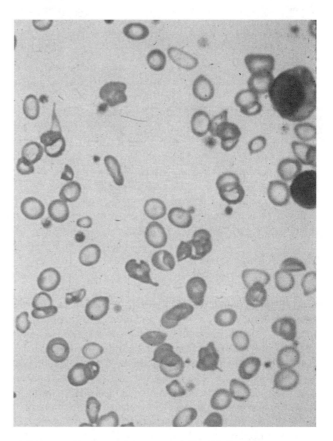

FIGURE 5-1 Healthy and Anemic Red Blood Cells

Source: Crowley LV. *An Introduction to Human Disease: Pathology and Pathophysiology Correlations.* 7th ed. Sudbury, MA: Jones & Bartlett; 2007. Reprinted with permission. Photograph courtesy of Leonard V. Crowley, M.D., Century College.

or total iron-binding capacity, and can be used as a clinical indicator of iron status. Iron loss is usually minimal, except through blood loss due to menstruation in females.

Recommendations

The RDA for adults older than 50 is 8 mg/day. This amount reflects the RDA for adult men of all ages, but a reduction in the RDA for women after menstruation and blood loss cease with menopause.

Typical Intakes of Older Adults

Mean intake for adults is 14.9 ± 36.9 mg/kg. Median intake has been reported to be 16 to 18 mg/day for men and 12 mg/day for women. Mean iron intake has been reported to be 11 mg for older women and 15 mg for older men who do not take supplements. Intakes of iron for older women and men who take supplements are 24 mg and 27 mg, respectively, when dietary iron and supplemental iron are combined. Intakes may be lower for those with lower animal protein intakes, such as those with limited income, vegetarians, and those with poor appetite and lower calorie intake.

Food Sources

Dietary iron is referred to as either heme iron or nonheme iron. Heme iron is that found in the hemoglobin or myoglobin of animal muscle products, that is, meat. Usually, the darker the meat, the higher the myoglobin or hemoglobin content, and therefore the richer it is in iron. Nonheme iron is found in cereals and vegetables. Many breakfast cereals are fortified with iron. The amount of iron in a food product can be found on the Nutrition Facts label as a percentage of 18 mg, which is the RDA for women between 19 and 50 years. Iron is often added to ready-to-eat breakfast cereal at levels of 25% to 90% of the 18-mg RDA.

Deficiency and Toxicity

There are three generally accepted stages of iron deficiency: depleted iron stores, early functional iron deficiency, and iron deficiency anemia. Hemoglobin and hematocrit levels are generally used to screen for anemia, although these measures are not specific to the causes of anemia. Anemia attributable to iron deficiency is characterized by low hemoglobin and hematocrit, with small, pale red blood cells. A low transferrin and ferritin level and a high iron-binding capacity also indicate iron deficiency. A limitation of using blood markers for iron deficiency identification is that ferritin levels may be elevated regardless of body iron stores in inflammation or malignancy, both of which occur frequently in the older adult.

Iron deficiency is not prevalent in older adults, but it can occur because of poor intake over a long period of time, because of gastrointestinal bleeding, or because of medical conditions. A reduction in stomach acidity, achlorhydria, occurs in about one-third of elderly people and may decrease absorption of iron. Iron deficiency prevalence is 3% to 4% in men older than 70 and 6% to 7% in women older than 70.

The UL for iron for adults is 45 mg/day and is based on the intake of supplemental iron that may produce gastrointestinal distress. Iron overload has been investigated for links to heart disease, and changes in iron metabolism may be associated with neurologic disorders.

Special Considerations

Iron reserves may be used quickly in persons receiving the chemotherapy medication recombinant erythropoietin, or epoetin, because the medication dramatically increases the production of red blood cells. Those receiving dialysis for kidney failure and those with intestinal blood loss, as seen in ulcerative colitis, are also at risk for iron deficiency and may also be treated with epoetin.

During inflammation, iron metabolism is altered. Iron is required for cell proliferation and differentiation of both immune cells and pathogens. The cells of the immune system have unique routes of acquiring iron in addition to those of most other cells. This is useful when iron deficiency may occur during infection or tumor development. In infection or inflammation, iron is rerouted for storage in the reticuloendothelial system rather than as ferritin, making iron unavailable for infectious cells. Infections increase the difficulty of assessing iron status because ferritin levels may be low as a result of the infection, not necessarily because of low total body iron.

Zinc

Zinc is required as a catalyst for about 100 enzymes, is a key structural component in many proteins, and is a regulator of gene expression. Zinc is essential for immune function and growth. Zinc is also required for normal smell and taste functions, as well as for skin integrity.

Absorption and Metabolism

Most zinc is absorbed in the jejunum in a saturable, transcellular manner. Zinc absorption is poor and could lead to zinc deficiency in malabsorption syndromes such as Crohn's disease or short bowel syndrome.

Zinc absorption from a diet rich in animal protein will be higher than from a diet low or devoid of animal protein, such as a vegetarian diet. This is especially true if the vegetable-based diet is high in phytic acid, which can bind to zinc and reduce absorption. Supplemental iron may decrease zinc absorption due to competition for protein transporters in the gastrointestinal lumen. There is no consistent evidence that aging affects zinc absorption or that requirements are higher in older adults.

Recommendations

The RDA for men older than 51 is 11 mg/day and for women is 8 mg/day. This recommended level of intake is the same as for younger adults.

Typical Intakes of Older Adults

Mean zinc intake is 9.4 ± 18.6 mg zinc per day for adults. A follow-up of men in a longitudinal study reported a mean dietary zinc intake of 11.2 mg/day (range: 3.4–29.8 mg/day). About 20% of the participants reported taking vitamin and mineral supplements that included zinc. Total daily zinc intake from the diet and supplements averaged 17.1 mg/day. A study of older men and women reported intakes of 11 mg and 8 mg zinc for men and women, respectively, who did not take supplements, and 19 mg and 15 mg total zinc intake, respectively, for those who did take supplements.

Food Sources

Zinc is found in meat, seafood, whole grains, and legumes, although the content can vary. Meat and seafood contain the highest amounts of zinc. Zinc is sometimes added to ready-to-eat cereals at a level of 2% to 10% of the RDA. The comparison RDA for the Nutrition Facts label for zinc is the 15-mg RDA for adults from a previous guideline.

Deficiency and Toxicity

Zinc deficiency in the older adult may result in alopecia, dermatitis, and impaired immune function. Mild zinc deficiency may result in distorted taste, losses of taste, or poor dark adaptation of the eyes. Plasma zinc is often used to assess zinc status, although plasma zinc does not necessarily reflect body reserves or recent zinc intake. Other methods are less reliable.

There have been no adverse events reported from dietary zinc intake. The Tolerable Upper Intake Level includes intake from food, fortified food, water, and supplements. For adults older than 19 years, the UL is 40 mg/day.

Chronic intake of high levels of supplemental zinc may result in suppression of the immune response, decreased high-density lipoprotein (HDL) level, and reduced copper and iron status. Acutely, gastrointestinal distress may occur with intakes of 50 to 150 mg/day of supplemental zinc. High supplemental levels of zinc intake can raise plasma zinc levels above the normal range.

Special Considerations

Vegetarianism and alcohol abuse may impair zinc absorption and increase zinc requirements. Studies investigating whether zinc supplementation of the older adult could be of benefit to immune function have concluded that supplementation only has a beneficial effect if zinc deficiency exists.

Copper

Copper's main function is as a cofactor in a number of enzymes, such as catalase, cytochrome oxidase, and peroxidases.

Absorption and Metabolism

The absorption of copper occurs primarily in the small intestine, with some absorption possible in the stomach. Copper absorption varies with intake, with a usual range of 20% to 50% of copper intake. At very low copper intakes, absorption may reach 75% of the ingested copper.

Most of the copper in the body circulates in the blood bound to the protein ceruloplasmin. Copper balance is achieved through intestinal absorption and excretion in the stool.

Recommendations

The RDA for both men and women aged 51 years or older is 900 mcg/day. This recommendation is the same as for adults of a younger age.

Typical Intakes of Older Adults

The intake of copper by adults is 1.3 ± 8.5 mg according to the Total Diet Study. Intakes for men older than 50 are 0.9 to 1.1 mg/day and for women are 0.7 to 0.8 mg/day.

Food Sources

Organ meats, seafood, nuts, and seeds are the main sources of copper in the diet. Liver is very high in copper, and mixed nuts and peanut butter are good sources of copper. Tea, potatoes, milk, and chicken are low in copper but eaten often, and therefore also contribute to dietary copper intake.

Deficiency and Toxicity

Copper deficiency is rare, but it may result in normocytic, hypochromic anemia and a reduced white blood cell count. Copper status can be assessed by plasma copper or ceruloplasmin levels, although these measures cannot reflect toxicity. An inherited neurologic disorder of copper malabsorption, Menkes disease, is usually diagnosed in childhood.

Copper toxicity is also rare, usually the result of contamination of food or beverages. This accidental acute toxicity results in gastrointestinal distress. More severe toxicity symptoms only occur in Wilson disease, which is a rare hereditary disease. The UL for copper has been set at 10 mg/day (10,000 mcg/day).

Special Considerations

Supplemental zinc intake or the medication penicillamine decreases copper absorption and can result in copper deficiency. However, copper deficiency remains rare and is usually associated with general malnutrition, parenteral nutrition without copper supplementation, and severe malabsorption or nephrotic syndromes.

Chromium

Research supports chromium's role in carbohydrate metabolism through interaction with insulin. The precise mechanism is not yet known.

Absorption and Metabolism

Although chromium absorption is responsive to varying intake levels, absorption is poor at all levels, constituting only 0.5% to 2% of intake. The exact mechanism of transport is not yet known, and different chemical forms of chromium appear to be absorbed in different ways. The most common form of chromium is trivalent chromium, which is bound to a serum protein for transport through the blood.

Recommendations

The AI for men 51 years or older is 30 mcg/day, and for women of similar age it is 20 mcg/day. This recommended intake is lower than that recommended for younger adults.

Typical Intakes of Older Adults

Dietary chromium intakes cannot be determined from any existing databases because the amount of chromium in various foods has not been quantified. Processing may increase or decrease the amount of chromium found in a food. In general, cereals, some beers, and some wines may be high in chromium. Intake from supplements has been estimated to be 30 mcg for men and women.

Food Sources

Dietary chromium has decreased in recent years due to the decrease in contamination of food sources by stainless steel containers and other metal cooking or storage ware. Foods high in chromium include bran cereals and some beer and wine. Good sources may include fruits and vegetables, eggs, and meat.

Deficiency and Toxicity

Chromium toxicity is very rare because chromium is so poorly absorbed. Similarly, chromium deficiency is also rare. Currently, no clinically useful indices of chromium status are available.

Special Considerations

Increased urinary chromium losses may occur in type 2 diabetes. Those with renal or hepatic disease may be susceptible to adverse effects from high chromium intake.

Selenium

Selenium forms complexes with certain proteins to become "selenoproteins." These selenoproteins have important roles in antioxidative functions and the regulation of thyroid hormone action. Selenium is also important to detoxification systems. Because of its function as an antioxidant and in detoxification, selenium is being investigated for a role in preventing cancer.

Absorption and Metabolism

Most selenium that is ingested is absorbed. After absorption, selenium circulates in the blood bound to plasma proteins. The body's reserve of selenium is either as selenomethionine or as glutathione peroxidase. Urine is the primary route of excretion, although selenium may also be excreted in the feces.

Recommendations

The RDA for men and women older than 55 is 55 mcg/day, the same value as for younger males and females.

Typical Intakes of Older Adults

The mean selenium intake for adults is 76 ± 124 mcg/day. For men aged 51 to 70, the mean selenium intake is 135 mcg/day; for men older than 70, it is 112 mcg/day. For women aged 51 to 70, the mean selenium intake is 94 mcg/day; for women older than 70, it is 83 mcg/day.

Food Sources

The amount of selenium in plants is quite variable, depending upon the selenium content of the soil. However, several species of garlic and broccoli accumulate a larger percentage of selenium from the soil than other plants. Meat and seafood are reliable sources of selenium, although actual content will vary with the selenium intake of the animal.

Deficiency and Toxicity

Plasma selenium levels can be used to assess selenium deficiency, as can whole blood selenium levels. The selenium deficiency disease called Keshan disease is a heart disease occurring primarily in China. Selenium deficiency is not common in the United States. One enzyme indicator of selenium status, glutathione peroxidase, has been found to decrease in the older adult. Institutionalized older adults with low selenium status respond to supplementation.

Selenium toxicity can result from food sources or supplement intake. Chronic selenium toxicity first results in changes in the fingernails, followed by the loss of the nails and hair. At higher levels of toxicity, diarrhea, nausea, tooth mottling, and eventually nervous system changes can result.

Special Considerations

Selenium has been linked to vitamin E in that they both can prevent lipid peroxidation, a reaction linked to the aging process. However, studies have not shown either selenium or vitamin E to have an effect on slowing the aging process.

Aluminum

No physiologic role has been found for aluminum. This suggests that aluminum is either neutral in the body, has a function that can be accomplished by a different mineral, or is a toxicant. In the latter regard, aluminum has been investigated for a possible role in the development of Alzheimer's disease.

Absorption and Metabolism

Very little aluminum is absorbed in the intestines. In fact, the intestine acts as a barrier to aluminum, although the barrier is not as effective in older adults as it is in younger adults.

Recommendations

Because aluminum has no known essential function, there is no recommended intake.

Food Sources

Aluminum is commonly added to water at municipal water treatment plants to decrease turbidity. Aluminum may be found in foods cooked in aluminum cookware.

Deficiency and Toxicity

There are no deficiency symptoms for aluminum. Aluminum has negative effects on several other minerals, such as calcium and magnesium, causing them to be ineffective in their respective functions. Although not conclusive or causal, scientific results support an association between aluminum and Alzheimer's disease. Aluminum has been reported in the autopsied brain tissue of people with Alzheimer's disease. It is hypothesized that aluminum physically and biochemically interferes with normal brain function.

Molybdenum

Molybdenum is a cofactor for at least three enzymes involved in oxidation and detoxification reactions.

Absorption and Metabolism

Molybdenum is absorbed by passive diffusion, although the exact mechanism and location have not been reported. Absorption rates range from 50% to 93%. Retention of molybdenum is low, with most being excreted in the urine.

Recommendations

The RDA for men and women older than 51 is 45 mcg/day, the same as for adults of a younger age. This level of intake is based on balance studies but not on prevention of deficiency, because no deficiency symptoms have been found.

Typical Intakes of Older Adults

Dietary intake of molybdenum is unknown. Mean intake of molybdenum by adults from supplements is 29 to 30 mcg/day.

Food Sources

Good sources of molybdenum include leafy vegetables, grains, legumes, kidneys, liver, and milk.

Deficiency and Toxicity

A molybdenum deficiency state has not been reported. There is no known toxicity of molybdenum in humans. The UL of 2 mg/day (2,000 mcg/day) is based on animal studies only.

Manganese

Manganese has a role in protein, fat, and carbohydrate metabolism as well as several enzyme reactions and bone formation. Manganese is required for normal immune function, reproduction, and digestion as well as blood clotting.

Absorption and Metabolism

Only a small percentage of ingested manganese is absorbed, and much of that becomes part of bile and is secreted back into the gastrointestinal tract. It is not clear whether absorption is active, passive, or both. Most manganese in the serum is bound to albumin, although levels in the blood are very low normally. Manganese is found in higher concentration in the mitochondria of cells, and therefore is higher in the liver, kidney, and pancreas than in the blood.

Recommendations

The AI for manganese for men older than 51 is 2.3 mg/day, and for women, 1.8 mg/day.

Typical Intakes of Older Adults

The mean dietary intake of manganese by adults is 2.4 ± 4.5 mg/day. Intake of supplemental manganese by adults is 2.6 to 2.7 mg/day.

Food Sources

Unrefined grain products, tea, nuts, and leafy vegetables are good sources of manganese. Refined grain products, dairy products, and meat have some manganese.

Deficiency and Toxicity

A clinical deficiency of manganese due to poor intake in healthy individuals has not been reported. Plasma manganese levels reflect dietary intake, both above and below normal range.

Toxicity is primarily related to inhaled manganese dust and is considered an occupational hazard. Manganese toxicity, called manganism, is associated with increased manganese brain levels. The effects are neurologic, with symptoms similar to Parkinson diseas. The UL for adults is 11 mg/day.

Nickel

Although nickel is an essential trace element in lower animals, no studies have shown nickel to have a biochemical role in higher animals and humans. Nickel may be involved in enzymatic reactions, gene expression, or iron metabolism.

Absorption and Metabolism

Nickel absorption from dietary sources is typically less than 10%. Absorption seems to be decreased with food, especially milk, coffee, tea, and orange juice. Nickel is transported in blood bound to albumin or, to a lesser extent, nickeloplasmin. Nickel does not accumulate in any tissue except in the lungs after environmental pulmonary exposure. Nickel is excreted through the urine.

Recommendations

There is no recommended intake for nickel because there have been no studies to support the nutritional importance or biochemical function of nickel.

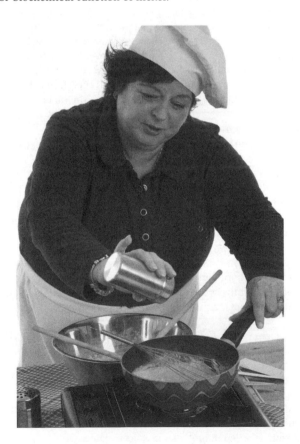

Typical Intakes of Older Adults

Data from the Total Diet Study indicate a median intake of 80 to 97 mcg of nickel per day for the older adult. More recent data for adults indicate higher levels of 131 ± 296 mcg nickel per day, although intake data specifically for older adults are not provided.

Food Sources

The major food sources of nickel are mixed dishes and soups, grain products, vegetables and legumes, and desserts. Meat may also be a significant source of dietary nickel.

Deficiency and Toxicity

Although nickel deficiency has been reported in animals, a nickel deficiency has not been found in humans. In addition, there is no evidence of toxicity of nickel from a normal diet. The UL is based on animal work with soluble nickel salts, which may be ingested in contaminated water. For adults older than 19, the UL is 1.0 mg/day of soluble nickel salts.

Special Considerations

Those who have nickel sensitivity from previous dermal exposure and those with renal disease may have lower tolerable intake levels than the UL for adults.

Iodine

Iodine is an essential part of the thyroid hormones. The two main thyroid hormones are thyroxine (T4) and triiodothyronine (T3). The T4 hormone has four iodine molecules in its structure, and the T3 has three. The thyroid hormones affect cell differentiation, metabolism, and growth.

Absorption and Metabolism

Most ingested iodine is almost completely absorbed. The iodine not used by the thyroid gland is excreted in the urine. Urine iodine is the marker for assessing iodine status, reflecting intake for the previous three to four days.

Recommendations

The RDA for men and women older than 50 is 150 mcg/day, the same as for younger adults. This recommendation was established based on the iodine accumulation in the thyroid gland.

Typical Intakes of Older Adults

The median intake of iodine for adults was reported to be 240 to 300 mcg/day for men and 190 to 210 mcg/day for women. For men and women 51 years and older, mean intake was 230 to 240 mcg iodine per day for each gender. Intake of iodine from supplements is 126 mcg/day for adult men and 137 mcg/day for adult women.

Food Sources

Iodine is found in dairy products, marine fish, and foods grown in iodine-rich soils. Seaweed is very high in iodine. Some salt is fortified with iodine, although fortification is not mandatory in the United States.

Deficiency and Toxicity

The earliest clinical symptom of iodine deficiency is thyroid enlargement, called goiter. The thyroid enlarging causes a bulge in the neck, but reflects a more serious lack of thyroid hormones secondary to a lack of iodine. The lack of thyroid hormones is called hypothyroidism. Iodine deficiency results in increased thyroid-stimulating hormone, and possibly triiodothyronine (T3), with a decrease in thyroxine. However, these increases or decreases may not be noticeable if the hormones remain within a normal range. Causes other than iodine deficiency may also be the reason for changes in thyroid function.

Acute cases of iodine poisoning result in burning of the mouth and throat, with gastrointestinal symptoms. Cardiac irregularities and coma may result, but acute poisoning is rare. Chronic excess iodine intake may increase stimulation of the thyroid gland, causing its enlargement (goiter), similar to effects seen with iodine insufficiency. This chronic overstimulation of the thyroid gland is associated with an increased risk of thyroid cancer.

Special Considerations

Iodine deficiency is relatively rare in the United States because of a sufficient amount of iodine in core foods. However, those with severe dietary restrictions may have reduced iodine status.

Fluoride

Fluoride is needed for bone and tooth structure and can help to prevent the development of cavities both before and after teeth emerge. Before teeth erupt, fluoride is important in increasing the resistance of the enamel structurally. After teeth have emerged, fluoride is important for reducing the acid produced by bacterial plaque.

Absorption and Metabolism

About one-half of ingested fluoride is absorbed. Absorption occurs throughout the intestine. For healthy adults, about one-half of the absorbed fluoride is retained, with the remainder being excreted by the kidneys.

Recommendations

The AI for adult men of all ages is 4 mg/day, and for women 3 mg/day. This recommendation is based upon reference weights for men and women.

Typical Intakes of Older Adults

Estimates of fluoride intake have not been reported because of the difficulty of determining the fluoride content of food and beverages that may or may not be processed with fluoridated water and their distribution to any number of locales.

Food Sources

The primary sources of fluoride are water and foods or beverages made with fluoridated water.

Deficiency and Toxicity

Fluoride toxicity is called fluorosis and occurs in tooth enamel and bone. Fluoride toxicity only affects teeth prior to eruption and results in mature teeth that have increased protein content and porosity. This can lead to stains and pitting of teeth. Once erupted, teeth are no longer susceptible to the toxic effects of fluoride. Skeletal fluorosis is related to the dose and duration of overconsumption. Most studies suggest that at least 10 mg/day for 10 years is required to produce even the mildest of skeletal fluorosis symptoms. Early symptoms include increased bone density and sometimes joint stiffness or pain. As more fluoride is deposited in bone, it, too, becomes more porous, and deformity, pain, and osteoporosis can develop. The UL for adults is 10 mg/day.

Table 5-3 summarizes the discussion of the trace minerals.

Conclusion

The major minerals include calcium, phosphorus, magnesium, sodium, chloride, and potassium. The usual diet of the older person is low in calcium, magnesium, and potassium; adequate in phosphorus and chloride; and excessive in sodium.

The trace minerals include iron, zinc, copper, chromium, selenium, aluminum, molybdenum, manganese, nickel, and iodine. The usual diet of the older person is adequate in iron, manganese, selenium, and iodine, and probably adequate in zinc and copper, although estimated intakes vary. More research is needed to assess the usual intake of chromium and fluoride. No recommended level of intake is established for aluminum, molybdenum, and nickel.

The mineral requirements for the older healthy person are the same as for younger adults for phosphorus, fluoride, potassium, sodium, chloride, copper, iodine, manganese, selenium, and zinc. Recommended intakes are slightly higher in older adults than young adults for magnesium. The guidelines for chromium and iron intake are lower for older adults than for younger adults.

Osteoporosis and hypertension are prevalent in the older adult. These chronic diseases increase recommended intakes of calcium and potassium for the older adult and decrease

TABLE 5-3 Summary Table for the Trace Minerals

Name	Main Functions	Food Sources	Toxicity	Deficiency	Special Considerations of Older Adults
Iron	Oxygen transport; energy metabolism	Meat and fortified products	Anemia	Rare	May require additional iron if receiving chemotherapy or dialysis; infection distorts body reserves.
Zinc	Immune function; growth; enzymes; smell, taste, and skin integrity	Meat, seafood, whole grains, and legumes; fortified breakfast products	Dermatitis; impaired immune function; distorted taste and smell; delayed wound healing	Rare	Supplemental zinc only helps immune function if zinc deficiency was present and is corrected.
Copper	Enzymes	Organ meats, seafood, nuts, seeds	Rare; anemia	Rare	—
Chromium	Carbohydrate metabolism	Cereals, some beers, and some wine	Rare	Rare	—
Selenium	Antioxidant and detoxification	Meat and seafood	Rare	Loss of nails and hair	—
Aluminum	Not known	Water or contaminant from aluminum cookware	None known	None known	May be associated with Alzheimer's disease.
Molybdenum	Enzyme cofactor	Leafy vegetables, grains, legumes, kidneys, liver, milk	None known	None known from dietary sources	—
Manganese	Enzyme cofactor, metabolism, normal immune function, reproduction	Unrefined grain products, tea, nuts, leafy vegetables	None known	None known from dietary sources	—
Nickel	None known	Mixed dishes and soups, grain products, vegetables and legumes, desserts	None known	None known from dietary sources	—
Iodine	Thyroid hormone	Dairy products, marine fish	Goiter	Goiter	—
Fluoride	Bone, teeth	Water	Porous teeth and bone	Fluorosis	—

recommended intakes for sodium. Diminished renal function and the use of diuretics for treatment of hypertension are common in the older adult and may alter recommendations for several mineral intakes.

Activities Related to This Chapter

1. Interview an older adult concerning his or her usual day's intake. Analyze the day's intake for adequacy in minerals.

2. Assess three vitamin–mineral supplements as to whether they provide minerals that are usually inadequate in an older adult's diet or ones that are usually adequate.

3. Make a poster depicting foods and their groups according to the MyPyramid graphic. Use words or periodic table symbols to indicate which foods are good sources of which minerals.

REFERENCES

American Dietetic Association. Position of the American Dietetic Association and Dietitians of Canada: women's health and nutrition. *J Am Diet Assoc.* 1999;99(6):738–751.

Anderson JJB, Sell ML, Garner SC, Calvo MS. Phosphorus. In: Bowman BA, Russell RM, eds. *Present Knowledge in Nutrition.* 8th ed. Washington, DC: International Life Sciences Institute; 2001:chap 27.

Andrews NC. Molecular control of iron metabolism. *Best Pract Res Clin Haematol.* 2005;18(2):159–169.

Aschner JL, Aschner M. Nutritional aspects of manganese homeostasis. *Mol Aspects Med.* 2005;26(4–5):353–362.

Atkinson SA, Ward WE. Clinical nutrition: the role of nutrition in the prevention and treatment of adult osteoporosis. *CMAJ.* 2001;165(11):1511–1514.

Barceloux DG. Chromium. *J Toxicol Clin Toxicol.* 1999;37(2):173–194.

Barceloux DG. Copper. *J Toxicol Clin Toxicol.* 1999;37(2):217–230.

Barceloux DG. Molybdenum. *J Toxicol Clin Toxicol.* 1999;37(2):231–237.

Barger-Lux MJ, Heaney RP. Caffeine and the calcium economy revisited. *Osteoporosis Int.* 1995;5(2):97–102.

Borak J. Adequacy of iodine nutrition in the United States. *Conn Med.* 2005;69(2):73–77.

Bronner F, Pansu D, Stein WD. An analysis of intestinal calcium transport across the rat intestine. *Am J Physiol.* 1986;250(5 pt 1):C561–C569.

Centers for Disease Control and Prevention. Iron deficiency—United States, 1999–2000. *MMWR.* 2002;51(40):897–899.

Chan GK, Duque G. Age-related bone loss: old bone, new facts. *Gerontology.* 2002;48(2):62–71.

Chernoff R. Micronutrient requirements in older women. *Am J Clin Nutr.* 2005;81(5):1240S–1245S.

Cook JD. Diagnosis and management of iron-deficiency anaemia. *Best Pract Res Clin Haematol.* 2005;18(2):319–332.

Dabeka RW, McKenzie AD. Survey of lead, cadmium, fluoride, nickel, and cobalt in food composites and estimation of dietary intakes of these elements by Canadians in 1986–1988. *J AOAC Int.* 1995;78(4):897–909.

Dawson-Hughes B. Interaction of dietary calcium and protein in bone health in humans. *J Nutr.* 2003;133(3):852S–854S.

Demigné C, Sabboh H, Remesy C, Meneton P. Protective effects of high dietary potassium: nutritional and metabolic aspects. *J Nutr.* 2004;134(11):2903–2906.

Dibley MJ. Zinc. In: Bowman BA, Russell RM, eds. *Present Knowledge in Nutrition.* 8th ed. Washington, DC: International Life Sciences Institute; 2001:chap 31.

Ervin RB, Kennedy-Stephenson J. Mineral intakes of elderly adult supplement and non-supplement users in the third National Health and Nutrition Examination Survey. *J Nutr.* 2002;132(11):3422–3427.

Eschbach JW. Iron requirements in erythropoietin therapy. *Best Pract Res Clin Haematol.* 2005;18(2):347–361.

Finley JW. Selenium accumulation in plant foods. *Nutr Rev.* 2005;63(6 pt 1):196–202.

Freeland-Graves JH, Friedman BJ, Han WH, et al. Effect of zinc supplementation on plasma high-density lipoprotein cholesterol and zinc. *Am J Clin Nutr.* 1982;35(5):988–992.

Goodman VL, Brewer GJ, Merajver SD. Copper deficiency as an anti-cancer strategy. *Endocr Relat Cancer.* 2004;11(2):255–263.

Gums JG. Magnesium in cardiovascular and other disorders. *Am J Health-Syst Pharm.* 2004;61:1569–1576.

Hambidge M. Biomarkers of trace mineral intake and status. *J Nutr.* 2003;133(suppl 3):948S–955S.

Hands ES. *Food Finder: Food Sources of Vitamins and Minerals.* 2nd ed. Salem, OR: ESHA Research; 2001.

He FJ, MacGregor GA. Potassium: more beneficial effects. *Climacteric.* 2003;6(suppl 3):36–48.

Heaney RP. Calcium absorption. *J Bone Miner Res.* 1989;4(5):795–796.

Heaney RP. Meta-analysis of calcium bioavailability. *Am J Ther.* 2001;8(1):73–74.

Hyun TH, Barrett-Connor E, Milne DB. Zinc intakes and plasma concentrations in men with osteoporosis: the Rancho Bernardo Study. *Am J Clin Nutr.* 2004;80(3):715–721.

Illich JZ, Kerstetter JE. Nutrition in bone health revisited: a story beyond calcium. *J Am Coll Nutr.* 2000;19(6):715–737.

Institute of Medicine. *Dietary Reference Intakes: Applications in Dietary Assessment.* Washington, DC: National Academies Press; 2000.

Institute of Medicine. *Dietary Reference Intakes for Calcium, Phosphorus, Magnesium, Vitamin D, and Fluoride.* Washington, DC: National Academies Press; 1997.

Institute of Medicine. *Dietary Reference Intakes for Vitamin A, Vitamin K, Arsenic, Boron, Chromium, Copper, Iodine, Iron, Manganese, Molybdenum, Nickel, Silicon, Vanadium, and Zinc.* Washington, DC: National Academies Press; 2001.

Institute of Medicine. *Dietary Reference Intakes for Vitamin C, Vitamin E, Selenium, and Carotenoids.* Washington, DC: National Academies Press; 2000.

Institute of Medicine. *Dietary Reference Intakes for Water, Potassium, Sodium, Chloride, and Sulfate.* Washington, DC: National Academies Press; 2004.

Kordas K, Stoltzfus RJ. New evidence of iron and zinc interplay at the enterocyte and neural tissues. *J Nutr.* 2004;134(6):1295–1298.

Kumar N, Crum B, Petersen RC, et al. Copper deficiency myelopathy. *Arch Neurol.* 2004;61(5):762–766.

Meneton P, Jeunemaitre X, de Wardener HE, MacGregor GA. Links between dietary salt intake, renal salt handling, blood pressure, and cardiovascular diseases. *Physiol Rev.* 2005;85(2):679–715.

National Research Council. *Recommended Dietary Allowances.* 10th ed. Washington, DC: National Academies Press; 1989.

Nielson FH. Boron, manganese, molybdenum, and other trace elements. In: Bowman BA, Russell RM, eds. *Present Knowledge in Nutrition.* 8th ed. Washington, DC: International Life Sciences Institute; 2001:chap 36.

Park YK, Yetley EA, Calvo MS. Calcium intake levels in the United States: issues and considerations. *FAO.* 1997;20:34–42.

Pennington JA, Jones JW. Molybdenum, nickel, cobalt, vanadium, and strontium in total diets. *J Am Diet Assoc.* 1987;87(12):1644–1650.

Pennington JA, Schoen SA, Salmon GD, et al. Composition of core foods of the US food supply, 1982–1991. III. Copper, manganese, selenium, and iodine. *J Food Comp Anal.* 1995;8:171–217.

Pennington JA, Young BE. Total Diet Study nutritional elements, 1982–1989. *J Am Diet Assoc.* 1991;91(2):179–183.

Schaefer TJ, Wolford RW. Disorders of potassium. *Emerg Med Clin North Am.* 2005;23(3):723–747.

Spencer H, Kramer L, Osis D, Norris C. Effect of phosphorus on the absorption of calcium and on the calcium balance in man. *J Nutr.* 1978;108(3):447–457.

Sunde RA. Selenium. In: Bowman BA, Russell RM, eds. *Present Knowledge in Nutrition.* 8th ed. Washington, DC: International Life Sciences Institute; 2001:chap 44.

Taylor GA, Moore PB, Ferrier IN, et al. Gastrointestinal absorption of aluminum and citrate in man. *J Inorg Biochem.* 1998;69(3):165–169.

Townsend MS, Fulgoni VL 3rd, Stern JS, et al. Low mineral intake is associated with high systolic blood pressure in the Third and Fourth National Health and Nutrition Examination Surveys: could we all be right? *Am J Hypertens.* 2005;18(2 pt 1):261–269.

Turnlund JR. Human whole-body copper metabolism. *Am J Clin Nutr.* 1998;67(5 suppl):960S–964S8.

U.S. Department of Agriculture, Agriculture Research Service. *Nutrient Intakes from Food: Mean Amounts Consumed per Individual, One Day, 2005–2006.* Available at: http://www.ars.usda.gov/SP2UserFiles/place/12355000/pdf/0506/Table_1_NIF_05.pdf. Accessed May 18, 2009.

U.S. Department of Agriculture, Center for Food Safety and Applied Nutrition. Total Diet Study statistics on element results. Revision 2. 2004. Available at: http://www.cfsan.fda.gov/~comm/tds-res.html. Accessed September 21, 2005.

U.S. Department of Health and Human Services and U.S. Department of Agriculture. *Dietary Guidelines for Americans 2005.* 2005. Available at: http://www.healthierus.gov/dietaryguidelines/. Accessed September 29, 2005.

Umbreit J. Iron deficiency: a concise review. *Am J Hematol.* 2005;78:225–231.

Vachharajani TJ, Zaman F, Abreo KD. Hyponatremia in critically ill patients. *J Intensive Care Med.* 2003;18(1):3–8.

Van den Heuvel EG, Muijs T, Van Dokkum W, Schaafsma G. Lactulose stimulates calcium absorption in postmenopausal women. *J Bone Miner Res.* 1999;14(7):1211–1216.

Vaquero MP. Magnesium and trace elements in the elderly: intake, status, and recommendations. *J Nutr Health Aging.* 2002;6(2):147–153.

Vincent JB. The biochemistry of chromium. *J Nutr.* 2000;130(4):715–718.

Vincent JB. Recent developments in the biochemistry of chromium(III). *Biol Trace Elem Res.* 2004;99(1–3):1–16.

von Muhlen DG, Greendale GA, Garland CF, et al. Vitamin D, parathyroid hormone levels and bone mineral density in community-dwelling older women: The Rancho Bernardo Study. *Osteoporosis Int.* June 1, 2005 [Epub ahead of print].

Weiss G. Modification of iron regulation by the inflammatory response. *Best Pract Res Clin Haematol.* 2005;18(2):183–201.

Zatta P, Lucchini R, van Rensburg SJ, Taylor A. The role of metals in neurodegenerative processes: aluminum, manganese, and zinc. *Brain Res Bull.* 2003;62(1):15–28.

Zeng H, Uthus EO, Combs GF Jr. Mechanistic aspects of the interaction between selenium and arsenic. *J Inorg Biochem.* 2005;99(6):1269–1274.

CHAPTER

6

Smell and Taste in Older Adults

Ann Schmidt Luggen, PhD, GNP and
Jacqueline Marcus, MS, RD, LD, FADA

CHAPTER OBJECTIVES   Upon completion of this chapter, readers will be able to:

1. Describe the anatomy and physiology of the oral cavity
2. State some of the problems of dentition that affect nutrition
3. Describe the physiologic changes of smell and taste that occur with age
4. List medical treatments and pharmacologic agents that are given to older people that can affect taste and smell
5. Describe techniques that the dietitian or other health professional can use to enhance eating

KEY TERMS AND CONCEPTS

Ageusia

Anosmia

Caries

Gingivitis

Limbic system

Mastication

Olfaction

Papillae

Periodontitis

Thresholds

Xerostomia

American baby boomers are predicted to live longer than their predecessors, and this increased longevity may increase the incidence of oral health disorders. With prolonged use and abuse of the oral cavity, few persons reach old age without a number of problems in this area. In addition, there are changes related to normal aging. For example, a newborn has approximately 10,000 taste buds; but by age 60, this number is significantly lower. Other changes to the oral cavity are thought to be caused by age-related changes in olfactory nerves and receptors, poor chewing and swallowing, declining sensitivities, medical conditions, medications, nicotine, caffeine, and alcohol. Elevated taste **thresholds** (or reduced sensitivity) for all the basic tastes seem to occur in healthy older individuals.

Oral Cavity

Increased longevity may have major ramifications on age-related diseases, including dental problems and taste and smell disorders. Chemosensory disorders may influence nutritional health.

Oral and pharyngeal cancers predominantly affect older adults and significantly affect function and quality of life for older adults suffering from them. The survival rate for these cancers is only 50% and has not changed for many years. Risk factors for oral and pharyngeal cancers include age, male sex, smoking tobacco, smokeless tobacco, drinking alcohol, sunlight

> **thresholds** Reduced sensitivity for taste that occurs in older adults.

89

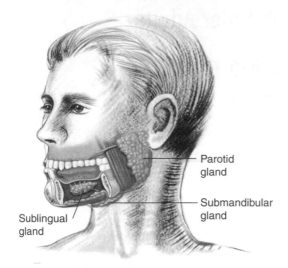

FIGURE 6-1 Anatomy of the Oral Cavity

Source: Insel P, Turner RE, Ross D. *Discovering Nutrition.* 2nd ed. Sudbury, MA: Jones & Bartlett; 2006, p. 117. Reproduced with permission.

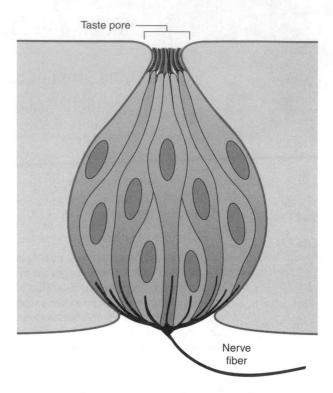

FIGURE 6-2 Taste Bud

Source: NIH SeniorHealth. Problems with taste. July 2005. Available at: http://nihseniorhealth.gov/problemswithtaste/toc.html. Accessed February 13, 2007.

exposure (lip cancers), a diet low in fruits and vegetables, and HPV (human papillomavirus).

Infections of the oral cavity in older patients, including those with dental procedures, can result in significant cardiac infections and infections in any artificial knee, hip, or shoulder joints. All health professionals should be aware that dental caries and periodontitis are infectious diseases and perform careful assessments for secondary prevention.

The anatomy of the oral cavity (**Figure 6-1**) includes the lips, teeth, cheeks, tongue, gingiva (gums), hard and soft palates, anterior and inferior pillars, uvula, tonsils, and posterior pharyngeal wall. The frenulum is beneath the tongue, the opening ducts of the submandibular and sublingual glands are at the base of the frenulum, and the opening for the parotid gland is inside the right cheek. All of these areas can cause problems in the older patient.

Tongue

The tongue has taste buds (**Figure 6-2**), or **papillae**, on its back, side, and tip (**Figure 6-3**). The number of taste buds begins to diminish after age 50. The physiologic role of the taste system is to trigger ingestive and digestive reflex systems that alter the secretion of oral, gastric, pancreatic, and intestinal juices. It also enhances the feelings of pleasure and satiety, and enables the determination of the quality of sampled foods. It distinguishes the nutrients that "taste good"

papillae Small bumps on the tongue. Some contain taste buds.

xerostomia Dry mouth due to inadequate saliva.

(often sweet) from potential toxins that "taste bad" (bitter). It is little appreciated in health care that taste dysfunction may alter food choices and patterns of consumption, which may result in weight loss or malnutrition, and may sometimes impair immunity and cause death.

The tongue is a common site of problems for the older adult with nutritional problems (**Box 6-1**). A tongue with deep longitudinal fissures is usually seen in the older adult with dehydration. An enlarged tongue should lead one to suspect hypothyroidism. A small, shrunken tongue may be indicative of malnutrition. A black tongue may indicate bismuth toxicity (e.g., caused by use of Pepto-Bismol® or similar over-the-counter medications). A smooth, red, shiny tongue with diminished papillae (geographic tongue) can indicate niacin or vitamin B12 deficiency or anemia.

Salivary Dysfunction (Dry Mouth)

The prevalence of **xerostomia** and hyposalivation is estimated to be 30% in adults older than age 65. It is thought that more than 70% of older adults in long-term care settings receive at least one drug that causes dry mouth.

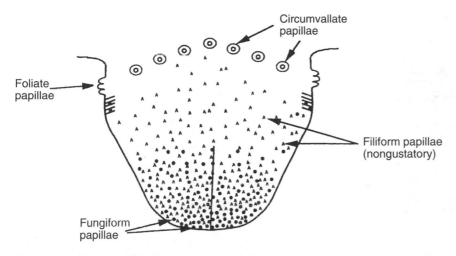

FIGURE 6-3 Tongue Papillae

Source: Chernoff R. *Geriatric Nutrition.* 3rd ed. Sudbury, MA: Jones & Bartlett; 2006, p. 119. Reproduced with permission.

Nearly 55% of older adults in the community setting take one drug that causes dry mouth. This dryness may cause the individual to stop taking the needed drug altogether. There are about 400 drugs that cause the salivary glands to produce less saliva. Many of these are for hypertension or depression. Some of the pharmacologic agents (anticholinergics) and cancer therapies taken by older adults cause dry mouth. (**Box 6-2**).

The three pairs of salivary glands are the submandibular, sublingual, and parotid glands. They secrete about 1 liter

---

◖ BOX 6-1 Problems of the Tongue

Black Hairy Tongue

Usually, this is a temporary, harmless condition caused by an overgrowth of bacteria or yeast on the papillae. The hairy appearance is due to a rapid growth of papillae or abnormal shedding of cells.

- **Causes:** Poor hygiene, bismuth-containing medications, mouthwashes with oxidizing agents (e.g., peroxide, witch hazel, and menthol), tobacco use, or excessive consumption of coffee or tea.

- **Management:** Brush tongue with toothbrush twice a day; rinse mouth with diluted peroxide (1:5 water) and then with water. Antibiotics.

Geographic Red Tongue

The papillae are missing in certain areas of the tongue, so that there are smooth red patches with a maplike appear-ance. These patches may change size day to day, and the condition may cycle between better and worse for months. It can be uncomfortable, especially when eating hot or spicy foods.

- **Causes:** Alcohol, tobacco, toothpastes, genetics, psoriasis, fissures, hormonal changes, stress, and allergies.

- **Management:** Avoid hot, spicy foods; acidic foods and drinks; alcohol; tobacco; and toothpastes with tartar control, strong flavoring, or whitening agents. Use a toothpaste for sensitive teeth. See dentist or health professional if the condition continues for longer than ten days.

Sources: Mayo Clinic. Geographic tongue. April 2006. Available at: http://www.mayoclinic.com/health/geographic-tongue/DS00819/DSECTION=all&METHOD=print. Accessed February 13, 2007; Mayo Clinic. Black hairy tongue. December 2006. Available at: http://www.mayoclinic.com/health/black-hairy-tongue/HQ00325. Accessed February 13, 2007.

of saliva each day. The function of saliva is to protect tissues in the oral cavity, maintain speech function, aid in chewing and swallowing, and assist in taste perception. Further, saliva contains antimicrobial factors and bicarbonate, which neutralize bacterial acids to a pH of about 7.4. This pH aids in prevention of tooth decay by controlling bacteria, viruses, and fungi in the mouth. It also helps heal sores in the mouth.

Although there is only a little diminution of saliva production with aging, many older adults suffer dry mouth. Saliva is not controlled by hormones, but rather by autonomic nervous system stimulation. Some chronic illnesses cause dry mouth. These include Parkinson's disease, diabetes, and Sjögren's syndrome (which also causes dry eyes). Diabetes, depression, and stress are also thought to cause dry mouth. Dehydration is a common cause of dry mouth and is often found by examination of the mouth.

In most cases, dry mouth cannot be cured, but an effort should be made to treat it through communication with a specialist, especially if the cause is unknown. Some methods of therapy include drinking or sipping more water or sugarless drinks (especially during meals), avoiding medications that cause dry mouth, and limiting drinks that cause dry mouth, such as coffee, tea, and some sodas with caffeine. Other treatments include sucking on sugarless candy or chewing sugarless gum. Tobacco and alcohol should be avoided (alcohol is very drying), as should salty or spicy foods, which may cause pain. At night, use of a humidifier may be helpful to avoid waking up unable to swallow or with a dry or sticky tongue.

At present, there is considerable ongoing research into managing this disorder. Gene therapy is being explored. The idea is to replace, manipulate, or supplement nonfunctional genes with healthy ones. At the National Institute of Dental and Craniofacial Research and Harvard University, efforts are under way to develop an artificial salivary gland for those who have lost all salivary gland function. The artificial gland would produce saliva-like fluid and be inserted inside the cheek.

Dental and Gingival Problems

Dental health is often a neglected area in older adults, especially among those who are debilitated or who have limited mobility. Many older adults are edentulous due to lack of fluoride and good dental care in their early years. In the 1960s, more than 70% of adults older than age 75 were edentulous. Currently, about 40% are edentulous; 25% have loss of tooth-supporting structures due to advanced periodontal disease.

Third-party reimbursement is inadequate for dental care for older persons. Most need to pay out of pocket for this expense, which is one reason for neglect. This population is less likely to go to the dentist compared with any other age group.

Periodontal disease occurs when colonies of bacteria, called *plaque*, form on the teeth at the gum line (**Figure 6-4**). Inflammation of the gum is called **gingivitis**. It can develop rapidly in older adults, even when they are very healthy. If the inflammation and infection continues upward to the tooth ligament and bone, it is termed **periodontitis**, which occurs in 20% to 40% of adults with teeth. The older adult may complain of bad breath, which is a symptom of periodontitis (**Box 6-3**). By the time adults are in their 50s, 90% have periodontal disease activity. As periodontal disease advances, the tooth becomes malpositioned, loosens, and is lost.

gingivitis Oral condition that causes red, bleeding gums. It is less serious than periodontal disorders, but it will lead to serious disease if neglected.

periodontitis A group of disorders affecting the gums and teeth in the mouth. The gums become reddened and painful and often bleed and recede from the teeth, exposing the root of the tooth. Part of the problem is the accumulation of plaque on the lower part of the tooth at the gum line, which changes into tartar when there is poor oral hygiene for a prolonged period of time.

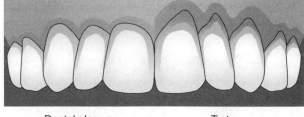

Dental plaque   Tartar

FIGURE 6-4 Gum Disease

Source: NIH SeniorHealth. Problems with taste. July 2005. Available at: http://nihseniorhealth.gov/problemswithtaste/toc.html. Accessed February 13, 2007.

▶ BOX 6-3 Bad Breath (Halitosis)

There are many causes of bad breath, which can be an important sign of periodontitis.

Causes

- Poor dental hygiene (poor brushing and flossing), which causes food particles to remain in the mouth that collect bacteria and emit hydrogen sulfur vapor. The sticky plaque remains on the teeth.

- Food breakdown, especially if the food contains volatile oils, such as onions and garlic. After digestion, the oils are carried to the lungs and given off in the breath. Alcohol does the same; although alcohol has no odor, the breath smell comes from other components of the drink.

- Dry mouth, with the accumulation and decomposition of dead cells in the gums, tongue, and cheeks. It often occurs during sleep and is termed "morning breath."

- Chronic lung infections produce foul smelling breath. Kidney failure causes urinelike odor. Liver failure causes a fishy odor.

- Acid reflux from the stomach can cause bad breath.

- Sinus infections can discharge to the posterior pharynx and cause bad odor.

- Tobacco use dries the mouth and promotes periodontal disease.

- Severe dieting produces unpleasant fruity odors (ketoacidosis) from fasting.

- Canker sores can be related to bad breath, especially when accompanying periodontal disease.

Management

Good dental hygiene is the key to improving or preventing bad breath. Keep a toothbrush with you to use after eating anything, and floss a minimum of once a day. Brush the tongue to remove dead cells, bacteria, and food debris, especially in the middle third of the tongue, where most bacteria are found. Clean dentures very well. Change your toothbrush every two to three months, and have regular dental checkups—a minimum of twice a year. Drink more water (not soft drinks, coffee, or alcohol) to stimulate saliva production.

Source: Mayo Clinic. Bad breath. June 2006. Available at: http://www.mayoclinic.com/print/bad-breath/DS00025/DSECTION=all&METHOD=print. Accessed February 13, 2007.

Management of periodontal disease is a job for the professional. Debriding the roots below the gingiva may include planning or scaling or surgery. Topical and systemic antibiotics may be used. At the personal level, good daily care with tooth brushing and flossing to remove the plaque is essential. Brushing or cleaning after each meal with fluoride toothpaste is preferred.

Dental **caries**, or tooth decay, is a major reason for tooth loss. Decay is demineralization and cavitation of the tooth enamel (outer surface), the dentin (inner layer), and the pulp (center). There may be caries on the root surface. When there is necrosis of the pulp, an abscess (infection) may occur. This can cause infections in virtually any area of the body if not treated. Any infection in this area can also increase the risk of myocardial infarction (heart attack) or stroke. Infection also makes it more difficult to control blood glucose levels in those with diabetes.

Loss of teeth usually means that the older adult will get dentures, or false teeth. Although these aid in speech and give the face the more usual contours, the user's ability to chew well is not predictable. Diminished oral intake often occurs. Older adults may change the type and consistency of foods they choose to eat, which can become unappetizing, monotonous, limited, and inadequate in nutritive value. If continuing weight loss occurs, the dentures will no longer fit, and obtaining new ones is difficult and expensive, especially for the older, more debilitated patient.

Chemosensory Perception

Both taste perception and **olfaction** decline with age, although taste is much less affected than smell. Further, both taste and smell cells are the only sensory cells that are regularly replaced throughout one's lifespan. When there is a taste problem, it is usually due to loss of smell. Many pharmaceutical agents interfere with both taste and smell. Certain pathophysiologic problems and diseases can alter taste and smell, for example, Alzheimer's

caries Tooth disease that causes cavities and tooth decay.

olfaction Sense of smell.

disease. The older adult may eat spoiled food without recognizing the bad smell or taste.

Taste

The true tastants are salt, sugar, sour, bitter, and umami (or savory like a meat smell; pronounced "ooh mommy"). Each stimulates specific receptors on the tongue, soft palate, pharynx, larynx, and epiglottis. The types of taste buds on the tongue are varied in number and in their ability to taste more or less well. Approximately 25% of Americans are nontasters, 50% are medium tasters, and 25% are supertasters.

As mentioned earlier, the number of taste buds begins to diminish at about age 50. Loss of taste is termed **ageusia**; diminished taste is *hypogeusia*.

Taste is a function of multiple nerves in the tongue, soft palate, uvula, pharynx, and upper esophagus. Cranial nerves VII (facial nerve), IX (glossopharyngeal nerve), and X (vagus nerve) are three of these nerves. They mediate sweet, sour, bitter, salty, and metallic sensations. Because of the number of nerves involved, it is rare for a person to have no sense of taste. Taste declines more gradually with age than does smell. The greatest amount of taste is lost in the fungiform papillae on the frontal third of the tongue, where the loss is about 50% by age 50. Because of this loss, there is a need for greater concentration of flavor.

Smoking, drinking hot drinks, nasal and sinus infections, antibiotics, exposure to chemicals and metals, periodontal problems, and inflammatory problems in the oral cavity can all damage taste buds. Damage to the hippocampus of the brain can also cause impaired taste, as can any head injury. Other conditions that can affect taste (and usually smell) include Parkinson's disease; Alzheimer's disease; stroke; chronic renal disease; hypothyroidism; chronic liver disease; localized ear, nose, and throat illness; and viral infections. Nutritional deficiencies implicated in the loss of taste include reduced levels of zinc, vitamin B3, vitamin B12, and nutrition problems related to cancer. Damage to the glossopharyngeal nerve (IX) causes the loss of the ability to detect bitterness. Damage to the facial nerve (VII) causes loss of sensation for sour, sweet, and salt tastes, leaving only bitter tastes. Older adults undergoing chemotherapy for cancer may have parageusia, or perverse taste, which is an unpleasant taste. In such cases, anorexia and malnutrition often occur because eating becomes a very negative experience. The loss of the older adult's third molar is one of the causes of ageusia (complete loss of taste).

Some older adults describe a metallic taste. This is fairly common. Some antibiotics, antidepressants, and antihypertensive drugs cause this phenomenon. In addition, oral infections, such as periodontitis or abscesses, can also cause a metallic taste. The occurrence is not serious. Good oral hygiene and brushing the tongue may help.

Older adults may experience a persistent salty taste. Dehydration is a common cause of this taste. It can also be caused by certain medications, such as antithyroid agents, and some chemotherapy drugs. Infections of the salivary glands or a disease such as Sjögren's syndrome that results in diminished salivation are also causative. The taste can also be caused by sinusitis with postnasal drainage or allergies. The salty taste can often be alleviated through management of the original underlying problem.

The loss of salivary gland function also affects taste in general. The enzyme amylase, found in saliva, aids in the perception of sweet tastes, and its production decreases with progressive aging. However, other authors state that the acuity of salt and bitter tastes diminishes with age, and that the perception of sweet and sour tastes does not.

Taste bud cells are constantly being renewed; turnover averages ten and a half days. Measurements of taste dysfunction in aging indicate a progressive decline in turnover with age. Decline in taste and smell acuity begins around age 60 and is more pronounced by age 70, but it may be noticeable earlier. Renewal of taste buds slows mainly after menopause as a result of estrogen deficiency. Protein and zinc shortages also can retard taste bud renewal.

Some taste researchers believe that chemosensory sensitivity to all the basic tastes decreases as people age. Others think this applies only to some tastes. Research is evolving. It may be that foods have to be more assertive to achieve the same sensations in older adults as in younger tasters. People might reach for the salt shaker or sugar bowl to compensate. Liberalized use of salt or sugar may be fine for a few; others may not be able to tolerate additional sodium or extra calories.

Smell

Many older adults fail to notice a loss of olfactory sensation or function. Most older adults underreport their loss of olfactory sensation when asked. Fifty percent of individuals aged 65 to 80 experience smell loss; approximately 75% of those aged 80 to 97 have olfactory impairment. Women appear to retain better function in smell and taste than do men. Only 1% to 2% of all Americans younger than age 65 experience loss of smell to any degree. Risk factors associated with increased impairment are smoking, stroke, epilepsy, pollutants, airborne toxins, nasal congestion, or upper respiratory infections from viruses and bacteria.

Like taste receptors, olfactory receptors are continually renewed, but they have a longer turnover time—between 30 and 120 days compared to every 10 days for taste cells. Although olfactory neurons can regenerate, they must do so by reinnervating the olfactory bulb, which is located within

ageusia Loss of taste.

the **limbic system**, or emotional brain center. The olfactory bulb shows considerable degenerative changes with aging. It has a moth eaten appearance due to losses of neurons, which becomes excessively pronounced in people with Alzheimer's disease.

Cranial nerve I, the olfactory nerve, carries odor. Odors reach the olfactory system in two ways: from the environment through the nostrils and from the mouth through the nasopharynx (the retronasal route). Both routes transport odors to the olfactory neuron receptors in the upper nasal cavity. These neurons transmit the identity, concentration, and duration of odors directly to the central nervous system by way of the olfactory bulb, bypassing the blood–brain barrier. To test the ability to smell, practitioners usually use coffee, cloves, peppermint, or other odors that are distinctive. Irritant smells (e.g., ammonia, vinegar) excite cranial nerve V, the trigeminal nerve.

This direct access to the brain from the environment allows olfaction to be very vulnerable. Some more virulent agents using this route include the polio virus, rabies virus, herpes simplex virus, and HIV (human immunodeficiency virus). Permanent smell loss can occur from upper respiratory infections including the common cold. Other causes include head trauma, rapid head movement forward or backward, and rhinosinusitus. Toxic agents may cause smell loss resulting in many lawsuits for exposure. Some of these agents include acrylates, methacrylates, and cadmium, although cadium smell loss is reversible after the removal of the toxin or change of work environment. Many neurological diseases, such as Parkinson's disease, Alzheimer's disease, and multiple sclerosis are also causes of permanent smell loss. However, they are far less common than respiratory infections.

Loss of smell is categorized by degree. Hyposmia is impairment of smell. Parosmia is faulty recognition of smell (e.g., identifying a beef smell as bacon). Cacosmia is the abnormal perception of unpleasant odors without an actual odor being present. **Anosmia** is total loss of smell.

Flavor

What is commonly called taste is really flavor. Flavor is composed of several perceptions: taste, smell, appearance, temperature, texture, sound, and the feel in the mouth. Foods are often rejected if they are rubbery, grainy, or slippery. If either taste or smell is impaired, flavor is altered.

The perception of flavor is often impaired in older adults because of changes in taste, olfaction, salivary dysfunction (hypofunction), dentures, and oral stereognosis (the ability to perceive an object in the mouth by feeling it). Dentures present physical and thermal barriers.

Boldly flavored ingredients, concentrated sauces, and flavor extracts may enhance flavor enjoyment. Likewise, sensory techniques, such as activation of smell memory, varying temperature and textures, and smelling food before tasting, may also enhance flavor enjoyment.

Causes of Chemosensory Losses in Older Adults

The olfactory anatomy makes olfaction more vulnerable to loss than taste. This is because olfaction depends on one nerve, whereas three nerves transmit taste. In addition, olfactory receptors are lodged in a small sinus region, whereas taste receptors are located in several places on the tongue, palate, and throat. Moreover, olfactory receptors are directly exposed to environmental toxins and agents through breathing, whereas neurons within taste receptors are protected within the mouth.

The ability to perceive the full olfactory flavor of a food also depends on adequate **mastication**, or chewing, to release olfactory volatiles and mouth and swallowing movements to pump volatiles retronasally to the olfactory epithelium. It has been hypothesized by some that older adults are not able to release food volatiles effectively and do not generate enough airflow to transport these volatiles. Conditions that impair mastication, and mouth or swallowing movements, including tooth loss, gum disease, and poor dentures can diminish retronasal perception, even if the olfactory system is intact.

Age-related impairment of taste and smell can be caused by factors other than aging, as has been mentioned earlier. These factors include a number of medical conditions such as allergic rhinitis, dementias, bronchial asthma, cancer, chronic renal failure, diabetes mellitus, epilepsy, hypothyroidism, liver disease and cirrhosis, niacin (vitamin B3) deficiency, numerous medications, tumors, and viral hepatitis.

Medical treatments such as radiation or chemotherapy may also impair taste and smell and cause food to lose appeal. Because flavor plays a role in stimulating proper digestion, older people who undergo these treatments may lose weight and their physical condition may deteriorate.

Adults 65 and older are prescribed the highest number of drugs of any age group. The older population (ages 65 and older), which is 12.6% of the U.S. population, buys 33% of all prescription drugs. This is critical knowledge in dietary management because numerous drugs have been implicated in altered taste sensations (**Table 6-1**). Medications may affect both taste and smell by altering the production or composition of saliva, causing oral discomfort, interfering with food flavors, or imparting a bitter taste. Lipid-lowering drugs, antihistamines, antimicrobials, anti-inflammatories, zinc

limbic system Area of the brain that controls emotion, behavior, and long-term memory. It is also associated with the olfactory system.

anosmia Loss of smell.

mastication Chewing.

TABLE 6-1 Common Pharmaceutical Agents Affecting Chemosensory Perception

Taste Perception	Olfactory Perception
Allopurinol	Amitriptyline
Acyclovir	Amphetamine
Ampicillin	Beclomethasone dipropionate
Baclofen	Codeine
Buspirone	Dexamethasone
Captopril	Enalapril
Diclofenac	Hydromorphone
Gemfibrozil	Morphine
Hydrochlorothiazide	Pentamidine
Labetalol	Tocainide
Nifedipine	
Phenytoin	
Procainamide	
Propranolol	
Sulfamethoxazole	
Sulindac	
Tetracyclines	

Source: Data from American Geriatric Society. *Geriatric Review Syllabus.* New York: American Geriatric Society; 2006.

deficiency medications, bronchodilators, antihypertensives and cardiac medications, muscle relaxants, antidepressants, anticonvulsants, and vasodilators have all been implicated. If an older adult is prescribed a new drug and his or her sense of taste or smell changes, it is easier to change the drug than if the sensory loss had been an ongoing problem.

Ingredients That Enhance Flavor and Sensory Enjoyment

The use of extracts to amplify flavor has been shown to stimulate aging taste buds and olfactory nerve endings. The extracts used should complement the base food served. Maple extract can be used to heighten the flavor of glazed vegetable or pork dishes, whereas almond or vanilla extracts can be used to enhance fruit sauces, mixed fruit cups, puddings, and baked goods. Start with ½ to 1 teaspoon of extract per recipe.

Umami is a Japanese term that describes food as savory; that is, having a delicious and meaty taste. The cause of this flavor is glutamate, an amino acid. Glutamate is found in chicken and meat broth and stock, in other meats, and in some cheeses. Glutamate is often added to foods as monosodium glutamate; however, many people are said to be allergic to this product.

Older adults who are limited to clear liquid diets, both in home and institutional settings, may benefit from the addition of fruit flavors to gelatins, juices, and popsicles. Vegetable and meat or poultry concentrates can be added to

broths. Full liquid diets may be enhanced by maple, fruit, chocolate, or vanilla flavors added to nutritional supplements or milkshakes. Meat, mushroom, or vegetable bases may be added to soups.

In one institutional study by Shahar, Kan, and Wan, nearly all older patients consumed insufficient quantities of food to meet their requirements for energy and nutrients, except for vitamin C. The patients preferred vegetables, fruits, and beans to red meat, milk, and dairy products. Food services in hospitals should consider food preferences among older patients in order to improve their nutrient intake.

Strongly Flavored Foods and Ingredients

Strongly flavored foods and ingredients, such as garlic, onions, olives, sun-dried tomatoes, flavored vinegars, citrus fruit, or ripe berries, impart a lot of flavor. However, they may not be tolerated by aging, sluggish, or sensitive digestive tracts.

Concentrated Fruit Sauces and Jams

Concentrated fruit sauces can be paired with nectars or jams. Pureed apricot, peach, or pineapple may be paired with protein foods for patients on chemotherapy, with good results.

Sour

One report of women with olfactory dysfunction found a lower preference for bitter or sour tastes such as citrus fruit. The sour taste in these foods becomes more highly apparent to the taster, and thus less appealing.

Herbs and Spices

The use of herbs and spices may be helpful for people with chemosensory disorders. However, this may not be effective with every seasoning. It is best to individualize. A planned diet is only successful when it is eaten.

Dry Rubs

Dry rubs are herb and spice combinations that may be rubbed directly onto raw meat, poultry, or fish. The dry rubs perform much the same functions that marinades do for grilled or roasted entrees without added liquid or oil.

Sugar

Putting sugar on vegetables may encourage increased consumption. Anecdotally, sugar cravings seem to occur in older adults. Many older adults add increased amounts of sugar and salt to meals.

Fat

Older adults prefer high-fat foods because they lend a creamy texture to foods that is pleasing to the taste. Older women consume a higher proportion of dietary fats than younger women.

Sharp-tasting greens such as mustard, turnip, and beet and vegetables such as broccoli, brussels sprouts, and cauliflower may be enhanced by a little fat, such as a creamy dressing, cheese sauce, cream, sweet butter, flavored oils, or bacon tidbits. Fat also promotes the absorption of fat-soluble phytochemicals and plant-based, disease-fighting agents such as lutein (in spinach), beta-carotene (in carrots), and lycopene (in tomatoes).

Monosodium Glutamate

Monosodium glutamate (MSG) may also reduce perceived bitterness or acidity. Flavor enhancers such as MSG do not depend on a person's ability to smell. In addition to helping people enjoy food, MSG can help people comply with sodium-restricted diets. When used in combination with a small amount of table salt, MSG is highly effective in reducing the total amount of sodium in the diet.

Wine

Wine has been known to enhance appetite. It may also affect food preferences because of its interaction with umami in foods. Low-tannin wines, such as burgundies, may be best matched.

Techniques That Enhance Flavor and Sensory Enjoyment

Compensating for taste or smell is within our control. Food professionals need to create meals that appeal to all the senses, not merely taste and smell. Foods must also vary in their visual appeal, the sounds they produce because of texture, and temperature.

Choose High-Quality Foods

To ensure that foods taste good, start with high-quality foods. Choose foods that are fresh, brightly colored, full-flavored, and seasonal.

Focus on Appearance

Food should be ethnically and culturally appropriate and attractively arranged and garnished. Foods with great eye appeal elicit more salivary, gastric, pancreatic, and intestinal secretions. Familiarity is appealing and pleasing.

Experiment with different shapes, colors, and textures to offset boredom. Place food in set layouts on plates that have simple patterns or solid colors so the older adult can see the food well and remember where to find it, "eating with the eyes."

Arouse Hunger

To stimulate hunger, lift the lid from a food tray or entrée to release concentrated aromas just before setting it in front of a diner. You can achieve this in a home setting by eating in the kitchen, from which smells emanate, or by taking a deep sniff before eating.

Activate Smell Memory

Take advantage of the human ability to remember smells. Although olfaction decreases with age, humans have a remarkable smell memory. Aromatic foods with a pleasant memory can soothe ("Remember, Mother used to make this pudding").

Contrast Texture, Size, and Shape

Combining foods with different sizes, shapes, and textures throughout a meal may add interest and reduce sensory fatigue. Start with hot, chunky soup; switch to a tender steak, creamy pasta, and crunchy steamed asparagus; and then finish with irregular berries. Switching foods (eating one bite of meat, vegetables, starch, and so forth) may also lessen fatigue. Clearly, problems with dysphagia will interfere with this strategy.

Vary Temperature

Some degree of temperature variation may be desirable to stimulate thermoreceptors; however, extreme temperatures of hot or cold tend to lessen flavor.

Liberalize Diets

Long-term care residents with olfactory impairments may benefit from a liberalization of some diet restrictions to stimulate appetite. Exceptions to this suggestion include renal patients or those with ascites, edema, or heart failure.

Encourage Good Mastication

Chewing food well breaks down food cells and releases flavor molecules to interact with taste and smell receptors. It sets up air currents that force odorants retronasally to reach more olfactory receptors and increase perceived odors. Good mastication requires healthy dentition or proper-fitting dentures. Loose dentures can interfere with chewing and retronasal processing. Those who wear complete or palatal-covering dentures have lower olfactory sensitivity.

Applications of Flavor Enhancement

Home and Institutional Menus

Flavor enhancement strategies can be used in home settings on a one-to-one basis or incorporated into food service menus. The menu in **Table 6-2** is one used in a long-term care facility and illustrates the addition of flavor enhancements.

Restaurant Menus

By examining trend data, one can see that Americans are experimenting with bolder, more aggressive flavors and

TABLE 6-2 Typical Food Service Menu with Suggested Flavor Enhancement

Sun.	Mon.	Tues.	Wed.	Thurs.	Fri.	Sat.
Cr. of Wheat	Oatmeal (1)	Malt O' Meal	Oatmeal (1)	Oatmeal (1)	Cr. of Rice	Oatmeal (1)
Sweet roll	Fruit or juice	Prunes	Bacon (6)	Fruit or juice	Prunes	Fruit or juice
Bacon (6)		Raisin toast			Raisin toast	
Soup of day	Soup of day	Soup of day	Soup of day	Soup of day	Soup of day	Soup of day
Pot roast (4, 6)	Chicken	Beef steak (4)	Sausage (1)	Pork chops	Pollock (1)	Swedish
Mashed	breasts (7)	Mashed	Conugue	(1, 7, 10)	Mashed	meatballs (4)
potatoes (12)	Potato (2, 6)	potatoes (12)	potatoes (12)	Baked potato	potatoes (1,12)	Mashed
Carrots (1, 3)	Zucchini (3, 4, 8)	Cauliflower (2, 4)	Broccoli (2,5)	(6, 12)	Spinach (2, 8)	potatoes (12)
Layer cake	Jell-O	Ice cream	Brownies	Red cabbage (3)	Pie	Yellow squash
Fruit mix (5)	Peaches	Applesauce	Fruit cocktail (5)	Frozen yogurt	Assorted. fruit	(3, 4)
				Peaches	(14)	Triple berry bar
						Fruit mix (5)
Cream of cauli-	Pasta fagioli (15)	Tomato soup (15)	Fr. onion soup	Minestrone soup	Chicken/Wild	Beef barley soup
flower soup (15)	Italian beef	Chicken lasagna	(15)	(15)	rice soup (15)	(15)
Hot dog on bun	sandwich	(15)	Chicken patty on	Beef tomato	Cottage cheese/	Spaghetti/Meat
Tomato salad	Tossed salad	French bread	bun	macaroni (4, 15)	Fruit	sauce (4)
(9, 10, 15)	(9, 10, 13)	Relish plate (13)	Tossed salad	Three-bean salad	Tossed salad	French bread
Lemon pudding	Banana	Pineapple	(9, 10, 13)	(3, 9, 10)	(9, 10, 13)	Cucumber salad
Mandarin	Fruit cup (14)	Fruit mix (5)	Fruited Jell-O	Banana	Cookie	(3, 9, 10)
oranges (5)			Sliced peaches	Mandarin	Fruit cocktail (5)	Dark red cherry
				oranges (5)		Applesauce

Key: (1) maple syrup flavor, (2) cheese sauce/flavoring, (3) sugar on vegetables, (4) ½ tsp MSG per pound of meat or four to six servings of vegetables, (5) vanilla/almond extracts, (6) bacon/bacon-flavored granules, (7) concentrated fruit sauces, (8) butter on green vegetables, (9) flavored vinegars, (10) flavorful oils (peanut, sesame), (11) dry rubs, (12) sweet butter on other vegetables, (13) creamy dressing on vegetables, (14) ripe berries, (15) contains natural glutamate.

seeking new taste experiences. Southwestern and Indian foods are found more frequently in grocery stores, and new restaurants are common all around the United States.

Hispanic-Inspired and High-Flavor Cuisine

Hispanic-inspired cuisine is on the rise in the United States, paralleling the growing Hispanic American population. Hispanic-inspired cuisine relies heavily on aromatic cinnamon, cumin, and fennel. Fruit salsas with mango and lime as a marinade contribute intense flavor and texture. Root vegetables such as yucca, baby bok choy, purple potato, jicama, and fennel have expanded the range of American palates.

Americans now expect flavor with every mouthful. Many older women eat not for pleasure, but to continue eating to find flavor. Rubs, brines, stocks, reductions, marinades, and foams help concentrate flavor by removing water or by infusing intensified flavors. Smoking, slow roasting, and toasting with aromatic woods or spices and seeds deepen flavor dimensions.

Appetizers as Entrees

Americans are seeking multiple taste experiences within the same menu. A variety of appetizers, tapas, handheld food, skewers, and sampler plates are being chosen instead of traditional meals.

Conclusion

As sensory scientists unmask the chemical mysteries that activate the taste buds and olfactory receptors, it behooves dieticians, nutritionists, and other health care professionals who influence older adults to pay heed. No food is nutritious unless it is consumed, and little food is consumed unless it tastes good. Improved consumption may affect health and longevity. With a significant portion of the U.S. population aging, sensory enhancement for the older adult makes good sense.

Activities Related to This Chapter

1. Test yourself on the meanings of the key terms located at the beginning of the chapter. Use each in a sentence.
2. Describe or make up a plate of food that would be appetizing to an older adult.
3. Search the Internet literature for a list of medications that change the flavor of foods.

4. Visit the National Institutes of Health (NIH) website and find research on malnutrition and chemosensory loss so that you can lead a discussion on this topic.

Case Study

Maria, 80, and her husband Rico, 88, live at home in an apartment, thanks to the fact that their doting children live nearby and help on a regular basis. In recent years, Rico has eaten less and less at mealtimes; he has lost 20 pounds over the past three years, although he has never been overweight. Maria is overweight, but recently has not been as interested in food as she usually has been. When the children come by, they often find uneaten food in the refrigerator. At a medical visit, you are called in to help.

Questions

1. What questions do you need to ask in the patient history?
2. What information do you need to have from the physician or nurse practitioner?
3. Will the patients' culture make a difference in your plan of care?
4. What kind of testing will you do with Maria and Rico?

REFERENCES

American Cancer Society. Oral cancers. 2008. Available at: http://www.cancer.org. Accessed March 30, 2009.

American Geriatric Society. *Geriatric Review Syllabus*. New York: American Geriatric Society; 2006.

Centers for Disease Control and Prevention. *CDC Fact Book 2000/2001*. Washington, DC: Department of Health and Human Services; 2000.

Chernoff R. *Geriatric Nutrition*. 3rd ed. Sudbury, MA: Jones & Bartlett; 2006.

Ham RJ, Sloane PD, Warshaw GA, Bernard MA, Flaherty E. *Primary care geriatrics*. 5th ed. St. Louis: Mosby; 2007.

Harvard Medical School. What's happened to my sense of taste? *Harvard Women's Health*, 2003;10(10):8.

Insel P, Turner RE, Ross D. *Discovering Nutrition*. 2nd ed. Sudbury, MA: Jones & Bartlett; 2006.

Luggen AS. Biologic maintenance needs. In: Ebersole P, Hess PMK, Luggen A. *Toward Healthy Aging*. 7th ed. Philadelphia: Elsevier Mosby; 2008.

Mackay-Sim A, Johnston A, Owen C, Burne T. Olfactory ability in the healthy population: reassessing presbyosmia. *Chemical Senses*. 2006;31(8):763–771.

Mayo Clinic. Loss of taste and smell: a normal part of aging? October 2007. Available at: http://www.mayoclinic.com/print/loss-of-taste-and-smell/AN01198/METHOD = print. Accessed March 30, 2009.

Mayo Clinic. Metallic taste in mouth: a cause for concern? July 2006. Available at http://www.mayoclinic.com/print/metallic-taste/AN01386. Accessed February 13, 2007.

Mayo Clinic. Salty taste in mouth: what causes it? August 2006. Available at: http://www.mayoclinic.com/health/salty-taste-in-mouth/AN01411. Accessed February 13, 2007.

McCance K, Huether S. *Pathophysiology*. 5th ed. Philadelphia: Elsevier Mosby; 2006.

Mumenthaler M, Mattle H, Taub E. *Neurology*. 4th ed. New York: Thieme; 2004.

Murphy C, Schubert C, Cruickshanks K, et al. Prevalence of olfactory impairment in older adults. *JAMA*. 2002;288(18):2307–2313.

National Institute of Dental and Craniofacial Research. Dry mouth. 2009. Available at: http://www.nidcr.nih.gov/OralHealth/Topics/DryMouth/DryMouth.htm. Accessed March 30, 2009.

National Institute of Dental and Craniofacial Research. 2009. Periodontal (gum) disease: causes, symptoms, and treatments. February 2009. Available at: http://www.nidcr.nih.gov/Oralhealth/topics/gumdiseases/periodontalgum-disease.htm. Accessed March 30, 2009.

National Institute on Aging. Dry mouth. 2005. Available at: http://www.nia.nih.gov/NewsAndEvents/PressReleases/PR20051007.htm. Accessed February 13, 2007.

National Institute on Deafness and Other Communication Disorders. Statistics on smell and taste. May 2008. Available at: http://www.nidcd.nih.gov/health/statistics/smell.asp. Accessed January 28, 2009.

National Institute on Deafness and Other Communication Disorders. Taste and smell statistics. 2008. Available at: http://www.nidcd.nih.gov/NidcdInternet/Templates/InternetTopicNavigation.aspx?NRMO. Accessed May 19, 2008.

NIH SeniorHealth. Problems with taste. July 2005. Available at: http://nihseniorhealth.gov/problemswithtaste/toc.html. Accessed February 13, 2007.

NIH Senior Health. Problems with taste: symptoms and diagnosis. 2008. Available at: http://nihseniorhealth.gov/problemswithtaste/symptomsanddiagnosis/03.html. Accessed March 30, 2009.

Shahar S, Kan YC, Wan CP. Food intakes and preferences of hospitalised geriatric patients. *BMC Geriatr*. 2002;2(2):3.

U.S. Department of Health and Human Services, Office of Disease Prevention and Health Promotion. Healthy People 2010. October 2006. Available at: http://www.nidcr.nih.gov/HealthInformation/StatisticsAndData.htm. Accessed February 13, 2007.

Weber J, Kelley J. *Health Assessment in Nursing*. 2nd ed. Philadelphia: Lippincott Williams & Wilkins; 2003.

Winkler S, Garg A, Trakol M, et al. Depressed taste and smell in geriatric patients. *J Am Dental Assoc*. 1999;130:1759–1765.

CHAPTER

7

The Aging Gastrointestinal Tract

Ann Schmidt Luggen, PhD, GNP

· ·

CHAPTER OBJECTIVES   Upon completion of this chapter, the reader will be able to:

1. Describe the components of the gastrointestinal (GI) tract and the major changes they undergo with aging
2. Discuss each of the problems that commonly affect the aging GI tract and describe how nutrition may affect these disturbances
3. List the ways that nutrition can compensate for or improve common GI problems in older adults

KEY TERMS AND CONCEPTS

Aspiration

Diverticulosis

Diverticulitis

Dysphagia

Fecal incontinence

Gastroesophageal reflux disease (GERD)

Gastrointestinal (GI) tract

Hiatal hernia

Irritable bowel syndrome (IBS)

Nonsteroidal anti-inflammatory drugs (NSAIDs)

Parkinson's disease

Peptic ulcer disease (PUD)

Steatorrhea

· ·

The ingestion and absorption of nutrients via a functioning digestive system are essential for health and well-being. The processes of digestion include ingestion of food; propulsion of food from the mouth; secretion of mucus, water, and enzymes; mechanical and chemical digestion of foods; absorption of digested food; and propulsion of wastes from the anus.

The **gastrointestinal (GI) tract** includes the oral cavity; the throat, or oropharynx; the esophagus, the stomach, the duodenum and small intestine, the gallbladder, the pancreas, the liver, the large intestine, the rectum, and the anus (**Figure 7-1**). The lining of the GI tract is composed of four layers, which vary in thickness: mucosa, submucosa, mus-

cularis, and serosa. The liver, gallbladder, and pancreas are the accessory organs of the GI tract.

The GI tract is innervated by the sympathetic and parasympathetic divisions of the autonomic nervous system. Some nerves originate in the brain, outside of the GI tract (extrinsic fibers). Intrinsic fibers originate within the GI tract and respond to local stimuli. Hormones and

> **gastrointestinal (GI) tract** The connected series of organs and structures used for digestion of food and absorption of nutrients; also called the *alimentary canal* or the *digestive tract*. The GI tract includes the mouth, esophagus, stomach, small intestine, large intestine (colon), rectum, and anus.

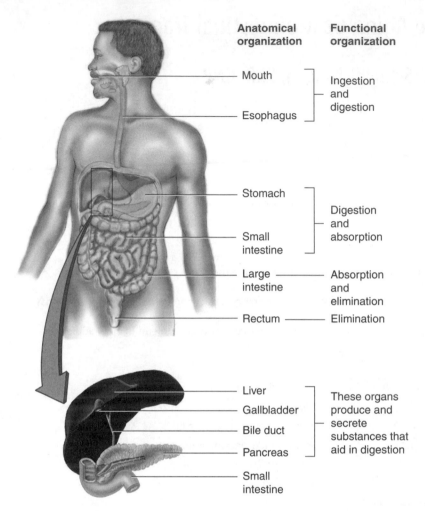

Anatomical organization   **Functional organization**

Mouth — Ingestion and digestion

Esophagus —

Stomach — Digestion and absorption

Small intestine —

Large intestine — Absorption and elimination

Rectum — Elimination

Liver — These organs produce and secrete substances that aid in digestion

Gallbladder —

Bile duct —

Pancreas —

Small intestine —

FIGURE 7-1 The Gastrointestinal Tract

Source: Insel P, Turner RE, Ross D. *Discovering Nutrition.* 3rd ed. Sudbury, MA: Jones & Bartlett; 2007; p.112. Reproduced with permission.

neurotransmitters also affect the GI tract. Digestive hormones are not secreted into the GI tract itself, but rather into the bloodstream, where they target special tissues.

Age-Related Changes in the Gastrointestinal Tract

In general, the GI tract, perhaps more than other body systems, retains normal functioning with increasing age. However, age-related changes do begin to occur prior to age 50. Aging affects the absorption and metabolism of foods, vitamins, and medications. The body has increased susceptibility to foodborne infections and other infections because of diminished immune function. **Table 7-1** summarizes the physiologic changes and their implications to the GI tract over time.

Gastrointestinal Tract Problems in the Older Adult

The Oral Cavity

Gum disease causes infections and loosens the tooth's structural support, resulting in tooth loss. Over time, teeth may become brittle and susceptible to fracture. The chewing teeth can become worn after many years of use, making it difficult for the older adult to chew foods well enough to swallow without harm. See Chapter 6 for greater detail on this topic.

Teeth

Dental caries and periodontal disease are the two most common oral diseases. Older adults are at risk for new and recurrent decay, which is left untreated in about 30% of those

TABLE 7-1 Age-Related Changes in the GI Tract

Area	Change	Implications	Contributors
Oropharynx	Dec. neuromuscular coordination, loss of tooth supports, dentin	Choking, dysphagia, aspiration	Stroke, other neuromuscular problems, alcohol
	Dec. taste buds	Loss of appetite	Advanced old age
	Dec. taste sensation	Impaired taste	Medications
	Loss of teeth	Impaired chewing	Poor care
	Sarcopenia	Dec. chewing	Dec. exercise, malnutrition
Esophagus	Dec. motility	Indigestion, GERD	Obesity, DM, HH
	Dec. LES function	Slow emptying, incr. acid, injury	Medications, Ca, Peppermints, stroke, PD
Stomach	Dec. acid response	Mucosa unprotected	Tobacco, alcohol,
	Dec. blood flow	Incr. injury—PUD	DM, CHF, herbals
	Slow emptying	Early satiety	NSAIDS, Meds,
	Dec. motility, volume		*H. pylori* infection
	Dec. absorption of some nutrients		
Small Intestine	Relaxed villi, atrophy mm fibers	Dec. absorption of most nutrients	Vascular disease
	Dec. mucosal surface		
	Dec. absorption of some nutrients		
Gallbladder	Dec. contractility	Cholelithiasis	Obesity, multiparity
	Incr. cholecystokinin	Dec. appetite	
Liver	Dec. size, blood flow, perfusion	Dec. effectiveness of function	Alcohol, herbals, meds
	Fibrosis, regeneration dim.	Dec. metabolism	
Pancreas	Dec. endocrine function	DM risk	DM
Colon	Dec. mucus production, elasticity	Constipation, loss of urge	DM, dementia
	Perception of distention		
Rectum/anus	Dec. resting pressure	Fecal incontinence	Dementia, neurologic disease

DM = diabetes mellitus; Dec = decreased; HH= hiatal hernia; LES = lower esophageal sphincter; Incr. = increased; GERD = gastroesophageal reflux disease; Ca = cancer; CHF = congestive heart failure; PD = Parkinson's disease; dim = diminished

Sources: Mayhew M, Edmunds M, Wendel V. *Gerontological Nurse Practitioner Review Manual.* Washington, DC: American Nurses Credentialing Center; 2001; Miller CA. *Nursing for Wellness in Older Adults.* 4th ed. Philadelphia: Lippincott; 2004; Huether S. Structure and function of the digestive system. In: McCance K, Huether S, eds. *Pathophysiology.* 4th ed. St. Louis: Mosby; 2002:1231–1337; American Geriatric Society. *Geriatrics Review Syllabus.* 6th ed. New York: American Geriatric Society; 2006.

who have teeth (**Figure 7-2**). In one public health study by the Centers for Disease Control and Prevention, more than 50% of older adults in 26 states reported having most of their teeth. However, those who were edentate (having no teeth) ranged from 42% in Kentucky to 13% in Hawaii. Hispanic and non-Hispanic Whites have similar rates of decay. Mexican Americans have higher rates of untreated caries. The rate of tooth decay is higher among smokers.

The severity of periodontal disease increases with age. Men are more likely than women to have severe periodontal disease. The poorest people have the most severe disease, a category into which many older adults fall. Approximately 23% of adults aged 65 to 74 have severe periodontal disease (6 mm of periodontal attachment loss).

Older adults often do not have dental insurance after retirement and must pay for dental services out of pocket. Medicare does not cover basic dental services, and Medicaid provides limited coverage in some states. Older adults pay three-fourths of their dental care out of pocket. Being disabled, homebound, or institutionalized increases the risk of poor oral health. **Box 7-1** discusses methods for maintaining good oral health.

Oral and throat cancers occur in 30,000 people in the United States each year; most of these cancers occur in older adults. Survival rates are poor, especially among African Americans; overall, oral and throat cancers cause 8,000 deaths each year. Major causes of these cancers are tobacco and alcohol.

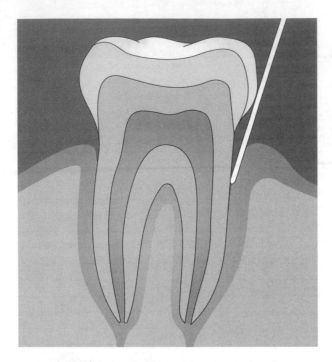

FIGURE 7-2 Periodontal Disease

Source: National Institute of Dental and Craniofacial Research, National Institutes of Health.

Dysphagia and Odonophagia

Dysphagia is difficulty with swallowing; *odonophagia* is pain upon swallowing. Either or both of these may be caused by gastroesophageal reflux disease (GERD), which is discussed later in this chapter. Dysphagia affects one in every 17 people. It predominantly affects older adults; more than 6.2 million people in the United States older than age 60 experience dysphagia. The causes of dysphagia are multifactorial and vary in severity. Some of the causes are stroke, Parkinson's disease, head, neck, and chest injuries, Zenker diverticulum, oropharyngeal tumors, and prominent cervical osteophytes (osteoarthritis of the cervical spine).

Dysphagia is the suggestive diagnosis if the patient complains of or assessment reveals pocketing of food in the cheeks, speech abnormalities with slurring of words, orofacial changes, facial weakness, abnormal tongue movements, and foods becoming stuck if swallowed. The patient may drool, regurgitate nasally, or become reluctant to eat certain foods or even eat at all.

dysphagia Difficulty swallowing. It may result from a neurological disorder that impairs esophageal motility or from a mechanical obstruction of the esophagus.

aspiration (1) Abnormal entry of food or fluid into the airway. (2) Withdrawal of fluid or substance by suction from the airway to promote breathing when the airway is obstructed.

Swallowing is very complex and utilizes 50 pairs of muscles and many nerves to move food from the mouth to the stomach. There are three stages of this process: (1) tongue movement, saliva, and preparation to swallow; (2) food (or liquid) pushed to the back of the mouth, triggering a swallowing reflex causing passage through the pharynx toward the esophagus (the larynx [voice box] closes and breathing stops, which prevents aspiration into the lungs); (3) food or liquid enters the esophagus and is carried to the stomach.

Management of dysphagia is primarily concerned with preventing **aspiration**. Aspiration pneumonia is associated with higher rates of morbidity and mortality than community-acquired pneumonia and should be prevented if at all possible.

The clinician should assess the patient's ability to swallow. It is best to observe swallowing of different kinds of liquids and foods to determine which are most problematic. A speech therapist, if available, is most proficient at this evaluation and can make recommendations. **Box 7-2** presents interventions for dysphagia.

To diagnose the cause of dysphagia, some factors should be considered. Those with oropharyngeal dysphagia will complain of foods or pills becoming "stuck" when they try to swallow. Swallowing hesitancy and tongue tremor usually point to Parkinson's disease as the cause. In esophageal dysphagia, the older adult will point to the sternum when describing where the problem is. When the patient has dysphagia with both liquids and solids at the same time, it is usually indicative of a motility disorder in the esophagus. However, if the patient has dysphagia with solids first and then later with liquids, a mechanical obstruction is probably the cause. When the dysphagia is progressive, such as this, one may suspect cancer or stricture. When it is inter-

BOX 7-2 Managing Dysphagia Symptoms

- Target the cause, when possible.
- Obtain a speech therapy consult.
- Begin appropriate food and liquid consistencies.
- Sit with the older adult to ensure proper eating habits are followed (e.g., not talking while eating).
- If esophageal spasm is present, calcium channel blockers may be prescribed.
- Monitor and control progression of symptoms.

mittent, the cause is probably esophageal spasm or a lower esophageal ring. When the patient has dysarthria and nasal regurgitation of foods, there may be a weakness of the soft palate. Zenker diverticulum or pharyngoesophageal diverticulum may be the cause when there is halitosis, a sense of fullness in the neck region, and food regurgitation. If the cause is not known, the patient should have an endoscopy or barium swallow.

In general, foods should be pureed, thickened, and homogenous. Exclude all raw foods except bananas. Cut tender meats to 1 cm or less. Avoid nuts; raw, crispy foods; and foods that are stringy (green beans, celery). Fluids may be thin or regular. They may be nectarlike so that they can be taken through a straw and are spillable (e.g., eggnog) or honeylike and not taken through a straw but rather eaten with a spoon (e.g., yogurt). Foods may be pudding-like (e.g., thickened applesauce).

Aspiration

Aspiration is a serious complication of dysphagia and dysphasia (difficulty speaking). It is common in older adults who have had a stroke and in those with **Parkinson's disease** and other neurologic problems. Although it can cause airway obstruction, it more commonly results in pneumonia. Diagnosis is made by patient self-report of difficulty breathing and cough, X-ray of the chest, elevated white blood cell count, abnormal lung sounds assessed via stethoscope, elevated temperature, and change in the character of sputum. The older adult will need antibiotics if pneumonia occurs.

Management of aspiration is multifactorial if malnutrition and dehydration are to be avoided. The older adult needs to concentrate at meals and avoid the social occasion that mealtime usually is. He or she should sit upright in a chair, rather than elevated in bed. Food should be taken and swallowed from the strongest side of the mouth in the

older adult with a paralysis or unilateral weakness. The older adult at risk for aspiration should sit upright for about 30 minutes following the meal.

Salivation is an important part of dysphagia management. Foods with strong taste increase salivation, which enhances bolus formation. Lemon, herbs, and seasonings of the patient's preference are desirable. Salivation is also enhanced with cold or warm foods rather than those at lukewarm temperatures. Water should be chilled and served separate from the meal—either before the meal or after.

Because large meals can be intimidating, smaller, more frequent meals are often preferable. Bite-size pieces that necessitate chewing are most desirable. The consistency of the food is important. An evaluation will be helpful to see what consistency works best for the particular problem. Usually, somewhat thickened foods, with honeylike consistency for drinks, works well.

Esophagus

Inflammation of the esophagus is often caused by viral infections, but it may be the result of a burn or from a pill stuck in the mucosa of the throat. Inflammation commonly is caused by acid reflux in older adults with GERD.

Heartburn

Heartburn is a symptom of acid reflux, or GERD. It manifests as substernal burning pain or pressure that may radiate to the throat and mouth or to the jaw and shoulders and occasionally the arms. The patient may complain of hoarseness. A burning, sour regurgitation may occur. Many people may not have heartburn as a symptom, but rather dry cough, asthma, and difficulty swallowing.

Gastroesophageal Reflux Disease

Gastroesophageal reflux disease (GERD) is the most common gastrointestinal disorder affecting older adults. GERD causes many of the symptoms of the upper GI tract problems discussed previously. These symptoms affect 40% of the older population in the United States. Persistent symptoms affect quality of life dramatically. Approximately 50% of cases will require medical management. If left untreated, severe problems may develop, such as erosive esophagitis, strictures with dysphagia, esophageal ulceration, and bleeding.

GERD is the retrograde movement of gastric contents into the esophagus as a result of an incompetent lower esophageal sphincter,

Parkinson's disease
A common neurological disorder characterized by bradykinesia, rigidity, resting tremor, and impaired righting reflex.

gastroesophageal reflux disease (GERD) A condition in which the gastric contents move backward (reflux) into the esophagus, causing pain and tissue damage.

TABLE 7-2 GERD Symptoms

Typical Symptoms	Atypical Symptoms	Complicated Symptoms
Heartburn	Retrosternal chest	Weight loss
Water brash	pain	Bleeding
Sour taste in mouth	Cough	Choking from acid-
Belching	Wheezing	caused cough
Indigestion	Hoarseness	Shortness of breath
Dysphagia	Throat clearing	Hoarseness
Regurgitation	Vomiting	Chest pain
	Halitosis	Anemia
	Sore throat	

Sources: Reuben D, Herr K, Pacala J, et al. *Geriatrics at Your Fingertips, 2009.* 11th ed. New York: American Geriatric Society; 2009; Hill C. Gastroesophageal reflux disease. In: Meiner S, ed. *Care of Gastrointestinal Problems in the Older Adult.* New York: Springer; 2004:23–46.

transient relaxation of the sphincter, or compromise of other antireflux mechanisms. When symptoms of GERD are present, they should be medically treated (**Table 7-2**).

First-line management of GERD is nutritional and includes avoidance of sympton-causing foods, most often citrus fruits, chocolate, drinks with caffeine or alcohol, fatty and fried foods, garlic and onions, mints, spicy foods, and tomato-based foods such as spaghetti and pizza. The older adult should stop eating large meals. Contributing factors include obesity, smoking, and hiatal hernia, which is otherwise normal in an adult of older than 50 years. Drugs commonly prescribed to older adults that may cause GERD and that may be discontinued with consultation with the primary caregiver include anticholinergics, benzodiazepines, calcium channel blockers, dopamine, estrogen, isoproterenol, nicotine gum or patches, nitrates (oral, SL, patch), and opioids. Smoking and chewing tobacco should be discouraged. See **Box 7-3** for other nonpharmacologic methods of management of GERD.

Medical management is pyramidal and starts with a plan to reduce the risk factors and contributors to GERD, such as alcohol, cigarettes, and mints (See **Box 7-4**). There is actually very little evidence that lifestyle and dietary interventions are effective. The second step is to use antacids such as Maalox, Mylanta, or Tums (which contribute calcium but are constipating). H2 antagonists such as cimetidine (Tagamet), famotidine (Pepcid), or ranitidine hydrochloride (Zantac) are also utilized for short-term relief. The third step occurs when the previous steps are unsuccessful and involves the use of proton pump inhibitors (PPIs), such as Prilosec/Nexium, Prevacid, and Protonix. These are most effective and can heal the esophageal lining.

BOX 7-3 Nonpharmacological Methods of GERD Management

- Avoid lying down for three hours after eating.
- Avoid tight-fitting clothes.
- Avoid alcohol and high-fat foods.
- Avoid spicy foods and pepper.
- Avoid chocolate, spearmint, and high-acid foods.
- Elevate head of bed 6 to 8 inches.
- Stop smoking.
- Lose weight if overweight.
- Drink 6 to 8 ounces of water with all medications.
- Stop drugs that precipitate reflux.
- Take antacids, such as Tums, or baking soda in water.
- Consider surgery.

Source: Reuben D, Herr K, Pacala J, et al. *Geriatrics at Your Fingertips, 2009.* 11th ed. New York: American Geriatric Society; 2009.

PPIs significantly reduce acid secretion, but they do not eliminate intragastric acidity completely. Further, most of PPIs have a relatively short serum half-life of two to four hours. Approximately 91% of those receiving PPIs in the morning and at bedtime have breakthrough nocturnal acid. Maximum benefit occurs when the PPI is taken 15 to 30 minutes prior to a meal, because this blocks the most pumps. Bedtime dosing of H2RAs should be considered to inhibit nocturnal acid breakthrough.

BOX 7-4 Medical Management of GERD

First-line efforts	Nutritional, positional
Second-line efforts	Histamine receptor antagonists, ranitidine (Zantac), famotidine (Pepcid)
Third-line efforts	Proton pump inhibitors, omeprazole (Prilosec), lansoprazole (Prevacid), etc.

Source: Reuben D, Herr K, Pacala J, et al. *Geriatrics at Your Fingertips, 2007–2008.* 7th ed. New York: American Geriatric Society; 2007.

Hiatal Hernia

Hiatal hernia is a diaphragmatic hernia in which there is protrusion of the fundus of the stomach through the hiatus, or opening of the diaphragm into the thorax. It is caused by weakened esophageal muscles around the opening of the diaphragm and is precipitated by heavy lifting, coughing, lying flat in bed, or performing a Valsalva maneuver or other cause of increased intra-abdominal pressure. The "sliding" hiatal hernia occurs in 60% of adults over the age of 60.

Upper Gastrointestinal Tract Problems

Peptic Ulcer Disease

Peptic ulcer disease (PUD) refers to both gastric and duodenal ulcers. Approximately 5 million cases of PUD occur each year in the United States. Approximately 80% of duodenal ulcers and 60% of gastric ulcers are caused by *Helicobacter pylori*. Older adults are much more likely than their younger counterparts to suffer the complications of PUD, including stress ulcers that occur with hospitalization.

The second most common cause of PUD is the use of **nonsteroidal anti-inflammatory drugs (NSAIDs)**, such as motrin, ibuprofen, naproxyn, and aspirin. The risk of ulcer complications is three times greater among those who use NSAIDs than among nonusers. It is highest in adults older than age 60. Older women are two to four times more likely to be hospitalized with PUD. NSAIDs are prescribed unfortunately to more than 40% of older patients. Of these, 8% are hospitalized for complications, often a GI bleed. Perforation and hemorrhage are the most common complications of PUD. Risk factors for adverse events in older adults treated with NSAIDs include age greater than 65, comorbid medical conditions, oral glucocorticoid use, history of PUD, history of upper GI bleed, and the use of anticoagulants. Aspirin is a common NSAID that causes gastrointestinal bleeding. It is widely used for the prevention of cardiovascular events, but it causes ulcers and bleeds, especially in older adults. PPIs are a useful adjunct to the medication regime as a mucosal protectant even in those on very low doses of aspirin.

Clinical signs of PUD include epigastric pain and hematemesis, or coffee-ground emesis. Approximately 50% of older adults do not have pain with PUD, making diagnosis difficult. The observation of blood in the stool or anemia in a blood test will give rise to suspicion.

Stress Ulcers

Risk factors for stress ulcers include a history of GI bleeding in the past year (most common risk factor), multiple organ failure, hypotension, use of mechanical ventilation for more than 48 hours, kidney failure, major trauma, shock or head injury, coagulopathy, 25% degree burns over the body, liver failure, spinal cord injury, and quadriplegia. A study

is currently in place by the National Institutes of Health to examine the use of Prevacid for treatment of stress ulcers. The drug is currently in use for treatment of gastritis and therapy for peptic ulcers. Prevention of stress ulcers in hospitalized older adults may be difficult and may occur despite efforts to prevent them.

Nausea and Vomiting

Nausea and vomiting have many possible causes, including motion sickness; intracranial lesions; chemotherapy drugs for cancer (40% to 70%); NSAIDs; opiates; antibiotics; digoxin; stomach inflammation; mechanical obstruction; gallbladder inflammation; motility disorders; dyspepsia or gastroparesis; viral or bacterial infections; hepatitis; meningitis; metabolic conditions such as uremia, acidosis, and adrenal insufficiency; alcohol intoxication; and psychiatric disorders.

The older adult with nausea and vomiting must be evaluated for dehydration and, if seriously ill, hospitalized. Drugs useful for stopping the nausea and vomiting include prochlorperazine, odansetron, diphenhydramine, meclizine, benzodiazepines, and scopolamine. Corticosteroids are said to enhance the effects of other antiemetics, especially in those with increased intracranial pressure. Caution must be used in prescribing these drugs for older adults because they cause confusion, sedation, and delirium.

Gastroparesis

The most common causes of gastroparesis are diabetes, idiopathic, and postsurgical. It is the medical term for delayed stomach emptying. Common presenting symptoms are nausea (93%), early satiety (86%), vomiting (68%), and pain (46% to 89%). Others complain of heartburn from reflux. Those with frequent vomiting experience malnutrition, but gastroparesis does not always restrict food intake. Many have phytobezoars, that is, concretions of indigestible food residue retained in the stomach.

Diabetes mellitus is the most common cause of gastroparesis; it occurs in 30% of those with type 2 and 27% to 58% of those

hiatal hernia A physical abnormality that allows the stomach to protrude through the diaphragm and up into the chest. Often caused by weakened musculature.

peptic ulcer disease (PUD) A duodenal or stomach ulceration or erosion often caused by the bacterium *Helicobacter pylori*, which lives in an acid environment. It is treatable with antibiotics.

nonsteroidal anti-inflammatory drugs (NSAIDS) Drugs used to treat pain, inflammation, and fever (antipyretic). They are not opiates nor steroids. Aspirin, ibuprofen, and naproxen are commonly used NSAIDs.

with type 1. It affects gastric motor function rather than small bowel transit, which indicates the sensitivity of the stomach to diabetic injury. Autonomic neuropathy is a contributing cause to gastroparesis in those with long-standing diabetes.

Idiopathic gastroparesis is also very common, especially in middle-aged women (90% of those affected are women). It often starts after a viral infection or following an injection of tetanus vaccination or hepatitis vaccine. Postsurgical gastroparesis complicates stomach surgery. The cause is damage to the vagal nerve in procedures such as those for ulcer disease or malignancy, gastrojejunostomy, esophagectomy, Whipple procedures for pancreatitis, heart or lung transplantation, gastric bypass, and fundoplication for GERD.

Often the treatment after GI surgery is inserting a nasogastric tube and specifying "nothing by mouth" for a period of time. A review of studies regarding recovery after gastric surgery examined a study by Lowenfels that compared two groups: one receiving the usual nasogastric tube and one in which patients were allowed to choose what they wanted to eat and when they wanted to eat it. No differences in outcomes were found between the two groups. Others have found no difference in giving a restricted diet to postsurgery patients. Postlaparotomy dysmotility predominantly affects the stomach and colon; the small bowel recovers normal function between four and eight hours. Feeding is tolerated and food is absorbed within 24 hours. Early feeding is associated with the risk of vomiting, but also with reduced length of hospital stay, fewer infections, and perhaps diminished risk of dehiscence.

Management of gastroparesis includes nutritional modifications and medications to stimulate gastric emptying. The patient may need drugs to reduce vomiting. Sometimes psychological and surgical interventions are required. Dietary recommendations include liquids to prevent dehydration and salt and mineral loss; avoiding milk products, vegetables, fruits, and meat, but eating saltine crackers and drinking Gatorade, and soft drinks sipped slowly during the day. Fat-free consomme is permitted.

A second diet could be ingestion of more calories, including a small amount of dietary fat (less than 40 gm/day); skim milk and yogurt; low-fat cheeses; fat-free bouillon and soups made with skim milk and with pasta; cream of wheat; white rice; eggs; peanut butter (2 Tb/day); vegetable juice; well-cooked vegetables without skins; apple juice; cranberry, grape, pineapple, prune juices and canned fruits without skins. Avoid citrus juices. The diet includes small amounts of fat; hard candies; puddings; ice milk; jelly; and soft drinks and Gatorade are all permitted.

For a third diet, for maintenance, the diet is the same as Diet 2 with the addition of poultry, fish, and lean ground beef, breads and cereals, coffee, tea, and water. However-

er, non-caloric beverages should be limited if the patient cannot maintain adequate caloric intake. Fat is limited to 50 gm/day and fiber is restricted due to indigestability. Low-fat meals are needed to compensate for the gastric motor impairment. Enteral and parenteral nutrition may be needed if there are symptom flares or for permanent support. Indications for this therapy are significant malnutrition (e.g., more than 10% weight loss over 6 months and responsiveness to dietary modification), essential mineral deficiencies, or electrolyte disturbances with frequent hospitalization.

Those with refractory gastroparesis may benefit from enteral or parenteral nutrition intermittently for symptom flares or for permanent support. In diabetic gastroparesis, jejunostomy placement for enteral feeding improves overall health status with reduced symptoms, enhanced nutrition, and decreased hospitalizations.

Medical treatment includes prescriptions of prokinetics that stimulate gastric emptying. These include erythromycin, metoclopramide, domperidone, and, less often, cisapride, bethanechol, and other macrolides, such as azithromycin. Drugs to inhibit vomiting include antiemetics such as phenothiazines (e.g., prochlorperazine, thiethylperazine), tricyclic antidepressants, and mirtazapine. Cannabinoids, ginger, and benzodiazepines are other unproved possibilities. Any medication that inhibits motility should be discontinued. Maintaining euglycemia may help avoid the inhibitory effects of hyperglycemia on gastric motor function.

Malabsorption

Malabsorption is a clinical term for some defects that occur during digestion and absorption of food nutrients and in infections of the GI tract. Malabsorption can occur when there is disruption of any of the three phases of digestion and absorption: (1) in the luminal phase, dietary fats, proteins, and carbohydrates are hydrolyzed and solubilized; (2) in the mucosal phase, the brush-border membrane of intestinal epithelial cells transport digested nutrients from the lumen into cells; and (3) in the postabsorptive phase, lipids and other key nutrients are transported from epithelial cells via the lymphatic system and portal circulation to other parts of the body.

Malabsorption has many causes. It often occurs in older adults with pancreatic insufficiency; for example, in those with chronic pancreatitis and pancreatic cancer. Pancreatic insufficiency is the cause in about 20% to 30% of cases of malabsorption in the older adult. Most have no history of pancreatic pain or alcoholism. Another 30% of cases are caused by anatomic abnormalities (e.g., small-intestine diverticulosis, strictures, partial obstruction), which promote stasis and predispose to bacterial overgrowth. Another 20% of patients develop the bacterial overgrowth syndrome without anatomic abnormalities. This occurs when gastric acid secretion is inadequate. Pernicious anemia and vitamin B12 deficiency are common, suggesting that gastric atrophy and achlorhydria allow proliferation of gastric and small intestinal bacteria. Motility disorders such as gastroparesis can also impair bacterial clearance, allowing overgrowth. Other causes include cirrhosis and biliary tract disease and diseases such as sprue, lymphatic obstruction, and parasitic infestation.

Malabsorption should be investigated when the older adult has weight loss or failure to maintain weight, causing debility. Other signs and symptoms include diarrhea; greasy, malodorous stools (steatorrhea); abdominal bloating; and gas (flatulence). Diarrhea is not always present, but chronic diarrhea is the symptom that most often prompts evaluation.

Steatorrhea, malabsorption of fat, is suspected when the stool is foul-smelling, bulky, and difficult to flush down the toilet. It occurs when more than 6% of dietary fat is excreted in stool. It is a hallmark of malabsorption.

Excessive flatus (gas) and bloating of the abdomen are often caused by maldigested carbohydrates. When advanced, severe vitamin and mineral deficiencies occur. Clinically, the health professional will see anemia secondary to deficiencies in iron, folate, vitamin B12, or a combination of these and easy bruising and bleeding secondary to vitamin K deficiency.

Diagnosis can be made by various general blood tests. Steatorrhea is confirmed by a quantitative 72-hour stool collection. If the fecal fat is 40 g or more, pancreatic insufficiency or small intestine mucosal disease is indicated. A d-xylose test can differentiate pancreatitis from mucosal disease. An endoscopic biopsy may also be done, looking for bacterial overgrowth and parasites.

Treatment objectives are to correct deficiencies of nutrients, vitamins, and minerals and to identify and treat underlying causes. Supplemental iron is given via ferrous sulfate or gluconate tablets. B12 injections are given monthly with cobalamin deficiency. Fat-soluble vitamin and calcium supplements are given. The diet is high protein, low fat, and high calorie for weight loss. Medium-chain triglycerides are given as a dietary supplement because they are hydrolyzed readily by pancreatic lipase. Parenteral nutrition is considered in those with severe malnutrition unresponsive to oral feeding and in rare situations in which the temporary avoidance of enteral feeding is necessary.

Lower Gastrointestinal Tract Problems in Older Adults

The function of the colon is to absorb fluid and electrolytes. The colon transports its contents and evacuates them via the rectum and anus. Dysfunction often is related to changes in transit time (normally about 72 hours) or to pelvic floor dysfunction.

Antibiotic-Associated Enteritis

Antibiotics often cause diarrhea. Occasionally, it may be severe, bloody, painful, with fever, and even life threatening. Much has been reported about the morbidity and mortality associated with antibiotic-associated diarrhea due to *Clostridium difficile*, which causes a pseudomembranous colitis. These problems are especially dangerous in older adults. Age is a major risk factor; it occurs 10 times more often in adults 65 and older. Outbreaks occur frequently in nursing facilities due to a lack of good hand washing. The bacteria are passed in feces and spread to food and objects, and the bacteria produce spores that may persist in a room for weeks or months. Variables associated with mortality in one study were hypoalbuminemia, impaired functional capacity, and elevated serum urea. The *C. difficile* toxin itself was not associated with mortality rates, although the bacteria seems to be worsening.

Risk factors for antibiotic-associated enteritis include parenterally administered antibiotics such as floroquinolones, cephalosporins, clindamycin, and penicillin, and some antineoplastic agents, such as cyclophosphamide, doxorubicin, fluorouracil, and methotrexate. Signs and symptoms include pain and cramping, nausea, loss of appetite, weight loss, dehydration, diarrhea (10–15 times a day and often bloody), hypovolemia, hypoalbuminemia, leukocytosis, fever, and fecal leukocytes. Complications include dehydration, kidney failure in severe sudden dehydration, bowel perforation which could lead to peritonitis, toxic megacolon with potential rupture of the colon, and even death with mild to moderate infection that progresses rapidly if not treated quickly.

Treatment involves stopping the offending agent and switching to metronidazole (Flagyl) or vancomycin. These drugs cause nausea and bitter taste in the mouth. The diarrhea is treated with cholestyramine resin (Questran). The use of probiotics, especially a natural yeast called Saccharomyces boulardii, in conjunction with antibiotics, prevents recurrence.

Lactose Intolerance (Hypolactasia)

Lactose, or milk sugar, is a disaccharide found in mammalian milk and dairy products. An enzyme, lactase (lactase-phlorizin hydrolase), splits lactose into two monosaccharides—glucose and galactose. The enzyme is found on the mucosal surface of epithelial cells of the small intestine. Small children and infants have the enzyme in abundance. Lactase is at its peak when it is most necessary for growth. It gradually declines with aging so that in adulthood, 30% of the population has continued lactase "persistence." Lactase is most deficient in American Indians (90% to 100%) and nearly all Asians

steatorrhea Production of stools containing an abnormally high amount of fat.

(93% to 98%); it is deficient in 79% of African Americans and in 12% to 20% of adult Whites.

Lactose maldigestion occurs when lactose is not absorbed in the small intestine. It then passes through the GI tract to the colon where, in those who are "intolerant," it leads to symptoms of lactose intolerance. Symptoms include abdominal pain, bloating, flatus, diarrhea, borborygmi (noisy, rumbling gut sounds), and sometimes nausea and vomiting. Occasionally, older adults present with constipation due to diminished gastric motility.

Lactose is necessary for the absorption of calcium and other essential nutrients. Without lactose, there is an increased risk for osteoporosis, hypertension, and colon cancer. We need only 50% of lactase activity for effective utilization of lactose.

Lactose is found in dairy foods and in nondairy foods such as instant breakfast mixes, cake mixes, mayonnaise, deli meats, vitamin supplements, breads, sausages, burgers, processed chicken, soft drinks, lager beers, and some medications. The following strategies can be used to include lactose in the diet without the symptoms of bloating, gas, abdominal pain, and diarrhea.

1. After excluding lactose-containing products for a period of time, take small quantities of lactose-containing foods such as milk (½ cup) and slowly increase until symptoms occur.
2. Eat lactose-containing foods with meals; for example, add milk to cereal or other foods to slowly improve tolerance.
3. Change the type of lactose-containing foods usually eaten. For example, whole milk is preferable to low-fat milk; chocolate milk is tolerated better than white milk. Many cheeses (e.g., parmesan, cheddar, Swiss, aged cheeses) contain less lactose than milk and yogurts and are good sources of protein and calcium and often cause no symptoms.
4. Lactose-reduced products, such as milk, are available (70% to 99% lactose free). Other lactose-free products include Boost Drink, Boost Plus, Ensure, Ensure Plus, Nu Basics, and Nu Basics Plus. Lactase enzymes, available as capsules or chewable tablets, can be taken with lactose-containing foods to aid digestion.

It is important to find other sources of calcium in a lactose-free diet. Calcium is found in broccoli, leafy greens, canned salmon, oranges, almonds, some tofus, calcium-fortified breads and juices, soy milk, and calcium supplements. Further, lactase enzyme tablets can be taken just prior to a meal with lactose.

Many of the myths about lactose intolerance diminish quality of life. Some believe that people with lactose intolerance cannot tolerate any milk or dairy products. This is not so. They may tolerate up to 12 g of lactose if consumed over a day. Another myth is that lactase deficiency is rare. However, up to 70% of the world population is known to be lactase deficient. A third myth is that goat milk is lactose-free. Goat milk contains 4% lactose, just slightly less than whole milk and low-fat milk. Lastly, a negative lactose breath test indicates that the patient can tolerate all dairy products. This test does not confirm lactose intolerance in all cases.

Lactase deficiency is difficult to diagnose and little was known about it until about 50 years ago. People have begun to self-diagnose themselves as having lactase deficiency, even though their abdominal discomfort may be due to other causes. Cow's milk protein allergy, ulcerative colitis, or irritable bowel syndrome, to name just a few conditions, may cause similar symptoms to lactose intolerance. In actual practice, some older adults with lactose intolerance are able to consume milk and dairy products without developing symptoms; however, others will need lactose restriction. Patients should have an antidiarrheal agent on hand. Medications such as loperamide (Imodium A-D) will reduce symptoms of lactose intolerance.

Irritable Bowel Syndrome (IBS)

About 75% of **irritiable bowel syndrome (IBS)** cases occur in women. Symptoms of IBS include intermittent or continuous abdominal pain and alterations in bowel patterns. For the diagnosis, the abdominal pain should occur at least 12 weeks out of the previous 12 months. Bowel pattern alterations may be episodic diarrhea and/or constipation, relief of pain after a bowel movement, mucus in stool, or bloating. The symptoms are worse during times of stress. IBS is often considered a disorder of young women, but it affects those of all ages and usually begins after the age of 35.

IBS is a functional disorder and is frequently seen with other functional disorders, such as fibromyalgia, chronic pelvic pain, and interstitial cystitis. The loss of quality of life in these patients is considerable. Symptoms occur in 10% of adults after viral or bacterial enteric infections. Risk factors include gender (female), longer duration of gastroenteritis, and the presence of psychosocial stresses. Warning signs of IBS are rectal bleeding, anemia, weight loss, fever, family history of colon cancer, symptom onset at 50+ years of age, and a major change in symptoms.

Treatment is aimed at reducing the symptoms of diarrhea, constipation, and pain. For diarrhea-predominant disease, low doses of alosetron may help alleviate symptoms, especially pain, and improve quality of life; however it has severe restrictions for use by the FDA. It is to be used only in the case of severe IBS. Osmotic laxatives are used for constipation, although they have not been studied in older

irritable bowel syndrome (IBS) A disruptive state of intestinal motility of unknown cause. Symptoms include constipation, abdominal pain, and episodic diarrhea.

people with IBS. Fiber and bulking agents can also be used, but they cause bloating. The FDA approved Lubiprostone for constipation-predominant IBS. Other antispasmodic agents, such as hyoscyamine or mebeverine, are also used.

Constipation and diarrhea are managed when they occur. A food diary can be useful in identifying those foods that precipitate the symptoms. Foods known to precipitate IBS symptoms include fried foods, caffeine, alcohol, milk products, foods high in sugar, fatty foods, gas-producing vegetables, and products that contain sorbitol and xylitol (chewing gum and sugarless candy). After the suspected foods are identified, they can be omitted from the diet one at a time to determine just which ones are causative.

Other methods of managing IBS include increased physical activity, development of regular defecation habits, management of pain associated with IBS, therapy that develops a perception of self-control of the problem, and combinations of these methods. Pharmacotherapy is used to control the symptoms, whether predominantly diarrhea or constipation. For diarrhea-predominant IBS, over-the-counter loperamide is available. Lomotil is used for more serious diarrhea. Constipation-predominant IBS is managed as constipation (see the discussion of constipation later in this chapter).

Intestinal Ischemia

Mesenteric ischemia is a result of diminished blood flow to the bowel. The resultant injury is from hypoxemia and associated nutrient deficiency. When blood flow is interrupted (mesenteric and hypogastric arteries), there is significant compromise in at least two main arterial trunks (**Figure 7-3**).

The situation can occur acutely or chronically, usually from atherosclerosis. It may occur in the small or large bowel, and it may be occlusive, as in an embolus, or nonocclusive, as in ischemia.

Mesenteric ischemia occurs in older people, and they present with postprandial abdominal pain. The pain may last several hours and often occurs after a heavy meal. Over time, the pain worsens, becoming severe and incapacitating. The individual fears eating, and significant weight loss may occur before the problem is diagnosed. Of course, this condition is much more difficult to diagnose in an older adult with dementia in the long-term care setting. Steatorrhea occurs in about 50% of patients. It can be fatal. See **Table 7-3** for signs and symptoms of acute intestinal ischemia and chronic intestinal ischemia.

The risk factors for ischemia include age older than 50, high blood pressure, diabetes, elevated levels of lipids, and smoking. A higher risk is indicated if atherosclerosis has been diagnosed in other areas of the body, such as the heart, legs, or brain. Other factors that increase risk are low blood pressure, heart failure, irregular heart, blood clotting disorder, hernia, and previous abdominal surgery.

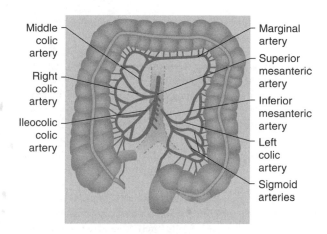

FIGURE 7-3 Blood Supply to Intestine

Source: National Institures of Health, 2008.

If the patient has many risk factors, dietary changes can stop the progression of atherosclerosis and lower blood pressure. The patient needs to become more physically active and lose weight. Quitting smoking will help reduce the risks. All of these changes will also help to prevent stroke, heart attack, and other serious disorders.

Acute mesenteric ischemia is a medical emergency and must be diagnosed correctly and quickly. Diagnosis may occur through exploratory surgery, colonoscopy, ultrasound, X-rays, or angiography. Management is surgical (bypass or endartectomy) after the cause of the ischemia is discovered. The individual may require an ostomy (opening in

TABLE 7-3 Signs and Symptoms of Acute and Chronic Intestinal Ischemia

Acute Intestinal Ischemia	Chronic Intestinal Ischemia
Sudden mild to severe abdominal pain	Cramps, fullness 30 minutes after eating, lasting 1 to 3 hours
Urgent feeling of need to move bowels	Abdominal pain that progressively worsens over weeks to months
Frequent forceful bowel movements	
Tender abdomen	Fear of eating due to pain
Distention, swelling of abdomen	Unintended weight loss
Blood in stool	Nausea, vomiting
Nausea, vomiting	Bloating
Fever	

Source: Mayo Clinic. Intestinal ischemia. 2006. Available at: http://www.mayoclinic.com/print/intestinal-ischemia/DS00459/METHOD=print&DSECTION=all. Accessed April 19, 2008.

the colon for digested contents to be excreted) if the colon tissue has infarcted and is necrosed.

The Role of Fiber in Lower Gastrointestinal Problems

Low intake of dietary fiber has a causative role in many of the dysfunctions discussed in the following sections. Management of these problems can include increasing the amount of fiber in an older person's diet. Fiber is a component of fruits, vegetables, and grains. Fiber is indigestible and softens stool. It also lowers intracolonic pressure so that stool is easy to pass.

The American Dietetic Association recommends 20 to 35 grams of fiber every day. Foods high in fiber include whole grain cereal and bread; fruits such as peaches and apples; vegetables such as carrots, squash, broccoli, cabbage; and starchy vegetables such as lima beans and kidney beans. See **Table 7-4** for a sampling of foods with high fiber content. When adding fiber to the older adult's diet, do so very slowly. If it is added in large amounts, the individual will have gas pains, a bloated abdomen, and probably diarrhea.

Diverticulosis and Diverticulitis

A diverticulum is a pouching out of the colon in a weak spot, usually in the sigmoid colon, although in people of Japanese descent it occurs most often in the right colic flexure. Approximately 10% of adults in the United States age 40 and older; 30% of those age 60 and older; and 65% of those 85 and older have **diverticulosis**. If these pouches become inflamed, the disorder is called **diverticulitis** (**Figure 7-4**). Diverticulitis occurs in 10% to 25% of people with diverticulosis, and 10% have bleeding. The incidence of diverticulitis is higher in developed countries, in which fiber intake is lower.

The cause of diverticulosis is thought to be a low-fiber diet. The disease is rare in countries where people eat high-fiber vegetable diets. The incidence is low in Western vegetarian diets, and in Africa and Asia it is nearly unknown. Straining at stool may contribute to the development of diverticula.

Diverticulitis can occur with infection. It can develop suddenly and without warning. Abdominal pain; tenderness in the left side of the abdomen; and fever, nausea, vomiting, chills, and cramping may occur. Perforations, tears, and blockages

diverticulosis Small outpouchings in the colon and large intestine. They increase with age, so that most 80-year-olds have diverticula. They may be asymptomatic or there may be cramping and bloating.

diverticulitis Infection and inflammation of the diverticula. The patient will have fever, left-sided pain, constipation, and diarrhea. The worst possibility is that it perforates the wall of the colon. The best preventative measure is eating fiber, which keeps the colon active.

TABLE 7-4 Foods with High Fiber Content

Food	Serving	Fiber Content (g)
All-Bran cereal	½ cup	9.6
Post Bran Flakes	¾ cup	5.3
Kidney beans	½ cup	5.7
Cooked spinach	1 cup	4.3
Raw broccoli	1 medium stalk	3.9
Apple	1	4
Cooked carrots	½ cup	2.5
Baked beans	½ cup	6.5
Baked potato	1	3
Whole wheat bread	1 slice	2
Tomato	1	1
Romaine lettuce	1 cup	1

Sources: National Digestive Diseases Information Clearinghouse. Fecal incontinence. NIH Publication No. 04-4816. March 2004. Available at: http://digestive.niddk.nih.gov/ddiseases/pubs/fecalincontinence/index.htm. Accessed September 27, 2004; U.S. Department of Agriculture (USDA) Nutrient Database for Standard Reference, Release 15. See http://www.nal.usda.gov/fnic/cgi-bin/nut_search.pi.

of the colon may occur. Considerable bleeding may occur if the small blood vessel in the diverticulum weakens and bursts. If the infection continues, an abscess can occur, then perforation, and even peritonitis—the leaking of pus and infection into the intra-abdominal area. Antibiotics are essential in management, as is surgery. Peritonitis can be fatal. Scarring from infection can cause partial or total blockage of the colon, which can back up the stool and become an emergency situation.

Treatment for diverticular disease is a high-fiber diet. Fiber keeps stool soft and lowers intra-colonic pressure so that stool can move through easily. The American Dietetic Association recommends 20–35 grams of fiber every day.

Foods high in fiber include whole grain cereal and bread; fruits such as peaches and apples; vegetables such as carrots, squash, broccoli, cabbage; and starchy vegetables such as lima beans and kidney beans. Antibiotics (rifaximin) plus dietary fiber supplements and laxatives such as methylcellulose and lactulose are recommended, but their usefulness remains unproven. Calcium antagonists have been found to have a protective effect.

Constipation

Constipation is a symptom of a problem, rather than a disorder or disease. The problem of constipation increases with age, and it is more common in women. The international definition of constipation includes two or more of the following symptoms for 12 months (without taking laxatives):

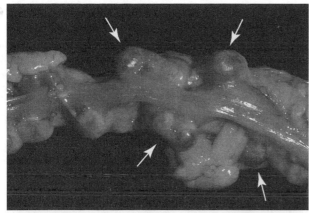

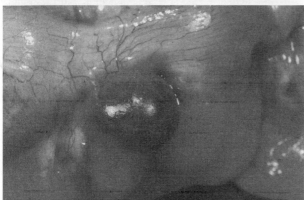

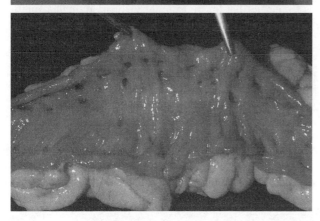

FIGURE 7-4 Diverticula of Colon

Reproduced from *An Introduction to Human Disease*. 7th ed. Photo courtesy of Leonard V. Crowley, M. D., Century College.

- Strains 25% of the time
- Hard stools 25% of the time
- Feeling of incomplete evacuation 25% of the time
- Two or fewer bowel movements per week

> **BOX 7-5 Commonly Used Drugs Associated with Constipation and Their Approximate Incidence**
>
> | | |
> |---|---|
> | Alprazolam (10–25%) | Ondansetron (10%) |
> | Bupropion (25%) | Oxybutynin XL (20%) |
> | Clonidine (10%) | Oxycodone (20%) |
> | Epoetin (40–50%) | Pamidronate (30%) |
> | Fentanyl transderm (10%+) | Tramadol (25–45%) |
> | Mirtazapine (12%) | Ursodiol (10–25%) |
> | Morphine (25–70%) | Venlafaxine (15%) |
> | Nefazodone (10–15%) | |
>
> *Source:* Thomas D. Clinical consensus: the constipation crisis in long-term care. *Ann Long-Term Care.* 2003;11(suppl):3–14.

Constipation can be caused by constipation-predominant IBS, inactivity, dehydration, and certain drugs, such as opiates and anticholinergics (see **Box 7-5** for drugs associated with constipation). Diets low in fiber and inadequate fluid intake put the individual more at risk. Older adults may experience constipation if they fail to attend to the feeling of needing to defecate (e.g., being out shopping and not going to the bathroom when the "signal" occurs) or because of incomplete defecation. Other risk factors include depression, Parkinson's disease, hypercalcemia, hypokalemia, hypothyroidism, Diabetes mellitus, tumor, stroke, spinal cord injury, and uremia.

In the assessment of constipation, patients should be asked how they define constipation in terms of frequency, character of stools, and associated symptoms such as straining. A diet assessment should follow, with a focus on appropriate fiber and fluid intake. The person's defecation habits should be assessed. Potential medical causes should be determined, when possible. The person should be screened for contributing factors, such as anxiety, depression, and dementia. In addition, a review of the person's medications should be reviewed for a possible cause. For example, iron supplements, narcotics, anticholinergics, antacids, and laxatives (stimulants) can all cause or contribute to constipation.

See **Box 7-6** for medical diagnoses that should be considered for chronic constipation.

Management of constipation includes adding fluids, consuming more dietary fiber, increasing physical activity, and identifying and stopping (with medical consultation) medications that may enhance constipation. Liquids that help manage constipation include water, prune, grape, and apricot juice. The power pudding recipe combines

BOX 7-6 Medical Diagnoses Associated with Constipation

Irritable bowel syndrome (IBS)	Uremia
Parkinson disease	Hypercalcemia (hyperparathyroidism)
Multiple sclerosis	Amyloid
Prior colon surgery	Cancers
Hypothyroidism	Volvulus
Diabetes mellitus	Strictures
Hypophosphatemia	Rectocele
Hypomagnesemia	Intussusception

Sources: Thomas D. Clinical consensus: the constipation crisis in long-term care. *Ann Long-Term Care.* 2003;11(suppl):3–14; Ali M, Lacy B. 2004. Abdominal complaints and gastrointestinal disorders. In: Landefeld C, Palmer R, Johnson M, et al., eds. *Current Geriatric Diagnosis and Treatment.* New York: McGraw-Hill; 2004:220–238.

on the size of the patient and the humidity. If humidity is low, more fluids will be needed. Also, if the individual has been perspiring, more fluids are needed. Further, many fluids are obtained through lettuce and other foods with a high percentage of water.

Additional interventions include bowel training—regularity, biofeedback, medications, and surgery. Nondietary management is also available. See **Box 7-7** for a list of constipation management techniques.

Impaction

Fecal impaction is a frightening occurrence for the older person and a difficult problem for the caregiver to manage. Impaction occurs when chronic constipation is not managed well, often when the individual is dehydrated or on opioids (e.g., morphine). It can also occur when the individual is on anticholinergic drugs and antidiarrhea medications. It occurs frequently in older adults who have become bedridden, such as in late dementia. The feces become extremely hard and stop moving. Watery diarrhea may occur, moving around the hard stool; this should raise suspicion rather than be treated, which would worsen the situation.

Usually, fecal impaction is managed by manual removal, by enemas, or both; however, it can require surgical removal or removal through colonoscopy or sigmoidoscopy. The patient should then be placed on a stool softener, such as docusate, and bulk-fiber laxatives, such as Metamucil, which add bulk and fluid to the stool. Dietary management is similar to that for managing constipation: increasing fiber intake from whole wheat grains, bran, and fresh fruits and vegetables will add bulk to the stool and promote bowel movements. Increasing fluid intake is important, too.

Diarrhea

Diarrhea is defined as bowel movements that are increased in number or frequency (more than three per day), more liquid in consistency, and more difficult to control. **Fecal incontinence** is the inability to control bowel movements. Diarrhea

bran, applesauce, and prune juice. This recipe has been very effective in the long-term care setting. Power pudding is quite palatable to older adults and is very effective. It is important to begin with small amounts of pudding to avoid cramping and discomfort. Start with a tablespoon a day and slowly advance on a daily basis until the desired effect occurs, then maintain that dose. No medications should be necessary with this dietary intervention, although sufficient fluid intake is essential. Six to eight glasses of water each day is the usual advice, although this is certainly dependent

fecal incontinence The inability to hold a bowel movement until one is able to get to the toilet. It may occur when passing gas. Occurs in those with dementia and those with neurological damage. It occurs more frequently in older adults and in women.

BOX 7-7 Constipation Management

I. Early Management	II. Next level	III. Needs PRN agents	IV. Severe constipation
Increase fluids	Stool softeners	Milk of Magnesia	Stimulants: senna, bisacodyl
Increased dietary fiber	Bulking agents	Lactulose	
Increase exercise	Suppositories (glycerin)	Sorbitol	
Bowel training			
Education			

Source: Ali M, Lacy B. 2004. Abdominal complaints and gastrointestinal disorders. In: Landefeld C, Palmer R, Johnson M, et al., eds. *Current Geriatric Diagnosis and Treatment.* New York: McGraw-Hill; 2004:220–238.

can be a symptom of an illness. Diarrhea is the second most common cause of death in the world and a sign of one of the four most common infectious illnesses in older nursing home patients in the United States. The most common infection is viral gastroenteritis, a mild viral infection that goes away on its own within a few days. It is often called the "stomach flu" (**Figure 7-5**). Food poisoning and traveler's diarrhea are caused from eating food or drinking water contaminated with bacteria or parasites. Acute diarrhea lasts less than two weeks; this is a very long time and a dangerous problem in the older adult. An individual experiencing loose stools for longer than four weeks has chronic diarrhea.

As mentioned earlier, diarrhea can be caused by constipation, or, more likely, fecal impaction. It is a component of IBS. It can be caused by malabsorption syndromes such as lactase deficiency (i.e., lactose intolerance). Lactase deficiency increases with age and is common worldwide. It is characterized by bloating, abdominal distention, and loose stools.

Diarrhea can be managed in a number of different ways. Foods that contribute to diarrhea should be limited. For many older adults, these foods include caffeinated drinks; chocolate and chocolate drinks; alcohol; carbonated drinks; dairy products; smoked and cured meats; fatty, greasy foods; and sweeteners—sorbitol, xylitol, mannitol, and fructose—found in fruit juices, diet drinks, sugarless chewing gum, and candy.

Another management technique is for the person with diarrhea to eat smaller meals more frequently. Large meals cause bowel contractions that may lead to diarrhea. Diarrhea may also result if fiber is added too quickly to the diet. In addition, the patient should eat and drink at different times. Digestion will slow if the individual drinks 30 minutes before or after a meal, but not with the meal.

A variety of foods are thought to slow digestion. These include bread, oatmeal, rice, potatoes, bananas, tapioca, yogurt, cheese, and smooth peanut butter. These foods also add bulk to the stool. Yogurt contains probiotics (beneficial bacteria) that can shorten the course of diarrhea and lessen its severity. Pectin, a form of dietary fiber found in apples and citrus peel, is also helpful. The person should consume foods high in potassium, if tolerated, to replace lost electrolytes. A diet of broth, tea, and toast and avoidance of the liquids, food, and sweeteners mentioned earlier can reduce diarrhea until it subsides.

Fluid replacement is necessary to prevent dehydration. Caffeinated beverages and milk, which may prolong loose stools, should be avoided. However, milk may be useful if the diarrhea is quite mild, because it contains needed fluids and nourishment.

Fecal Incontinence

Fecal incontinence is the inability to control bowel movements. Similar to urinary incontinence, the individual may feel the urge to evacuate but cannot get to the toilet in time. In addition, stool may leak unexpectedly from the anus. Fecal incontinence is more common in older women than other age groups. It is less common in younger men, but becomes more common as men age.

Constipation is the most common cause of fecal incontinence. Large, hardened stools lodge in the rectum and watery stools leak out around them. Foods that contribute to diarrhea may also contribute to fecal incontinence by relaxing the internal anal sphincter. Other causes of fecal incontinence include anal sphincter muscle damage, nerve damage to the nerves of the anal sphincter or rectum, a loss of storage capacity in the rectum, diarrhea, and pelvic floor dysfunction. A major cause of fecal incontinence in women is damage to the nerves around the anus caused by trauma during childbirth. Other causes of nerve damage include diabetes and multiple sclerosis.

The individual with fecal incontinence is usually referred to a proctologist; however, some management efforts should be tried before referral is made. Management of constipation is a priority, if that appears to be a problem. High-fiber foods will add bulk and make stools easier to control. However, if constipation is not the problem, high-fiber foods may cause diarrhea and contribute to the problem.

Hemorrhoids

This is a condition in which the veins of the anus or lower rectum are swollen and inflamed because of increased pressure in the veins in that area. Approximately 50% of

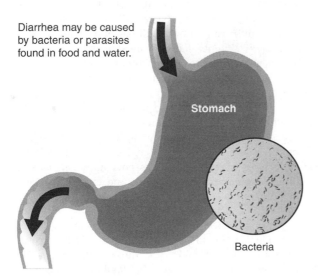

Diarrhea may be caused by bacteria or parasites found in food and water.

Stomach

Bacteria

FIGURE 7-5 Stomach Diarrhea, Bacteria That Helps Form It

Source: National Institutes of Health, 2008.

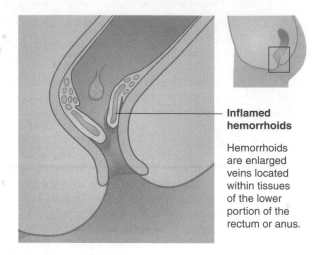

Inflamed hemorrhoids

Hemorrhoids are enlarged veins located within tissues of the lower portion of the rectum or anus.

FIGURE 7-6 Inflamed Hemorrhoids

Source: National Institutes of Health, 2008.

the population has had hemorrhoids by age 50. In younger people, hemorrhoids often develop because of straining at stool and after childbirth. Hemorrhoids in older adults can be caused by chronic constipation, an anal canal that slides downward, prolonged sitting, and anal intercourse. Hemorrhoids may be internal (inside the anus) or external (under the skin around the anus) (**Figure 7-6**).

Complications of hemorrhoids include fissures, abscesses, fistulae, and itching, which is called *pruritus ani*. The hemorrhoid may also become thrombosed, which occurs when a blood clot forms in the hemorrhoid's blood vessel. One symptom of hemorrhoids is bleeding, which can produce a bright red spot of blood on the toilet tissue. Occasionally, blood clots may also be seen.

Without treatment, hemorrhoids may disappear in a few days. However, hemorrhoids can become a cycle of straining, itching, rubbing, and bleeding. When there is bleeding, the anal area should be evaluated by a health care professional.

Clearly, it makes good sense to maintain regularity of stools and a soft consistency. A high-fiber diet and sufficient fluids are essential. Management of any constipation is essential as well (see the previous discussion of constipation). Warm tub baths in warm water several times a day for 10 minutes is helpful for managing an acute hemorrhoid problem. If the individual is bed-bound, soothe the affected area with warm moist cloths. Hemorrhoid creams and suppositories can be useful, and bulking agents can help to minimize straining. Nonsurgical treatments for hemorrhoids include injection sclerotherapy, electrocoagulation, cryotherapy, and laser therapy. Surgery should only be considered if nonsurgical treatments are not successful.

Gastrointestinal Tract Cancers

Chronic GERD is a known risk factor for esophageal cancer, and GERD is on the rise. Today, esophageal cancer is six to eight times more prevalent than it was in the 1970s, and its incidence is increasing more rapidly than any other cancer in the United States. The 5-year survival rate is 12%. Those with significant reflux have 10 times the risk of those without significant GERD. Men have 4 times the risk of developing this cancer compared to women. Risk factors include age; most people who get esophageal cancer are older than age 60. The American Cancer Society states that the majority of people with esophageal cancer are between 70 and 84 years of age. Nearly 80% are between the ages of 55 and 84.

Other risk factors include male sex, race, lifestyle choices, and preexisting conditions. African Americans are twice as likely to develop it compared to White Americans. Other risk factors are tobacco use and alcohol use, and those who use both alcohol and tobacco are at an especially high risk for esophageal cancer. Long-term gastric acid reflux may lead to Barrett's esophagus, a chronic irritation to the lower esophagus, which may become malignant over time. A history of another head or neck cancer increases risk for esophageal cancer. Obese men are 50% more likely to die of this cancer. Dietary risk factors include low intake of fruits and vegetables and vitamins A, B$_2$, and C.

Esophageal cancer does not present with early symptoms, and when symptoms do occur it is usually quite late in the course of the disease. The symptoms and signs of esophageal cancer are difficulty swallowing; severe weight loss; pain in the throat or back behind the breastbone or between the shoulder blades; hoarseness or chronic cough; vomiting; and coughing up blood. All of these signs and symptoms can be caused by conditions other than esophageal cancer, so a proper diagnosis must be made.

Treatment is similar to other methods of cancer care (see the chapter on cancer and nutrition). The individual with esophageal cancer must consume enough calories and protein to control weight loss and maintain strength. Many older adults with this type of cancer find it difficult to eat well because of difficulty swallowing. They do not feel like eating if they are uncomfortable and tired. Also, common side effects of treatment, such as poor appetite, nausea, vomiting, dry mouth, mouth sores, and change in taste, make it difficult to consume enough calories.

Following surgical treatment, nutrition may be parenteral or through a feeding tube, usually nasogastric, until the individual is able to eat. Individuals should be encouraged to eat small meals and snacks throughout the day. The patient may be able to manage soft, bland foods moistened with sauces or gravies. Pudding, ice cream, and soup are nourishing, easy to swallow, and may feel good. The use of a blender is helpful to process solid foods. A booklet from the National Cancer Institute, *Eating Hints for Cancer Patients*, which can be found at the institute's website, offers a number of valuable suggestions.

Prevention is based on decreasing or preventing risk factors. Risk may be decreased nutritionally through a diet high in cruciferous foods such as cabbage, broccoli, and cauliflower. Green and yellow vegetables and fruits have also been found to diminish risk.

Stomach Cancer (Gastric Cancer)

Stomach cancer occurs mainly in adults older than age 65. Two-thirds of people who have it are over 65 years old. It occurs more frequently in those who have had *H. pylori* infections of the stomach or gastric inflammation. It is more common in men; smokers; those with a family history of stomach cancer; and those who frequently consume pickled, salted foods. See **Box 7-8** for additional risk factors for stomach cancer.

Early symptoms of stomach cancer are vague, such as indigestion or stomach discomfort. Once symptoms do appear—blood in the stool, vomiting, unexplained weight loss, and jaundice—it is late in the disease course and the cancer is difficult to treat (**Figure 7-7**). Treatments include surgery, radiation, chemotherapy, antiangiogenesis therapy, bone marrow and blood stem cell transplantation, gene therapy, photodynamic therapy, hyperthermia, lasers, and compassionate drug use in the latest stage.

Colorectal Cancer

Colorectal cancer is the third most common cancer of men and women in the United States and occurs equally in older men and women. Deaths also occur equally in men and women. Indeed, patients older than age 65 are the fastest growing segment of the cancer population. It is estimated that within 20 years, over 75% of cases and 85% of deaths from colorectal cancer will be in this age group. However, the incidence of this cancer has been decreasing over the last 2 decades, which is thought to be due to the increase in screening. See Chapter 12 on cancer and nutrition in older adults.

Risk factors in addition to age include inherited genetic mutations (familial adenomatous polyposis and others), family history of colorectal cancer, and personal history of chronic inflammatory bowel disease. Modifiable factors associated with increased risk for this cancer include smoking, obesity, physical inactivity, a diet high in processed or red meats, and inadequate intake of fruits and vegetables. Studies do indicate that obese men and women are more likely to develop and die of colorectal cancer.

Chemoprevention of colorectal cancers in those who have familial adenomatous polyps of the bowel that will later be-

---

BOX 7-8 Risk Factors for Stomach Cancer

Infection	*Helicobacter pylori*
Gender	Greater for men
Aging	Greater in adults older than age 50, especially 60s through 80s
Geography	Greater in Japan, China, Southern and Eastern Europe, South and Central America
Ethnicity	Greater for Hispanic Americans, Asian/Pacific, Islanders, African Americans, less for non-Hispanic Whites
Diet	Smoked foods, salted fish, meat; pickled vegetables, nitrates, and nitrites in cured meats
Tobacco	Use doubles incidence of stomach cancer, especially near the esophagus
Obesity	Probably increases risk of cancer near the esophagus
Previous stomach surgery	E.g., ulcer surgery for as long as 15 years after surgery
Pernicious anemia	Slight risk with this disease, but worth screening
Hypertrophic gastropathy (Menetrier disease)	Excess growth of stomach lining leads to large folds and low levels of stomach acid (rare)
Type A blood	Higher risk of stomach cancer (reason unknown)
Inherited cancer syndromes	Rare, genetic, but risk is 70% to 80%; family history of stomach cancer increases risk
Stomach polyps	Some types of polyps, noncancerous, adenomas, can develop into cancer
Epstein-Barr virus infection	Causes stomach cancer in 5% to 10% of those with virus; a less aggressive cancer
Occupations	Coal, metal, rubber industries

Source: American Cancer Society. What are the risk factors for stomach cancer? 2007. Available at: http://www.cancer.org/docroot/CRI/content/CRI_2_4_2X_What_are_the_risk_factors_for_stomach_cancer_40.asp. Accessed June 11, 2009.

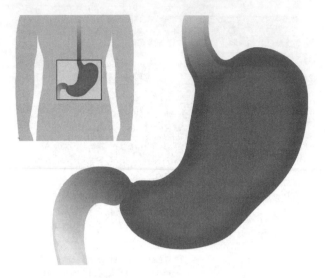

FIGURE 7-7 The Stomach

Source: National Institutes of Health, 2008.

come cancerous has been demonstrated by the use of Sulindac and Celicoxib (a COX-2 inhibitor) NSAIDS, and hormones such as estrogen and progesterone, although these drugs are not recommended for prevention at this time. These agents may actually prevent or reverse the development of colorectal cancer. Because the survival rate of this cancer is so poor, the emphasis is on prevention.

Flavonoids have been tested to prevent the recurrence risk of neoplasia in patients with resected colorectal cancer and after adenoma polypectomy. In one study by Hoensch, Groh, Edler, and Kirch, one group of patients was treated with a flavonoid mixture every day and another was not. After 3–4 years, there was no recurrence and only one polyp in the flavonoid group. In the control group, 20% experienced recurrence and adenomatous polyps appeared in four patients. Although this was a small study, the authors concluded that the recurrence rate of this cancer can be reduced with sustained long-term treatment with a flavonoid mixture.

In terms of chemotherapy treatment for the cancer, bowel mucosal injury associated with 5-fluorouracil frequently results in severe diarrhea and, probably, lactose intolerance. This results in a poor nutritional status in these patients. In one study by Osterlund and colleagues, *Lactobacillus* cap-

sules provided no benefit to patients. This may be due to inadequate dosage, but the researchers recommend lactose dietary restriction in these patients.

Activities Related to This Chapter

1. Test yourself on the key terms and concepts introduced in this chapter.
2. Search the Internet for topics related to this chapter. Report your findings to your classmates.
3. Visit the Nutrition Screening Initiative website (www.aafp.org/afp/980301ap/edits.html).
4. Visit the American Cancer Society website (www.cancer.org) for information on nutrition and cancer.
5. In a small group, discuss the processes of digestion and causes of age-related problems.
6. Discuss how to manage constipation in older adults.

Case Study

Mrs. Williams, age 80, has been widowed for two years. Recently, her vision has worsened and her osteoarthritis keeps her in her chair much of the day. She has stopped many of her social activities. She has a son and daughter who live within an hour driving time, but they visit only on weekends. She enjoys her grandchildren at that time, also. She receives Meals on Wheels for lunch and supper, but a review of her refrigerator shows that they have piled up, uneaten for the most part. She has lost 15 pounds in the past six months.

Questions

1. What are the areas of Mrs. Williams' life that are risk factors for malnutrition?
2. What are other risk factors for poor nutrition in older adults living in the community?
3. What problems can occur in a woman who is sedentary, lacking in social activities, and eating poorly?
4. What can a health professional do to change this situation? What would you do?
5. Are there any assessment tools that can be used to help identify all the problems in an individual with possible malnutrition?

REFERENCES

A.D.A.M. Medical Encyclopedia [online]. Diarrhea. 2006. Available at: http://www.nlm.nih.gov/medlineplus/ency/article003126.htm. Accessed April 20, 2008.

A.D.A.M. Medical Encyclopedia [online]. Esophageal cancer. 2006. Available at: http://www.nlm.nih.gov/medlineplus/ency/article/003126.htm. Accessed April 20, 2008.

Akhtar A. Acute diarrhea in frail elderly nursing home patients. *J Am Med Dir Assoc.* 2003;4(1):34–39.

Ali M, Lacy B. 2004. Abdominal complaints and gastrointestinal disorders. In: Landefeld C, Palmer R, Johnson M, et al., eds. *Current Geriatric Diagnosis and Treatment.* New York: McGraw-Hill; 2004:220–238.

American Cancer Society. 2008. Cancer facts and figures. Available at: http://www.cancer.org/downloads/STT/2008CAFFfinalsecured.pdf. Accessed January 30, 2009.

American Cancer Society. Milk may lower colon cancer risk. July 26, 2004. Available at: http://www.cancer.org/docroot/NWS/content?NWS_1_1x_Milk_May_Lower_Colon_Cancer_Risk.asp?sitearea = NWS&viewmode = print&. Accessed October 23, 2004.

American Cancer Society. What are the risk factors for stomach cancer? 2007. Available at: http://www.cancer.org/docroot/cri/content/cri_2_4_2x_what-are-the-risk-factors-for_stomach_cancer_40.asp?sitearea = . Accessed April 20, 2008.

American Geriatric Society. *Geriatric Nursing Review Syllabus.* New York: American Geriatric Society; 2007.

American Geriatric Society. *Geriatrics Review Syllabus.* 6th ed. New York: American Geriatric Society; 2006.

Andrews CN, Shaffer E. Diverticular disease of the colon: review and update. *Geriatrics Aging.* 2002;5(10):11–16.

Arber N, Levin B. Chemoprevention of colorectal neoplasia: the potential personalized medicine. *Gastroenterology.* 2008;134(4):1224–1237.

Beverley L, Travis I. Constipation: proposed natural laxative mixtures. *J Gerontol Nurs.* 1992;18:5.

Bhala N, Lanas A. Low-dose acetylsalicyclic acid and the use of gastroprotectors among older adults. *Geriatrics Aging.* 2008;11(1):53–58.

Bishara J, Peled N, Pitlik S, Samra Z. Mortality of patients with antibiotic-associated diarrhoea: the impact of *Clostridium difficile. J Hosp Med.* 2008;68(4):308–314.

Centers for Disease Control and Prevention. Public health and aging: retention of natural teeth among older adults—United States, 2002. *MMWR.* 2003;52(50):1226–1229. Available at: http://www.cdc.gov/mmwr/preview/mmwrhtml/mm5250a3.htm. Accessed September 27, 2004.

Clarren S. (2004). Diverticular disease. In: Meiner S, ed. *Care of Gastrointestinal Problems in Older Adults.* New York: Springer; 2004:177–200.

Dupee RM. Acute intestinal ischemia in the elderly. *Ann Long-Term Care.* 2008;16(4):34–36.

Dysphagia Institute at Froedtert Hospital, Medical College of Wisconsin. Dysphagia Institute focuses on swallowing disorders. 1999. Available at: http://www.mcw.edu/gastro/dys.htm. Accessed December 2, 2000.

Finlay E, Straton J, Gavrin J. Nausea and vomiting: an overview of mechanisms and treatment in older patients. *Geriatrics Aging.* 2007;10(2):116–121.

Folden S, Backer J, Maynard F, et al. Practice guidelines for the management of constipation in adults. 2003. Available at: http://www.guideline.gov/summary/summary.aspx?view_id = 1&doc_id = 3687. Accessed February 5, 2004.

Fraunfelder M. Dysphagia Institute. October 17, 2007. Available at: http://www.froedtert.org/SpecialtyAreas/Gastroenterology/ProgramsandServices/Programs/DsyphagiaInstitute.htm. Accessed March 20, 2008.

Galvan T. Dysphagia: going down and staying down. *Am J Nurs.* 2001;101(1):37–44.

Gunter D. A nursing guide to the assessment of GERD in long-term care. *The Director.* 2004;12(4):221–228.

Harrison R, Marrie TJ. Aspiration pneumonia among older adults. *Geriatrics Aging.* 2008;11(2):111–115.

Hasler WL. Gastroparesis: current concepts and considerations. *Medscape J Med.* 2008;10(1):16.

Hill C. Gastroesophageal reflux disease. In: Meiner S, ed. *Care of Gastrointestinal Problems in the Older Adult.* New York: Springer; 2004:23–46.

Hoensch H, Groh B, Edler L, Kirch W. Prospective cohort comparison of flavonoid treatment in patients with resected colorectal cancer to prevent recurrence. *World J Gastroenterol.* 2008;14(14):2187–2193.

Huether S. Alterations of digestive function. In: McCance K, Huether S, eds. *Pathophysiology.* 5th ed. Philadelphia: Elsevier; 2006:1385–1446.

Huether S. Structure and function of the digestive system. In: McCance K, Huether S, eds. *Pathophysiology.* 4th ed. St. Louis: Mosby; 2002:1231–1337.

Humes D, Simpson J, Spiller R. Colonic diverticular disease. *BMJ Clinical Evidence* [online]. 2007. Available at: http://clinicalevidence.bmj.com.

Insel P, Turner RE, Ross D. *Nutrition.* 3rd ed. Sudbury, MA: Jones & Bartlett; 2007.

Jackson/Siegelbaum Gastroenterology. 2008. Gastroparesis diet for delayed stomach emptying. Available at: http://www.gicare.com/Diets/Gastroparesis.aspx. Accessed February 2, 2009.

Kaltenbach T, Crockett S, Gerson LB. Are lifestyle measures effective in patients with gastroesophageal reflux disease? *Arch Intern Med.* 2006;166:965–971.

Klapproth JA, Yang VW. 2008. Malabsorption. Available at: http://emedicine.medscape.com/article/180785-print. Accessed February 2, 2009.

Lomer MC, Parkes GC, Sanderson J. Lactose intolerance in clinical practice: myths and realities. *Aliment Pharm Ther.* 2008;27(2):93–103.

Lowenfels AB. Recovery after abdominal surgery: is early feeding preferable? A best evidence review. January 22, 2008. Available at: http://www.medscape.com/viewarticle/568983. Accessed January 30, 2008.

Luggen AS. Pharmacology update: GERD. *Geriatric Nurs.* 2005;26(1):5.

Mayer EA. Irritable bowel syndrome. *New Engl J Med.* 2008;358(16):1692–1741.

Mayhew M, Edmunds M, Wendel V. *Gerontological Nurse Practitioner Review Manual.* Washington, DC: American Nurses Credentialing Center; 2001.

Mayo Clinic. December 2008. C. difficile. Available at: http://www.mayoclinic.com/print/c-difficile/DS00736/METHOD = print&DSECTION = all. Accessed February 2, 2009.

Mayo Clinic. Intestinal ischemia. 2006. Available at: http://www.mayoclinic.com/print/intestinal-ischemia/DS00459/METHOD = print&DSECTION = all. Accessed April 19, 2008.

Mayo Clinic. February 2008. Lactose intolerance. Available at: http://www.mayoclinic.com/print/lactose-intolerance/DS00530/METHOD = print&DSECTI. Accessed February 2, 2009.

Medical Association Communications. *Symposium Highlights for Nurse Practitioners.* Anaheim, CA: Medical Association Communications; 2003.

Meiner S. *Care of Gastrointestinal Problems in the Older Adult.* New York: Springer; 2004.

Merck Manual of Geriatrics. Malabsorption. 2006. Available at: http://www.merck.com/mrkshared/mmg/sec/ch111/ch111a.jsp. Accessed March 23, 2006.

National Cancer Institute. April 2008. Esophageal cancer prevention. Available at: http://www.cancer.gov/cancertopics/pdq/prevention/esophageal/healthprofessional. Accessed February 2, 2009.

National Cancer Institute. 2008. Gastric cancer. Available at: http://www.nlm.nih.gov/medlineplus/stomachcancer.html. Accessed February 2, 2009.

National Cancer Institute. Nausea and vomiting. Available at: http://www.cancer.gov/cancertopics/pdq/supportivecare/nausea/healthprofessional. Accessed March 30, 2009.

National Center for Chronic Disease Prevention and Health Promotion. Oral health for older Americans. December 18, 2003. Available at: http://www.cdc.gov/OralHealth/factsheets/adult-older.htm. Accessed September 27, 2004.

National Digestive Diseases Information Clearinghouse. Diverticulosis and diverticulitis. NIH Publication No. 04-1163. April 2004. Available at: http://digestive.niddk.nih.gov/ddiseases/pubs/diverticulosis/index.htm. Accessed April 30, 2004.

National Digestive Diseases Information Clearinghouse. Fecal incontinence. NIH Publication No. 04-4816. March 2004. Available at: http://digestive.niddk.nih.gov/ddiseases/pubs/fecalincontinence/index.htm. Accessed September 27, 2004.

National Digestive Diseases Information Clearinghouse. 2007. Heartburn, gastroesophageal reflux (GER), and gastroesophageal reflux disease (GERD). Available at: http://digestive.niddk.nih.gov/ddiseases/pubs/gerd/. Accessed March 30, 2009.

National Digestive Diseases Information Clearinghouse. Hemorrhoids. NIH Publication No. 02-3021. February 2002. Available at: http://digestive.niddk.nih.gov/ddiseases/pubs/hemorrhoids/index.htm. Accessed September 27, 2004.

National Institute of Diabetes, Digestive, and Kidney Diseases. Irritable bowel syndrome. NIH Publication No. 07-693. September 2007. Available at: http://digestive.niddk.nih.gov/ddiseases/pubs/ibs/. Accessed February 2, 2009.

National Institute on Deafness and Other Communication Disorders. Dysphagia. Available at: http://www.nidcd.nih.gov/health/voice/dysph.asp. Accessed January 29, 2009.

National Institutes of Health/National Library of Medicine. January 2009. Researchers zero in on GI cancers. Available at: http://www.nlm.nih.gov/medlineplus/news/fullstory_73825.html. Accessed February 2, 2009.

Nordenstedt H, Zheng Z, Cameron A, et al. Postmenopausal hormone therapy as a risk factor for gastroesophageal reflux symptoms among female twins. *Gastroenterology.* 2008;134(4):921–928.

Osterlund P, Ruotsalainen T, Peuhkuri K. Lactose intolerance associated with adjuvant 5-fluorouracil-based chemotherapy for colorectal cancer. *Clin Gastroenterol Hepat.* 2004;2(8):696–703.

Resnick B. Nutrition and gastrointestinal diseases. In: Meiner S, ed. *Care of Gastrointestinal Problems in the Older Adult.* New York: Springer; 2004.

Reuben D, Herr K, Pacala J, et al. *Geriatrics at Your Fingertips, 2007–2008.* 7th ed. New York: American Geriatric Society; 2007.

Rhodes M. May 2008. Irritable bowel syndrome: controlling symptoms with diet. Available at: http://www.webmd.com/ibs/guide/controlling-irritable-bowel-syndrome-with-diet. Accessed February 2, 2009.

Rosati G, Bilancia D. Role of chemotherapy and novel biological agents in the treatment of elderly patients with colorectal cancer. *World J Gastroenterol.* 2008;14(12):1812–1822.

Saad R, Chey WD. Irritable bowel syndrome with constipation among older adults. *Geriatrics Aging.* 2007;10(2):84–90.

Stanley M, Blair K, Bear P. *Gerontological Nursing.* 3rd ed. Philadelphia: FA Davis; 2005.

Thomas D. Clinical consensus: the constipation crisis in long-term care. *Ann Long-Term Care.* 2003;11(suppl):3–14.

U.S. Department of Health and Human Services. *Oral Health in America: A Report of the Surgeon General.* Washington, DC: U.S. Department of Health and Human Services; 2000.

Aging and the Cardiovascular System

Ann Schmidt Luggen, PhD, GNP

· ·

CHAPTER OBJECTIVES   Upon completion of this chapter, the reader will be able to:

1. Describe the major cardiovascular problems in older adults
2. Delineate the risk factors for the major cardiac problems
3. Plan the nutritional management of hypertensive older adults
4. Describe the nutritional prevention of cardiac problems
5. Distinguish types of fat that are included in the healthy diet from those to be restricted
6. Review the foods that interact with warfarin therapy

KEY TERMS AND CONCEPTS

Arteriosclerosis

Atherosclerosis

Cholesterol

Heart failure (HF)

High density lipoproteins (HDL)

Hypertension

Low density lipoproteins (LDL)

Monounsaturated fats

Myocardial infarction (MI)

Polyunsaturated fats

Prehypertension

Saturated fats

Triglycerides

· ·

One in three (80,700,000) American adults have cardiovascular disease (CVD) (disease of the blood vessels of the heart), and one-half of these are age 60 and older. As the aged population increases, this number will also increase. **Heart failure (HF)**, the end stage of CVD, is the number one cause of hospitalization and rehospitalization in older adults and its incidence increases following age 65.

The most common problems of older adults affecting the cardiovascular system are **atherosclerosis** and **arteriosclerosis**, the accumulation of fatty materials that line the blood vessels of the body and block blood flow. They affect the arteries, including those at the periphery, as well as

heart failure (HF) A progressive disorder of the heart in which the heart is unable to pump sufficient blood for the body's metabolic demands. Results from such disorders as hypertension, rheumatic heart disease, coronary artery disease, and valve insufficiency.

atherosclerosis Deposition of fatty plaques within artery walls. Medium and large arteries acquire yellowish deposits (atheromatous plaques) composed of cholesterol, fat, cellular debris, and calcium. These plaques cause vessel walls to become thick and hardened.

arteriosclerosis Blood vessel walls become hardened and thickened with lipid deposits and lose their natural elasticity. This causes an increase in blood pressure and narrowing of the arteries of the heart and legs.

the brain and heart. Atherosclerotic cardiovascular disease (ASCVD) is the leading cause of death in the United States.

Morbidity and mortality can be managed and reduced with nutritional guidance. Many nutritional plans are provided by the National Institutes of Health (NIH), the Centers for Disease Control and Prevention (CDC), and other major groups, such as the American Heart Association (AHA).

Nutrition Epidemiology of Heart Disease

Caloric intake has been increasing among all age groups. The mean intake of calories as fat is 33% in men and 33.2% in women. Caloric intake of **saturated fat** is 10.8% for both men and women. White men are more likely to have elevated **cholesterol** from intake of saturated fats than African American men; however, Mexican American men have the highest rates of elevated cholesterol (**Table 8-1**). Mexican American men are more likely to be overweight than their White and African American counterparts. However, African American men have the highest rates of obesity followed by White men and then Mexican American men. Overweight is defined as a BMI of at least 25 kg/m2, whereas obesity is a BMI of at least 30 kg/m2.

Meat consumption is also rising. Today, it is 200 pounds per person per year, compared to 177 pounds in 1970.

The recommended intake of dietary fiber each day is 20–35 g, but American adults consume a daily average of 15.6–17.8 g for men and 13.6 g for women.

The highest proportion of adults who consume fruits and vegetables at least five times a day is White adults aged 65 and older with college degrees who do not smoke and who engage in leisure activities. Approximately 33% of U.S. adults consume fruit twice a day, and 27% consume vegetables three or more times a day. Children consume far less. One-third of infants and toddlers consume no fruits or vegetables on any given day, but 62% consume desserts and 20% eat candy and sweet beverages.

Each year, over $33 billion in medical costs and $9 billion in productivity is lost due to conditions associated with poor nutrition, such as heart disease, cancer, stroke, and diabetes. It is obvious that there is a need for more education about nutrition and cardiovascular health.

saturated fats Fatty acids found in animal products, palm oil, coconut oil, and cocoa butter. It is recommended that not more than 10% of calories come from saturated fats every day (per the 2005 Dietary Guidelines for Americans). The American Heart Association recommends less than 7% of energy per day from saturated fats.

cholesterol A waxy lipid (sterol) whose chemical structure contains multiple hydrocarbon rings.

Research on Heart Disease Prevention Through Diet

The Women's Health Initiative (WHI), an epidemiological study of nearly 50,000 older women (ages 50–79), proposed that a long-term intervention diet to reduce cancer that was low in fat and high in vegetables, fruits, and grains would also reduce cardiovascular risk. Over the eight years of the study, there was no significant reduction in heart disease, stroke, or cerebrovascular disease in postmenopausal women, which suggests that a more focused diet and lifestyle intervention may be necessary to achieve the desired results.

The prevention of heart disease through diet is a major focus of research. One study, OmniHeart (Optimal Macronutrient Intake Trial to Prevent Heart Disease), tested the effects of a controlled feeding trial of three healthy diet patterns on blood pressure, lipid levels, and estimated cardiovascular risk. The 164 subjects, who all had prehypertension or hypertension, followed the prescribed diet for 19 weeks. One diet was similar to the DASH diet, in that it was composed of 58% carbohydrate (CHO), 15% protein, and 27% fat. The second diet had 10% more protein, 10% less CHO, and more unsaturated fat. The third diet was higher in unsaturated fat and 10% less CHO (i.e., 48% CHO, 15% protein, 37% fat). Each diet had 6% saturated fat and 100–200 mg of cholesterol. Sodium was 2,300 mg, and calcium, magnesium, and potassium were consistent with the DASH diet. The researchers concluded that these dietary patterns offer flexibility in macronutrient intake that should make it easy for anyone to eat a heart-healthy diet and reduce the risk of cardiovascular disease.

A study by Katcher and colleagues in 2008 examined the influence of a whole-grain-enriched hypocaloric diet on cardiovascular risk factors in men and women with metabolic syndrome. The positive results included a moderate improvement in weight loss in the abdominal region in the whole-grain group compared to a refined-grain group; the CRP (C-reactive protein) diminished 38% in the whole-grain group, but remained unchanged in the refined-grain group. Both grain diets decreased LDL (the "bad" cholesterol) significantly.

A study by Wang and colleagues in 2008 following more than 28,000 middle-aged and older women found that the higher the amount of low-fat dairy product intake, calcium,

TABLE 8-1 Prevalence of Risk Factors Among Men for Heart Disease

	African American	White	Mexican American
High cholesterol	47.9%	44.8%	49.9%
Overweight	67.0	71.0	74.6
Obesity	30.8	30.2	29.1

Source: Data from American Heart Association (AHA). Heart disease and stroke statistics—2008 update. Available at: http://www.americanheart.org. Accessed February 19, 2008.

and vitamin D, the lower the risk for hypertension. However, the risk of high blood pressure did *not* change with calcium or vitamin D supplements. Other foods that can make a difference in avoiding heart disease can be found in **Table 8-2**.

In 2007, the American Heart Association updated its guidelines for preventing cardiovascular disease in women. The newer guidelines have expanded recommendations on lifestyle factors, including nutrition. Unregulated dietary

monounsaturated fats Fatty acids found in nuts; avocados; popcorn; whole-grain wheat products; oatmeal; and olive, canola, peanut, safflower, flaxseed, and sunflower oils. Lowers low density lipoproteins (the 'bad' lipids) and possibly raises the high density lipoproteins (the 'good' lipids). Protective against heart disease.

TABLE 8-2 Recommended Foods to Maintain a Healthy Heart

Food	Rationale: Lower high blood pressure to reduce high risk factors for heart disease.
Swiss chard	High in potassium, which then lowers sodium. Has 1,000 mg of potassium per cup; requirements are 4,000 mg/day. Rich in calcium and magnesium; helps prevent high blood pressure. Rainbow variety (yellow, red, pink stalks) is less bitter.
Herbs	Good salt substitute; salt has 2,400 mg sodium/tsp. Suggest chives, rosemary, parsley, sage, and thyme.
Nonfat/low-fat yogurt	Calcium and potassium are 50% higher than in low-fat milk. These minerals lower blood pressure, both systolic and diastolic.
Extra-virgin olive oil	Rich in **monounsaturated fats**. Lowers LDL cholesterol when it replaces saturated fats, such as butter, in the diet.
Almonds	Contain polyphenols that keep LDL cholesterol from adhering to artery walls. An ounce a day as part of a healthy diet may lower LDL cholesterol by 13% to 20%. Almonds are the most heart-healthy nut, but all nuts are healthy and protect against atherosclerosis. Almonds are a good source of calcium; heating them brings out the most flavor.
Salt	If one cannot avoid eating salt, use a mortar and pestle and crush *kosher* salt, which has only *one-half* the sodium as table salt.
	Rationale: Lower high blood sugar, which is a high risk factor for heart disease.
Carrots	Eating ½ cup of crunchy carrots or other dark yellow vegetable every day cuts the risk of diabetes by 27%. To enhance absorption, serve with a little fat, such as olive oil.
Barley	This grain is the least likely to spike the blood sugar. Contains a soluble fiber, beta-glucan, which is digested slowly. It lowers cholesterol levels. Barley flour can be substituted for all-purpose flour. Hulled barley has more fiber than pearl barley, but both are excellent grains.
Cayenne chili	The capsaicin in this product may lower blood sugar. The spice can be added in small quantities to many main or side dishes.
	Rationale: Weight loss—overweight or obese are high risk factors for heart disease.
Broccoli	Filling food: ½ cup has 27 calories and 3 g of fiber. Chop and season before cooking.
Pork, lean	A high-protein meal burns twice the number of calories as a high-carbohydrate one. Lean pork tenderloin has 122 calories; 3 ounces of pork top loin has 147 calories and 5 g fat.
Oranges	Only 65 calories and nearly always in season. Contains pectin, which stimulates fullness and helps control cholesterol.
	Rationale: Decreases inflammation—a high risk factor for heart disease if overweight or obese.
Salmon	A major source of omega-3-fatty acids, which help control inflammatory conditions. It contains three to six times the amount as other seafood. For those complaining of a fishy taste, poach it in milk or white wine or stock.
Black beans	Contain high amounts of magnesium. Magnesium lowers CRP (C-reactive protein, which is thought to be indicative of heart disease when elevated).
Dried cherries	Contain anthocyanins that help neutralize enzymes that cause plaque to break apart. Fresh cherries can do the same thing, but are less available year round.

Source: Adapted from Cicero K. 15 foods that can save your heart. Heart Health Center. February 1, 2008. Available at: http://www.webmd.com/heart/features/ 15-foods-can-save-your-heart. Accessed February 20, 2008.

supplements, such as folic acid, are not recommended. See **Box 8-1** for highlights of these changes.

Recent research has focused on the relationship of flavonoids and cardiovascular disease. Over 34,000 older women free of CVD were followed for 16 years in the Iowa Women's Health Study. Diets were evaluated over time. Researchers found an inverse relationship between foods rich in flavonoids (e.g., citrus such as grapefruit, strawberries, apples, pears, tea, wine, bran added to foods, and dark chocolate) and CVD and mortality. Interestingly, there was no association between the foods and stroke mortality.

Risk Factors for Cardiovascular Disease

Risk factors for cardiovascular disease in older adults include increasing age, male gender, heredity (including race), smoking, dyslipidemias, high blood pressure, physical inactivity, obesity and overweight, and diabetes. Diabetes is the most important risk factor and is discussed at length in Chapter 11.

Risk factors are identified by physicians by category of low to very high risk of morbidity and mortality to determine how aggressive treatment needs to be (**Table 8-3**). The "lower" category has 0–1 risk factors; "moderate" has 2 or more risk factors and a 10-year coronary artery disease (CAD) risk of less than 10%; "moderately high" has 2 or more risk factors and a 10-year CAD risk of 10–20%; "high" is cardiovascular disease (CVD), diabetes, peripheral artery disease, stroke, transient ischemia attack (TIA), or abdominal aortic aneurysm, diabetes mellitus (DM), or a 10-year CAD risk greater than 20%. The "very high" category is DM plus CVD, acute coronary syndrome, and multiple severe or poorly controlled risk factors. The 10-year risk of a myocardial infarction (MI) can be calculated by age and cholesterol levels.

As mentioned earlier, cardiovascular heart disease is the leading cause of death of men and women 65 years of age and older, and its incidence increases with age. Heart disease is the leading cause of death in women, killing nine times as many women as breast cancer. Each year, 60,000 more women than men die from heart disease. Women have a greater incidence of ischemic heart diseases (IHD), which is a microvascular dysfunction, and not just coronary artery disease, which is larger vessel dysfunction. Women's coronary arteries are smaller than men's and do not dilate to accommodate increased blood flow when needed. The prevalence of hypertension in older women is highest in

> **BOX 8-1** **American Heart Association Updated Guidelines for Preventing Cardiovascular Disease in Women**
>
> - Lifestyle changes to manage blood pressure: weight control, increased physical activity, alcohol moderation, sodium restriction, emphasis on fresh fruits and vegetables and low-fat dairy products.
> - Stop smoking; counsel, utilize nicotine replacement or other cessation therapy.
> - To lose weight, engage in a minimum of 60–90 minutes of moderate-intensity activity (brisk walks) on most to all days of the week.
> - Reduce saturated fats to less than 7% of calories when possible.
> - Increase omega-3 fatty acid intake: eat oily fish two times a week and/or consider a capsule supplement of 850–1000 mg of EPA and DHA in women who have heart disease; 2–4 g for women with high triglycerides.
> - No hormone replacement therapy or SERMS for prevention of heart disease.
> - *Do not use* antioxidant supplements (e.g., vitamin E, C, beta-carotene) for primary or secondary prevention of heart disease.
> - Do not use folic acid for prevention of heart disease, even in high risk women.
> - Consider routine low-dose aspirin in women 65 and older, whatever the CVD risk status, if benefits may outweigh risks.
> - Upper dosage of aspirin is 325 mg/day, not 162 mg/day.
> - Consider lowering LDL-c to less than 70 mg/dL in very high risk women with heart disease.
>
> EPA = eicosapentaenoic acid
>
> DHA = docosahexaenoic acid
>
> SERMS = selective estrogen receptor modulators
>
> *Source:* Data from American Heart Association (AHA). Updated guidelines advise focusing on women's lifetime heart risk. Journal Report. February 19, 2007. Available at: http://www.americanheart.org/presenter.jhtml?identifier=3045524. Accessed February 19, 2008.

TABLE 8-3 Risk Factors for 10-Year Survival

	Very Low Risk	Very High Risk
HBP	120/80	140/90
Cholesterol	200	240
HDL	50	40
DM	No	Yes
Cigarettes	No	Yes

Source: Data from American Heart Association (AHA). Heart disease and stroke statistics—2009 update. Available at: http://www.americanheart.org. Accessed July 13, 2009.

TABLE 8-4 Prevalence of Heart Disease and Hypertension by Race/Ethnicity

Ethnic Group	Heart Disease (%)	Hypertension (%)
Whites	12.0	21.0
African Americans	10.2	31.2
Hispanics/Latinos	8.3	20.3
Asians	6.7	19.4
Native Hawaiians/Pacific Islanders	22.4	—
American Indians/Alaska Natives	13.0	25.5

Source: Data from American Heart Association (AHA). Heart disease and stroke statistics—2008 update. Available at: http://www.americanheart.org. Accessed February 19, 2008.

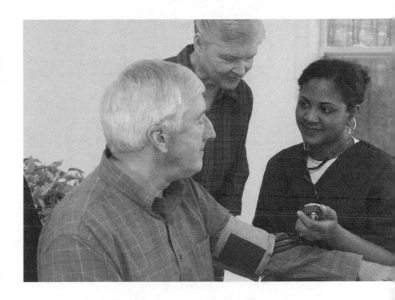

women over 75 (76.4%). The second highest prevalence is also in women, for those ages 65–74. Premenopausal high blood pressure (HBP) is a major risk factor for IHD, as is anemia. In addition, younger women with polycystic ovarian syndrome, which has many components of the metabolic syndrome, are also at increased risk of developing IHD.

The risk of cardiovascular disease (CVD) increases as blood pressure increases. Because African Americans often have elevated blood pressure, they have a higher mortality rate from CVD. African Americans are 1.3 times more likely to suffer a fatal stroke than their White counterparts, 1.5 times more likely to die from heart disease, and 4.2 times more likely to experience end-stage kidney disease. African American men also have a considerably higher death rate from high blood pressure (hypertension) than White males (49.7% vs. 14.9%). American Indians, Alaska Natives, Native Hawaiians, and Pacific Islanders share similar risks. See **Table 8-4** for data about heart disease and hypertension.

Risk Factors for Cardiovascular Disease

As cited in the introduction to this chapter, one in three American adults have CVD, and one-half of those with CVD are age 60 and older. The National Institutes of Health (NIH) National Heart, Lung, and Blood Institute (NHLBI) has developed programs, including Heart Truth Partners, to reach women of different ethnic and racial minorities in order to sound a "red alert" about the number one killer of women in an effort to inspire women to take action to reduce their risk for heart disease.

The initiative hopes to communicate that heart disease is more prevalent in African American women than White women and that the risk factors—hypertension, overweight, and diabetes—are higher in African American women. More than 80% of middle-aged African American women are overweight or obese, 52% have hypertension, and 14% have been diagnosed with diabetes. Latinos also have high

rates of diabetes, overweight and obesity, and physical inactivity. The prevalence of CVD is much higher in African American females than among White or Mexican American females (49%, 35%, and 34.4%, respectively). These differences are echoed in the prevalence of coronary heart disease, stroke, and heart failure. African American men are comparable to African American women in the high prevalence of CVD, coronary heart disease, and stroke.

Both normotensive and hypertensive older adults experience cardiovascular changes with aging. However, these changes occur in hypertensive adults at a much younger age and the changes may be exaggerated (**Figure 8-1**).

Hypertension

More than 25% of the world population and 27% of the U.S. population has **hypertension,** or high blood pressure (HBP). Recent data suggests that this number is higher—33%. In adults older than 50 years of age, 90% have a lifetime risk of having hypertension. Its prevalence in older adults in the United States is 50% to 70%. Hypertension has reached epidemic proportions in the United States. Hypertension is a major risk factor for stroke, coronary artery disease, heart attack (myocardial infarction), and heart failure. Adults with hypertension are at a greater risk for heart attack. This is especially true of people of South Asian ethnicity. In a longitudinal study conducted in Great Britain over a five-year period, the researchers found a significantly higher risk of heart attack in South Asians compared to Whites. This may be due to the higher prevalence of diabetes in this population.

> **hypertension** When resting blood pressure persistently exceeds 140 mm Hg systolic or 90 mm Hg diastolic.

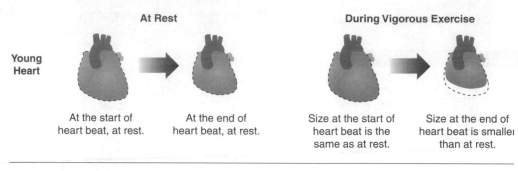

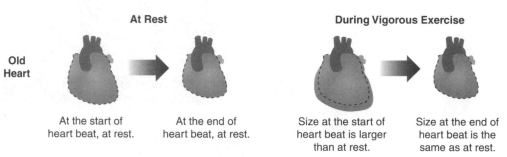

FIGURE 8-1 Young Heart and Old Heart

Source: National Institute on Aging/National Institutes of Health, 2008.

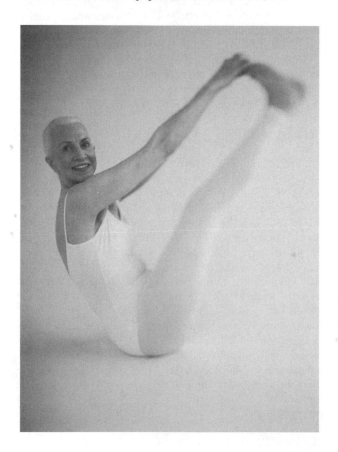

Hypertension is defined as a systolic blood pressure (SBP) of 140 mm Hg (millimeters of mercury on a sphygmomanometer) or higher and/or diastolic blood pressure (DBP) of 90 mm Hg or higher. Hypertension can be of two types: diastolic or systolic.

Diastolic hypertension occurs most often in middle-aged and older adults. The diastolic pressure is the second number in a blood pressure reading; for example, 130/**90** mm Hg. Diastolic pressure measures the force in the blood vessels when the heart is at rest (between heartbeats). In this example, 90 is an elevated diastolic blood pressure. Normal blood pressure is a SBP below 120 and a DBP below 80.

Systolic hypertension is most common in older adults. Systolic pressure (SBP) is the first number in a blood pressure reading; for example, **140**/70 mm Hg. In this example, 140 is an elevated systolic pressure. High SBP is a risk factor for stroke. This pressure is the measure of the force applied against the inner walls of arteries as the heart pumps blood around the body. The goal of management of systolic hypertension is to prevent coronary artery diseases (CAD). Successful management of systolic hypertension reduces the incidence of stroke, heart attack, heart failure, and mortality. In fact, maintaining a BP of 130/80 mm Hg decreases risk for stroke in hypertensive adults by half. To see some of the effects of aging on arteries, see **Figure 8-2**.

According to the Senior Hypertension and Physical Exercise (SHAPE) Study, exercise, weight loss, and diet can help to reduce high blood pressure. In this study, the partici-

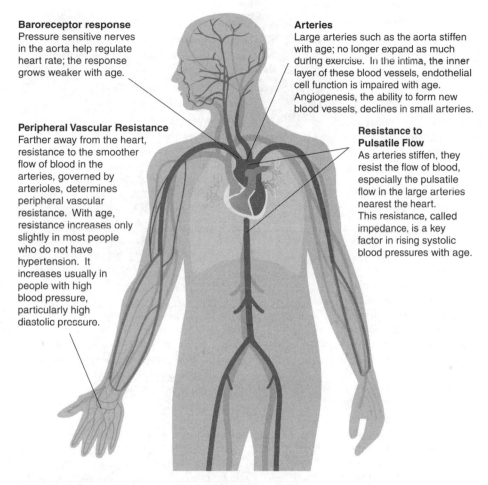

Baroreceptor response
Pressure sensitive nerves in the aorta help regulate heart rate; the response grows weaker with age.

Arteries
Large arteries such as the aorta stiffen with age; no longer expand as much during exercise. In the intima, the inner layer of these blood vessels, endothelial cell function is impaired with age. Angiogenesis, the ability to form new blood vessels, declines in small arteries.

Peripheral Vascular Resistance
Farther away from the heart, resistance to the smoother flow of blood in the arteries, governed by arterioles, determines peripheral vascular resistance. With age, resistance increases only slightly in most people who do not have hypertension. It increases usually in people with high blood pressure, particularly high diastolic pressure.

Resistance to Pulsatile Flow
As arteries stiffen, they resist the flow of blood, especially the pulsatile flow in the large arteries nearest the heart. This resistance, called impedance, is a key factor in rising systolic blood pressures with age.

FIGURE 8-2 Aging Arteries

Source: National Institute on Aging/National Institutes of Health, 2008.

pants engaged in supervised aerobic exercises (treadmill, cycling) and strengthening (weight lifting) three times a week for 90 minutes.

Prehypertension

Approximately 69 million adults (about 25% of the population) in the United States have prehypertension. **Prehypertension** is an untreated systolic pressure of 120–139 mm Hg or an untreated diastolic pressure of 80–89 mm Hg and "*not* being told by a health professional on two occasions that the patient has hypertension." These adults are more likely to have above normal cholesterol levels, be overweight or obese, and have diabetes.

Gender and Ethnic Factors for Hypertension

Hypertension appears to be different in older women and older men. Until age 45, a higher percentage of men than women have high blood pressure. From ages 45 to 54, the percentage of men and women with high blood pressure is similar. After age 54, more women have hypertension. Among those aged 65 to 74, 64.7% of men and 69.6% of women have hypertension. In the 75 and older age group, 64.1% of men have and 76.4% of women have hypertension. Women taking oral contraceptives are two to three times more likely to have hypertension.

African Americans have the highest incidence of hypertension. In fact, the prevalence of hypertension in African Americans is among the highest in the world, and it continues to increase. African Americans develop high blood pressure earlier

prehypertension A systolic blood pressure equal to or greater than 120 mm Hg and a diastolic blood pressure equal to or greater than 80 mm Hg. It is a new category of risk indicating a greater risk for hypertension.

in life, and their average blood pressure is much higher. The prevalence of hypertension is very high in African American women compared to White and Mexican American women (42.0%, 26.7%, and 24.3%, respectively).

Dietary Factors and Hypertension

Increased salt intake has long been known to be a factor in hypertension, and reducing intake is one of the lifestyle modifications recommended for treatment. One major study examined the effects on BP of reduced dietary sodium and the DASH (Dietary Approaches to Stop Hypertension) diet. Reducing sodium intake lowered BP in hypertensive and nonhypertensive subjects, in African Americans and other races, and in men and women. In those hypertensive subjects taking the DASH diet and reduced sodium intake, the BP was diminished the most (11.5 mm Hg).

African Americans are more sensitive to reduced salt and increased potassium intake, and engage in less exercise than older White adults. One cultural challenge is that African Americans find it difficult to follow diets such as the DASH diet, which is a dramatic change from their normal diet. Another cultural challenge is that African Americans report a larger ideal body image and BMI and have little outside pressure to lose weight.

Much research has been conducted on the influence of diet on hypertension. Some dietary modifications include reducing saturated fat and salt intake, losing weight, moderating alcohol consumption, increasing potassium intake, and consuming more fruits and vegetables. The American Heart Association has updated its nutritional guidelines for blood pressure management. Many dietary modifications are included in the DASH diet. Nonpharmacologic approaches such as decreased sodium intake, weight reduction, and exercise are more effective in older adults than in younger patients.

There is evidence that low potassium stores and the ratio of potassium to sodium are involved in the causation of hypertension. As our diets have changed over the years (by increasing the amount of sodium in processed foods), the previous ratio of 1:1 of sodium to potassium is now 20:1. Total body potassium stores are not reflected in blood potassium levels. Greater amounts of potassium-rich foods are needed in the diet.

See **Box 8-2** for guidelines and for proteins recommended for hypertension management.

A prospective study by Wang and colleagues linking whole- and refined-grain intake with hypertension risk was published in 2007. The study examined nearly 30,000 U.S. women older than age 45 who were free of cardiac disease and hypertension, and followed them for 10 years. The researchers concluded that high whole-grain intake was associated with a reduced risk of hypertension.

BOX 8-2 American Heart Association Updated Guidelines for Hypertension Management

Weight	Lose weight if overweight; maintain normal weight. Increase physical activity.
Sodium	Reduce to 1.5 g/day. Check food labels.
Fruits, vegetables	Eat eight to ten servings each day, which will increase K+ (potassium), which reduces blood pressure in normal and hypertensive older adults. In older adults with kidney dysfunction or heart failure, potassium should be less than the otherwise recommended 4.7 g/day.
Alcohol	Moderate intake. Alcohol use increases BP, especially in those taking more than two drinks/day. Women should consume no more than one drink/day and men two drinks/day or fewer.
Proteins	Skim or 1% (low fat) milk; fat-free or low-fat dairy products; yogurt; fish from cold waters, such as cod, tuna, halibut, salmon, mackerel, herring; poultry, white meat, skinned; peas, beans, and legumes; soy products.
DASH Diet	In addition to fruits and vegetables, emphasize low-fat dairy products. Consume whole grains, fish, nuts, and poultry. Restrict fats, red meats, sweets, and sugar-containing drinks. Substitute some carbohydrates with plant proteins, such as soy, or with monounsaturated fat. The DASH diet is not recommended for those older adults with kidney failure. Older adults without kidney failure derive great benefit from the diet.

Source: Data from Appel L. Dietary approaches to prevent and treat hypertension (AHA Scientific Statement). *Hypertension,* 2006;47: 296–308.

Tobacco

Secondary prevention of coronary heart disease can improve survival in adults older than age 75. Of primary importance is smoking cessation. Smokers are two to four times more likely to develop coronary heart disease than nonsmokers. Nearly 21% of adults continue to smoke. However, smoking has declined 50% since 1965. American Indian/Alaska Natives have the highest rate of tobacco use, followed by Whites, African Americans, Hispanic/Latinos, and Asian Americans (33.8%, 31.4%, 27.3%, 23.3%, and 11.7%, respectively).

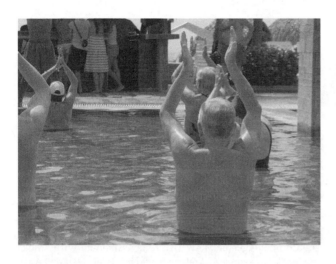

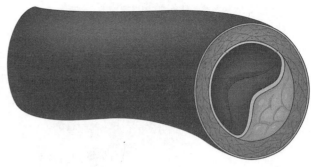

FIGURE 8-3 Development of Atherosclerosis

Source: Insel P, Turner RE, Ross D. *Nutrition.* 3rd ed. Sudbury, MA: Jones & Bartlett; 2007, p. 405. Reproduced with permission.

Exercise

Another method of prevention is to exercise regularly and to maintain that level with aging. However, physical activity declines with aging. The prevalence of inactivity in those 45 to 64 is 16.3% in men and 17% in women. The prevalence of inactivity in adults 66 to 74 is 21.4% in men and 24.5% in women. Inactivity in adults 75 and older is 29.7% in men and 39.6% in women. The amount of *some* exercise is 68.6% in adults 18 to 44. The amount in those 75 and older is 40.2%.

The prevalence of physical inactivity during leisure time is greatest among Mexican Americans. Those adults whose main language is Spanish have the highest prevalence of inactivity (38% of men and 58% of women). Among English-speaking Mexican Americans, 15% of men and 28% of women are physically inactive, which is similar to that of the general population. Health professionals can do a lot more to educate older adults on the importance of activity.

African Americans and American Indian/Alaska Natives have a very high prevalence of *never* engaging in any vigorous physical activity (71.7% and 71.1%). This compares with Asian adults, 66.6% of whom never engage in vigorous physical activity, and White Americans, 60.0% of whom never engage in vigorous physical activity.

Dyslipidemias

An important step in reducing the risk of coronary artery disease is to reduce cholesterol levels. Dyslipidemias, (high blood cholesterol, high triglycerides, high LDLc, and low HDLc), leads to deposition of plaques of fat and calcium (atherosclerosis), which narrow the intima (lining) of arteries and disturb blood flow, thus increasing the risk of myocardial infarction (MI) and stroke (**Figure 8-3**).

See **Table 8-5** for criteria for dyslipidemias. An expert treatment panel on detection, evaluation, and treatment of high blood cholesterol in adults, the Adult Treatment Panel

(ATP III), has published recommendations for management of cholesterol problems (**Box 8-3**).

Cholesterol

A cholesterol-lowering diet is the initial therapy for dyslipidemias if the older adult is not at risk for malnutrition. Low or dropping cholesterol levels can be seen in malnutrition. A cholesterol level under 160 is considered low and is a marker for malnutrition, an indication for increased mortality. The cholesterol-lowering diet should be adequate nutritionally, with sufficient calories, protein, calcium, iron, and vitamins. The diet should be affordable and easily understood by the patient and family.

Low Density Lipoprotein

Diet alone can lower **low density lipoprotein** cholesterol (LDL-c) (the "bad" cholesterol) by 10% to 15%. Statin drugs can lower LDL-c

> **low density lipoprotein (LDL)** Cholesterol-rich lipoproteins generated from the breakdown and removal of triglycerides from intermediate-density lipoprotein in the blood.

TABLE 8-5 Criteria for Dyslipidemia

Cholesterol	Optimal	Desirable	Low	Borderline	High
Total cholesterol	—	<200	—	200–239	>240
LDL	<100	—	—	130–159	>190
TG	—	<150	—	130–159	160–189
HDL	—	>45	<40	>60	

Source: Data from Expert Panel on Detection, Evaluation, and Treatment of High Blood Cholesterol in Adults. Executive Summary of the Third Report of the National Cholesterol Education Program (NCEP) Expert Panel on Detection, Evaluation, and Treatment of High Blood Cholesterol in Adults (Adult Treatment Panel III). *JAMA.* 2001;285:2486–2497.

BOX 8-3   A Summary of ATP III Recommendations for Cholesterol Management, 2004 Update from 2001 Recommendations

Risk Category	Recommendations
High, Very High Risk	Drug therapy for those with LDL >100 mg/dL
	Optional treatment until LDL level is <70 mg/dL
	Overall management goal of LDL level <100 mg/dL
Moderately High Risk	Drug therapy for those with LDL >130 mg/dL
	Overall management goal of LDL level <130 mg/dL
	Optional treatment for those with LDL level 100–129 mg/dL
Moderate Risk	Drug therapy for those with LDL >160 mg/dL
	Overall management goal of LDL level <130 mg/dL
Lower Risk	Drug therapy for those with LDL >190 mg/dL
	Overall management goal of LDL <160 mg/dL
	Optional treatment for those with LDL level 160–189 mg/dL

Sources: Data from Expert Panel on Detection, Evaluation, and Treatment of High Blood Cholesterol in Adults. Executive Summary of the Third Report of the National Cholesterol Education Program (NCEP) Expert Panel on Detection, Evaluation, and Treatment of High Blood Cholesterol in Adults (Adult Treatment Panel III). *JAMA.* 2001;285:2486–2497; Grundy S, Cleeman J, Merz C. Implications of recent clinical trials for the National Cholesterol Education Program Adult Treatment Panel III Guidelines. *Circulation.* 2004;110: 227–239.

high density lipoprotein (HDL) Blood lipoproteins that contain high levels of proteins and low levels of triglycerides. Synthesized primarily in the liver and small intestine, HDL picks up cholesterol released from dying cells and other sources and transfers it to other lipoproteins.

polyunsaturated fat Fatty acids found in sunflower, corn, soybean, and cottonseed oils. A healthy fat found in grains and seafood, such as herring, mackerel, salmon, and halibut. Protects against heart disease and insulin resistance.

triglycerides Fats composed of three fatty acid chains linked to a glycerol molecule.

by 61%. The following dietary fats should be limited when trying to lower LDL-c: butter, margarine, hydrogenated shortening, cream sauces, bacon, meat gravy, lard, coconut oil, cocoa butter (in chocolate), and partially hydrogenated palm and soybean oils. See **Table 8-6** for types of fats and **Table 8-7** for recommendations of dietary fats. Cholesterol-lowering margarines are available that can lower cholesterol by 10% to 15% (e.g., Take Control and Benecol).

High Density Lipoprotein

One to two glasses of red wine each day can improve **high density lipoprotein** cholesterol (HDL-c) (the "good" cholesterol) in men, or one glass per day in women. Low HDL-c is a strong indicator of CAD risk. The cause of the low value should be identified and appropriate lifestyle changes should be suggested. Low HDL-c is associated with smoking, lack of exercise, and overweight. High HDL-c levels seem to be protective against atherosclerosis. Few pharmacologic agents are useful in increasing HDLs; two of these are fibrates and nicotinic acid, which are not well tolerated. It has been found that regular consumption of berries, a rich source of polyphenols, mono and **polyunsaturated fats** such as almonds and vitamin C, significantly raise HDL-c.

Triglycerides

Triglycerides (TG) is the chemical form that fat exists in food and in blood plasma. With cholesterol, it forms blood plasma lipids. Ingested carbohydrates exist as TG and are transported to cells for storage. When energy is needed, hormones transport them for use. When there is excessive TG in the blood plasma, hypertriglyceridemia exists. It is linked to heart disease in many people. It is seen in those with DM. Normal blood levels are less than 150 mg/dL and very high levels are greater than 500. Management includes weight loss, cutting calories, reducing saturated fat content, reducing alcohol consumption, eating low fat dairy products, eating high omega 3 fatty acid foods such as fish, and omitting red meats. Pharmacologic therapies for high triglycerides include fenofibrate, clofibrate, and gemfibrozil.

Other Cardiovascular Diseases

Arrhythmias

Many types of irregular heartbeats are common and harmless. However, atrial fibrillation (AF) may occur when the heart does not receive enough blood, which affects the heart's ability to conduct impulses properly. Thrombi may form and cause a stroke to occur; with AF the incidence of stroke is seven times that of the general population of that age. The median age of patients with atrial fibrillation is 75 to 80 years. However, the incidence of AF begins to increase in adults over age 60. It is more common in men than women, but it becomes more common in women with

TABLE 8-6 Healthy and Unhealthy Fats

Healthy
Monounsaturated fats
Liquid at room temperature.
Found in olive oil, peanut oil, canola oil, avocados, and nuts.
Polyunsaturated fats
Liquid at room temperature.
Found in vegetable, safflower, corn, sunflower, soy, and cottonseed oils.
Omega-3 fatty acids
A polyunsaturated fat found in seafood, such as salmon, mackerel, and herring; flaxseeds, flax oil, walnuts, soybeans, and canola oil.

Unhealthy
Saturated fats
Solid or waxy at room temperature.
Found in animal products, such as red meat, poultry, butter, and whole milk. Also found in coconut oil and palm oil.
Trans fats
Solid, less likely to spoil, hydrogenated.
Found in baked goods, crackers, cookies, cakes, fried foods, donuts, French fries, shortening, some margarines.
Dietary cholesterol
Found in animal products such as meat, poultry, seafood, eggs, dairy products, lard, and butter. Cholesterol is also made in the body.

Source: Adapted from Mayo Clinic. Dietary fats: know which types to choose. 2007. Available at: http://www.mayoclinic.com/health/fat/NU00262. Accessed February 7, 2007.

advancing age. Initially, AF may not be serious, but over time it can cause systemic embolization, which can cause serious problems such as stroke, heart attack, infarction of abdominal viscera, and impaired circulation to the extremities. It can cause death.

AF can be caused by hyperthyroidism; electrolyte disorders involving potassium, sodium, calcium, and magnesium, which are involved in electrical impulses to the heart; alcoholism; stimulant abuse, such as caffeine, and nicotine, or illicit drugs (amphetamines and cocaine); obstructive sleep apnea; uncontrolled diabetes; obesity; hypertension; over-the-counter drugs such as pseudoephedrine; or other problems in CAD. The patient may report palpitations, shortness of breath, dizziness, or feel no symptoms at all. It is often an incidental finding without symptomatology.

Atrial fibrillation is found by checking the pulse. With AF, the pulse will be irregularly irregular. If the pulse is very fast, 130–180 beats per minute (and it can be much faster), the AF must be treated urgently, because the older patient may go into heart failure if this heart rate continues for an extended time.

Management of AF often includes warfarin therapy, which keeps the blood "thinned." Patients often die of stroke without anticoagulation. However, warfarin interacts adversely with many medications and some foods. For example, cauliflower, broccoli, and dark green leafy vegetables high in vitamin K antagonize the effects of warfarin. See **Table 8-8** for management of older adults taking warfarin therapy. Other therapies for AF include cardioversion; heparin; aspirin for anticoagulation; beta blockers for slowing the

TABLE 8-7 Recommendations for Fat Intake

Type of Fat	Recommended Intake
Cholesterol	<300 mg/day
Monounsaturated fats	<15% of total daily calories
Polyunsaturated fats	<10% of total daily calories
Saturated fats + trans fats	<10% of total daily calories

TABLE 8-8 Foods, Vitamins, and Medicinals That Interact with Warfarin Therapy

Diminish Warfarin's Effect	Enhance Warfarin's Effect
Broccoli	Vitamin E (>400 IU)
Brussels sprouts	Salicylates (aspirin)
Green leafy vegetables	Binge ethanol intake
Greens	Acetaminophen
Cabbage	Flu vaccine
Cucumber with peel	Potassium products
Endive	Garlic
Kale	Gingko
Red lettuce	Celery
Mint (raw)	Dandelion
Parsley (raw)	Horseradish
Spinach	Horse chestnuts
Swiss chard	Licorice
Green tea	Chamomile
Turnip (raw)	Sweet woodruff
Watercress	Red, sweet clover
Vitamin K supplements	Clove
Ascorbic acid	Onion

Source: Data from Neighborcare. *Geriatric Drug Therapy Handbook, 2004–2005.* Hudson, OH: Lexi-Comp; 2004; Aschenbrenner DS, Venable SJ. *Drug Therapy in Nursing.* Philadelphia: Lippincott; 2006.

heart rate; and others, all of which may have serious side effects. A study by Fauchier, de Labriolle, et al. in 2008 has shown that statin drugs, which are useful in the treatment of LDL-c, can reduce the incidence of AF 61% compared with placebo.

Peripheral Arterial Disease (PAD)

Atherosclerosis is the evolving damage to arterial walls from plaques deposited in the walls' lining (see Figure 8-3). The damage occurs in the arteries of the legs, heart, kidneys, and other areas. It is part and parcel of dyslipidemias and hypertension and other problems of the vascular system. It can also result from exposure to lead and cadmium, which come from cigarette smoke. Older adults with renal insufficiency have a high prevalence of peripheral artery disease (PAD), according to government studies. It occurs more often in Hispanic and African American adults than in Whites.

Atherosclerosis can result in lower extremity arterial disease, or LEAD. Approximately 15% of adults older than 55 years have demonstrable LEAD. Two-thirds of those with LEAD have no demonstrable symptoms. However, symptoms in those with LEAD may include pain and muscle fatigue of the lower extremities with exercise. This is known as intermittent claudication. As the disease progresses, the older adult may have pain even at rest. This is caused by ischemia, extreme narrowing of the arteries, and in some cases the affected limb may be lost.

With PAD, the practitioner may see signs of thin skin at the periphery; loss of hair, especially on the toes; cold extremities; and ulcers that do not heal. Peripheral pulses may be absent. Skin may be red, toenails thickened, and the older adult may experience pain and cramping at night when resting with the feet elevated. As the disease progresses, limb-threatening ischemia can occur and, late in the course, can occur even at rest. Nonhealing ulcers occur at this time and gangrene may be present.

The risk factors and management for PAD are the same as those in coronary artery disease. Disease in one area suggests disease in other areas, such as the heart, the brain's vessels, and in the periphery, which includes all areas outside the heart and brain (e.g., arms, legs, kidneys, stomach). High lipid levels speed the process of atherosclerosis; smoking causes spasm of the blood vessels and aggregation of the platelets; both worsen the disease. **Figure 8-4** shows a healthy artery with a lumen where blood flows freely and a narrowed artery in which blood flows sluggishly.

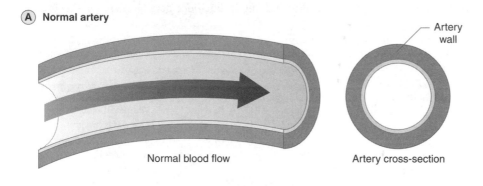

(A) **Normal artery**

Normal blood flow

Artery wall

Artery cross-section

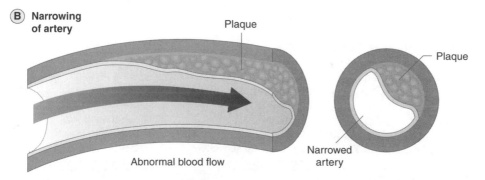

(B) **Narrowing of artery**

Plaque

Abnormal blood flow

Plaque

Narrowed artery

FIGURE 8-4 Healthy Artery and Unhealthy Artery

Source: National Institute of Aging, National Heart, Blood and Lung Institute, 2008.

BOX 8-4   Risk Factors for Myocardial Infarction

- Increasing age
- Male sex
- Elevated LDL-c
- Low HDL-c
- Elevated blood pressure
- Smoking
- Diabetes
- Family history of cardiovascular disease
- Obesity
- Sedentary lifestyle

Source: Data from *BMJ Clinical Evidence Handbook, Summer 2007.*
London: BMJ Publishing Group; 2007.

Statins can reduce the incidence of intermittent claudication (the pain or cramping on walking or other exercise) and can improve exercise duration. Many other drugs are available for treatment of PAD and CAD; some prevent blood clots from forming or relax and widen the blood vessels. In extreme cases, threatening ischemia may occur at rest. Non healing ulcers and gangrene may be present. At this time, a surgeon may consider angioplasty or bypass surgery.

Myocardial Infarction (MI)

Approximately 25% of people who have an acute heart attack, or **myocardial infarction** (more recently called acute coronary syndrome), will die from it. Half of these will die within one-half hour from the onset of symptoms. Myocardial infarctions occur more often in men older than 65 years, and in African American men more often than White men. African American postmenopausal women have MIs more often than postmenopausal White women. The incidence increases with advancing age (**Box 8-4**). Women are much less likely to survive the crisis than men. Poorer, less educated people are more likely to die than those with higher incomes and higher education.

The symptoms of a myocardial infarction are different in older adults compared to younger adults. Fewer than 50% experience chest pain. Approximately 21% are "silent" MIs. The MI in the much older adult often presents as acute shortness of breath. Other symptoms include gastrointestinal upset, fatigue, dizziness, confusion, and/or stroke. Other, more common symptoms include crushing chest pain, nausea and vomiting, and diaphoresis (extreme sweating), which are seen with frequency in younger adults.

An MI is caused by the sudden rupture or erosion of an atheromatous plaque in the blood vessel lining (Figure 8-3). When the heart is deprived of oxygen-rich blood, the area surrounding the blocked blood supply becomes necrotic or dies. Also, the heart requires more blood during exertion or at times of stress.

The management of an acute MI is urgent care. Management following an MI is both medical and surgical. Coronary artery bypass and stent placement in occluded coronary arteries are common. Later management includes dealing with the risk factors—hypertension, hyperlipidemias, diabetes, and smoking. Other areas of management include thyroid disorders, anemias, and heart failure. These risk factors can be limited through prevention.

Heart Failure (HF)

Heart failure is the end stage of cardiac disease. It is a consequence of hypertension, CHD, diabetes mellitus, and/or cardiomyopathy. It is when the heart is unable to deliver a sufficient blood supply to meet the body's needs. The cause may be systolic or diastolic dysfunction. Systolic heart failure is the abnormal pumping function of the heart. Diastolic heart failure is the heart's inability to relax so that it can fill with blood. Heart failure can also be described as "left-sided failure," when fluid backs up into the lungs, causing shortness of breath, or "right-sided failure," when fluid backs up into the abdomen, legs, and feet causing swelling, or edema.

Women tend to develop heart failure at an older age than men. White men and White women have a higher rate of HF than do African American men and women. After a certain age, most cases of heart failure are preceded by heart attacks, which in turn are preceded by hypertension in 75%. Following a myocardial infarction, 22% of men and 46% of women will be disabled by heart failure within 6 years. The rates change when this is broken into older age groups (**Table 8-9**). The prevalence of diabetes (DM) is increasing among older adults with HF, and DM is a risk factor for death of these people.

Those with mild to moderate HF symptoms have a 50% mortality over three to four years. Mortality reaches 50% within 12 months in those with severe HF. Women survive longer with heart failure than do men. Nearly 30% to 40% of those with HF die suddenly, probably from arrhythmias associated with HF. However, new data indicates an increase in the incidence of HF and also an improved survival rate among older adults, especially among older men.

myocardial infarction (MI) Death of muscle tissue in the heart due to the loss of blood flow from either a blood clot or progressive narrowing of the coronary arteries. The patient feels nausea; sweating; midsternal chest pain, which may radiate to the arms and neck; weakness; and possible loss of consciousness.

TABLE 8-9 Heart Failure Within Six Years of Heart Attack by Age and Race

Age	Group			
	Non-African American Men	African American Men	Non-African American Women	African American Women
75–84	43.3%	52%	26.3%	33.5%
85 and older	73.1%	66.7%	64.9%	48.4%

Sources: Data from American Heart Association (AHA). Heart disease and stroke statistics—2006 update. 2006. Available at: http://www.americanheart.org/downloadable/heart/113535864858055-1026_HS_Stats06book.pdf. Accessed December 28, 2008; American Heart Association (AHA). Heart disease and stroke statistics—2008 update. Available at: http://www.americanheart.org. Accessed February 19, 2008.

Heart failure is the most common cause of hospitalization of Medicare-eligible older adults. Nearly 77% of the one million hospitalizations for HF involve those older than age 65. The condition is very costly and a major cause of chronic disability. Management involves the prevention of the primary causes of HF—hypertension and coronary heart disease.

Risk factors and predictors of heart failure among women with CHD include diabetes. Diabetic women with elevated BMIs or low creatinine clearance are at highest risk for HF. In nondiabetic women without risk factors, the annual incidence rate is 0.4% (**Box 8-5**).

Assessment

When assessing the older adult with heart failure, one frequently finds edema in the feet and legs; edema in the lower back of a bedridden patient; rales, or crackling sounds, in the lungs, indicating fluid buildup; jugular venous distention in the neck above the clavicle; and an abnormal heart sound called an S3 gallop. A blood test called a BNP (*b-natriuretic peptide*) is useful in diagnosing HF when the diagnosis is not clear. A chest X-ray will often show cardiomegaly (enlarged heart, usually the left ventricle) and pleural effusions (fluid in the base of the lungs). An electrocardiogram (ECG) will demonstrate HF. Other assessment methods include echocardiograms and cardiac catheterizations. See **Table 8-10** for signs and symptoms of heart failure.

Women have more symptoms with heart failure, for example, shortness of breath and more difficulty during exercise. Depression with heart failure is seen more often in women. Women also have more peripheral edema than do men (**Figure 8-5**).

▶ BOX 8-5   Risk Factors for Heart Failure

- High blood pressure
- Coronary artery disease
- Past history of MI
- Irregular heart rhythm
- Diabetes
- Sleep apnea
- Congenital structural heart defects
- Viral infection, which damages heart muscle
- Alcohol abuse, which weakens heart muscle
- Kidney disease

Source: Data from Mayo Clinic. Heart failure. January 3, 2008. Available at: http://mayoclinic.com/print/heart-failure/DS00061/DSECTION=all&METHOD=print. Accessed December 28, 2008.

TABLE 8-10 Signs and Symptoms of Heart Failure

Signs	Symptoms
Peripheral edema	Dyspnea on exertion or at rest
Weight gain	Orthopnea (requires pillows for sleep)
Bilateral rales in lungs	
Tachycardia	Paroxysmal nocturnal dyspnea
Third heart sound	Fatigue
Increased jugular venous pressure	Diminished exercise tolerance
Positive hepatojugular reflux	Unexplained cough, often at night
Apical impulse of heart displaced laterally	Acute confusion state (delirium)
	Nausea, abdominal pain, distention
	Diminished food intake
	Decline in functional status

Source: Data from Lewis L. New ways to manage heart failure in the nursing home. *Caring for the Ages.* 2002;3(3):25-26.

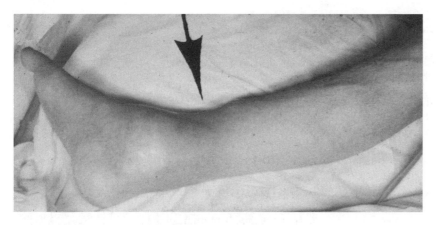

FIGURE 8-5 Peripheral Edema

Source: Reproduced from *An Introduction to Human Disease.* 7th ed. Photo courtesy of Leonard V. Crowley, M.D., Century College.

Management

An important management tool for older adults with HF is a weekly weight. Older adults with severe failure should be weighed daily. A weight gain of 2 pounds or more should be reported to the primary care provider. Fluid-volume overload is a major problem in HF, because the fluid accumulates in the periphery and in the lungs. Regular weighing will demonstrate early weight gain so that medical intervention can be given to attending to and preventing an exacerbation of the condition.

Medications, including diuretics, ACE-inhibitors, ARBs (angiotensin II receptor blockers), beta blockers, calcium channel blockers, and nitrates, can be used to manage heart failure.

Sodium management is very important because sodium can exacerbate HF. Older adults with HF should be on a no-added-salt diet and possibly even more stringent salt restrictions, such as consuming no more than 1.5 to 2 g/day of sodium. Some recommend limiting sodium intake to 3 to 4 g/day, stopping or limiting alcohol intake, and measuring serum potassium and magnesium and replacing as indicated by the results. The latter might be accomplished by giving 400-mg magnesium oxide supplements once or twice a day. Magnesium-rich foods include halibut, dry roasted almonds, cashews, whole-grain cereals, spinach, avocados, raisins, and bananas. If hyponatremia occurs, easing the sodium restriction or lowering the diuretic dosage will help.

Some professionals substitute table salt with a potassium salt. A study by Chang et al. in 2006 that examined this substitution found that those consuming potassium salt had lower blood pressure, increased survival from cardiovascular death, and lower medical costs for in-patient care. A baseline potassium level should be obtained before and during this substitution.

Families must understand the need to exclude salty food gifts. However, at the end of life if the older adult desires special treats such as bacon or ham, this should probably be considered in terms of increasing quality of life.

A number of over-the-counter drugs can cause fluid and sodium retention. These include sodium-based antacids, high-dose aspirins, NSAIDs (nonsteroidal anti-inflammatory drugs), ginseng, gingko, echinacea, and decongestants. These should be avoided by older adults with HF.

Anorexia of Cardiac Disease

Weight loss often occurs in late-stage heart failure and cardiovascular disease. Some of the medications used to manage cardiovascular disease suppress the appetite. In the older adult with HF and CVD, and especially in those who are institutionalized, cholesterol may no longer be a problem, and, indeed, they should not be given cholesterol-lowering drugs. Those who plan the menus should not try to improve the patient's lipid status, but rather maintain the patient's weight and current cholesterol levels and preserve the pleasure of eating and quality of life. An effort should be made to follow the government food pyramid, MyPyramid. These foods can be appetizing and provide a heart-healthy diet.

Conclusion

Cardiovascular disease is an important area of concern for older adults. Good nutrition is vital and can mean the difference between poor health and good health, or life and death. Good nutrition can prevent heart disease to a great extent, except in the person who has inherited severe hypercholesterolemias, which causes severe disease, even in children. Every adult with cardiovascular problems should have a dietary evaluation by a health professional.

Activities Related to This Chapter

1. Search the Internet for the Seventh Report of the Joint National Committee on Prevention, Detection, Evaluation, and Treatment of High Blood Pressure (JNC 7).
2. Develop a diet for an older adult with dyslipidemia.
3. Develop a diet for an older adult with low cholesterol and a teaching plan to help the person understand why cholesterol is important.
4. Develop a week's diet for an older adult who is on diuretic therapy for heart failure.
5. List foods that are contraindicated when an older adult is on warfarin therapy.
6. Test yourself on all the key words in this chapter.

Case Study

Joe, 72, was recently diagnosed with dyslipidemia. Before putting Joe on a medication, the nurse practitioner recommended that he try and make lifestyle changes to reduce his cholesterol. She gave him educational materials about the Mediterranean diet.

Questions

1. What is dyslipidemia?
2. What lipids might be elevated or too low?
3. What is the Mediterranean diet?
4. How might the Mediterranean diet be helpful to Joe?
5. Joe thinks he is too busy to make lifestyle changes, although his wife is willing to work on making this diet possible for them both. What else should he prioritize?
6. How often would you follow up with Joe?

REFERENCES

AHA 2009 Update. http://www.americanheart.org/presenter. jhml?identifier = 10865. 2/11/2009.

American Dietetic Association (ADA). Liberalized diets for older adults in long-term care. Available at: http://www. eatright.org/cps/rde/xchg/ada/hs.xsl/home_3772_ENU_ HTML.htm. Accessed January 21, 2008.

American Geriatric Society (AGS). *Geriatric Review Syllabus.* 6th ed. New York: American Geriatric Society; 2006.

American Heart Association (AHA). AHA Scientific Statement: Secondary prevention of Coronary Heart Disease in the elderly (with emphasis on patients > 75 years of age). *Circulation.* 2002;105:1735.

American Heart Association (AHA). Heart disease and stroke statistics—2006 update. 2006. Available at: http://www.americanheart.org/downloadable/heart/ 113535864858055-1026_HS_Stats06book.pdf. Accessed December 28, 2008.

American Heart Association (AHA). Heart disease and stroke statistics—2008 update. Available at: http://www. americanheart.org. Accessed February 19, 2008.

American Heart Association (AHA). Risk factors and coronary heart disease. 2009. Available at: http://www. americanheart.org/presenter.jhtml?identifier = 4726. Accessed February 11, 2009.

Appel L. Dietary approaches to prevent and treat hypertension (AHA Scientific Statement). *Hypertension.* 2006;47:296–308.

BMJ Clinical Evidence Handbook, Summer 2007. London: BMJ Publishing Group, 2007.

Bosworth HB. The relationship of hypertension control with race, ethnicity, and age. *Long-term Care Interface.* 2006;7(9):30–37.

Bruckert E, Hansel B. HDL-c is a powerful lipid predictor of cardiovascular diseases. *Int J Clin Prac.* 2007;61(11):1905–1913.

Centers for Disease Control and Prevention (CDC). Heart disease. November 15, 2007. Available at: http://www. cdc.gov/heartdisease. Accessed February 6, 2008.

Centers for Disease Control and Prevention (CDC). Promoting active lifestyles among older adults. 2001. Available at: http://www.cdc.gov/nccdphp/dnpa/physical/pdf/ lifestyles.pdf. Accessed January 27, 2009.

Chang HY, Hu YW, Yue CSJ, Wen YW, Yeh W, Tsai SY, et al. Effect of potassium-enriched salt on cardiovascular mortality and medical expenses of elderly men. *Am J Clin Nutr.* 2006;83:1289–1296.

Cicero K. 15 Foods that can save your heart. Heart Health Center. February 1, 2008. Available at: http://www. webmd.com/heart/features/15-foods-can-save-your-heart. Accessed February 20, 2008.

Cleveland Clinic, 2006. Heart attack. http://myclevelandclinic. org/disorders/Heart_Attack/hic/Heart_Attak.aspx Retrieved 2/11/2009.

Coll PP. Myocardial infarction and angina. In Ham RJ, Sloane PD, Warshaw GA, *Primary Care Geriatrics.* 4th ed. St. Louis: Mosby; 2004.

Dunbar R, Szapary PO. Inflammation, metabolic syndrome, and CV risk reduction. *Cardiology Review,* supplement. University Pennsylvania School of Medicine, April 2004.

Ebersole P, Hess P, Luggen A. *Toward healthy aging.* St. Louis: Mosby; 2004.

Erlund I, Koli R, Alfthan G, Marniemi J, Puukka P, Mustonen P et al. Favorable effects of berry consumption on platelet function, blood pressure and HDL cholesterol. *Am J Clin Nutr.* 2008;87(2):323–331.

Fauchier L, de Labriolle P, et al. Antiarrhythmic effect of statin therapy and atrial fibrillation. *J Am Coll Cardiol.* 2008;51:828–835.

Harvard Medical School. New view of heart disease in women. *Harvard Women's Health Watch.* 2007;14(6):1–3.

Hollingsworth PW. CHF: systolic vs. diastolic. Presentation, Kentucky Nurse Practitioners and Nurse Midwives, Northern Kentucky Convention Center, Covington, Kentucky, April 2005.

Howard B, Van Horn L, Hsia J, Manson J, Stefanick M, Wssertheil-Smoller S et al. Low-fat dietary pattern and risk of cardiovascular disease: the Women's Health Initiative randomized controlled dietary modification trial. *JAMA.* 2006;295(6):655–666.

Katcher H, Legro R, Kunselman A, Gillies P, Demeres L, Bagshaw D, Kris-Etherton P. The effects of a whole grain enriched hypocaloric diet on caradiovascular disease risk factors in men and women with metabolic syndrome. *Am J Clin Nutr.* 2008;87(1):79–90.

Kearney PM, Whelton M, Reynolds K. Global burden of hypertension: analysis of worldwide data. *Lancet.* 2005;356:217–223.

Lewis L. New ways to manage heart failure in the nursing home. *Caring for the Ages.* 2002;3(3):25–26.

Luchi RJ, Taffet GE. Congestive heart failure. In Ham RJ, Sloane PD, Warshaw GA, *Primary Care Geriatrics.* 4th ed. St. Louis: Mosby; 2004.

Mayo Clinic. HDL cholesterol: how to boost your 'good' cholesterol. 2008. Available at: http://mayoclinic .com/health/hdl-cholesterol/CL00030. Accessed April 3, 2009.

Mayo Clinic. Heart arrhythmias. February 16, 2007. Available at: htp://mayoclinic.com/print/heart-arrhythmias/ DS00290/DSECTION = all&METHOD = print. Accessed February 20, 2008.

Mayo Clinic, 2008. Heart failure. http://mayoclinic.com/print/heart-failure/DS00061/DSECTION = all&METHOD = print. Accessed Dec 28, 2008.

Mayo Clinic. Peripheral arterial disease (PAD). May 2, 2006. Available at: http://mayoclinic.com/print/peripheral-arterial-disease/DS00537/DSECTION = all&Meth. Accessed February 20, 2008.

McCance,K, Huether S. Pathophysiology 5th ed., 2006. Phila: Elsevier/Mosby.

Merck Manual of Geriatrics, 3rd ed. Online Update, Beers M, 2006 Cardiovascular diseases. http://www.merck.com/cvd.

Mink P, Scrafford C, Barraj L, Harnack L, Hong C, et al. Flavonoid intake and cardiovascular disease mortality: a prospective study in postmenopausal women. *Am J Clin Nutr.* 2007;85(3):895–909.

National Heart, Lung, and Blood Institute, National Institutes of Health. No date, The seventh report of the Joint National Committee on Prevention, Detection, Evaluation, and Treatment of High Blood Pressure. www.nhlbi.nih.gov/gideliines/hypertension/index.htm., retrieved 2, 2008.

Patel J, Lim H, Gunarathne A, Tracey I, Durrington P, Hughes E, Lip G. Ethnic differences in myocardial infarction in patients with hypertension: effects of diabetes mellitus. *QJM.* 2008;101(3):231–236.

Reuben D, Herr K, Pacala J, Pollock B, Potter J, Semla T. *Geriatrics at Your Fingertips, 2006–2007.* 8th ed. New York: American Geriatric Society; 2006.

Rich MW. Cardiac disease. In Landefeld CS, Palmer RM, Johnson MA, Johnston CB, Lyons WL, *Current Geriatric Diagnosis and Treatment.* New York: McGraw-Hill; 2004, pp. 156–182.

Richie R. Updating the latest in hypertension therapy. *Clinical Advisor.* Oct 2008;48–55.

Sacks FM, Svetkey LP, Vollmer WM, Appel LJ, Bray GA, et al. Effects on blood pressure of reduced dietary sodium and the dietary approaches to stop hypertension (DASH) diet. *N Engl J Med.* 2001;344(1):3–10.

Stewart, KJ, Bacher AC, Turner KL, Fleg JL, Hees PS, Shapiro EP et al. Effect of exercise on blood pressure in older persons. *Arch Int Medicine.* 2005;165:756–762.

Vega-Lopez S, Ausman LM, Jalbert SM, Erkkila AT, Lichtenstein AH. Palm and partially hydrogenated soybean oils adversely alter lipoprotein profiles compared with soybean and canola oils in moderately hyperlipidemic subjects. *Am J Clin Nutrition.* 2006;84(1):54–62.

Wang L, Gaziano J, Liu S, Manson E, Buring J, Sesso H. Whole- and refined-grain intakes and the risk of hypertension in women. *Am J Clin Nutr.* 2007;86(2):472–479.

Wang L, Manson J, Buring J, Lee I, Sesso H. Dietary intake of dairy products, calcium, and vitamin D and the risk of hypertension in middle-aged and older women. *Hypertension.* 2008;51:1073–1079.

World Health Organization. Technical report 894: Obesity: Preventing and managing the global epidemic. 2000. Geneva: WHO.

Wooley DC. Peripheral vascular disease. In Ham RJ, Sloane PD, Warshaw GA, *Primary Care Geriatrics.* 4th ed. St. Louis: Mosby; 2004.

Zagaria M. Issues in pharmacotherapy: ACE inhibitors in hypertension. *Am J for Nurse Pract.* 2008;12(11–12):26–31.

The Renal/Genitourinary Systems in Aging

Ann Schmidt Luggen, PhD, GNP

CHAPTER OBJECTIVES   Upon completion of this chapter the reader will be able to:

1. Describe the anatomy of the genitourinary system
2. Discuss common problems that occur in the kidney and genitourinary system with aging
3. List the ways that nutrition can compensate or improve problems with the aging or compromised kidney
4. State some of the dietary methods used to manage electrolyte imbalance
5. Relate some of the issues in chronic renal failure

KEY TERMS AND CONCEPTS

Acute renal failure

Benign prostatic hyperplasia (BPH)

Calculi

Chronic renal failure (CRF)

Electrolytes

Erythropoietin

Hyperkalemia

Hypernatremia

Hypokalemia

Hyponatremia

Incontinence

The Kidney

Over 20 million U.S. adults—one in nine—have kidney disease. The incidence of kidney disease is rising. This may be a consequence of the increasing prevalence of obesity, diabetes, and hypertension.

The kidneys are vital to the maintenance of blood volume and blood nutrients and the excretion of waste via the urinary tract (**Figure 9-1**). They are able to excrete excess water, nitrogenous wastes, organic acids, toxic substances, drugs, electrolytes, and sulfates. The kidneys regulate blood pressure. They participate in red blood cell production via **erythropoietin**. Vitamin D is activated by the kidneys. All of these are vital processes to maintaining life.

A number of medical conditions affecting the renal system change or occur with greater frequency in aging

adults. The literature suggests that the most common medical conditions affecting the renal/genitourinary system are urinary incontinence, urinary tract infections (UTIs), prostate disease, genitourinary malignancies, sexual dysfunction, stone disease (**calculi**), electrolyte imbalances, and renal disease/failure. These conditions will be discussed in the following pages.

erythropoietin Produced by the kidney and essential for normal erythropoiesis. It regulates red blood cell production in the bone marrow.

calculi Urinary stones composed of crystals, protein, and other substances that may form and obstruct the urinary tract. The most common minerals in the stones are calcium phosphate and calcium oxalate. They occur more frequently in men than women and in warmer climates over colder ones.

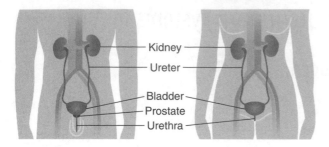

FIGURE 9-1 Renal System Anatomy

Source: National Institute of Diabetes and Digestive and Kidney Diseases (NIDDK), National Institutes of Health, 2004, NIH Public. No. 04-4807. Washington, DC: U.S. Department Health and Human Services.

With increasing age, the kidneys shrink in weight and size. At age 30, the kidney weighs 150 to 200 grams. At age 90, the kidney weighs 110 to 150 grams. The number of glomeruli diminishes by 30% to 40% by age 90 as a result of glomerulosclerosis (**Figure 9-2**).

Nephrons, the structural and functional unit of the kidneys, also diminish in size and number with age (**Figure 9-3**). The nephron is the combination of the Bowman's capsule and the renal tubule, and it functions via an ultrafiltration process. Blood flow through the kidneys declines by approximately 50% from young adulthood to old age because of changes in the kidney's arteries and capillaries. The decline of the glomerular filtration rate (GFR) with age is the cause of most of the functional disability that occurs in the kidney. This change in GFR indicates that harmful substances and waste that once were excreted are now accumulating in the body or are being excreted slowly. Uric acid and medications may remain in the body for a significant period of time. Estimating GFR in older adults is essential so that the dosage of medications may be altered to avoid harm. Despite these age-related changes, the kidney is well able to remain healthy and provide homeostasis, although it is less able to respond when stressed.

One of the primary roles of the kidneys is waste excretion. Only the kidneys can excrete urea, a protein metabolite. They regulate water and mineral balance by excreting excess fluid and conserving it, as needed. The kidneys also produce and regulate erythropoietin, which regulates red blood cell production in the bone marrow. The anemia that develops during chronic renal failure is probably related to decreased production of erythropoietin. The kidneys regulate renin and sodium, which play a role in blood pressure maintenance. The kidneys also help regulate and maintain the body's pH. Kidneys produce active vitamin D hormone, which helps to maintain the calcium–phosphorus ratio in bone. The kidneys are neuroregulated, which causes a thirst response when water loss occurs, for example, from sweating.

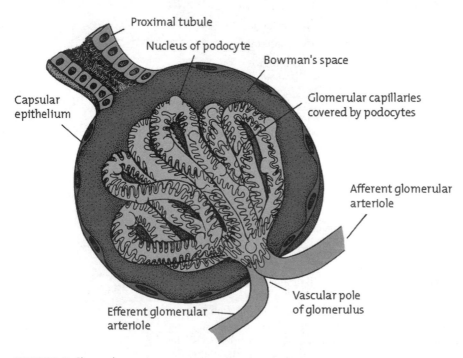

FIGURE 9-2 Glomerulus

Source: Reproduced from *An Introduction to Human Disease.* 7th ed. Courtesy of Leonard V. Crowley, M.D., Century College.

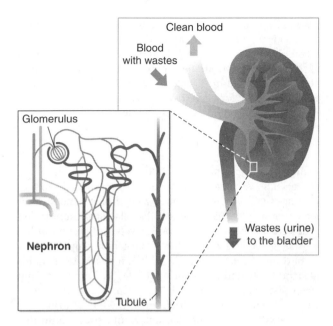

FIGURE 9-3 Nephron and Kidney

Source: National Institutes of Diabetes and Digestive and Kidney Diseases (NIDDK), 2008.

Urinary Tract Problems

Many problems can arise in the urinary tract of older adults, including urinary incontinence. Other problems seen in older adults include bladder cancers, prostate disease and cancers, and urinary tract infections.

Urine is normally clear, light yellow, but it becomes turbid in the presence of other substances. The urine may contain blood (abnormal), bacteria (abnormal), cells (shedding of lining of urinary tract [normal], white blood cells (indicate bacterial infection), casts (form in the renal tubule; indicate inflammation), or crystals (form when urine cools; indicate inflammation or infection). Protein is not normally present in urine; however, if proteins are present the urine will foam when shaken and be yellow or orange from bile pigments.

Urine pH is normally 5.0 to 6.5, but it can range from 4.5 to 8.0. It is alkaline after a meal and more acidic prior to the next meal. It is believed that a more acidic urine helps to prevent UTIs.

Incontinence

Urinary **incontinence** is not a natural consequence of aging. It is, however, very common in older adults, especially if there is a neurologic problem or if dementia is present. This troublesome problem occurs more frequently with advancing age. It is more common in women until age 85, after which it affects men and women equally. It is estimated

that 15% to 35% of community-dwelling adults in the United States older than age 60 and that at least 50% of older adults in long-term care facilities suffer from incontinence. According to one government survey, 38% of women older than age 60 suffer incontinence and 17% of men older than 60 do. It is one of the major factors leading to nursing home admissions.

In women, risk factors for incontinence include pregnancies; vaginal childbirth; cough with pulmonary disorders; mobility problems, such as arthritis; obesity; neurologic disorders, such as Parkinson's disease or stroke; diabetes; and cognitive impairment. In men, additional risk factors include prostate hypertrophy, and prostatectomy. In addition, as shown in **Box 9-1**, a number of medications are associated with incontinence.

There are four types of urinary incontinence: stress, urge, overflow, and functional. Two or more of these may be present at the same time, which is called mixed incontinence.

Incontinence may also be transient. It can be caused by delirium—an acute confusional state—which, in turn, may be caused by infection, dehydration, or another acute medical problem. Other causes of transient incontinence are drugs (see Box 9-1); severe depression or psychosis; restricted mobility; excessive fluid output from high fluid intake; stool impaction; diuretics such as furosemide, caffeine, and alcohol; hyperglycemia; diabetes insipidus; peripheral vascular disease; heart failure; or less often, hypercalcemia.

At present, no evidence-based approach to the prevention of urinary incontinence is available. Avoiding caffeine and alcohol is helpful. Staying close to a toilet after taking a diuretic is another strategy. Management of constipation and avoiding high fluid intake are other methods to avoid the problem.

Urinary Tract Infections (UTIs)

Inflammation of the urinary tract caused by infection is a common problem among older adults, especially those residing in nursing home facilities. Urinary tract infections are one of the top 10 principal hospital diagnoses of older adults. Invasion of

incontinence Loss of the ability to control the elimination of urine. May be occasional or consistent loss of control. Very common in older adults. *Stress* incontinence, which is common in older women, occurs when intra-abdominal pressure exceeds urethral resistance. Urethral muscles become weakened and small amounts of urine are passed. *Urge* incontinence, which is more common in younger women, is an overactive bladder. It is caused by urinary tract infections or central nervous system lesions. The woman feels that she must urinate but cannot control the urine until the time it takes to reach the toilet. *Functional* incontinence occurs when the urinary tract is intact but incontinence occurs due to dementia, musculoskeletal disability, or environmental factors. *Overflow* incontinence is caused by spinal cord abnormalities that affect the detrusor muscles of the bladder.

BOX 9-1 Common Medications/Drugs Associated with Incontinence

Medication/Drug	Effect
Alcohol	Urgency, sedation, frequency
Anticholinergics (ex.) Antihistamines Anti-Parkinson's Antidiarrheals Antiarrhythmics Antispasmodics	Retention, impaired emptying
Antidepressants	Sedation, anticholinergic effects
Antipsychotics	Sedation, anticholinergic effects, rigidity
Calcium-channel blockers	Retention, impaired detrusor contractility, peripheral edema, and nocturnal urination
Diuretics (loop)	Frequency, urgency
Narcotic analgesics	Fecal impaction, urinary retention, sedation
NSAIDs	Peripheral edema and nocturnal urination
Sedative hypnotics	Sedation

Source: Data from DuBeau CE. Urinary incontinence. In: Landefeld CS, Palmer R, Johnson MA, Johnston CB, Lyons W, eds. *Current Geriatric Diagnosis and Treatment.* New York: McGraw Hill; 2004; American Geriatric Society. *Geriatrics Review Syllabus.* 6th ed. New York: American Geriatric Society; 2006.

normal gram-negative bacterial bowel flora (e.g., *Escherichia coli*) is the most common cause of UTIs in older adults. Uncomplicated UTIs occur in healthy older adults and are easily managed. Complicated UTIs occur in frail, debilitated older adults who have decreased immune resistance. Older women with diabetes, an immunosuppressive disorder, or an indwelling catheter are more likely to have recurrent or ongoing infections. Often the first symptom is urinary incontinence, although in frail older adults a new onset of confusion is often the signal of a UTI.

Asymptomatic UTIs do not require antibiotic treatment. Nearly 15% of women in the community and 40% in long-term care settings have asymptomatic bacteriuria. Cranberry products reduce the incidence of UTIs because of the product's acidity. A recommendation for dosage is 300 mL of cranberry juice each day; however, studies continue at this date to fully clarify this. Vitamin C tablets are also useful, because it is more difficult for bacteria to flourish in an acid environment. Estrogen replacement is another option for prevention of UTIs.

benign prostatic hyperplasia (BPH) Enlarged prostate gland of the male. Very common in older men. May be problematic when it causes compression of the urethra. This can result in urinary retention, incomplete emptying of the bladder, urinary overflow incontinence, nocturia (waking up at night to urinate), and hesitancy.

Prostate Disease

Benign prostatic hyperplasia (BPH) is very common, almost universal, in very aged men. It affects approximately 36% of men aged 60 to 79, 44% of men 70 and older, and 90% of men over age 80. BPH seems to be related to diminishing testosterone levels or the estrogen levels still present in the prostate gland with diminishing testosterone (**Figure 9-4**).

BPH interferes with quality of life. It necessitates multiple trips to the bathroom during the day and night, causing sleep disturbances. The older man fears prostate cancer. Other symptoms include dribbling at the end of urination, diminished urine stream, hesitancy, and straining to urinate. As the disorder progresses, the bladder fails to empty, leading to postvoid residual volume of urine. This leads to urge incontinence, requiring a quick run to the bathroom.

Management of BPH is mainly pharmacologic; however, surgery may be performed if there are recurrent UTIs, hematuria, bladder stones, or renal insufficiency. BPH can be managed with alpha-1 blockers, such as terazosin, which relaxes the smooth muscle of the bladder neck, allowing urine to pass more easily. Usually, two types of medications are given to manage this problem: alpha blockers (such as doxazosin, alfazosin, and terazosin) and 5α-reductase inhibitors (such as finasteride dutasteride). Dietary considerations in BPH management include eating whole, fresh, unrefined, and unprocessed foods.

Impotence and Erectile Dysfunction

Impotence or erectile dysfunction is very common among older men; 20% to 46% of men between the ages of 40 to 69 experience it to some degree. The dysfunction can be moderate to severe and is managed with pharmacologic agents, such as sildenafil.

Stones

Urolithiasis is a general term indicating stones present at any location in the urinary tract. *Nephrolithiasis* is the presence of stones in the kidney. Stones may be present in the renal pelvis, renal calyces, ureter, bladder, or urethra. Stones may be sand- or gravel-sized or very large and branching.

Stones are very common and affect men more than women by a ratio of 3:1. It is estimated that one in five persons will experience urolithiasis. Older adults who have incontinence often decrease their fluid intake, thus increasing the propensity for stone formation.

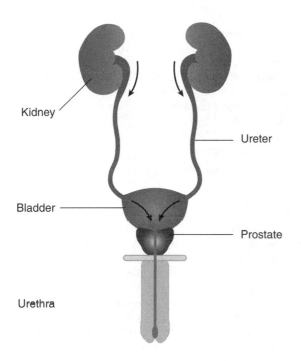

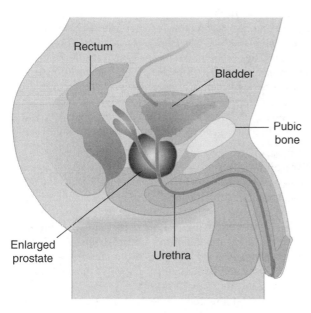

FIGURE 9-4 Front and Side View of the Prostate Gland

Source: National Institutes of Diabetes and Digestive and Kidney Diseases (NIDDK), 2008.

The most common stones are composed of calcium oxylate (70%). These stones have a recurrence rate of 10% in one year and 50% at five years after the first episode of kidney stones. The second most common stone is struvite (10%), which contains a mixture of magnesium, ammonium, and phosphate. These stones usually occur with an infection caused by urease-producing organisms. Uric acid stones (10%) occur in some instances; cysteine (an amino acid) stones and xanthine stones are rare.

Stones develop when crystals separate from the urine and then aggregate within the ureter, the renal pelvis, or other area. It is not clear why stones develop. The incidence is higher in those with small bowel dysfunction, UTIs, anatomical/structural abnormalities of the kidney and ureter, a ureterocele, vesicoureteral reflux, a ureteric stricture, or hyperparathyroidism. Uric acid calculi (stones) occur in those with gout and with chronic metabolic acidosis. Women who have had a surgical menopause are at high risk because of increased bone resorption and excretion of calcium via the urinary tract. Diuretics and some anticonvulsants are associated with stone formation. In addition, people with hypercalcuria, which is inherited, are at greater risk of developing stones. People with hypercalcuria lose calcium whether their intake of calcium is high or low.

Older adults who are dehydrated and those who perspire a lot are more likely to form stones. Interestingly, those who live in the Southeastern United States (the stone belt!) are more vulnerable. Further, the incidence of kidney stones in the United States is increasing and continues to increase with aging. Once a person has a kidney stone, it is likely that he or she will have more.

Older adults who eat protein, sodium, calcium, and oxalate to excess may be more vulnerable to stone formation. Proteins increase the urinary excretion of calcium, oxalate, and uric acid and reduce urinary pH. The excess sodium intake is then excreted via the urine. High urinary sodium increases excretion of calcium and uric acid.

Excessive intake of certain oxylates (found in spinach, beets, peanuts, chocolate, black tea, okra, wheat bran, and strawberries) will increase excretion of oxalates. Other high-oxalate foods (grits, wheat germ, whole wheat flour, blackberries, gooseberries, red currants, tangerines, sweet potatoes, eggplant, cocoa, leeks, summer squash) do not seem to cause the problem. However, the conservative advice is to avoid high-oxalate foods.

The dietary prescription (**Box 9-2**) is to eat the RDA for calcium every day, mainly from calcium-rich foods. When calcium comes from supplements, the risk for stones is higher.

Diagnosis of stones is not difficult and can be made clinically. The pain is often excruciating. The area over the kidneys is tender. There may be blood in the urine. Nausea, vomiting, and diarrhea occur, and the older adult is restless.

Most stones pass within 48 hours. Analgesics are given and the patient is encouraged to consume fluids. If the stones do not pass (10% to 20% of cases), other medical/surgical interventions may be required. If stones block urine flow, hydronephrosis of the kidney may occur, with

BOX 9-2 Prescription for Urolithiasis

- Increase fluid intake to dilute the urine (3 L per day).
- Increase fluids in hot weather and if perspiring.
- Drink fluids in the evening, because urine concentrates overnight.
- 50% of fluid intake should be water.
- Coffee, tea, and wine may lower risk for stones.
- Grapefruit juice may increase risk for stones.
- Avoid high intake of protein.
- Avoid high intake of sodium.
- Avoid high doses of vitamin C if susceptible to oxalate stones (oxalate is synthesized from vitamin C).
- Maintain adequate calcium intake.
- Avoid high-oxalate foods.
- For uric acid stones:
  - Consider a low-purine diet (low in red meats, organ meats, scallops, and sardines).
  - Eat protein in moderation (it acidifies urine).
  - Limit alcohol intake.

Source: Data from Dudek S. *Nutrition Essentials for Nursing Practice.* 5th ed. Philadelphia: Lippincott; 2006.

subsequent renal atrophy, abscess, infection, and/or sepsis. This will compromise renal function. All older adults who have stones, who have had stones, or who are at potential risk should increase their fluid intake.

Genitourinary (GU) Malignancies

Genitourinary malignancies are more common in older adults. Such malignancies include cancers of the prostate, bladder, kidney, ovary, and uterus.

acute renal failure Acute renal failure is an abrupt decrease in renal function usually associated with lessened urine output (oliguria). It may be caused by vascular obstruction, hypotension, or after administration of radiocontrast media when doing X-rays. It is reversible if diagnosed early.

chronic renal failure Chronic renal failure is an irreversible loss of renal function. It is progressive to end-stage renal disease. It is usually caused by long term hypertension and diabetes mellitus.

electrolytes Substances that dissolve into charged particles (ions) when dissolved in water or other solvents and thus are capable of conducting an electrical current. The terms electrolyte and ion are often used interchangeably.

Kidney Cancer

Early symptoms of kidney cancer are vague, but may include anemia, weight loss, hypercalcemia, hypertension, or fever. Advanced signs are flank pain, microhematuria, and a mass on the affected kidney. Surgery is the only option for kidney cancer; radiation and chemotherapy have not proven effective.

Prostate Cancer

African American men are almost twice as likely to develop prostate cancer than White men. Mortality is very high in this group, also. The median age of diagnosis is 68 years of age.

PSA (prostate-specific antigen) laboratory studies are performed annually with digital rectal exam (DRE) in middle-aged and older men. If the PSA is elevated (>4 ng/mL), or elevates over time, a biopsy may be performed. A PSA greater than zero is strongly indicative of prostate cancer.

Many treatment options are available for prostate cancers. Some urologists watch and wait; some do radical prostatectomy; others utilize radiation therapies, hormonal therapy, and chemotherapies. See Chapter 17 on cancers and nutrition.

Bladder Cancer

Bladder cancer is common in older adults. Men are four times more likely to develop this cancer than are older women. Older White males have a higher incidence of bladder cancer compared to other groups; however, older African American men are more likely to die from it. Risk factors for bladder cancer include tobacco use and chemical exposure in the workplace. If the older male has hematuria on urinalysis, a cystoscopy should be considered.

Kidney Problems

Kidney problems in older adults are usually related to other concomitant health problems. Some of these include hypertension, atherosclerosis, fluid and electrolyte problems, sequelae from drugs that affect the renal system, **acute renal failure**, **chronic renal failure**, and diabetes. An elevated serum creatinine level is often used to identify renal problems. An elevated level in males is greater than 1.4 mg/dL, in women, greater than 1.2 mg/dL.

Loss of renal function affects the body's metabolism, nutritional requirements, and nutrition status. If urine output decreases, fluids and **electrolytes** accumulate in the blood. Uremia occurs when nitrogenous wastes accumulate. Metabolic acidosis occurs when the kidneys can no longer excrete acids that are produced in normal metabolism. Many nutrients that should be reabsorbed are excreted in the urine instead. Abnormal or loss of synthesis of renin (needed to sustain normal blood pressure), erythropoietin (needed for red blood cell production), and vitamin D may lead to hypertension, anemia, and osteopenia.

Anemia is common with kidney disease. The National Kidney Foundation Workgroup states that any work up of a patient with this disease should include a complete blood count (CBC) analysis, at least annually. In addition, the absolute reticulocyte count, serum ferritin level, and serum transferrin saturation should be evaluated. The lower limit for hemoglobin is 11. If the patient is on erythropoietin-stimulating agents, the hemoglobin should be maintained at 13, if possible, and the patient tested monthly. See Chapter 10 on hematological problems for more detail.

Hypertension

Systolic blood pressure (SBP) increases with advancing age. See Chapter 10 for more on hypertension and cardiovascular diseases. The prevalence of elevated blood pressure, systolic and diastolic, is 50% to 70%, and highest in older African Americans and in women. Most (about two-thirds) of older adults with hypertension have sodium-sensitive hypertension. That is, blood pressure increases with increased sodium intake.

Older adults have both orthostatic hypotension (blood pressure drops when standing from a sitting or lying position) and postprandial hypotension (drop in blood pressure after eating a meal). These changes are most likely related to a decline in baroreflex sensitivity and changes in the sympathetic nervous system without adequate compensation. Renovascular disease is the most common secondary form of hypertension in older adult patients, after essential hypertension.

The treatment goal is 135/85 mm Hg or 130/80 mm Hg or lower in older adults with diabetes. Many pharmacologic agents are available for management of hypertension. Lifestyle modifications are also very useful in blood pressure management in older adults. Weight reduction, stopping smoking, exercise programs, moderation of alcohol intake, and diet changes that include diminution of sodium, cholesterol, and saturated fats are effective. Adequate intake of potassium, magnesium, and calcium are also important in this regimen. **Box 9-3** describes a number of nonpharmacologic strategies for the management of hypertension.

Fluid and Electrolyte Problems

Hyponatremia

Hyponatremia is an excess of fluids as indicated by a serum sodium level less than 132 mmol/L. This can occur with diminished extracellular fluids (ECF); increased ECF, as in heart failure; or with normal ECF caused by SIADH (syndrome of inappropriate antidiuretic hormone), which can be brought on by SSRIs (a class of antidepressants), other antidepressants, carbamazepine, NSAIDs (e.g., naprosyn), barbiturates, psychosis, meningitis, postoperative state, pneumonias, asthma, and tumors of the lung, pancreas, and thymus. Other causes include increased osmolality and hyperglycemia. It may be caused by normal osmolality from severe hyperlipidemia and hyperproteinemia (e.g., multiple myeloma, a common disorder in older adults). Other causes include decreased

> **BOX 9-3 Nonpharmacologic Interventions for Hypertension**
>
> *By the Practitioner*
> - Evaluate caloric intake at each visit.
> - Evaluate weight at each visit.
> - Assess time spent exercising days/week; recommend 30 to 45 minutes most days of the week.
> - Evaluate sodium intake at each visit.
> - Assess fat intake; recommendation is that less than 30% of total calories should be from fat and less than 10% should be from saturated fat.
> - Assess potassium intake; recommendation is 3,500 mg/day (90 mEq/day).
> - Assess magnesium intake; recommendation is 280–350 mg/day.
> - Assess calcium intake; recommendation is 800–1,200 mg/day.
> - Ask about alcohol consumption at each visit.
>
> *By the Patient*
> - If overweight, lose weight; sustain healthy weight.
> - Begin exercise program or maintain exercise.
> - Stop smoking, if smoking.
> - Avoid secondhand smoke.
> - Drink alcohol in moderation, if at all.
> - Decrease sodium intake; no added salt to meals.
> - Avoid saturated fats.
> - Reduce cholesterol; attain normal blood lipid levels.
> - Eat potassium-rich foods such as bananas, yogurt, halibut, apricots, cantaloupes, tomato juice, spinach, potatoes, acorn squash.
> - Eat magnesium-rich foods, such as almonds, cashews, sesame seeds, halibut.
> - Eat calcium-rich foods, such as milk, yogurt, almonds, tofu, calcium-fortified juices, and greens and take additional calcium tablets.
>
> *Source:* Data from American Geriatric Society. *Geriatrics Review Syllabus.* 6th ed. New York: American Geriatric Society; 2006; Insel P, Turner RE, Ross D. *Discovering Nutrition.* 2nd ed. Sudbury, MA: Jones & Bartlett; 2006; National Guideline Clearinghouse. *Hypertension, Nutrition Management for Older Adults*; 2002.

> **hyponatremia** Abnormally low sodium concentrations in the blood due to excessive excretion of sodium (by the kidney), prolonged vomiting, or diarrhea.

plasma osmolality from increased extracellular fluid from kidney failure, heart failure, hepatic cirrhosis, and nephrotic syndrome. Symptoms occur when the sodium is less than 125 mmol/L and include somnolence, cognition deficits, seizures, and then coma from edema of the brain.

Management is to find and treat the underlying cause. One should increase sodium slowly; eliminate water excess; replace urine output with saline or isotonic saline; and monitor the sodium until resolution occurs and symptoms disappear. If the disorder is chronic, eliminate the precipitating causes (medications, illness); restrict water to 1,000 to 1,500 mL a day; and liberalize salt intake.

Hypernatremia

Older adults, especially those in nursing homes, are often dehydrated. Dehydration, or **hypernatremia**, is caused by water loss, hypotonic sodium loss, hypertonic sodium gain, and impaired thirst, which is common in elders and sometimes is caused by lack of access to fluids.

Water loss may be a result of increased sweating and respiration, very high temperatures without relief, hypercalcemia, or lithium intake. Hypotonic sodium loss occurs with vomiting and diarrhea; nasogastric (NG) drainage; osmotic cathartics, such as lactulose; hyperglycemia with osmotic diuresis; or from acute tubular necrosis in the kidney. Hypertonic sodium gain is caused by treatment with hypertonic saline by health providers. Impaired thirst can occur normally with hypertonicity, delirium, and/or intubation. It can also occur in those who have no or difficult access to water. It is important to teach older adults that in hot weather, especially without air conditioning, increased fluid intake is essential, even if they do not feel thirsty.

Management includes measuring intake & output; obtaining urine osmolality; treating any underlying causes; and correcting the imbalance slowly over 48 to 72 hours with pure water. In cases of severe volume depletion, the older adult should be provided with normal saline and then switched to hypotonic fluids when stable. See **Figure 9-5** for the formula to estimate the effect of 1 L of infusate on serum sodium.

Fluid Replenishment in Hypernatremia

Use this formula when estimating the effect of one liter of any infusate on serum sodium (Na).

$$\text{Change in serum Na} = \frac{\text{infusate Na} - \text{serum NA}}{\text{Total body water} + 1}$$

- Infusate Na (mmol/L): D5W = 0; ¼ NS = 34; ½ NS = 77; NS = 154
- Total body water calculated as a fraction of body weight (0.5 kg in older men, and 0.45 in older women)
- Divide the treatment goal (often use 10 mmol/L/d) by change in serum Na/L (in the formula) to determine amount of solution to be given over 24 hours
- Compensate for normal fluid losses, about 1–1.5 L/d
- To determine rate/hour, divide the amount of solution for repletion plus the amount for compensation of normal fluid losses, by 24 (hours/day).

Na = sodium   L = liter   d = Day

FIGURE 9-5 Formula for Fluid Replenishment in Hypernatremia

Source: Data from Reuben D, Herr K, Pacala J, et al. *Geriatrics at Your Fingertips, 2009.* 11th ed. New York: American Geriatric Society; 2009.

B12 therapy; kidney problems, such as renal artery stenosis; and from hypomagnesemia from diuretic use.

Low potassium results in ventricular arrhythmias in the heart, muscle weakness, cramping, myalgias, muscle tenderness, and fatigue. Rhabdomyolysis, a breakdown of muscle mass, can occur. This causes a metabolic alkalosis in the kidneys, but with a low urine pH (aciduria).

Management includes potassium replacement with potassium chloride (KCl) (additional chloride), except in older adults with renal tubular acidosis. In this event, the patient should receive potassium with alkaline salts.

Hypokalemia

A low potassium (K) lab report usually indicates depletion of total body potassium. Causes include vomiting, diarrhea, laxative use, and nasogastric suction. **Hypokalemia** commonly occurs with diuretics and usually is easily avoided through the use of potassium supplements. It can also result from medications (e.g., antibiotics, steroids); vitamin

Hyperkalemia

Hyperkalemia can be caused by renal failure, renal tubular acidosis, metabolic acidosis, diabetic hyperglycemia, hyponatremia, hemolysis, rhabdomyolysis, constipation, drugs (e.g., ACE inhibitors, B-adrenergic blockers, NSAIDs, tetracycline), and gastrointestinal bleeding. Other, less common causes include pseudohyperkalemia from extreme thrombocytosis and leukocytosis.

Laboratory demonstration of hyperkalemia may vary by lab, but it is usually greater than 5.5 mEq/L. A laboratory value greater than 6 mEq/L should be treated with or without electrocardiogram (ECG) changes. See **Box 9-4** for management of elevated potassium.

hypernatremia Abnormally high sodium concentrations in the blood due to increased kidney retention of sodium or rapid ingestion of large amounts of salt.

hypokalemia Inadequate levels of potassium in the blood.

hyperkalemia Abnormally high potassium concentrations in the blood.

BOX 9-4 Management of Serum Potassium

Minor Elevation of Serum Potassium (<6 mEq/L) Without ECG Changes

- Diet low in potassium
- Oral diuretics: torsemide, bumetanide, loop + thiazide diuretics
- Avoid potassium-saving diuretics: triamterene and spironolactone
- Avoid NSAIDs
- Avoid ACE inhibitors
- Oral $NaHCO_3$ (650–1,300 mg twice a day)

Serum Potassium of 6–6.5 mEq/L Without ECG Changes

- All of those listed for minor serum elevation, plus those listed below.
- Sodium polystyrene sulfonate (SPS, Kayexelate): 15 to 30 grams by mouth q 6–24 hours/day or as an enema (30–50 grams in 100 mL of dextrose) once a day or as needed; will take hours to days for change on labs to occur.

Serum Potassium of 6.5 mEq/L with ECG Change (Peaked T Waves)

- May require hospitalization depending on the cause.

Serum Potassium of 8.0 mEq/L and ECG Changes (Peaked T Waves, Prolonged PR Interval, Loss of P Waves, Wide QRS)

- Hospitalization; acute deterioration of kidney function occurs; requires IVs and cardiac monitoring.

Source: Data from Reuben D, Herr K, Pacala J, et al. *Geriatrics at Your Fingertips, 2009.* 11th ed. New York: American Geriatric Society; 2009; American Geriatric Society. *Geriatrics Review Syllabus.* 6th ed. New York: American Geriatric Society; 2006.

BOX 9-5 Classification of Renal Dysfunction/Failure

Region of Dysfunction/ Failure	Causes
Prerenal	Loss of fluid (hypovolemia): vomiting, diarrhea, diuretics, intestinal obstruction, diabetes mellitus (uncontrolled); blood hemorrhage, blood plasma loss (peritonitis, burns) Hypotension: septic shock, heart failure, pulmonary embolus, renal artery stenosis
Intrarenal	Acute tubular necrosis (ATN), coagulation defects, bilateral acute pyelonephritis, renal artery or vein occlusion, glomerulopathy, malignant hypertension
Postrenal	Obstructive uropathy: stones, blood clots, edema, tumor; bladder neck obstruction from prostatic hypertrophy

Source: Data from McCance K, Huether S. *Pathophysiology.* 5th ed. Philadelphia: Elsevier Mosby; 2006.

Renal Disease and Failure

Kidney dysfunction in the older adult is often chronic, progressive, and irreversible. In some cases, however, it can be acute, rapid, progressive, and reversible. Renal failure is the inability to remove nitrogenous waste from the body and an inability to regulate fluids and electrolytes. A classification of renal dysfunction/failure is provided in **Box 9-5**. It is a worldwide problem and is increasing in prevalence.

Lung cancer, the most common cancer cause of death in the United States, is followed closely by kidney failure as a cause of death. Kidney failure is predictive of cardiovascular disease and is a risk factor for cardiovascular mortality as well as morbidity. Common kidney diseases in older adults are nephrotic syndrome from diabetes mellitus and membranous nephropathy (MN), possibly arising from NSAIDs, antibiotics, cancer, and/or hepatitis B infection.

Acute renal insufficiency/failure (ARF) is a common kidney dysfunction. It is an acute, sudden deterioration of renal status defined by diminished urine output or increased laboratory values such as hematuria and proteinuria, high urea and creatinine, and pyuria with WBCs or even normal urine. It is a medical emergency. It presents with a change in mental status and is usually reversible. ARF occurs in those with acute tubular necrosis, most commonly due to nephrotoxins or hypoperfusion, medications such as aminoglycosides and gentomycin, NSAIDS, and radiocontrast materials in some X-rays, obstruction from BPH, and collagen vascular diseases. Other causes include multiple myeloma (cancer) and cirrhosis with redistribution of extracellular fluid. ARF occurs in 8% to 10% of hospitalized older adults. **Figure 9-6** shows a cross-section of the glomerulus.

In younger adults, ARF presents as oliguria, or diminished urine output. In older patients, this may not occur, and the presenting symptom may be postural hypotension. Dependent edema of the ankles and legs may be present. The BUN (blood urea nitrogen) is elevated, as is the serum creatinine (Cr). A laboratory study to determine the

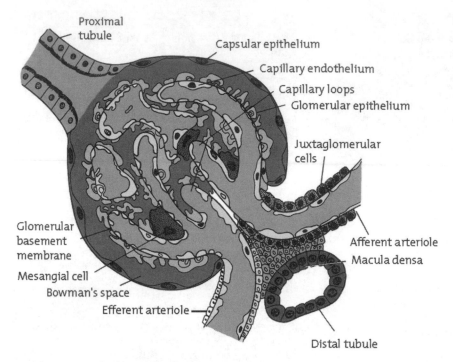

FIGURE 9-6 Cross-Section of the Glomerulus

Source: Reproduced from *An Introduction to Human Disease*. 7th ed. Courtesy of Leonard V. Crowley, M.D., Century College.

fractional excretion of urea (FEun) is done if the older adult is on diuretics. If the older adult is not on diuretics, a fractional excretion of sodium (FEna) is calculated (**Box 9-6**). If a urinalysis (UA) is normal, the cause of ARF is usually prerenal or postrenal. The bladder may need catheterization to determine the postvoid residual for an accurate assessment of output.

ARF is a difficult problem to manage, and the care team must include a nutritionist, a nurse, and a nephrologist (renal specialty physician). The patient may lose up to 1 pound a day during the management of ARF. Fluid loss must be monitored so that the patient does not go into heart failure. Further, nutritional supplements, which are high in calories, may be contraindicated in the patient with ARF.

◗ BOX 9-6 Formulas for Determining Severity of Acute Renal Failure

Formula for Older Adult on Diuretics	Results
$FEun = \dfrac{[\text{urine urea nitrogen / BUN}]}{\text{Urine Cr / plasma Cr}} \times 100$	<35% = prerenal azotemia >50% = ATN 35–50% = nondiagnostic

Formula for Older Adult Not on Diuretics	Results
$FEna = \dfrac{[\text{urine Na / plasma Na}]}{\text{Urine Cr / plasma Cr}} \times 100$	<1% = prerenal cause >3% = ATN

ATN = acute tubular necrosis

BUN = blood urea nitrogen

Na = sodium

Cr = creatinine

FE = fraction excretion

Source: Data from Reuben D, Herr K, Pacala J, et al. *Geriatrics at Your Fingertips, 2006–2007.* 8th ed. New York: American Geriatric Society; 2006.

Acute tubular necrosis (ATN) is caused by hypoperfusion of the kidney (ischemia) or nephrotoxins. Approximately 40% to 50% of cases caused by ischemia occur after surgery. ATN is also associated with trauma or sepsis (infection in the blood).

ATN is a precipitant of acute renal failure. Urinalysis will demonstrate epithelial cells and granular and epithelial cells casts. Management of ATN requires daily monitoring of the patient's weight. A good record of intake and output is important, as is frequent monitoring of electrolytes. Fluid replacement should equal urine excretion (and any other fluid losses), plus 500 mL for insensible losses (respiration, perspiration, etc.).

Dialysis is necessary if severe hyperkalemia (greater than 6.5 mEq/L), acidosis, or volume overload is not manageable with therapy. If uremia occurs (signs include coagulopathy, encephalopathy, pericarditis), dialysis is needed. Other, less urgent signs of uremia include nausea and vomiting and fatigue. With uremia, wound healing diminishes and the risk of pneumonia and other infections are anticipated. If the ATN is reversible, the goal is to maintain life until the kidney repairs itself, which may take up to 12 months.

Chronic Renal Failure

Chronic renal failure (CRF), or chronic kidney disease (CKD), is the irreversible loss of renal function. It affects nearly all the body's organ systems. CRF is progressive to the point of end-stage renal disease (ESRD). CRF commonly occurs with diabetes mellitus and hypertension—two very common problems of older adults. The goal of therapy is to slow the progression of kidney failure. This is best accomplished by keeping the blood pressure to 125/75 mm Hg or lower if there is proteinuria or elevated Cr (creatinine) and the diabetes to a HbA1c of less than 7. Although controversial, moderating the protein intake to 1 g per kilogram of body weight per day is often recommended.

Many older adults have chronic kidney disease and do not know it. Approximately 6 million people in the United States have as little as 60% of their kidney function. Minorities and those with high blood pressure and/or diabetes are most at risk for developing chronic kidney disease. If early treatment is begun when patients have no symptoms, kidney failure can be delayed.

Early diagnosis is possible by measuring serum creatinine levels in those older adults most at risk. The serum creatinine level is a measure of kidney function. However, even in the normal range, those at high risk should have creatinine clearance calculated. Older adults who are at risk for chronic kidney failure should be counseled to maintain recommended blood pressure and blood glucose levels. These older adults also need to avoid NSAIDs and other nephrotoxic agents that could increase the risk for acute renal failure.

Chronic kidney disease (CKD) is defined as kidney damage of at least three months or longer in duration with or without a decrease in GFR or a GFR less than 60 mL/min/1.73 m² for three months or longer with or without kidney damage. In CKD, renal function declines as the numbers of nephrons (the structural and functional unit of the kidney) decline. This occurs somewhat with normal aging, but more markedly with hypertension and diabetes.

Markers for CKD are proteinuria (albumin), abnormal urine sediment, abnormalities in imaging studies, and diagnostic values in blood and urine chemistry. Using a urine dipstick, the total protein will be greater than 1+; the albumin-specific dipstick will be positive. The urine albumin/creatinine ratio will be greater than 30 mg/g, and the urine total protein/creatinine ratio will be greater than 200 mg/g.

The GFR affects the excretion of water-soluble drugs and results in high serum levels of others. Consequently, it is necessary to estimate the GFR in *all* elderly patients who require medications. The GFR is low in older adults with CKD (<20 mL/min). Decline in GFR is determined by estimating the creatinine clearance through a 24-hour urine collection or through a mathematical estimation via the Cockcroft-Gault formula (**Box 9-7**).

A number of problems occur with CRF that require management. Anemia of chronic kidney disease is one such condition, and it requires very expensive drug management in order to be managed well. Two of the most often used drugs to manage this condition are darbepoetin alfa and epoetin alfa. These drugs reduce the need for red blood cell replacement by transfusion and can dramatically improve quality of life. Other problems include hyperphosphatemia, restless legs syndrome (RLS), uremic pruritus (itching), iron deficiency anemia, metabolic acidosis, and vitamin loss. See **Table 9-1** for management strategies for these problems.

Another problem in CKD is "the silent crippler," or renal osteodystrophy, which is now called CKD-MBD (MBD standing for mineral and bone disorder). This disorder is associated with extremely high cardiovascular disease morbidity and mortality. Renal osteodystrophy is the result of a calcium problem caused by the parathyroid glands, which release parathyroid hormone (PTH). The hormone draws

> **BOX 9-7 Cockcroft-Gault Formula for Estimating Creatinine Clearance**
>
> $$\text{Creatinine Clearance mL/min} = \frac{(140 - \text{age}) \times \text{weight (kg)} \times (0.85 \text{ in women}; 1.0 \text{ in men})}{72 \times \text{serum Cr (mg/dl)}}$$

TABLE 9-1 Management of Problems Associated with Chronic Kidney Disease

Problem	Management
Iron deficiency anemia	Parenteral iron (iron sucrose or sodium ferricgluconate, if on hemodialysis; ferrous sulfate, ferrous gluconate acceptable by mouth)
Anemia of CKD	Epoetin alfa, darbepoetin alfa
Hyperphosphatemia	Phosphate binders (e.g., calcium-based binders such as calcium carbonate or calcium acetate); sevelamer (if elevated serum calcium)
Hyperkalemia	Restrict orange juice, bananas, potatoes, cantaloupes, and tomatoes; diuretics, oral bicarbonate
Renal osteodystrophy due to secondary hyperparathyroidism	Pulse IV calcitriol; paracalcitol, doxercalciferol (if elevated serum calcium or phosphate levels); cinacalcet (lowers parathyroid level)
Bleeding (uremia)	Parenteral desmopressin (may need blood products if hemoglobin is greater than 1 g/dL/day)
Pruritus (uremia) and malodorous perspiration	Gabapentin, oral antihistamines, parenteral lidocaine with dialysis
Vitamin deficiencies (hemodialysis-removed)	Vitamin B complex, vitamin C (prescriptions, not OTC); folic acid; intact parathyroid hormone for vitamin D deficiency
Restless leg syndrome	Gabapentin, ropinirole, clonazepam
Metabolic acidosis (HCO$_3$ <20 mEq/L) (hemodialysis)	Citric acid plus sodium citrate; if GI upset occurs, use sodium bicarbonate tablets
"Feeling sick"	Between dialysis sessions, waste builds up in blood, causing "sick" feeling. Dietitian can help plan meals to avoid this problem.

Source: Data from Omnicare. *Geriatric Pharmaceutical Care Guidelines.* Covington, KY: Omnicare; 2006; Neighborcare. *Geriatric Drug Therapy Handbook.* Hudson, OH: Lexicomp; 2004; Reuben D, Herr K, Pacala J, et al. *Geriatrics at Your Fingertips, 2006–2007.* 8th ed. New York: American Geriatric Society; 2006; National Institutes of Diabetes and Digestive and Kidney Diseases (NIDDK), 2008.

calcium from the bones and raises blood calcium levels. This continues slowly over time, destroying the bones and causing extraskeletal calcifications. Further, phosphorus helps regulate calcium in the bones. In CKD, phosphorus levels rise, which decreases calcium levels, thus drawing more calcium from the bone.

Renal osteodystrophy often begins many years prior to the appearance of symptoms. Often the symptoms appear after a patient has been on dialysis for several years. If left untreated, the bones become weakened and at risk for fracture and may even cause pain.

Older patients and postmenopausal women are at greater risk for renal osteodystrophy, because they are already vulnerable to osteoporosis. Renal osteodystrophy can be managed by dietary changes. Reducing dietary intake of phosphorus is one of the most important steps in prevention of bone disease. Nearly all foods contain phosphorus, but it is particularly high in milk, cheese, dried beans, peas, nuts, and peanut butter. It is also wise to limit drinks such as cocoa, dark sodas, and beer. Medications such as calcium carbonate (Tums) can be prescribed with meals. The calcium carbonate will bind phosphorus in the bowel and decrease absorption of phosphorus into the blood. The binder should be free of aluminum, because aluminum can be toxic to these patients and cause anemia. It is a good idea for people with renal osteodystrophy to consult a renal dietitian.

Medical management of CKD-MBD is in its infancy. Because treatment should reduce cardiovascular mortality, research is ongoing. Recent novel approaches include active vitamin D analogues, noncalcium-containing phosphate binders, and cinacalcet.

End-Stage Renal Disease

End-stage renal disease (ESRD) is most commonly associated with diabetes and/or hypertension and occurs when the kidneys can no longer function normally on their own. The incidence of ESRD has nearly doubled in the past 10 years. Cardiovascular disease is the main cause of death in those with ESRD, and the CVD mortality is 5 to 30 times higher in dialysis patients than in the general population. ESRD is usually caused by diabetes, hypertension, and glomerulonephritis; these three account for 80% of all cases.

Many older adults die before they have dialysis. Secondary hyperparathyroidism (SHPT) occurs frequently in patients with CKD and is associated with complications, including bone disease, uremic pruritus, and higher cardiovascular morbidity and mortality. In a study by Kovesdy, Ahmadzadeh, Anderson, and Kalantar-Zadeh of over 500 older men, veterans with late-stage CKD but predialysis, one-half received calcitriol, the activated vitamin D analogue. The results showed that those in the treatment group had less need for dialysis and a lower incidence of mortality.

Dialysis

Those who are prepared emotionally and medically are better able to achieve long-term success with dialysis than those who are not. Dialysis is usually started once the GFR has dropped to 10 to 15. The older adult should be asked if he or she would prefer peritoneal dialysis versus hemodialysis. Few older adults are considered for transplant.

African Americans are four times more likely to develop kidney diseases requiring dialysis than any other ethnic group in the United States. Kidney disease often occurs in African American men at a very young adult age. It most cases it does not present with signs or symptoms, and thus it is less likely to be diagnosed. The main causes of kidney disease in African Americans are hypertension and diabetes.

According to the National Kidney Foundation, protein nutrition cannot be evaluated by a single assessment tool. When the older adult is undergoing dialysis, care should focus on the predialysis serum albumin, the percent of usual body weight, percent of NHANES II (National Health and Nutrition Evaluation Survey II) body weight, subjective global assessment, dietary interviews and diaries, and protein equivalent of total nitrogen appearance normalized to body weight. Such an assessment should be done monthly to every 6 months.

Patients undergoing hemodialysis lose bone mineral density (BMD), especially if the patient is underweight. Researchers found a significant positive relationship between BMD, weight, height, BMI, fractures, dialysis time, and intact PTH. This has important implications for the nutritionist.

Additional assessment tools include measurement of skin-fold thickness, mid-arm circumference, serum creatinine, cholesterol, blood urea nitrogen, and creatinine index. Predialysis serum albumin is a measure of future mortality risk. The lower limit of the normal range is 4.0 mg/dL; a value lower than 30 mg/dL is a risk factor for mortality. Those with low predialysis albumin should be evaluated for protein energy malnutrition. The prealbumin level is probably equally good as albumin as a measure of the visceral protein pool.

Serum creatinine is a commonly used measure of renal function. Low or declining cholesterol levels signify a mortality risk. Those with serum creatinine levels of 150 to 180 mg/dL should be evaluated for nutritional deficits.

The recommended daily energy intake for older adults on chronic peritoneal dialysis is 30 to 35 kcal per kilogram of bodyweight per day. Recommended daily protein intake is 1.2 to 1.3 grams per kilogram of body weight per day. At least 50% of dietary protein should be of high biological value. Older adults who are sedentary should have a total energy intake of 30 to 35 kcal per kilogram of body weight per day.

Nutritional counseling should be intensive and offered at least monthly at the start of dialysis. Nutritional supplementation will need to be considered for older adults who are unable to meet their nutritional goals. Their oral diet may need to be fortified with energy and protein supplements. If this is not adequate, tube feeding should be considered, as appropriate. If this is not adequate, the next step is intradialytic peritoneal nutrition or amino acids. If all of this is insufficient, consider parenteral nutrition.

In patients with kidney disease, five nutrients must be controlled: protein, sodium, potassium, phosphorus, and fluids (**Box 9-8**). However, individual needs vary; for example, if the patient is retaining fluids and sodium, the patient's blood pressure and body weight will increase. If sodium is too low, the patient's blood pressure and weight will decrease. See **Table 9-2** for food restrictions for patients undergoing hemodialysis.

BOX 9-8 Five Nutrients Requiring Control in Chronic Kidney Disease

1. **Sodium.** Limit to 1,500–3,000 mg/day

2. **Potassium.** No food source restrictions. Renal patients should not use potassium chloride as a salt substitute.

3. **Phosphorus.** If dietary protein is reduced, dietary phosphorus also falls. No further restriction needed unless the serum phosphorus level is high. With progression of renal disease, diet will not control phosphorus, and phosphate binders will become necessary. Do *not* use aluminum-based binders.

4. **Protein.** The lowest recommended level is 0.6 grams per kilogram of body weight plus 24-hour urinary protein loss. If the older adult cannot maintain this diet or a patient is at nutritional risk, the protein allowance should be raised to 0.7–0.8 grams per kilogram bodyweight.

   Older adults with insulin-dependent diabetes mellitus need 0.8 grams per kilogram body weight of protein because insulin deficiency increases protein degradation. Most (75%) protein should come from high biological value proteins (e.g., eggs). These proteins should be distributed over 24 hours.

5. **Fluid.** Calculate intake. Calculate urine output, estimating 500 mg for insensible water loss in addition to the 24-hour urine output. This amount determines fluid needs.

TABLE 9-2 Dietary Knowledge for Hemodialysis

Topic Area	Knowledge Need
Fluids	Calculate daily intake of fluids; include fluids in soups, ice cream, fruits, and vegetables. Fluids build up between dialysis sessions, which can lead to swelling and weight gain, increased blood pressure, and possible heart failure.
Potassium (K)	Increases between dialysis sessions; too much potassium is dangerous for cardiac status and may cause death. Avoid foods such as bananas, kiwis, and dried fruits; eat small portions of high-potassium foods (e.g., half a pear, orange, or melon). Soak potatoes to remove some potassium. Reduce intake of other high-potassium foods: apricots, beets, brussels sprouts, clams, dates, figs, lima beans, milk, peanuts, prune juice, raisins, sardines, spinach, tomatoes, winter squash, yogurt.
Phosphorus	Too much phosphorus leaches calcium from bone, causing bone weakness and possible fracture. Can also cause itching. Avoid foods high in phosphorus: milk, cheese, dried beans, peas, colas, nuts, peanut butter. Phosphate binders—Renagel, PhosLo, Tums, calcium carbonate—cause phosphorus to be excreted in the stool.
Protein	Prior to dialysis, patients are on a low-protein diet. On dialysis, patients are encouraged to eat high-quality protein in large amounts. Many older adults lose their taste for protein/meats, so this may be difficult. Protein will help retain muscle and repair tissue. It helps maintain resistance to infection and recover from surgeries more quickly. The following are sources of high-quality protein: meat, fish, poultry, and eggs, especially egg whites, which can be added to many recipes without much taste change.
Sodium	Sodium intake increases thirst; thirst causes increased fluid intake. Patients look for "low sodium" labels on foods. Advise patients not to use salt substitutes, because many contain potassium. Some salt substitutes do not include potassium.
Calories	If advised to gain weight, oils are a good way to add nutrient-dense calories. Vegetable oils such as olive oil, canola oil, and safflower oil are good on breads, rice, and pasta. Avoid butter and margarines, which may contribute to heart disease. Hard candy, sugar, honey, jams, and jellies also provide calories and energy without damage to arteries; however, if diabetic, this might not be advisable.
Vitamins/Minerals	Because so many foods have to be avoided, a supplement may be necessary. Nephrocaps is one. Advise the patient and family not to buy any over-the-counter supplements, which may contain vitamins and minerals that are harmful. Any supplement should be by prescription.

Source: Data from National Institutes of Diabetes and Digestive and Kidney Diseases (NIDDK), Eat Right to Feel Right on Hemodialysis. Available at: http://kidney.niddk.nih.gov/kudiseases/pubs/eatright/index.htm. Accessed June 30, 2009.

Conclusion

The kidney is a miraculous organ with many functions. When the kidneys fail, for whatever reason, there are serious consequences for the elderly patient. The same is true of failure of the genitourinary tract, especially with regards to urinary incontinence, which leads to loss of quality of life for many older adults. Diet and nutrition therapy can help in the management of many of these problems.

Activities Related to This Chapter

1. Draw the anatomy of the kidney and genitourinary system.
2. Lead a discussion of the problems that occur in the aging kidney and genitourinary system and how dietary management can make a positive difference.
3. List some of the important electrolytes and the abnormalities that can occur with abnormal kidney status and how dietary management can help.
4. Go online and visit the National Institute on Aging website and obtain up-to-date information on erythropoietin and its use in renal disease in older adults.

Case Study

Mr. Peters is a 68-year-old retiree who lives with his wife of 45 years in their own home. Mr. Peters, who is an African American, has had diabetes mellitus for ten years and his weight has fallen from 180 pounds (he is 5' 9") to 150 pounds. He and his wife eat a "good" diet. Recently, his physician has told him that his kidneys are not doing so well and that he has had an MI sometime in the recent past, as shown by electrocardiogram. His physician has advised Mr. Peters to seek further counseling, and he comes to you today.

Questions

1. What additional information should you provide to Mr. Peters?
2. How will you obtain good information?
3. Should his wife come with him to other visits?
4. What laboratory studies will you want to see?

REFERENCES

Agency for Healthcare Research & Quality. Primary care. Available at: www.ahrq.gov/research/dec01/1201RA16. hrm. Accessed August 9, 2006.

American Geriatric Society. *Geriatrics Review Syllabus*. 6th ed. New York: American Geriatric Society; 2006.

Bloom R, Bress J. Chronic kidney disease: a primary-care guide. *Clin Advis*. 2007;4;31–38.

British Medical Journal. *Clinical Evidence*. (14).

Burke MM, Laramie JA. *Primary Care of the Older Adult*. 2nd ed. St Louis: Mosby; 2004.

Castillo RF, Esteban de la Rosa RJ. Relation between body mass index and bone mineral density among haemodialysis patients with chronic kidney disease. *J of Renal Care*. 2009;35(S1):57–64.

Crowley L. *Introduction to Human Disease*. 6th ed. Sudbury, MA: Jones & Bartlett; 2004.

DuBeau CE. Urinary incontinence. In CS Landefeld, R Palmer, MA Johnson, CB Johnston, W Lyons, eds. *Current Geriatric Diagnosis and Treatment*. McGraw-Hill: New York; 2004.

Dudek, S. *Nutrition Essentials for Nursing Practice*. 5th ed. Philadelphia: Lippincott; 2006.

Ebersole P, Hess P, Luggen A. *Toward Healthy Aging*. St. Louis: Mosby; 2004.

Griebling TL. Geriatric urology. New frontiers in geriatrics research: an agenda for surgical and related medical specialties. American Geriatric Society. Available at: www.frycomm.com/ags/rasp/chapter.asp?ch = 10. Accessed March 28, 2006.

Neighborcare. *Geriatric Drug Therapy Handbook*. Hudson, OH: Lexicomp; 2004.

Kovesdy C, Ahmadzadeh S, Anderson J, Kalantar-Zadeh K. Association of activated vitamin D treatment and mortality in chronic kidney disease. *Arch Int Med*. 2008;168(4):397–403.

Landefeld CS, Palmer RM, Johnson MA, Johnston CB, Lyons WL. *Current Geriatric Diagnosis and Treatment*. Chicago: McGraw-Hill; 2004.

Love K. Early recognition and treatment of chronic kidney disease (CKD). Kentucky Nurse Practitioner Annual Conference, April 2007, Lexington, Kentucky.

Mohammed I, Hutchison AJ. Oral phosphate binders for the management of serum phosphate levels in dialysis patients. *J of Renal Care*. 2009;35(1)65–70.

National Institute of Diabetes and Digestive and Kidney Diseases (NIDDK), National Institutes of Health. Kidney and urologic diseases statistics for the U.S. NIH Public. No. 02-3895. Washington DC: US Dept. Health and Human Services; 2001.

National Institute of Diabetes and Digestive and Kidney Diseases (NIDDK), National Institutes of Health. Kidney and urologic diseases statistics for the U.S. NIH Public. No. 02-3895. Washington DC: US Dept. Health and Human Services; 2007.

National Institute of Diabetes and Digestive and Kidney Diseases (NIDDK), National Institutes of Health. What I need to know about urinary tract infections. NIH Public. No. 04-4807. Washington DC: US Dept. Health and Human Services; 2004.

National Institutes of Health, National Kidney and Urologic Diseases Information. Nutrition for later chronic kidney disease in adults, 2005. Available at: http://kidney.niddk.nih.gov/kudiseases/pubs/renalosteodystrophy/index.htm. Accessed February 26, 2008.

National Institutes of Health, National Kidney and Urologic Diseases Information. Renal osteodystrophy, 2005. NIH Public. No. 05-4630. Available at: http://kidney.niddk.nih.gov/kudiseases/pubs/NutritionLateCKD/index.htm. Accessed February 26, 2008.

National Kidney and Urologic Diseases Information Clearinghouse (NKUDIC). Kidney stones in adults. Available at: http://kidney.niddk.nih.gov/kudiseases/pubs/stones-adults/index.htm. Accessed February 26, 2008.

Ogata H, Koiwa F, Kinugasa K, Akizawa T. CKD-MBD: impact on management of kidney disease. *Clin Exp Nephrol*. 2007;11(4)261–268.

Reuben D, Herr K, Pacala J, Pollock B, Potter J, Semla T. *Geriatrics at Your Fingertips*. 8th ed. New York: American Geriatric Society; 2006–2007.

Stanfield P, Hui Y. *Nutrition and Diet Therapy*. 4th ed. Boston: Jones & Bartlett; 2003.

Svara F. Chronic kidney disease-mineral and bone disorder (CKD-MBD): a new term for a complex approach. *J of Renal Care*. 2009;35(1);3–6.

U.S. Renal Data System. Reference tables. 2006. Available at: http://www.usrds.org/reference_2006.htm. Accessed February 2008.

Urology Channel. Benign prostatic hyperplasia (BPH)/ enlarged prostate treatments. January 2009. Available at: http://www.urologychannel.com/prostate/bph/treatments.shtml. Accessed February 10, 2009.

CHAPTER
10

Nutritional Aspects of Management of Hematological Disorders in Older Adults

Kathy J. Shattler, MS, RD and
Ann Schmidt Luggen, PhD, GNP

CHAPTER OBJECTIVES   Upon successful completion of this chapter the reader will be able to:

1. Describe the process of hematopoiesis
2. Explain how aging affects the process of hematopoiesis
3. List the most common nutritional elements that affect the aging hematopoetic system
4. Define the different types of anemia
5. List the most common causes of anemia in older adults
6. Discuss the most common treatments for the various anemias
7. Describe the role of nutrition in the etiology of various anemias
8. Describe the role of nutrition in the treatment plan for various anemias

KEY TERMS AND CONCEPTS

Anemia	Lymphocytes
Apoptosis	Mean cell volume
Erythrocytes	Methylmalonic acid
Ferritin	Platelets
Folic acid	Pyridoxine
Granulocytes	Red blood cell
Hematopoiesis	Stem cell
Hemoglobin	Stroma
Iron	Vitamin B12

The reserve capacity of **hematopoiesis** (the formation of blood cells in the body, especially in the bone marrow) diminishes with advancing age. This renders the older adult more susceptible to **anemias**, age-related hematologic abnormalities in both men and women. Older adults are four to six times more likely than younger adults to have anemia. In many studies, the rates of anemia in older adults are even higher. This is particularly true of men aged 75 and older, who have significantly lower blood hemoglobin

hematopoiesis Production of blood cells in the bone marrow. It is a two-stage process of mitosis (division) and maturation (differentiation). The cells undergo these stages prior to entering the blood system. Each blood cell has a parent cell called a stem cell that determines what kind of blood cell it will be.

Anemia Abnormally low concentration of hemoglobin in the bloodstream; can be caused by impaired synthesis of red blood cells, increased destruction of red cells, or significant loss of blood.

values than men 65 years of age and younger. The decrease in hematopoiesis may be due to comorbid illnesses, diminished erythropoietin (EPO) drive, or both, or because of diminished androgen concentration with aging.

Hematological deficiencies are common in older adults. The adult may have an iron-deficiency anemia and a vitamin B-12 deficiency concomitantly. The laboratory diagnosis is complex. Combined deficiencies are common, so it is useful to look for B12, folate, and iron deficiencies in all cases.

Because older adults often have multiple comorbidities and inflammation-causing disorders, the usual laboratory values of **iron**, total iron-binding capacity, and **ferritin** are less reliable. Anemia of chronic disease (ACD) is particularly common in older adults, especially in those with acute and chronic infection, malignancy, protein-calorie malnutrition, unidentified chronic disease, and chronic inflammatory conditions such as rheumatoid arthritis. When ACD is combined with iron deficiency anemia (IDA), the anemia is often much more severe than in chronic disease alone. Further, older adults have a blunted neutrophilic response to infection. This contributes to increased infection-caused morbidity.

Although blood **platelets** do not diminish with age, concentrations of coagulation enzymes increase, leading to increased hypercoagulability. Fibrin increases, as do factors VII, VIII, IX, X and thrombin–antithrombin complexes. Hyperhomocysteinemia also increases with aging, contributing to hypercoagulability.

Physiology

The hematopoietic system involves a complex interplay between proliferating **stem cells**, the **stroma**, and a series of diffusible molecules that regulate production by the erythroid, myeloid, and lymphoid pathways. The term *hematopoiesis* refers to the formation and development of blood cells. All of the cellular components of the blood are derived from hematopoietic stem cells. Stem cells are pluripotential, meaning they can give rise to myeloid (monocytes, macrophages, neutrophils, basophils eosinophils, **erythrocytes**, megakaryocytes/platelets, dendritic cells) and lymphoid lineages (T-cells, B-cells and NK cells) and can self-renew. A progenitor cell, often confused with a stem cell, is an early descendant of a stem cell; such cells can differentiate, but they cannot renew themselves. The term *stroma* refers to the lipid-protein framework within a **red blood cell (RBC)**, to which **hemoglobin** molecules are attached.

Because of the high cellular turnover and the microenvironment, the entire hemapoietic process is at risk for compromise due to nutritional deprivation. Therefore, the aging hematopoietic system is extremely susceptible to environmental stressors that adversely affect bone marrow. The effect of age on hematopoiesis is one of diminished reserve.

Blood Components

The blood delivers substances for metabolism in tissue; defends against microorganisms that cause harm; and maintains the body's acid-base balance. Blood consists of cells and plasma.

Blood plasma, which supplies the blood's volume, is about 90% water and 10% dissolved substances. It totals about 6 quarts in younger adults, less in older adults (**Box 10-1**).Proteins constitute approximately 7% of the plasma

---

iron A trace element incorporated into the heme complex that carries oxygen to parts of the body. It is heavily regulated because it is toxic.

ferritin A complex of iron and apoferritin that is a major storage form of iron.

platelets Tiny disk-shaped components of blood that are essential for blood clotting.

stem cell A formative cell whose daughter cells may differentiate into other cell types.

stroma Connective tissue cells that are associated with the bone marrow and the rest of the hematopoietic system. They make up the support structure of cells.

erythrocytes or **red blood cells (RBCs)** Derived from erythroblasts in the bone marrow. Production is stimulated by the glycoprotein erythropoietin. An erythrocyte enters the blood as a reticulocyte after losing its nucleus. It then matures in the bloodstream. The number of reticulocytes is used as a clinical index of erythropoietic activity to determine whether new red blood cells are being produced.

hemoglobin The oxygen-carrying protein in red blood cells. Consists of four heme groups and four globin polypeptide chains. The presence of hemoglobin gives blood its red color.

▶ BOX 10-1 Components of Arterial Plasma

Water (93%)

Electrolytes: Na^+, K^+, Ca^{++}, Mg^{++}, Cl^-, HCO_3^-, HPO_4^-, SO_4^-

Proteins: Albumins, globulins, fibrinogen, transferring, ferritin

Gases: CO_2, O_2, N_2

Nutrients: Glucose and other carbohydrates (CHO), total amino acids, total lipids, cholesterol, individual vitamins, individual trace elements, iron

Waste: Blood urea nitrogen (BUN), creatinine, uric acid, bilirubin

Individual hormones

Source: Data from McCance K, Huether S. *Pathophysiology.* 5th ed. Philadelphia: Elsevier Mosby; 2006.

TABLE 10-1 Cellular Components of Blood

Cell	Function
Erythrocytes, red blood cells	Gas transport to lungs and tissues
Leukocytes, white blood cells	Body defense
Lymphocytes (a type of leukocyte)	Humoral, cell-mediated immunity
Monocyte (a type of leukocyte)	Phagocytosis
Eosinophil (a type of leukocyte)	Phagocytosis, antibody-mediated defense against allergic reactions, parasites, aids in recovery phase of infection
Neutrophil (a type of leukocyte)	Phagocytosis, early phase of inflammation
Basophil (a type of leukocyte)	Secretes vasoactive amines—histamine, bradykinin, serotonin, and heparin Anticoagulant; function not well understood
Platelet (fragment of cytoplasm)	Hemostasis after vascular injury for normal clot formation, coagulation

Source: Data from McCance K, Huether S. Pathophysiology. 5th ed. Philadelphia: Elsevier Mosby; 2006.

by weight. Blood proteins are classified as albumins, globulins, and clotting factors (e.g., fibrinogen). The albumin concentration is about 4 g/dL; it regulates diffusion and osmotic or oncotic pressure of water and solutes in the microcirculation of arterioles, venules, and capillaries. The globulins, or antibodies, come from plasma cells (**lymphocytes**). They are critical in protecting against pathogens. Fibrinogen is converted into the clotting factors that promote coagulation and stop bleeding in damaged blood vessels.

The cellular components of blood are essential for the functions just described (**Table 10-1**). Problems with these components cause loss of homeostasis. Some of these problems, for example, the various anemias, are very common in elderly people.

Bone Marrow

The bone marrow consists of myeloid tissue and is contained within the bone. Within the bone marrow are blood vessels, nerves, phagocytes, stem cells, the various blood cells, and stromal and fatty tissue. The most active bone marrow is in the pelvic bones, vertebrae, cranium, mandible, sternum, ribs, and proximal parts of the humerus and femur. The marrow in other bones is primarily inactive. The stem cells mature to all the different cells within the hematopoietic system, including the lymphoid system.

See **Figure 10-1** for a summary of hematopoiesis and the different cell components.

Initial differentiation of pluripotent stem cells occurs along one of two major pathways: lymphoid or myeloid. For example, when a pluripotent stem cell gives rise to a myeloid stem cell, the progenitor cells for each cell type are the neutrophils, monocytes, eosinophils, erythrocytes, megakaryocytic, mast cells, and basophils.

RBC Production

Under normal conditions, red blood cells (RBCs) are produced in the bone marrow. The bone marrow contains a small number of stem cells that are both pluripotential and self-perpetuating. Although morphologically similar to stem cells, the stem cells in the marrow are committed to either lymphoid or myeloid development. After this commitment to a certain pathway, the cells are referred to as *committed progenitor cells*. These cells have now lost the unlimited capacity for self-renewal.

The body requires adequate amounts of proteins, vitamins, and minerals to produce RBCs and hemoglobin. Nutrient deficiencies can cause a number of different hematologic problems, which will be discussed in this chapter. Some of the vitamins essential for erythropoiesis include vitamins B12, B6, and E; folate (**folic acid**); riboflavin; pantothenic acid; niacin; and ascorbic acid. Because B12 is a large molecule, it requires intrinsic factor to be absorbed through the gastrointestinal mucosa, although there is a small amount of passive diffusion.

B and T-cells

Lymphoid stem cells give rise to progenitor cells: T, B, and null cells. B cell development and maturation to a B cell lymphocyte occurs in the bone marrow. Further differentiation does not occur until the mature B lymphocyte encounters a specific antigen. T cell development and complete maturation occurs in the thymus. Further differentiation of the T cell occurs when it is presented with an antigen.

The lymphoid pathway subdivides into the B cell, T cell, and null cell pathways. B lymphocytes differentiate further into plasma cells that secrete immunoglobulins. T lymphocytes play critical rolls

lymphocytes White blood cells. Include T cells, B cells, and killer cells, all of which are important in immunity. Killer cells defend the body from tumors and viruses. T and B cells work against antigens, which are foreign substances in the body. They produce antibodies that fight the antigen.

folic acid (folate) A form of vitamin B9. Required for production and maintenance of new cells and DNA synthesis. Deficiency causes slowed red blood cell production. Appears in laboratory tests as a macrocytic anemia.

Lymphoid stem cells These give rise to progenitor cells: T, B, and null cells.

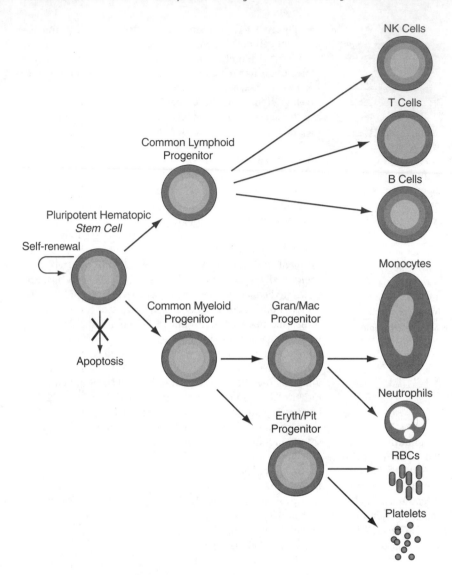

FIGURE 10-1 Hematopoiesis

Source: Printed with permission of CEU40.com

in cell-mediated immunity. The null cell pool contains the natural killer (NK) cells and a variety of immature lymphoid cells. Because hematopoetic stem cells and committed progenitor cells from the bone marrow cannot be morphologically distinguished from lymphocytes, they masquerade as null cells in the peripheral blood supply.

Myeloid Stem Cells

The myeloid pathway has three major branches: the erythroid, the megakaryocytic, and the phagocytic. The erythroid pathway, which does not branch any further, yields red

blood cells. Erythropoietin has a certain growth-promoting effect on the early precursor cells.

The proliferation and maturation of the erythroid precursor cells generally takes about four to five days, but many factors can affect this internal programming. Folic acid and **vitamin B12** are required coenzymes for the synthesis of DNA. Their absence causes abnormal DNA synthesis, and patients with a deficiency of these nutrients may have normal or even increased proliferation of progenitor and precursor cells, resulting in a hyperplasia but ineffective erythropoiesis. Iron is needed for the synthesis of hemoglobin, and a deficiency of this nutrient typically produces microcytic, hemoglobin-deficient red blood cells. However, in this case, fewer cells are produced. Other vitamins and trace metals contribute to the fact that nutritional deficiencies are a major cause of red cell precursor failure and anemia.

The Aging Hematopoetic System

The "aging" hematopoetic cell line is characterized by a decline in reserve capacity that makes it more susceptible to the adverse affects of stress on the system. This chapter covers the role of nutrition in the hematopoetic system and the effects of age on the process of hematopoiesis. In general, the normal changes that occur with aging include the diminution of the amount of bone marrow in the long bones steadily over time from age 70. The following are some other age-related changes:

- Erythropoietin is less effective in stimulating red blood cell development.
- Diminished cellular immunity.
- Diminished lymphocyte function.
- An increase in platelet stickiness
- Slightly diminished hemoglobin and hematocrit laboratory values (low normal range).

Aging stem cells may play a critical role in determining the effect of aging on organ function, and eventually on the lifespan. Cell division and differentiation during hematopoiesis are balanced by **apoptosis** (cellular death) to maintain a steady state. **Box 10-2** is a list of the changes that occur during apoptosis. If apoptosis fails, a leukemic state can occur.

The capacity for lymphopoiesis appears to diminish with age. The mechanisms remain elusive although they cause decline in immunity.

Aging appears to be an inevitable process that includes a dysregulation of the immune system, low grade inflammation, and other contributing changes. The challenge for the future is to identify nutritional and therapeutic strategies that will allow for successful aging.

Anemia in Older Persons

The prevalence of anemia increases with age, especially among those older than 80 years. Older men have higher rates of anemia than women. Anemia is more common in African Americans and in those with low incomes. Hispanics, especially Hispanic women, have been found to have anemia and poor iron status, probably due to cultural variations in dietary patterns, thus potentiating the possibility of the aging Hispanic elderly woman to be at greater risk for anemia. The annual incidence of anemia has been seen to rise with age.

In 80% of older adults, the anemia is normocytic (normal size RBCs). The complaint is "tired blood." In fact, in anemia the number of healthy RBCs is insufficient to carry adequate oxygen to tissues, which contributes to the

> ### BOX 10-2   Steps in Apoptosis
>
> - Decrease in cell volume
> - Modification of the cytoskeleton
> - Condensation of chromatin
> - Degradation of DNA into oligonucleosomal fragments
> - Shedding of apoptotic bodies
> - Quick phagocytosis to prevent inflammation
>
> *Source:* Data from Tabloski P. *Gerontological Nursing.* Upper Saddle River, NJ: Prentice Hall; 2006.

fatigue. The following are the most common anemias affecting older adults:

- Normocytic anemia: Caused by anemia of chronic disease (ACD) or multifactorial in nature.
- Microcytic anemia: Most often caused by iron deficiency and/or chronic blood loss.
- Megaloblastic anemia (macrocytic anemia): Most commonly caused by a B12 and/or folic acid deficiency.
- Sideroblastic anemia.

The prevention and treatment for each type of anemia differs, thus the correct clinical diagnosis of the particular type of anemia is important. See **Box 10-3** for classification of the different anemias. Sometimes it is difficult to determine the kind of anemia present in order to provide the correct management. For example, anemia of chronic disease (ACD) is a potential confounder in the assessment of iron status because it can mimic the hematological profile of iron deficiency anemia (IDA). The problem of distinguishing between IDA and ACD assumes greater importance among older patients due to the high prevalence of disease in this population. Confounding the problem is that IDA and ACD are often found together in the older adult. When this occurs, the anemia is more severe than either one alone.

Anemia can also occur when an older adult has slow blood loss perhaps, from aspirin administration, and thus has protein malnutrition and vitamin B12 deficiency—at the same time. However, in up to 25% of cases of anemia, no cause is identified.

vitamin B12 Essential for blood formation and the maintenance of the brain and nervous system. It is involved in the metabolism of every cell in the body as well as synthesis of DNA and fatty acids. A synthetic form, cyanocobalamin, can be given for deficiency.

apoptosis Programmed cell death. In humans, about 50 to 70 billion cells die each day. When apoptosis is excessive, cancers may occur.

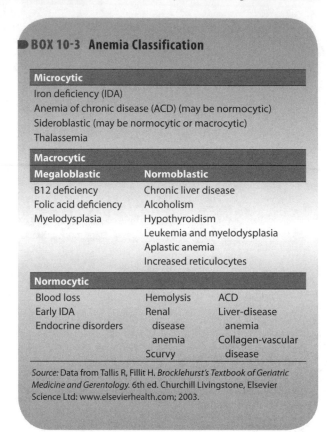

BOX 10-3 Anemia Classification

Microcytic
Iron deficiency (IDA)
Anemia of chronic disease (ACD) (may be normocytic)
Sideroblastic (may be normocytic or macrocytic)
Thalassemia

Macrocytic	
Megaloblastic	**Normoblastic**
B12 deficiency	Chronic liver disease
Folic acid deficiency	Alcoholism
Myelodysplasia	Hypothyroidism
	Leukemia and myelodysplasia
	Aplastic anemia
	Increased reticulocytes

Normocytic		
Blood loss	Hemolysis	ACD
Early IDA	Renal	Liver-disease
Endocrine disorders	disease	anemia
	anemia	Collagen-vascular
	Scurvy	disease

Source: Data from Tallis R, Fillit H. *Brocklehurst's Textbook of Geriatric Medicine and Gerentology.* 6th ed. Churchill Livingstone, Elsevier Science Ltd: www.elsevierhealth.com; 2003.

Signs and Symptoms of Anemia

Fatigue is often the presenting symptom of anemia, but it is vague and often goes unnoticed for a long time. Other signs and symptoms that may begin to cause concern include pale skin, mainly in the mucous membranes; weakness; rapid heartbeat; shortness of breath; dizziness; peripheral edema; headache; numbness or cool extremities; worsening chest pain if the older adult has angina; and cognitive problems, such as confusion, depression, agitation, and apathy. These symptoms are not hallmarks of anemia, but they will bring the older patient into the health care system.

Anemia doubles the risk that an older person will develop serious physical decline that can be a risk factor for loss of independence. Older adults with anemia have a greater physical or functional decline than those who do not. Even those with borderline anemia have diminished function.

Older people have twice the risk of a physical decline with anemia. Older adults with anemia have a 150% increased chance of hospitalization and a 200% increased chance of being admitted to a nursing home. Even mild anemia can reduce the ability of the older adult to function at his or her highest potential. The incidence of falls increases dramatically in the older adult, both those living in the community and those in nursing homes.

Untreated anemia in older adults has been associated with increased mortality and increased presence of comorbidities and may even predict early death. For example, in one study low hemoglobin was found to predict early death in 63 residents aged 70 to 99 years. In individuals aged 70 to 79 years, the five-year survival was 67% in adults without anemia and 48% in those with anemia.

A report issued by the American Heart Association states that heart failure worsens with anemia and increases the risk of death. Low hemoglobin levels are a predictor of increased risk of death and complications among heart failure patients. Further, the study reported that as many as 25% to 60% of patients with heart failure have anemia. The AHA states that studies have shown that in those with both anemia and heart failure, the risk of death and complications are increased by as much as 30% to 60%. Recent literature reiterates that the relationship between untreated anemia and patients with heart failure is great and there is a marked decline in health status, whereas health status improves with improved anemia status.

Some authors for the American Geriatrics Society recommend that an investigation for anemia not be pursued until blood hemoglobin is lower than 10 g/dL because a work-up with higher hemoglobin may show a poor yield of identifiable causes. This waiting, however, must rest on clinical judgment. When there are multiple chronic illnesses, the decision becomes more critical.

The Comprehensive Assessment

Assessment for anemia includes the usual history and physical examination, paying particular attention to the following:

- Physical indicators of anemia, such as pallor of the mucous membranes
- Indication of protein and/or energy malnutrition
- Weight change
- Review of medications for possible drug–nutrient concerns
- Diet history or review of food intake records

A registered dietitian or clinician will obtain a diet history (see Chapter 16) as part of the multidisciplinary assessment. The diet history will also assess for dietary habits, consumption of heme and nonheme iron, vitamin and mineral deficiencies, vegan/vegetarian lifestyle, protein/calorie intake, and fluid intake. In some cases, a review of food intake records may reveal information that the older patient is not able to provide. A diet history also screens the older patient for possible uses of botanicals and/or other supplements.

The Diagnosis

Most diagnoses of hematologic disorders begin with a complete blood count, or CBC, which includes RBC, hemoglo-

TABLE 10-2 Testing for Hematologic Disorders

Cell	Cause of abnormal test (possible)
RBC (red blood cell)	Anemias, hemorrhage, altered erythropoiesis, blood cancers
MCV (mean corpuscular volume)	Size of RBCs, anemias, thalassemias
MCH (mean corpuscular Hb)	Amount of Hb in RBC, anemias
MCHC (mean corp. Hb conc.)	Conc. of Hb in RBC, anemias
Hb (hemoglobin)	Anemias
HCT (hematocrit)	Percent of blood with RBCs; anemias, hemorrhage, blood cancers, erythrocytosis
Reticulocyte count	Hemorrhage, RBC destruction
Serum ferritin	Iron deficiency anemias (IDA)
TIBC (total iron-binding capacity)	Anemias, hemorrhage, IDA, iron overload, thalassemia
Transferrin saturation	Acute hemorrhage, hemochromatosis, hemosiderosis, sideroblastic anemia, IDA, iron overload, thalassemia
WBC count (white blood cells)	
Neutrophil count	Infection, myeloproliferative disorders, hematopoietic disorders, hemolysis
Lymphocyte count	Infection, anemias, cancers, hematopoietic disorders
Monocyte count	Polycythemia vera, Hodgkin disease
Eosinophil count	Hematopoietic disorders, allergy
Basophil count	Hemolytic anemias, Hodgkin disease, polycythemia vera, blood cancers

Source: Data from McCance K, Huether S. *Pathophysiology.* 5th ed. Philadelphia: Elsevier Mosby; 2006; Reuben D, Herr K, Pacala J, et al. *Geriatrics at Your Fingertips, 2006–2007.* 8th ed. New York: American Geriatrics Society; 2006.

bin, hematocrit, WBC and types of leukocytes, platelets, and iron studies (see **Table 10-2** for a complete list).

Basically, blood counts do not change with age. However, as noted, anemias are more common in older adults, especially in men aged 75 and older. Some potential effects of altered androgen levels in older men may affect hematologic parameters. Older men have significantly lower laboratory levels of androgen compared to men of 65 or younger.

Generally, the laboratory assessment for any type of anemia starts with the evaluation of hemoglobin (Hb).

If the Hb is low, the MCV (mean corpuscular volume) is evaluated (usually these are performed at the same time with one blood drawing [phlebotomy]). This lab result confirms whether the anemia is microcytic, normocytic, or macrocytic. However, keep in mind that RBCs, Hb, and hematocrit (HCT) can be elevated in people who are obese, who smoke, who live at high altitude, are stressed, or who exercise. Further, HCT and Hb are dependent on plasma volume, which changes throughout the day. Older patients who are more sedentary have a higher plasma volume and lower Hb levels. Other lab tests/assessments that the primary provider or other health provider or dietitian may order or recommend include: platelets, serum creatinine, BUN, total iron-binding capacity (TIBC), ferritin levels, serum vitamin B12, folic acid levels, serum erythropoietin, homocysteine (Hcy), **methylmalonic acid** levels (MMA), reticulocyte count, ANA (antinuclear antibody), Coomb's Test, indirect bilirubin, pre-albumin levels, and a current weight, with a history of weight changes over time. Additional tests may include a thyroid function assay, bone marrow studies, erythropoietin levels, and protein electrophoresis.

Serum ferritin is the appropriate noninvasive test if infection or inflammatory conditions do not exist and notwithstanding the use of homocysteine and methylmalonic acid levels. However, note that serum iron does not decline with healthy aging, and diagnosis of iron deficiency warrants identification of its etiology. It is well known that the absorption of iron decreases in the older adult—primarily because of gastric achlorhydria. More often, though, it is because of blood loss that occurs with the use of aspirin, nonsteroidal anti-inflammatory drugs (NSAIDS), anticoagulants, and the loss of blood that occurs with peptic ulcer (see **Figure 10-2**), diverticulitis, vascular malformations, and cancer.

What is the "normal" Hb for a definition of anemia? According to the World Health Organization (WHO), a Hb less than 13 g/dL in males and than 12 g/dL in females is consideration for anemia. A normal hematocrit in males is 40.7% to 50.3%; in women it is 36.7% to 44.3%. Hb measures the amount of oxygen-carrying proteins in the blood, and the hematocrit measures the amount of space red blood cells take up in the blood. Lab values often differ from lab to lab.

CBC panels used in the interpretation of anemia include, but are not limited to, the following:

MCV Mean corpuscular volume. Will help determine whether the anemia is microcytic, macrocytic, or normocytic (see Table 10-2). For example, the MCV may be increased

> **methylmalonic acid (MMA)** A laboratory test, rarely performed today, that is elevated in persons with vitamin B12 deficiency.

	with vitamin B12 and folate deficiency and decreased with iron deficiency.
RDW	Red blood cell (RBC) width. It is a calculation of the variation in the size of the RBCs. In some anemias, such as pernicious anemia, the amount of variation in RBC size causes an increase in the RDW.
MCHC	Calculation of the concentration of Hb inside the RBCs. Decreased MCHC values are seen in conditions where the hemoglobin is abnormally diluted inside the red cells, such as in iron deficiency anemia. Increased MCHC values are seen in conditions where the hemoglobin is abnormally concentrated inside the red cells.
Serum ferritin	A separate test from the CBC. Ferritin is an iron–protein complex found in most tissues, but particularly in the bone marrow and reticuloendothelial system. Serum ferritin is closely related to the amount of iron in the body. A high ferritin level can indicate iron overload, whereas a low fer-

ritin level can indicate low iron stores. It is also an acute phase protein that needs to be interpreted in light of inflammation and liver disease which may manifest in anemia of chronic disease.

Total Iron-Binding Capacity (TIBC) or Transferrin

The total iron-binding capacity (TIBC) and transferrin are typically used (along with serum iron) to evaluate persons suspected of having too much or too little iron. Usually, about one-third of the transferrin measured is being used to transport iron. In iron deficiency, iron is low, but TIBC is increased. In iron overload, such as in hemochromatosis, iron will be high, and TIBC will be low or normal. Ferritin levels will be high in hemochromatosis.

Because transferrin is made in the liver, TIBC and transferrin will also be low in the presence of liver disease. Transferrin levels can be used to monitor nutrition trends, but are not useful in iron deficiency anemia (IDA) that is complicated by anemia of chronic disease (ACD).

Data from NHANES III indicate that 11% of men and 10.2% of women between the ages of 65 and 85 have ane-

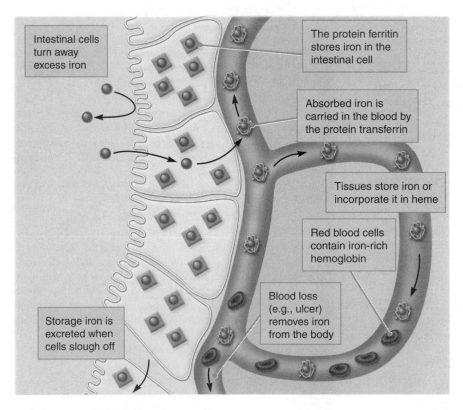

FIGURE 10-2 Iron Absorption

Source: Insel P, Turner RE, Ross D. *Nutrition.* 3rd ed. Sudbury, MA: Jones & Bartlett; 2007, p. 500. Reproduced with permission.

mia and that 20% of those older than age 85 are affected. Two recent studies, one by Dharmarajan, Pais, and Norkus, found that one-quarter of examined medical records from older adults identified a form of anemia. Clearly, anemia is a problem for the older adult.

Iron Deficiency Anemia

Iron deficiency anemia (IDA) is the most common form of anemia worldwide. It may be the second most common cause of anemia in older adults in the United States. In the older adult with IDA, one should consider it to be caused by blood loss or malignancy until proven otherwise. In one endoscopic study by Coban, Timuragaoglu and Meric of 1,388 patients aged 65 and older, 25% were found to have anemia. Of those with anemia, 30.5% of them had IDA. Out of those 30.5% who had IDA, 15.6% had a gastrointestinal malignancy.

Iron stores increase with age because the body is unable to eliminate excessive iron. Thus, signs of iron deficiency are almost never normal in the older adult despite the fact that it is common in this age group. Because iron is poorly

absorbed, many older adults barely get in their 8 mg/day, the current Dietary Recommended Intake (DRI) for this age group. Thus, even modest losses, increased requirements, or decreased intake may produce a deficiency.

Iron malabsorption generally occurs in older adults only with severe generalized malabsorption, after total gastrectomy, with erosive esophagitis, ulcers, colon cancer, or *H. pylori* infection, which impairs iron uptake. Therefore, iron deficiency equates to blood loss, usually from the gastrointestinal (GI) tract or the genitourinary (GU) tract. Evaluation is essential. Medications commonly causing this condition via blood loss include corticosteroids, aspirin, and NSAIDS.

Advanced heart failure in older adults can also cause IDA. A prospective investigation by Nanas and colleagues into the causes of "clinically significant anemia" in patients with advanced heart failure found that iron deficiency was a frequent cause of anemia. The mean age of the group was 57.9 years, plus or minus 10.9 years. Although the sample size was small, the conclusion was that the anemia should be thoroughly evaluated before considering therapeutic options.

A

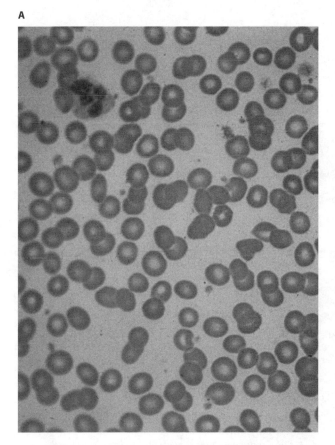

B

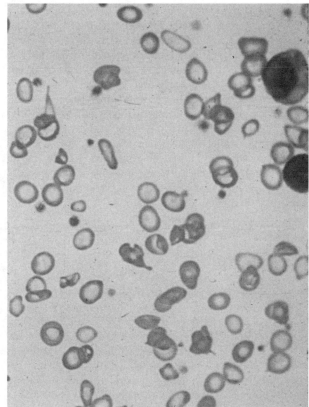

FIGURE 10-3 (A) Normal Red Blood Cells and (B) Abnormal Red Blood Cells

Source: Reproduced from *An Introduction to Human Disease.* 7th ed. Photos courtesy of Leonard V. Crowley, M.D., Century College.

In addition, a deficiency of vitamin A limits the body's ability to use stored iron. Vitamin A helps mobilize iron from its storage sites, so a deficiency of vitamin A may result in an "apparent" iron deficiency because Hb levels are so low.

Inhibitors of Iron Absorption

Phytates, polyphenols, soybeans, tannins, calcium, eggs, zinc, copper, tea, fiber, phosphorous, oxalate, and coffee all decrease the availability of iron. It is difficult for older adults to meet their dietary iron requirements without also consuming substances that impair its absorption. Probiotics may reduce the effect that phytates have on the inhibition of iron absorption.

Enhancers of Iron Absorption

Meat, poultry, fish, vitamin C, alcohol (not wine), and citric, malic, and tartaric acids all enhance the absorption of iron. Host-mediated enhancers include iron deficiency anemia, low body stores of iron, gastric acid, bile and pancreatic secretions, and hypoxia.

Stages to Disease Progression

There are three stages to disease progression. In the first stage, the demand for iron exceeds the supply, and the body's iron stores become depleted. The hemoglobin content in RBCs is normal at this time (**Figure 10-4**). In the second stage, iron transport to the bone marrow is diminished, which results in an iron deficiency erythropoiesis (development of RBCs). These new, small, Hb-deficient cells enter the blood and replace the older mature erythrocytes. In stage three, symptoms become evident, and there is little oxygen transport to tissues and damage begins.

Morphologically, iron deficiency is an example of microcytic hypochromic anemia. The diagnosis of IDA can be difficult in the older adult with other chronic (especially inflammatory) illnesses, because the laboratory tests for iron, TIBC, and ferritin are less reliable. Soluble transferrin receptors help differentiate ACD from IDA, with IDA having elevated receptors.

Presentation of Iron Deficiency Anemia

Mild IDA may be asymptomatic. Early symptoms include fatigue, weakness, and shortness of breath. Some symptoms give clues to the cause, for example, melanotic stools (blood in stool), acid reflux, and weight loss. When the hemoglobin is 7 g/dL or less, more severe symptoms occur. For example, the fingernails may become brittle, thin, ridged, and spoon-shaped due to poor capillary circulation. The tongue may become red and sore from glossitis, and it will be more or less painful based on the degree of anemia. Dryness at the mouth corners—angular stomatitis—may occur. Swallowing problems may occur due to hyposalivation and a questionable web formation at the area of the hypopharynx and esophagus.

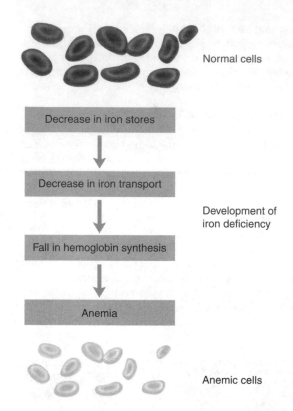

FIGURE 10-4 Normal and Anemic Red Blood Cells

Source: Insel P, Turner RE, Ross D. *Nutrition.* 3rd ed. Sudbury, MA: Jones & Bartlett; 2007, p. 506. Reproduced with permission.

Because iron is essential for compounds other than Hb, for example, enzymes and cytochromes, other abnormalities will occur. These include gastritis, irritability, neuromuscular alterations, numbness, tingling, and vasomotor disturbances. These may be caused by hypoxia in cerebral blood vessels. Further, confusion and other mental disturbances attributed to "aging" may actually be caused by IDA.

Some of the causes of IDA include the following:

- Crohn's disease
- Vitamin A deficiency
- Advanced heart disease
- Decreased absorption
- Gastric surgery
- Pernicious anemia with achlorhydria
- Celiac or tropical sprue
- Increased blood loss
- NSAID therapy
- Inflammatory bowel disease
- Intestinal parasites
- Malignancy, especially gastrointestinal
- Gastric or duodenal ulcer disease

Laboratory Iron Tests

Serum ferritin, serum iron, iron saturation, and serum iron-binding capacity are the usual measurements for diagnosis of IDA. A newer lab procedure is the serum transferrin receptor test. Because body ferritin is equal to stores, this serum value should provide an estimate of total body iron stores. In normal iron stores, the serum concentration is about 100 mcg/L. Serum ferritin, iron, and transferrin saturation will be very low in IDA, but the iron-binding capacity will be very high, reflecting the attempt to "capture" the little amount of iron available.

It is worth repeating that serum ferritin is not reliable if the older adult has an inflammatory disease or condition or has liver disease, alcoholism, or a malignancy. In a situation where the diagnosis is not made and further assessment is warranted, a bone marrow biopsy can be performed. With IDA, you may see a low MCV, MCH, and if acute, low RBCs. The following are some additional laboratory tests:

- **Fasting serum iron.** Free or unbound iron in serum; ideal range is 40–180 mcg/dL. Measurement is best done while fasting, because serum iron is too sensitive to recently consumed food or supplements and time of day.
- **Hemoglobin.** Low levels are seen with a variety of conditions, including IDA. Smoking may artificially elevate Hb levels as may dehydration.

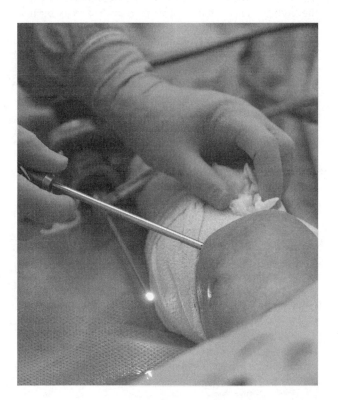

- **Ferritin.** This is not a reliable indicator of iron status in infection or inflammatory conditions. Ferritin measures stored iron. Low ferritin levels *can indicate* depletion of iron stores.
- **Transferrin.** A transport protein that usually will carry two molecules of iron to the bone marrow, liver, and ferritin. Transferrin is generally not used by health professionals anymore, rather TIBC is used in its place.
- **TIBC.** Tsat% is calculated by taking the serum iron and dividing by TIBC times 100%. This is also called *iron saturation*. A good Tsat% is 25% to 35%. If a higher percentage is obtained, one must consider iron loading. Low numbers are suggestive of iron deficiency.
- **Soluble transferrin receptor levels.** The most sensitive serum biomarker for the identification of iron deficient erythropoiesis. Normal bone marrow iron stores can coexist with an elevated receptor level and decreased MCV and MCHC. This is a useful marker of iron-deficient erythropoiesis due to both absent iron stores and restricted iron supply due to anemia of chronic disease. It does not discriminate between these two causes of iron-deficient erythropoiesis, however.
- **Ratio of soluble transferrin receptors/log ferritin (sTfR).** This test can be used to help differentiate coexisting IDA with ACD. If the ratio is greater than 2, consider IDA. If the ratio is less than 1, consider ACD. Alternatively, treat with ferrous sulfate, 325 mg/day, and recheck reticulocyte count after one to two weeks of therapy.

Management of Iron Deficiency Anemia

The first step in managing IDA is to determine and eliminate its cause, focusing on blood loss. Depending on the urgency of the bleeding situation, a blood transfusion may be required or other therapeutic measures utilized. This is the most potentially hazardous method of administration of iron and the most expensive. Each milliliter of transfused RBCs delivers 1 mg of iron. A study by Grey and Finlayson conducted on 615 older adult patients with severe iron deficient anemia stated that although rare to need or receive a transfusion (2.5% patients), the single red cell transfusions may be appropriate.

Iron replacement therapy is very effective if the anemia is due to nutrition problems. Oral iron therapy is inexpensive, safe, and convenient. Ferrous iron salts should be used; enteric-coated or sustained-release tablets should be avoided. One 325-mg tablet of ferrous sulfate contains approximately 97.5 mg of elemental iron. One dose each day will provide sufficient iron and diminish the likelihood of constipation, nausea, vomiting, and gastric distress. Frail older adults may not be able to tolerate this dose due to gastric upset or constipation. Giving the medication with meals will alleviate some of these problems, which are common causes for cessation of the medication. A reticulocyte response should

TABLE 10-3 Food Sources of Iron

Beef and red meat (liver)	Fish
Enriched cereals (Cheerios, corn flakes, All Bran)	Eggs
	Enriched grains (spaghetti)
Shellfish (oysters, clams, shrimp)	Tofu
Legumes (soybeans, lentils, lima beans)	Dried fruit
	Dark green vegetables
Poultry (dark meat)	(spinach)

begin in one to two weeks. Therapy should continue for 6 to 12 months to replenish iron stores. Iron-containing liquids can temporarily stain teeth. However, drinking through a straw or diluting the liquid may help avoid this effect.

Table 10-3 provides a list of foods containing high amounts of iron. Heme iron in foods is better absorbed than nonheme iron. Heme sources of iron include meat and meat by-products. Nonheme iron is plentiful in vegetables such as spinach, lentils, and lima beans.

Parenteral iron is used in those with severe malabsorption, in those who cannot tolerate oral iron at all, or in those whose iron loss is greater than that which can be replaced orally, for example, when bleeding. Parenteral iron can be given as iron dextran for deep intramuscular injection (IM) into the buttocks (maximum 2 mL/day = 100 mg elemental iron), or intravenous (IV) administration 2 mL/day at 1 mL/minute. When given IV or IM, a small test dose is administered, because some patients have suffered anaphylactic reactions. The older adult should be prepared for the possibility of pain at the site of injection, fever, and/or muscle aches. The calculation for IV iron replacement is:

$$[(0.3 \times \text{weight in lbs}) \times 100] \times (14.8 - \text{Hb})/14.8$$

For IDA of chronic kidney disease (CKD), sodium ferric gluconate complex and iron–sucrose complex are approved when the older adult is receiving supplemental erythropoietin and undergoing hemodialysis. Iron–sucrose complex has recently been approved for those who are predialysis.

An adequate response to iron therapy is an increase in Hb concentration of approximately 0.5 grams per week. Older patients respond as quickly as younger ones with oral supplementation therapy.

The patient may fail to respond to oral iron supplementation for a number of reasons, including an inability to absorb the iron. This may be confirmed by measuring the serum iron level at two and four hours after an oral dose of 325-mg ferrous sulfate.

Drug Interactions Associated with Treatment Success and Potential Complications

Essentially, any medication that decreases acidity may decrease the absorption of iron. The following medications may decrease the absorption of iron:

- Antihistamines
- H2 receptor antagonists (e.g., cimetidine, ranitidine)
- Proton pump inhibitors (omeprazole, lansoprazole)

Conversely, iron can decrease the absorption of some medications, such as:

- Levodopa
- Synthroid
- Cholestyramine resin
- Penicillamine
- Bisphosponates
- Tetracyclines
- Methyldopa

This is not an exhaustive list. Many medications should be taken two to three hours apart from iron supplementations for best absorption. This includes the avoidance of supplement usage in conjunction with iron, because many minerals interact with each other. For example, calcium and iron interact and should not be taken together. However, consuming foods high in vitamin C with iron-containing foods or supplements will increase absorption of the iron.

Iron Overload

Iron in excess of the body's needs is deposited in tissues as hemosiderin. When this results in tissue damage or when the body's iron content is greater than 5 g, it is termed *hemochromatosis*. It may occur as a result of a hereditary disorder that manifests in middle or late middle age or due to disorders of iron metabolism that release iron or deposit iron. The liver peptide, hepcidin, plays the role of negative regulator of systemic iron homeostasis. Deficiency of hepcidin, whether absolute or relative to iron overload, is the hallmark of hemochromatosis. It binds the transmembrane iron exporter ferroportin, inducing internalization and degradation. Excess iron can accumulate in nearly any tissue. Most damage occurs when it deposits in the liver, thyroid, pituitary, hypothalamus, heart, pancreas, and joints.

Hemosiderosis

Hemosiderosis may occur from recurrent hemorrhage within an organ. Deposits of iron from RBCs accumulate within the organ. Often the lung is affected due to recurrent pulmonary hemorrhage from chronic pulmonary hypertension, pulmonary fibrosis, and severe mitral stenosis. Sometimes this results in IDA because the iron deposited in the tissue cannot be reused.

Primary Hemochromatosis

Primary hemochromatosis is a hereditary disorder that is similar to hemosiderosis in that it deposits iron in tissues.

The disorder is characterized by increased iron absorption from the gastrointestinal tract and deposition in tissues. It can damage organs severely, causing premature death.

The disorder is autosomal recessive with a homozygous frequency of 1:200 (83%) and a heterozygous frequency of 1:8 in Northern Europeans. It does not often occur in Blacks and is rare in Asians. Symptoms are uncommon before middle age. It is the most commonly inherited disorder.

In this disorder there is increased iron absorption from the gastrointestinal tract and deposition in tissues. The total body content of iron can be as high as 50 g when normally it is 2.5 g in women and 3.5 g in men. Symptoms develop once there is already considerable tissue damage, when total body stores are more than 10 g. Usually cirrhosis or diabetes is the presenting sign. In women, symptoms develop after menopause. Symptoms include fatigue; hepatomegaly; arthralgias; manifestations of cirrhosis, diabetes, or cardiomyopathy; loss of libido; congestive heart failure; and bronze skin pigmentation.

Diagnosis is based on serum iron studies. Often there is a family history of the disorder to assist in diagnosis. Labs include serum iron, which is greater than 300 mg/dL; serum transferrin of more than 50% to 90%; and increased serum ferritin. A gene assay can definitively show the diagnosis, but other disorders, such as thalassemia must be discarded first.

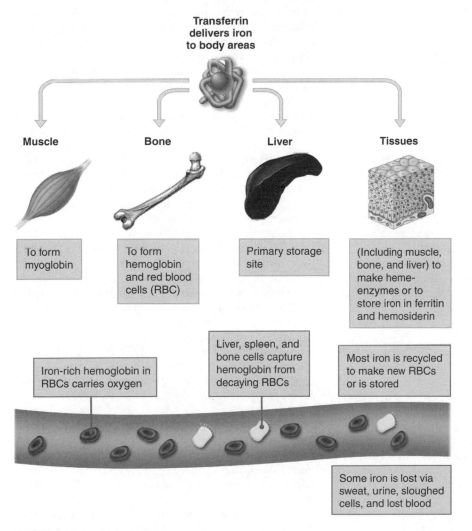

FIGURE 10-5 Iron in the Body

Source: Insel P, Turner RE, Ross D. *Nutrition.* 3rd ed. Sudbury, MA: Jones & Bartlett; 2007, p. 503. Reproduced with permission.

The onset of cirrhosis markedly affects the disease prognosis. A liver biopsy is performed if the serum ferritin is very high—more than 1,000.

Management of Iron Overload

In many cases, serial phlebotomies can be performed to rid the body of excess iron. The weekly phlebotomies, which remove approximately 500 mL of blood, may last for years, in order to prolong survival. Complications such as diabetes and cardiac problems should be treated as indicated. A low-iron diet is not currently recommended. If excess iron intake is a problem, discontinue supplements with iron in them (such as multivitamins) and fortified foods, such as iron-fortified cereal. Nutrition education should include the principles of getting adequate protein, folate, and other B vitamins that are at risk for depletion.

Other Disorders

Other disorders are associated with increased iron storage, but the reason for this is unknown. These disorders include alcoholic liver disease, nonalcoholic steatohepatitis, and chronic hepatitis C infection.

Anemia of Chronic Disease

Anemia of chronic disease (ACD) is the most common normocytic (and usually normochromic [normal amounts of iron in the RBC]) anemia in the older population. It is second in prevalence to IDA in the younger age groups. Anemia occurs in 11% of men and 10.2% of women older than 65. Two-thirds of these have ACD or other unexplained anemia. ACD can be mild or moderate, and its severity is related to the underlying causative disease.

Certain chronic diseases common in older people interfere with RBC production and result in chronic anemia. Cancers, cancer therapies, acute and chronic hepatitis, inflammatory bowel disease, protein-calorie malnutrition, and rheumatoid arthritis are examples. It is also often seen in chronic heart failure. Chronic kidney failure can also cause anemia. The kidneys produce erythropoietin, a hormone, which stimulates the bone marrow to produce RBCs. If there is a shortage, there is anemia.

As ACD progresses, it becomes microcytic and hypochromic. If Hb levels drop significantly, clinical manifestations of IDA appear. The sTfR values are generally low.

In ACD, iron stores are normal or even increased (ferritin more than 100 ng/mL). In addition, labs show mild anemia, low to normal serum iron, normal or reduced (TIBC), and low transferrin saturation. Older adults have increased concentrations of inflammatory cytokines, which play a significant role in the development of ACD. When the cause of ACD is not known, it is important to look for the cause (see above). It should not be assumed to be IDA and the older adult begun on iron therapy or subjected to major testing looking for blood loss.

ACD developing from rheumatoid arthritis responds to erythropoietin at usual dosages—50 to 150 U/kg subcutaneously every week. ACD resulting from cancer may respond to higher doses, although in 2009 the FDA updated its 2007 Boxed Warning section to emphasize that there may be an increase in mortality and a shorter time to tumor progression in patients with cancer receiving erythropoietin-stimulating agents (i.e., Procrit, Aranesp). The FDA further stated that, in the interim, health care professionals should consider the risk of tumor progression and decreased survival observed in recent clinical trials with the supportive care of anemic patients with cancer. Other warnings include that ESAs have not been shown to improve symptoms of anemia, quality of life, fatigue, or well-being in cancer patients. Patients may get blood clots while taking an ESA.

In chronic renal failure (CRF)—usually end-stage renal disease (ESRD)—there is diminished erythropoietin (EPO) production, diminished RBC survival, and impaired delivery of iron to the bone marrow. Cancer patients may have low EPO levels, also. Serum iron stores are normal. EPO therapy is considered first-line treatment in CRF patients. Starting doses are 80 to 120 units/kg subcutaneously 2 to 3 times a week (Omnicare, 2006). The Hb rise is 0.2 to 0.5 g/dL/week. If the increase after four weeks is less than 1 g/dL, then the dose is increased by 50%. If the increase is less than 3 g/dL in four weeks, then the dose is decreased by 25%. The target Hb is 11 to 12 g/dL. After the target is achieved, the therapy is individualized. Therapy can be given every week or every other week. Once-weekly EPO treatments given subcutaneously can improve quality of life, exercise capacity, and cognition. EPO is a very expensive therapy, but Medicare pays for it in those older adults with CRF and anemia from chemotherapy.

Nutrition should focus on providing enough protein divided into six small meals per day. Counsel on the need to avoid iron overload by avoiding iron-fortified foods and iron supplements if testing determines that the anemia is not IDA or IDA complicated by ACD. Use fewer heme sources of protein where possible by using milk, cheese, or other dairy sources of protein. If corticosteroids are used, monitor for high blood sodium, decreased potassium and calcium levels, hyperglycemia, and negative nitrogen balance.

Megaloblastic Anemias—Vitamin B12 and Folic Acid Deficiency

Megaloblastic anemias in the older population usually result from vitamin B12 (cyanocobalamin) and folate deficiency (**Figure 10-6**). Causes include poor dietary intake of folate or B12 (such as malnutrition or vegan diets), problems with absorption such as atropic gastritis or lack of intrinsic factor or stomach removal surgery. Other causes include chronic liver disease; hemolytic anemia; or drugs such as antibiotics, metformin for diabetes, nicotine, excess vitamin C and potassium. Other causes of inadequate B12 levels include

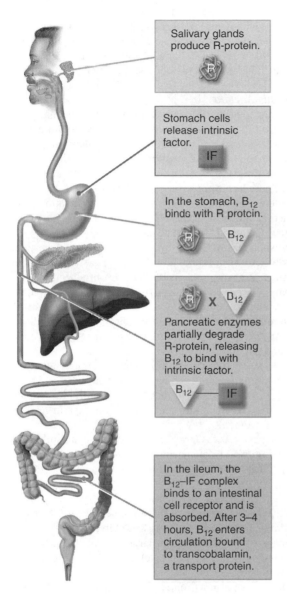

FIGURE 10-6 Vitamin B12 Absorption

Source: Insel P, Turner RE, Ross D. *Nutrition.* 3rd ed. Sudbury, MA: Jones & Bartlett; 2007, p. 444. Reproduced with permission.

Heliobacter pylori infection, which reduces production of intrinsic factor; celiac disease; Crohn's disease; h2 blockers such as Pepcid and Tagmet; and PPIs (proton pump inhibitors) with hypochlorhydria, anticonvulsants, and chemotherapeutics. Many of these deficiencies will only occur from protein-bound B12 and not that found in supplements. Vitamin B12 deficiency occurs in nearly 30% of older adults and is often unrecognized because of the disease's subtle manifestation and/or a masking effect from folic acid supplementation, which can improve the laboratory studies

while the neurological damage of vitamin B12 deficiency continues. Megaloblastic anemias are potentially serious, especially neurologically, and can be deadly.

Note that excessive folate may interfere with the function of vitamin B12 and delay or ameliorate the diagnosis of vitamin B12 deficiencies. With excessive folate you cannot look at the MCV and find a macrocytic state, so the macrocytosis becomes "masked". Testing for vitamin B12 deficiency may involve the Shillings test (which is expensive and frequently unavailable) or measuring homocysteine (Hcy) and methylmalonic acid levels (MMA). B12 fortification of foods with folic acid began in 1998 in both Canada and the United States to address the problem of neural tube defects. However, the risk fortification plays in individuals with marginal vitamin B12 status is troublesome and needs to be addressed in the nutritional assessment of the older patient.

Two markers that provide additional input on macrocytic anemias are homocysteine and methylmalonic (MMA) acid levels. In folic acid deficiency, both may be elevated or just Hcy may be out of range. Furthermore, it has been suggested that MMA elevation is a specific marker for vitamin B12 deficiency, with levels greater than 243 nmol/L being used as a cutoff for deficiency. In addition, the prevalence of anemia and incidence of cognitive impairment among older adults who are vitamin B12 deficient is much worse if accompanied by a high folate level. When B12 levels are normal, high serum folate is protective against cognitive impairment.

Deficiencies can occur because of inadequate intake of vitamin B12 or folic acid. Pathologic deficiencies occur with decreased intake and increased requirements. See **Table 10-4** for foods high in vitamin B12 and **Table 10-5** for foods high in folic acid.

Clinical Presentation of the Two Types of Vitamin B12 Anemia

The two types of vitamin B12 anemia discussed here are vitamin B12 deficiency and pernicious anemia (PA). Vitamin B12 deficiency is, as the name implies, an inadequate

TABLE 10-4 Foods High in Cobalamin/Vitamin B12

Very High	High	Fairly High
Beef liver	Salmon	Cod
Crab meat	Sardines	Milk
All Bran cereal	Ground beef	Cottage cheese
Wheat bran flakes	Tuna fish	Beef frankfurter
Chicken liver	Plain yogurt	Pork loin chops
Clams	Soymilk, fortified	Beef bologna
Oysters	Shrimp	Squid
Herring	Halibut	

Source: Data from Insel P, Turner RE, Ross D. *Discovering Nutrition.* 2nd ed. Sudbury, MA: Jones & Bartlett; 2006.

TABLE 10-5 Folic Acid-Rich Foods

Very High	High	Fairly High
Chicken liver	Beef liver	Crab (Alaskan king)
All Bran cereal	Spinach	Tomato juice
Wheat bran cereal	Lentils	Artichokes
Product 19 cereal	Cheerios cereal	Wheat germ
	Broccoli	Oranges
	Oatmeal, instant	Romaine lettuce
	Pinto beans	Kidney beans
	Spaghetti, enriched	Beets
	Asparagus	Sunflower seeds

Source: Data from Insel P, Turner RE, Ross D. *Discovering Nutrition.* 2nd ed. Sudbury, MA: Jones & Bartlett; 2006

level of vitamin B12. Pernicious anemia (PA) is a rare blood disorder that is characterized by the inability of the body to properly use the vitamin B12, which is essential for development of the RBCs.

Signs for both types of vitamin B12 anemia are subtle. Early signs include mood swings, infections, and gastrointestinal, kidney, and cardiac complaints. When the anemia has progressed to a Hb of 7 to 8 g/dL, the classic symptoms of anemia occur—muscle weakness, fatigue, spasticity, urinary incontinence, hypotension, vision problems, paresthesias of feet and fingers, and difficulty walking with abnormal gait and ataxia (shaky movement). Mental status may be affected, with cognitive impairment, depression, and mania. Neurologic problems occur, such as peripheral neuropathies and ataxia. Many or most of these occur *prior* to the anemia. They are not always reversible. It should be noted that many of these signs and symptoms can occur when the serum B12 level is just slightly below what is considered normal and much higher than that usually associated with anemia.

Vitamin B12 deficiency eventually leads to ineffective hematopoiesis. Signs of vitamin B12 deficiency may not occur for five to six years. In the early stages of a total body deficit of vitamin B12, serum levels of MMA and Hcy will rise. Following that, the serum B12 level will decrease. Afterwards, the MCV may or may not increase. If the deficiency is allowed to progress, anemia will eventually develop.

Discovering and treating the vitamin B12 deficiency may halt its progression, but it usually does not alter the damage that has been done unless caught very early. Dietary deficiency of vitamin B12 can cause hyperhomocysteinemia, as mentioned earlier, which can lead to heart disease and dementia. Homocysteine levels need to be normalized as soon as possible to avoid these conditions. No "normal" range has been established for serum B12. What is used is a *reference range*, which may vary from lab to lab and typically ranges from 122–600 pmol/L (159 to 780 pg/mL). Serum vitamin B12 is of limited value to diagnose a deficiency state when it is at the lower end of the reference range,

because the body will preserve serum levels at the expense of tissue stores. There is some consensus, however, that a serum value less than 230 pmol/L (300 pg/mL) represents a deficient state and that further testing may be performed.

Pernicious Anemia

Pernicious anemia (PA), as mentioned earlier, is characterized by the body's inability to properly use vitamin B12, which is needed for RBC development. PA develops slowly over 20 to 30 years. The result is ineffective erythropoiesis. There are three types of PA: congenital, juvenile, and adult-onset. These forms are based on age of onset and the nature of the defect causing impaired vitamin B12 utilization (e.g., absence of intrinsic factor). If there is no intrinsic factor, extrinsic factor (B12) is not absorbed.

PA usually is not caused by a vitamin B12 deficiency, but rather by chronic atrophic (autoimmune) gastritis and poor vitamin B12 absorption. Antibodies are produced against the parietal cells in which intrinsic factor (IF) is synthesized or against IF itself. PA is often associated with other autoimmune disorders, including vitiligo, thyroid disorders, Addison's disease, Sjogren's syndrome, Graves' disease, and hypopituitarism.

PA occurs primarily in adults older than age 60 and is more common in women than men and in those of Northern European descent. It occurs frequently in African Americans and Hispanics and at an earlier age in African American women.

In the past, PA was fatal. Today, PA is treated similarly to other vitamin B12 deficiencies, with oral or IM (intramuscular) administration of vitamin B12.

Pathology of Pernicious Anemia

Defective DNA synthesis results in ineffective erythropoiesis of large megaloblasts (young RBCs) in the bone marrow. The megaloblasts mature into large macrocytes (RBCs) in the blood circulation. Hemoglobin increases proportionately to the size of the RBC, so that the MCHC is normal and the cell is normochromic (normal amount of Hb in the cell).

Ineffective erythropoiesis contributes to premature cell death of *all* cell lines in the bone marrow, including RBCs, WBCs, and platelets. In addition, there is an increase in LDH (lactic dehydrogenase), which reflects cell destruction. There is an increase in indirect bilirubin, indicating breakdown of heme. Both can be measured in the blood via lab studies.

Diagnosis of Vitamin B12 Deficiency and Pernicious Anemia

Macrocytic or megaloblastic anemia is defined by a mean corpuscular volume (MCV) greater than 100 femtoliters. Megaloblasts are larger than normal RBCs and have small nuclei. High levels of MMA in the urine and serum, an abnormal marrow deoxyuridine suppression test, and increased excretion of formiminoglutamic acid are indicative of functional abnormalities from low vitamin B12. Older adults with vitamin B12 deficiency and PA may *not* necessarily have macrocytic anemia. However, this finding usually points to the diagnosis, and further investigation may be warranted, as indicated earlier. Other findings on the blood smear in addition to the macrocytic RBCs include hypersegmentation of polymorphonuclear leukocytes, and enlarged platelets. LDH, bilirubin, and ferritin may be elevated, and serum B12 is diminished. There may be a leukopenia (diminished WBCs). Diminished levels of vitamin B12 often are accompanied by increases in homocysteine and MMA, as stated earlier.

Management of Vitamin B12 Deficiency and Pernicious Anemia

Lifelong administration of vitamin B12 is indicated in PA and other types of vitamin B12 deficiencies. In most cases the regimen is 1 mg/day the first week. During the first weeks' injections, potassium levels must be monitored. These levels are reduced within 48 hours of the first injection. After the first week, the regimen is 1 mg/week for four to six weeks or until the stores are replenished or the HCT is normal, and then 1 mg/every three months for life. An oral form is available at high cost. Nasal vitamin B12 is also effective at 500 to 1,500 mcg per day of cyanocobalamin or hydroxycobalamin, and again, at high cost, because they are newer agents. The anemia is usually corrected by one month's time, and laboratory assessment should be done to confirm this. However, some peripheral blood smear abnormalities may continue for up to a year's time.

Folic Acid Deficiency

Folic acid deficiency in older adults may result from inadequate intake. The body stores folate for only four to six months. However, rapid deficiency can occur with malabsorption, malnutrition, alcoholism, and states of increased folate utilization, such as cancer or hemolytic anemia. In addition, certain medications, such as anticonvulsants, trimethoprim, triamterene, and nitrofurantoin, can cause folate deficiency (**Figure 10-7**).

Folic acid deficiency is probably not a common disorder in older adults who are well nourished. In past years, it was one of the most prevalent of all vitamin deficiencies. In the United States, many foods are mandated to be fortified with folate, thus this problem is diminishing.

Clinical Presentation

Folate deficiency results in neurological problems similar to those in vitamin B12 deficiency. It may be due, at least in part, to the homocysteine levels that accompany low levels of B12 and folate. Some of the neuropsychiatric changes that occur with folate deficiency include intellectual im-

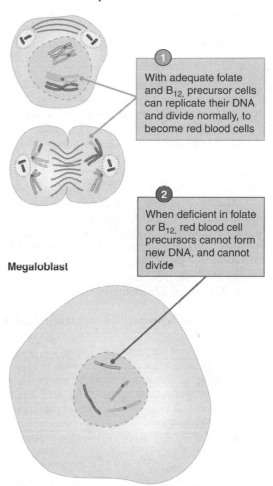

Normal red blood precursor

1 With adequate folate and B$_{12}$, precursor cells can replicate their DNA and divide normally, to become red blood cells

2 When deficient in folate or B$_{12}$, red blood cell precursors cannot form new DNA, and cannot divide

Megaloblast

FIGURE 10-7 Folate Deficiency

Source: Insel P, Turner RE, Ross D. *Nutrition.* 3rd ed. Sudbury, MA: Jones & Bartlett; 2007, p. 442. Reproduced with permission.

pairment, confusion, psychosis, depression, stupor, coma, cerebral ischemia, and paraplegia.

Diagnosis

Folate deficiency is confirmed by the presence of macrocytic RBCs and hypersegmented neutrophils in the blood smear, a normal serum vitamin B12 (unless both occur), and a low serum folate level less than 2 ng/mL or a RBC folate level less than 100 ng/mL. Serum folate levels are not stable and are less reliable than the RBC folate level. Serum homocysteine

Folic acid deficiency Lack of folic acid. Folic acid is found naturally in dark green leafy vegetables, citrus fruits, beans, and whole grains.

levels are elevated in 90% of patients with folate deficiency. MMA levels may be normal. If MMA levels are high, there is probably a coexisting B12 deficiency. However, kidney failure can artificially increase the MMA level.

Management

The deficiency can be managed by taking 1 mg of folic acid by mouth daily. The results are followed with laboratory tests. If the labs do not show improvement, the dosage is increased. A parenteral form of folic acid is available for older adults who have severe malabsorption. These management prescriptions, as with vitamin B12, will inhibit further destruction but will not reverse problems that are already present.

Anticonvulsants may pose a drug–nutrient interaction, decreasing absorption of folic acid. It is common to have meals or a tube feeding for 1 hour before and after administration of drugs such as Dilantin, primidone, or phenobarbitol. Vitamin C promotes the absorption of folic acid. As with vitamin B12 deficiency, a bland, liquid, or soft food diet may be needed until a sore mouth or tongue is healed.

Myelodysplastic Syndromes: Sideroblastic and Other Anemias

Myelodysplastic syndromes are a group of stem cell disorders with altered hematopoiesis causing anemia. They occur primarily, and rather commonly, in older adults. They are the most common hematologic cancer in the older adult. The course may be indolent or rapidly progressive to an acute myelogenous leukemia.

These stem cell disorders have a refractory anemia with ringed sideroblasts and account for 25% to 30% of these syndromes. Up to 20% of older adults may have unexplained refractory anemia. These syndromes are more common in men and are very rare in those younger than age 40 unless previously treated with chemotherapy or radiation therapy. Risk factors in addition to age of over 60 years and cancer therapy exposure include being White, male sex, exposure to tobacco smoke, pesticides, heavy metals such as mercury or lead and solvents such as benzene, family history of hematologic disorders, and pre-existing bone marrow conditions such as aplastic anemia.

Sideroblastic Anemia

Sideroblastic anemia (SA) in older people is a primary acquired form. Secondary sideroblastic anemia is usually caused by chronic alcohol use or secondary to malignancies of the hematologic system, for example, from leukemia or multiple myeloma. It may occur with vitamin B12 and/or folate deficiencies; rheumatologic disorders; from some drugs, for example, phenytoin and isoniazid; and from exposure to lead or other toxins. Primary pyridoxine deficiency, usually secondary to malnutrition, may also cause sideroblastic anemia (see **Table 10-6** for pyridoxine-rich foods). Idiopathic forms of SA are part of the myelodysplastic syndrome (MDS).

Presenting Signs of Myelodysplastic Syndromes

Fatigue, shortness of breath, decreased exercise tolerance, weakness, pale skin, easy bruising with petechiae purpura, epistaxis, and bleeding gums; fever, arthralgias, and frequent infections are common presenting symptoms. The clinician finds anemia (in 80%), thrombocytopenia, or leukopenia. Enlarged liver is present in 5%; spleen enlargement in 10%. Pallor is seen in 50% of cases. Interesting to this picture is the manifestation of peripheral neuropathy and dermatitis that also dominate this disorder.

Diagnosis

The diagnosis of SA is often made incidentally. The development of the cytopenias is very slow, and many patients are asymptomatic for some time. The anemia is attributed to aging. Laboratory findings include increase in serum iron, transferrin saturation, and ferritin. TIBC is often decreased. The hematocrit is about 20–30%. The MCV is normal or increased slightly, although occasionally is low which confuses it with IDA. The hallmark of diagnosis is reticulocytopenia. RBCs are microcytic and hypochromic; others are normochromic and normocytic or macrocytic. The blood smear shows abnormalities such as nucleated RBCs, basophilic stippling, target cells, and schistocytes. Leukopenia is mild to moderate—1,000 to 4,000 per mm^3, and neutropenia is more pronounced than lymphopenia. The patient may have a high or low number of platelets and presents with functional deficits.

Sideroblastic anemia (SA) Blood disorder in which there is sufficient iron but it is not used appropriately and does not function properly.

pyridoxine Also known as *vitamin B6*. Promotes red blood cell production and helps balance sodium and potassium. Diminished B6 causes seizures, nerve damage (numbness in hands and feet), anemia, skin problems, and mouth sores. It can be administered orally as a pill.

TABLE 10-6 Foods Rich in Pyridoxine and Vitamin B6

Excellent Sources	Good Sources
Sunflower seeds	Meats
Avocado	Poultry
Banana	Fish
Yeast	Whole grains
Wheat germ	Nuts
Wheat bran	Liver

Source: Data from Insel P, Turner RE, Ross D. *Discovering Nutrition.* 2nd ed. Sudbury, MA: Jones & Bartlett; 2006.

Nutrients involved in the biosynthesis of heme include **pyridoxine** and copper, among others. The role of copper is more complex, however, but this cause of SA is rare. Copper enhances intestinal iron absorption, modulates reticuloendothelial activity, facilitates cellular iron uptake from transferring, and promotes iron incorporation into heme. Copper deficiency from all causes (malnutrition, prolonged total parenteral nutrition, gastric surgery, prematurity, zinc supplementation, excessive chelation) can result in acquired sideroblastic anemia.

Management
The prognosis is variable. It may be a few months to 10 to 15 years. Most patients have increased iron stores with clinical hemochromatosis and diabetes, cirrhosis, heart disease, and pituitary dysfunction. However, many patients (50%) will have a relatively benign course and die of other causes.

In severe cases (50%), the goal is to induce a partial or complete remission and minimize the number of transfusions. Continual transfusions run the risk of alloimmunization and transfusion reactions. The mainstay of therapy is blood transfusion for the refractory anemias. However, this presents the risk of iron overload. Chelating agents such as desferrioxamine may be used, which decreases the risk of organ damage from iron deposits. Other blood products are also given. Nutrition support involves eating foods high in vitamin B6 and taking pyridoxine supplements, as needed. There is some disagreement in the literature regarding the amount of vitamin B6 to administer, because dosages greater than 100 mg/day may cause neurological side effects. According to the National Academy of Sciences, dosages of up to 100 mg/day are safe. Vitamin B6 is necessary for processing amino acids and for forming melatonin, serotonin and dopamine. The only curative therapy is allogenic stem cell transplantation, which is used in only 5% of patients at this time.

Patients with ringed sideroblasts are sometimes given 100 to 300 mg/day of pyridoxine, with variable results. Side effects to dosages of vitamin B6 at this level should be monitored and evaluated regularly, as noted earlier. A complete response to vitamin B6 generally occurs in cases resulting from the abuse of alcohol or the ingestion of pyridoxine antagonists. If vitamin B6 supplementation is successful, the Hb level will increase over the next few months. The appropriate maintenance dose of pyridoxine is the one that maintains a steady Hb level. If microcytosis persists, it is not of clinical importance. Folic acid and copper may also be needed. Protein and carbohydrate should be adequate, and energy should also be adequate enough to spare protein.

Refractory Anemia
Refractory anemia usually presents as macrocytic anemia, modest leukopenia, and normal or high platelets. It is more common in women. In rare instances it can become an acute leukemia. If the patient develops acute nonlymphocytic leukemia, the result is nearly always fatal. This is a disorder purely of the RBC lineage of cells and has no sideroblasts.

Thalassemia Minor
Thalassemia minor is an asymptomatic disorder that is often overlooked or misdiagnosed as iron deficiency. It occurs in people who originally came from areas around the Mediterranean Sea. Alpha thalassemia is most common in African, American Indian, and Asian populations, whereas beta thalassemia is most common in those of Greek and Italian ancestry. The most common form is beta thalassemia minor. It causes microcytosis with or without mild anemia. There may be splenomegaly, bronze coloring of the skin, and hyperplasia of the bone marrow. Iron studies are normal. A Hb electrophoresis may reveal the diagnosis. No treatment is required. Iron therapy is not indicated, because it could cause iron overload. Nutritional interventions for thalassemia minor are limited. If the patient is receiving blood transfusions, offer treatment for iron overloading. The patient will benefit from a diet high in quality protein, energy, B-complex vitamins (especially folic acid and vitamin B12), and zinc. The patient will need to avoid multivitamin and mineral supplements that contain large amounts of iron and vitamin C. The patient should also maintain adequate fluid intake. Future therapy may include iron-binding agents capable of preventing dietary iron absorption.

Vitamin and Mineral Considerations in Hematologic Problems

Hyperhomocysteinemia
Homocysteine is a medical problem in which there are abnormally large levels of homocysteine in the blood. It is implicated in myocardial infarction (arterial thrombosis) and venous thromboembolism as well as dementia (**Figure 10-8**). It can be inherited as a defect in methionine metabolism or acquired via vitamin B6 and B12 and folate deficiencies. Because healthy older adults often have low levels of B12 and folate, this is clinically significant. The disorder is also seen in those with chronic renal failure and with some drug use (methotrexate, anticonvulsants). This hypercoagulable state can be managed with folic acid 1 mg/day by mouth, with a goal of less than 10 umoles/L. Attention should be given to vitamin B12 status concurrently by administering an MMA test. Vitamin B6 deficiencies are rare, but when they occur they manifest as microcytic, hypochromic anemia accompanied by seborrhea, depression, confusion, and convulsions. Meat, bananas, carrots, potatoes, and corn are good sources of vitamin B6. The Daily

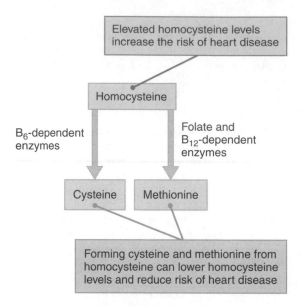

FIGURE 10-8 Homocysteine and Heart Disease

Source: Insel P, Turner RE, Ross D. *Nutrition.* 3rd ed. Sudbury, MA: Jones & Bartlett; 2007, p. 442. Reproduced with permission.

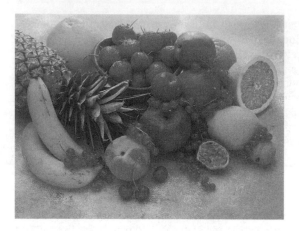

FIGURE 10-9 Fruits Containing Vitamin C

Recommended Intake (DRI) for this B vitamin is 1.5 mg/day. Supplements of these vitamins will decrease levels of homocysteine in the blood.

Vitamin C

Ascorbic acid promotes the absorption of iron and promotes prothrombin formation (involved in blood clotting), and helps to maintain the elasticity of the blood vessels and capillaries. Anemia will occur if ascorbic acid and iron intake are low. Some foods rich in vitamin C include chili peppers, green peppers, broccoli, parsley, strawberries, cantaloupe, watermelon, and citrus fruits (**Figure 10-9**).

Vitamins B1 and B2

Thiamin (B1) can create a shortage of other B vitamins if taken to excess. Good sources of vitamin B1 include liver, kidney, pork, peanuts, soybeans, and sesame seeds. The RDI for thiamin for older adults is 1.1 mg/day. Riboflavin (B2) helps in the production of RBCs. Achlorhydria in older adults may promote deficiency (see **Table 10-7** for riboflavin-rich foods).

Vitamin K

Vitamin K is a fat-soluble vitamin necessary for the regulation of blood coagulation. The most common reason for vitamin K deficiency is the use of broad-spectrum antibiotics that destroy normal GI flora, a source for vitamin K. Foods containing vitamin K or menadione, a vitamin K precursor, include dark green vegetables, cauliflower, tomatoes, soybeans, wheat bran, egg yolks, organ meats, and cheese. Deficiency is rarely caused by insufficient dietary intake. Clinical manifestations of deficiency range from an abnormal laboratory value to significant hemorrhaging. Management is parenteral administration of vitamin K with a correction of labs in 8 to 12 hours. Fresh frozen plasma can be given in the event of a hemorrhage or if immediate surgery is required.

Calcium

Calcium absorption is regulated by the parathyroid gland. Calcium absorption decreases with age primarily due to a lack of vitamin D receptors in the gut. Calcium should not be taken with iron or fiber, because they interfere with absorption. The tolerable upper limit for calcium is 2,000 mg/day. The DRI varies with age, but for older adults the DRI is 1,200–1,500 mg for calcium and 600 IU for vitamin D each day. Many older people have a low intake of dairy foods, causing inadequate dietary intake of calcium and vitamin D. Calcium citrate is absorbed more efficiently than calcium carbonate or gluconate. Calcium aids in the clotting of blood.

TABLE 10-7 Foods Rich in Riboflavin/Vitamin B2

Excellent Sources	Good Sources
Milk	Meat, poultry
Cheese	Fish
Wheat germ	Eggs
Yeast	Dark green leafy vegetables
Liver and kidney	Dry beans and peas
	Nuts

Source: Data from Insel P, Turner RE, Ross D. *Discovering Nutrition.* 2nd ed. Sudbury, MA: Jones & Bartlett; 2006.

Copper

Copper aids in the formation of Hb. It promotes absorption of iron from the GI tract. Copper deficiency can prevent the release of iron from storage sites, resulting in what appears to be iron-deficiency anemia. This condition does not respond well to iron supplementation and occurs even though the body has iron available. Electron microscopy shows dense deposits in the mitochondria and cytoplasm of erythroid and myeloid cells, which disappear after supplementation.

The typical diet includes 2 to 3 mg of copper per day, about half of which is absorbed. If a deficiency is found, supplemental copper of 3 to 6 mg/day should be given, along with a protein intake of at least 1 g per kilogram of bodyweight. Tube-fed patients need to be monitored closely to ensure that they are receiving sufficient copper.

Copper deficiencies occur with protein–energy malnutrition (PEM), chronic kidney disease, iron-deficiency anemias, prolonged total parenteral nutrition and tube feeding, or prolonged zinc intake. Signs of deficiency include poor wound healing, weakness, joint ache, osteoporosis, petechial hemorrhaging, and arterial aneurysms—all are related to the vital role copper plays in collagen formation.

Good food sources of dietary copper are shellfish, nuts, raisins, oyster, liver, legumes, corn oil, and lobster. Protein intake should be 1 g per kilogram of bodyweight. The use of multivitamins and minerals should be monitored to ensure that the patient does not receive large doses of zinc. Large doses of vitamin C are also not recommended in copper deficiency.

Zinc

Blood cells are especially vulnerable to zinc deficiency. One of the major functions of zinc is its assistance in linking oxygen to Hb. Because it is vital to the immune response, even the mildest deficiency increases the risk of infection. Zinc also has an important role in taste. A deficiency reduces taste perception, which often leads to poor appetite and poor nutrition.

A plasma zinc level can determine zinc deficiency. Supplementation will vary according to severity of deficiency. However, keep in mind that giving zinc for an excessive period of time—longer than three months, for example—can have an adverse effect on the immune system and cause other alterations in the nutrition of the body. One of the most classic conditions caused by excessive zinc supplementation is copper deficiency. Large amounts of phytate and fiber in vegetarian diets can depress zinc absorption significantly. Calcium supplements combined with a high phytate meal also depress zinc absorption.

Zinc deficiency is not common in the United States and Canada. Foods rich in zinc include red meat, seafood, dark meat poultry, and whole grains.

Protein-Calorie Malnutrition

Protein calorie malnutrition is a common syndrome of older adults. It occurs in nearly 25% of community older adults. The clinical manifestations of protein-calorie malnutrition (PCM) relate to the duration of the malnutrition, the extent of the malnutrition, and prior health status. PCM is diagnosed by assessing lab values, weight trends, and visceral protein status. The patient may look well nourished or chronically starved, depending on whether the patient has stress related protein-malnutrition (kwashiorkor) or compensated malnutrition (marasmus) (**Box 10-4**). The patient may have easily

> **Copper** Along with iron, it helps form RBCs. Good sources include dried fruits such as prunes, dark green leafy vegetables, cocoa, and black pepper.

▶ BOX 10-4 Classification of Malnutrition

Kwashiorkor	
ICD .9 code 260	Patient appears well nourished with protein intake insufficient to maintain visceral protein stores.
	Pitting edema may be present.
	Hair may be easily plucked.
	Takes place over a few weeks to months
	Delayed wound healing; development of decubitus ulcers
	Albumin is usually lower than 2.8.
	Transthyretin may be < 17.
	Total lymphocyte count < 1,500 mm^3
	TIBC < 200 mcg/dL
	BUN/Creatinine low
	Anemia may be present.

Marasmus	
ICD .9 code 261	Weight < 80% of standard for height
	Weight loss of 5% in 30 days; 10% in 180 days (unplanned)
	Patient looks chronically starved.
	May have normal albumin, transthyretin
	Glucose may be low.
	Cholesterol may be < 160 mg/dL.
	Other labs may vary.
	Anemia may be present.
	Absence of subcutaneous fat; muscle wasting
	Eats poorly (< 75% of meals)

Source: Data from Escott-Stump S. Hematology: Anemias and Blood Disorders. In: *Nutrition and Diagnosis-Related Care.* Baltimore: Lippincott Williams & Wilkins; 2008, pp. 624–656.

pluckable hair, and there may be an absence of subcutaneous fat. Glucose and cholesterol may be low. The total lymphocyte count (TLC), BUN, and creatinine may be low. Regardless of the type of PCM, anemia may develop.

The nutritional objectives for the older adult diagnosed with PCM include correcting weight loss (if present), providing adequate micronutrients and macronutrients, correcting dehydration, and avoiding refeeding. If the PCM (marasmus) is severe, tube feeding may be appropriate. Start IV glucose and gradually reintroduce soft, easily tolerated solids and provide sufficient calories to use nitrogen effectively. Provide 20 to 25 kcal/kg/day to avoid overfeeding and progress to 35 to 40 kcal/kg/day. In protein malnutrition, give 1.4 to 2.2 g/kg/day depending on the severity of depletion. Include thiamin in the multivitamin regime. Screen for zinc and copper deficiencies. Infection and sepsis may be major risks. Monitor the patient's weight, electrolytes, and transthyretin (prealbumin) trends. Follow nutrition-care plans monthly.

Conclusion

The assessment and subsequent treatment of anemias is complicated. It must take into account the process of hematopoiesis, changes with aging, and the various types of anemias. Each type of anemia has its own impact on metabolic processes and in provision of adequate nutriture for the micronutrient environment in which hematopoiesis occurs. Clearly, this is an area that needs more study.

Of particular interest is the effect of the aging process on the nutrient needs of the aging stem cell, the provision of nutrients, and the cycle of hematopoiesis. Future directions for research on anemia should include a more detailed examination of the importance of aging or age-related diseases on the pathogenesis of anemia, an assessment of the importance of anemia on outcomes such as physical function and cognitive function, and an analysis of whether impairments associated with anemia are amenable to correction by improving hemoglobin concentration.

Activities Related to This Chapter

1. Discuss the main concepts identified in this chapter and apply concepts to a case study.

2. Define the different types of anemia discussed in this chapter.
3. Visit the Women's Health.gov website (*www.4women.gov*) for more information on anemia and women's health.
4. List the treatments for each anemia identified in this chapter.

Case Study

Mrs. G is a 65-year-old woman with chronic rheumatoid arthritis. Lately she has been complaining that she is tired all the time and that her chest hurts. A past medical history reveals that she has not been eating well, has angina, and is taking NSAIDs for pain and inflammation associated with arthritis. A physical examination shows pallor of the mucous membranes and spoon-shaped nails as well as heart palpitations. She has not lost weight despite her poor appetite. You decide to run a CBC. The CBC shows that she has microcytosis and that her fasting serum iron, Tsat%, and ferritin are all low and her soluble transferrin receptor test was high. Her Hb is 9.5 g/dL. Her transthyretin is 15, and she is developing a decubitus ulcer on her right heel.

Questions

1. What type(s) of anemia does Mrs. G have?
2. What other information would be beneficial in diagnosing Mrs. G's nutritional state?
3. Mrs. G has rheumatoid arthritis. What test(s) would you run to differentiate between the different types of anemia Mrs. G may have?
4. After determining the type of anemia, how would you treat it?
5. What foods would you encourage Mrs. G to eat as part of the treatment plan?
6. How would you follow Mrs. G to see if your treatment plan is successful?

REFERENCES

American Geriatric Society. *Geriatric Review Syllabus*. 6th ed. New York: American Geriatric Society; 2006.

American Heart Association. 2005.

Camaschella C. Treating iron overload with hepcidin. *Blood*. 2006:107(7);2595.

Chang J, Bird R, et al. Clinical utility of serum soluble transferrin receptor levels and comparison with bone marrow iron stores as a index for iron-deficient erythropoiesis in a heterogeneous group of patients. *Pathology*. 2007:39(3);349–353.

Chenn, CC, Takeshima F, Miyazaki T, et al. Clinicopathological analysis of hematological disorders in tube fed patients with copper deficiency. *Intern Med*. 2007;46(12):839–844.

Chernoff R. *Geriatric Nutrition*. Sudbury, MA: Jones & Bartlett; 2006.

Coban E, et al. Iron deficiency anemia in the elderly: prevalence and endoscopic evaluation of the GI tract in outpatients. *Acta Haematol*. 2003:110;25–28.

Da Silva I., Shattler K. B12 status linked to dementia and CVD. Available at: http://www.ceu4u.com. Accessed January 2008.

Dharmarajan TS, et al. Does anemia matter? Anemia, morbidity, and mortality in older adults: need for greater recognition. *Geriatrics*. 2005:60(12);22–29.

Ebersole P, Hess P, Luggen A. *Toward Healthy Aging*. St. Louis: Mosby; 2004.

Encylopedia of Surgery. Hemoglobin test definition. Available at: http://www.surgeryencyclopedia.com/Fi-La/Hemoglobin-Test.html. Accessed February 3, 2008.

Escott-Stump, S. Hematology: anemias and blood disorders. In *Nutrition and Diagnosis-related Care*. Baltimore: Lippincott Williams & Wilkins; 2008; 624–656.

Federal Drug Administration. Communication about an ongoing safety review. Erythropoiesis-stimulating agents (ESAs): epoetin alfa (marketed as Procrit, Epogen) darbepoetin alfa (marketed as Aranesp). January 3, 2008. Available at: http://www.fda.gov/cder/drug/early_comm/ESA.htm. Accessed February 6, 2008.

Feldblum I, German L, Castel H, Harman-Boehm I, Bilenko N, et al. Characteristics of undernourished older medical patients and the identification of predictors for undernutrition status. *Nutr J*. 2007;6:37.

Grey DE, Finlayson J. Red cell transfusion for iron deficiency anaemia: a retrospective audit at a tertiary hospital. *Vox Sang*. 2008:94(2);138–142.

Insel P, Turner RE, Ross D. *Discovering Nutrition*. 2nd ed. Sudbury, MA: Jones & Bartlett; 2006.

Insel P, Turner RE, Ross D. *Nutrition*. 3rd ed. Sudbury, MA: Jones & Bartlett; 2007.

Iron Disorders Institute. Iron tests. Available at: http://www.irondisorders.org/Forms/irontests.pdf. Accessed February 3, 2008.

Iron Overload Association. Iron tests. Available at: http://www.irondisorders.org/Forms/irontests.pdf. Accessed February 3, 2008.

Kaplan K, et al. *Heliobacter pylori*—is it a novel causative agent in vitamin B12 deficiency? *J Internal Med*. 2000:160;1349.

Kennedy-Malone L, Fletcher KR, Plank LM. *Management Guidelines for Nurse Practitioners Working with Older Adults*. 2nd ed. Philadelphia: FA Davis; 2004.

Leukaemia Research. Myelodysplastic syndromes. 2009. Available at: http://www.lrf.org.uk/en/1/infdispatmye.html. Accessed February 4, 2009.

Mayo Clinic. Anemia. 2005. Available at: www.mayoclinic.com/print/anemia/DS00321/DSECTION = all&METHOD. Accessed February 16, 2007.

McCance K, Huether S. *Pathophysiology*. 5th ed. Philadelphia: Elsevier Mosby; 2006.

Merck Manual of Aging. 3rd ed. Update. Whitehouse Station, NJ: Merck Research Labs; 2000–2007.

Merck Manual Professional. Primary and secondary hemochromatosis. November 2005. Available at: www.merck.com/mmpe/sec11ch145/ch145a.html. Accessed February 18, 2007.

Morris M, Jacques PF, et al. Folate and vitamin B12 status in relation to anemia, macrocytosis, and cognitive impairment in older Americans in the age of folic fortification. *Am J Clin Nutrition*. 2007:85(1);3–5.

Nanas JN, Matsouka C, Karageorgopoulos D, et al. Etiology of anemia in patients with advanced heart disease. *J Am Coll Cardiol*. 2006;48(12):2485–2489.

Nardin RA, Amick AnH, et al. Vitamin B12 and methylmalonic acid levels in patients presenting with polyneuropathy. *Muscle and Nerve*. 2007:36(4);532–535.

National Cancer Institute. Myelodysplastic syndromes treatment. 2008. Available at: www.cancer.gov/cancertopics/pdq/treatment/myelodysplastic/patient. Accessed February 4, 2009.

National Institute on Aging (NIA). Anemia elevates risk of physical decline in older people. 2003. Available at: www.nia.nih.gov/NewsAndEvents/PressReleases/PR20030725. Accessed February 16, 2007.

National Institutes of Health. Dietary supplement sheet: iron. Available at: http://dietary-supplements.info.nih.gov/factsheets/iron.asp. Accessed January 12, 2008.

National Institutes of Health. Medline Plus herbs and supplements: vitamin B12. 2008. Available at: http://

www.nlm.nih.gov/medlineplus/druginfo/natural/patient-vitaminb12.html. Accessed February 4, 2009.

Omnicare. *Geriatric Pharmaceutical Care Guidelines*. Covington, KY: Omnicare; 2006.

Rajan S, Wallace JI, Beresford SAA, et al. Screening for cobalamin deficiency in geriatric outpatients: prevalence and influence of synthetic cobalamin intake. *J Am Geriatr Soc*. 2002;50:624–630.

Reuben D, Herr K, Pacala J, Pollock B, Potter J, Semla T. *Geriatrics at Your Fingertips*. 9th ed. New York: American Geriatric Society; 2007–2008.

Rimon E, Levy S, Sapir A, et al. Diagnosis of iron deficiency anemia in the elderly by transferrin receptor-ferritin index. *Arch Intern Med*. 2002;162:445–449.

Rush University Medical Center. Proportion of individuals with low serum vitamin B12 concentrations without macrocytosis is higher in the post-fortification period than in the pre-folic acid fortification period. *Am J Clin Nutr*. 2007;86(4):897–898.

Sandhu SK, Sekeres MA. Myelodysplastic syndromes: more prevalent than we know. *Geriatrics*. 2008;63(11):10–17.

Seaverson E, Buell J, Fleming D, Bermudez O, Potischman N, et al. Poor iron status is more prevalent in Hispanic than in non-Hispanic white older adults in Massachusetts. *J Nutr*. 2007;137:414–420.

Shils M, Shike M. Nutrition in the life cycle. In: *Modern Nutrition in Health and Disease*. Lanham, MD: Lexington Books; 2006; 832–835.

Signer RA, Montecino-Rodriguez E, Witte ON, McLaughlin J, Dorshkind K. Age-related defects in B lymphopoiesis underlie the myeloid dominance of adult leukemia. *Blood*. 2007;110(6):1831–1839.

Stanfield P, Hui YH. *Nutrition and Diet Therapy*. Sudbury, MA: Jones & Bartlett; 2003.

Tabloski, P. *Gerontological Nursing*. Upper Saddle River, NJ: Prentice Hall; 2006.

Tallis R, Fillit H. *Brocklehurst's Textbook of Geriatric Medicine and Gerontology*. 6th ed. Philadelphia: Churchill Livingstone, Elsevier Science Ltd.; 2003.

U.S. Food and Drug Administration, Center for Drug Evaluation and Research. Questions and answers on medication guides for erythropoiesis-stimulating agents (ESAs). January 2009. Available at: http://www.fda.gov/CDER/DRUG/infopage/RHE/qa2008.htm. Accessed February 4, 2009.

CHAPTER 11

Endocrine and Metabolic Alterations and Nutrition in the Older Adult

Mary B. Neiheisel, BSN, MSN, EDD, CNS, APRN-FNP, FAANP

Ardith L. Sudduth, PhD, GNP, FNP-BC and

Ann Schmidt Luggen, PhD, GNP

CHAPTER OBJECTIVES   Upon completion of this chapter the reader will be able to:

1. Describe physiological changes related to diabetes mellitus (non–insulin-dependent, type 2 diabetes) in the older adult
2. Identify the components of the dietary management of diabetes mellitus, type 2, in the older adult
3. Discuss the importance of diet, exercise, and medication in the management of diabetes mellitus, type 2, in the older adult
4. List the endocrine glands, describe their hormones, and explain the function of each hormone
5. Discuss disorders resulting from increases/decreases in hormone production
6. Identify age-related changes that occur in the endocrine gland
7. Discuss the nutritional deficits/excesses associated with changes in the production of hormones
8. Explain the management of specific endocrine disorders
9. Describe the ADA Standards of Care for diabetes
10. Discuss the role of nutrition in the prevention and management of osteoporosis

KEY TERMS AND CONCEPTS

Adrenal glands

Calcitonin

Diabetes mellitus, types 1 and 2

Endocrine glands

Glucogneogenesis

Glucose intolerance

Glycosylated hemoglobin

Hemoglobin A1C

Hypercalcemia

Hyperthyroidism

Hypocalcemia

Hypoglycemia

Hyponatremia

Hypothyroidism

Insulin sensitivity

Parathyroid glands

Pituitary (anterior and posterior)

Thyroid gland

Trophic hormones

This chapter discusses diabetes mellitus, osteoporosis, and other endocrine disorders that occur frequently in older adults. The endocrine system is a complex system made up of a number of **endocrine glands,** which produce numerous hormones. The hormones have many functions and are important in the maintenance and balance of life.

Diabetes Mellitus

Diabetes mellitus is a complex of metabolic alterations that are known collectively as *diabetes*. **Type 1 diabetes mellitus (T1DM)** is a chronic illness resulting from a lack of insulin production. **Type 2 diabetes mellitus (T2DM)** is a complex, chronic metabolic illness that results from a resistance to insulin by the tissues, leading to progressive beta cell failure (see the discussion immediately following). In older adults, diabetes can be an insidious illness that may take years to develop and be detected. Older adults often do not show the same symptoms of the disease as younger individuals. Multifactorial interventions for at-risk older adults with T2DM can provide sustained benefits with respect to the prevention of vascular complications, common in this disorder, and on death rates from cardiovascular causes.

Epidemiology

The prevalence of T2DM is 180 million and the World Health Organization projects the prevalence will double by 2030. Diabetes mellitus is the sixth most frequent disease-specific cause of death in the United States and about 65% of diabetes-related deaths result from heart disease or stroke. It is the fourth leading cause of death by disease in the world. The highest prevalence is in the Western Pacific, followed by the eastern Mediterranean, Middle East, and North America. Some racial and ethnic minorities are particularly affected by the disease, such as African Americans, Hispanics, Native Americans and Alaska Natives, Asian Americans, and Pacific Islanders.

Type 1 diabetes mellitus is generally diagnosed in a younger population and accounts for only about 5% to 10% of all diagnosed cases of diabetes; T2DM comprises approximately 90% to 95% of cases. Nearly 12 million adults in the United States have type 2 diabetes, and approximately 50% of these are undiagnosed. Older adults have T2DM with a long-term prediabetic syndrome.

In 2005, the prevalence of diagnosed diabetes among older adults aged 65 to 74 was about 12 times that of people younger than 45 years of age. A more recent study by Boschert has found that 33% of older adults in nursing homes have diabetes, which is much higher than previous reports of 11% to 27%. It is estimated that at least 20% of the population over age 65 has diabetes; the number of people with diabetes will only grow as the baby boomers reach retirement. Among older adults, the highest prevalence of diabetes is in younger of the older adults, those aged 65 to 74 years, followed by those 75 and older (**Figure 11-1**).

Types of Diabetes Mellitus

Diabetes mellitus is classified according to four clinical findings. Type 1 is the result of beta cell destruction or dysfunction, which usually leads to absolute insulin deficiency. Type 2 diabetes occurs over time as the B cells of the pancreas progressively produce less insulin at the same time that the tissues develop resistance to insulin. As a result, there is an excessive increase in hepatic glucose production, a decrease in the ability of insulin to regulate hepatic **gluconeogenesis**, and an impaired insulin-mediated glucose uptake in peripheral muscle and adipose tissue.

Research suggests that vitamin D plays a role in the pathogenesis of T2DM. A deficiency in vitamin D alters insulin synthesis and secretion and predisposes a person to **glucose intolerance**. Glucose intolerance occurs frequently in older adults as a result of the aging process and other factors. Recent research has revealed another contributing factor in the development of diabetes, that of diminished incretin effect, which is discussed at greater length later in this chapter.

endocrine glands Glands of the endocrine system that synthesize and release special chemical messengers known as *hormones*. The endocrine glands include the thyroid, parathyroid, pancreas, adrenal, pituitary, hypothalamus, pineal, thymus, ovaries, and testes.

diabetes mellitus, types 1 (T1DM) and 2 (T2DM) A chronic disease in which uptake of blood glucose by body cells is impaired, resulting in high glucose levels in the blood and urine. Type 1 is caused by decreased pancreatic release of insulin. In type 2, target cells (e.g., fat and muscle cells) lose the ability to respond to insulin.

gluconeogenesis Formation of glucose by the liver from non-carbohydrate sources.

glucose intolerance Impaired glucose tolerance; prediabetes state; associated with insulin resistance and increased risk of cardiovascular pathology.

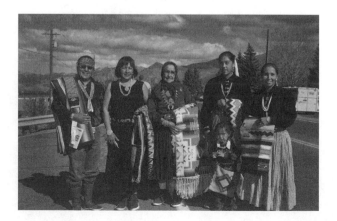

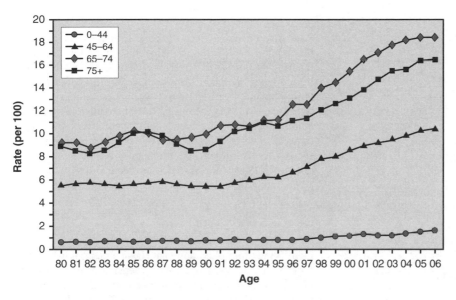

FIGURE 11-1 Prevalence of Diagnosed Diabetes by Age in the United States, 1980–2005

Source: Centers for Disease Control and Prevention. Prevalence of diagnosed diabetes by age in the United States, 1980–2005. Available at: http://www.cdc.gov/Diabetes/statistics/prev/national/figbyage.htm. Accessed February 12, 2008.

The third type of diabetes stems from a number of possible causes: injury to the exocrine pancreas; endocrinopathies from excessive hormones, such as epinephrine, which antagonize insulin activity; infections with subsequent destruction of the beta cells of the pancreas; genetic defects; and drugs or chemicals, such as those used in the treatment of cancer, AIDS, or organ transplantation. Drug- or chemical-induced diabetes is also common in older adults. The fourth category of diabetes is gestational diabetes. The focus of this chapter will be on T2DM.

Risk Factors

Diabetes mellitus is highly correlated with several risk factors that have been known for many years. Newer research has indicated additional risk factors for the development of diabetes in the older adult, such as metabolic syndrome. See **Box 11-1** for a summary of risk factors for T2DM.

Metabolic Syndrome

Approximately 42% of older adults in the United States are believed to have metabolic syndrome. It has been estimated that over 20% of the U.S. adult population, or more than 47 million U.S. residents, meet the criteria for metabolic syndrome. Metabolic syndrome is a group of risk factors, including hypertension (130/85 mm Hg or higher), dyslipidemia (triglyceride 150 mg/dL or higher; low high density lipoproteins [HDLs] 40 mg/dL or less in men and 50 mg/dL or less in women); hyperglycemia (110 mg/dL or higher);

and central obesity, which are associated with insulin resistance. These symptoms are highly correlated with risk for cardiovascular disease and T2DM. Metabolic syndrome is a complex, poorly understood disorder and treatment will depend on a more complete scientific understanding of it. However, it is known that the risk factors promote proinflammatory and prothrombic states, which occur in cardiovascular diseases.

The obese older adult is at higher risk for metabolic syndrome than one of normal weight. In one study of adults aged 70 to 79, reported by the American Dietetic Association, women had higher rates of metabolic syndrome than men. Older African Americans adults had higher rates of hypertension and abnormal glucose metabolism. Whites had higher rates of dysregulated lipid metabolism.

Older adults often have health-decline weight loss related to the loss of skeletal muscle and subcutaneous adipose tissue. Therefore, the older adult of normal weight may still be at risk for metabolic syndrome. The American Dietetic Association reported that visceral adipose tissue was associated with metabolic syndrome in men who were of normal weight most often, then in those who were overweight, and lastly, those who were obese. In women, metabolic syndrome was most often associated with normal weight, then overweight, and then obese older females. Subcutaneous abdominal adipose tissue was only associated with metabolic syndrome in men of normal weight. Subcutaneous thigh adipose tissue was inversely associated

▶ **BOX 11-1** **Risk Factors for Type 2 Diabetes Mellitus**

- Blood pressure ≥ 140/90 mm Hg
- First-degree relative with diabetes (parent, sibling, child)
- Obesity: BMI ≥ 35; waist circumference greater than 35 inches in women and 40 inches in men
- Physical inactivity
- Member of a high-risk ethnic population (African American, Hispanic, Native American, Asian American, Pacific Islander)
- Previous gestational diabetes or child with a birth weight ≥ 9 pounds
- Undesirable lipid levels: HDL ≥ 35 mg/dL or triglycerides > 250 mg/dL
- Clinical conditions associated with insulin resistance, such as polycystic ovary syndrome
- History of vascular disease
- History of impaired fasting glucose (100 to 125 mg/dL)
- History of impaired glucose-tolerance test (2-hour plasma glucose 140 mg/dL)
- Metabolic syndrome
- Sleep disorders
- Prediabetes
- Age: Older than 45 years

Source: Data from American Diabetes Association. Standards of medical care in diabetes—2006. *Diabetes Care.* 2006 Jan; 29 Suppl 1:S4-42; Mayo Clinic Staff. Type 2 diabetes. June 13, 2009. Available at: http://www.mayoclinic.com/health/type-2-diabetes/DS00585/. Accessed July 6, 2009.

Sleep Disorders

Sleep disorders have been linked to the development of diabetes. It has been found that altered sleep patterns result in insulin resistance and a decrease in carbohydrate tolerance. In one study by Yaggi, Aravjo, and McKinlay, researchers found that men reporting 6 or fewer hours of sleep per night were twice as likely to develop T2DM as those sleeping 6 to 8 hours; men sleeping over 8 hours were found to be three times as likely to develop T2DM. Lack of sleep may increase cortisol levels, which may predispose the body to insulin resistance. Sleep deprivation has been found to increase sympathetic tone, which inhibits pancreatic function that may contribute to reduced glucose tolerance.

Prevention of Diabetes

Identifying those older adults at risk is essential in diabetes prevention. Diabetes is a very expensive disease in terms of dollars spent and loss of health and well-being. By the time that diabetes mellitus is diagnosed, much damage has already been done to the body in terms of micro- and macrovascular damage to the eyes, kidneys, blood vessels, nervous system, heart, and brain.

Prediabetes

Diagnostic criteria are impaired fasting glucose of 100–125 mg/dL and/or impaired glucose tolerance 140–199 mg/dL (2-hour post 75g glucose challenge). Other risk factors include: 45 years of age or older; a BMI of 25 or higher; a triglyceride level of 150 mg/dL or higher; and family history of glucose intolerance (39% of patients with T2DM have at least one parent with it); gestational diabetes; or high infant birth weight. Recognizing a patient's risk for development of prediabetes can help the health professional plan the intervention to avoid the onset of diabetes. The longer and more supportive the relationship of the health professional with the older adult, the better the chance of reducing the onset of diabetes (See **Box 11-1**).

Significant lifestyle changes are essential to avoid diabetes. Patients who receive intense individualized instruction on weight reduction, nutrition, and physical activity are better able to delay the onset of diabetes mellitus. Noninstitutionalized older adults at high risk for type 2 diabetes should:

- Take part in a structured program emphasizing lifestyle changes with moderate weight loss through reduction of caloric intake and dietary fat and regular physical activity.
- Achieve USDA recommendations for dietary fiber intake (14 g fiber/1,000 kcal) and whole-grain foods (one-half of daily grain intake).
- Consume low-glycemic-index foods rich in fiber and important nutrients.

with metabolic syndrome in obese men and women. Therefore, the distribution of body fat is independently associated with metabolic syndrome in older men and women, particularly when they are of normal weight.

One of the easiest screening methods for metabolic syndrome is measuring waist circumference. A waist circumference of 35 inches (88 cm) for women and 40 inches (102 cm) for men should be a routine measure for identification of the person with diabetes. Further, weight circumference also has a strong association with hyperlipidemia and hypertension. Physical inactivity, obesity, and poor diet are risk factors for development of metabolic syndrome.

TABLE 11-1 Signs and Symptoms of Type 1 and Type 2 Diabetes

Signs and Symptoms of Type 1	Signs and Symptoms of Type 2
Age of onset younger than 30 years; however, can occur at any age.	Can emerge at any age.
Sudden onset, severe symptoms. Disease process may be present for several years.	Gradual onset; many older adults with type 2 do not show symptoms until in the later stages of the disease when complications develop.
Thirst, increased urination.	Thirst, increased urination. Hyperglycemia; may have significant increase in hyperglycemia before glycosuria.
Increased appetite, hunger.	Decreased appetite.
Rapid weight loss.	Gradual unexplained weight loss.
Thin.	Usually obese and sedentary.
Blurred vision.	Blurred vision.
Fatigue, weakness.	Fatigue, mood swings.
Glycosuria.	Glycosuria may not be present. Ability of the kidneys to reabsorb filtrated glucose increases with age.
Elevated blood glucose.	Elevated blood glucose; often asymptomatic to levels >200 mg/dL.
Nausea and vomiting.	Nausea and vomiting are rare.
Vaginal itching.	Recurrent vaginitis, urinary tract infections.
Ketones in urine.	Protein in urine.
Dry flaky skin.	Frequent fungal infections; wounds do not heal readily.
Sensation intact.	Evidence of complications: Feeling of "pins and needles" in feet Leg cramps when walking Chest pain Gum disease Impotence Hypertension

- Avoid high intake of alcohol; some studies have found that moderate intake may reduce the risk for diabetes and heart disease.
- Exercise 30 minutes every day.
- If overweight, decrease weight 5–10%.

The United Nations Resolution on Diabetes states that preventative measures for those at high risk for T2DM should include antidiabetic pharmacotherapy as well as lifestyle changes. The Global Partnership for Effective Diabetes Management, an expert group, also advocates aggressive early intervention. It recommends a HbA1c of less than 6.5% be obtained within 6 months of diagnosis through the use of oral medications, physical activity, diet, and supplemental insulin. The Canadian Diabetes Association also advocates aggressive management; its HbA1c goal is less than 7%.

Symptoms and Diagnosis of Diabetes

The differences in symptoms of diabetes mellitus type 1 and type 2 are found in **Table 11-1**.

Screening criteria for a diagnosis of diabetes mellitus are based on the American Diabetic Association's Standards of Medical Care in Diabetes. Because type 2 diabetes can easily remain undetected for many years, older adults who have at least one risk factor should be screened (see **Box 11-2**). Older adults who are symptomatic must be screened and treatment started immediately if they meet the criteria for type 1 or type 2 diabetes. Some experts suggest that older adults be screened for diabetes every three years using the criteria outlined in Box 11-2. One good screening tool is the hemoglobin A1C blood test.

Hemoglobin A1C, also known as *glycated hemoglobin* or **glycosylated hemoglobin**, is formed when glucose in the blood binds irreversibly to hemoglobin to form a stable glycated hemoglobin complex that lasts the life of a red blood cell, which is 90 to 120 days. It is a stable value over the lifespan of the red blood cell. It does not fluctuate like the daily blood glucose monitoring. It gives the health professional an overview of the blood sugars over a 3-month period of time.

Complications of Diabetes

Older adults often are not diagnosed with type 2 diabetes until complications appear. Older adults with diabetes experience a higher rate of complications than do younger individuals. They experience higher rates of premature death, functional disability, and coexisting illnesses, such as hypertension, coronary heart disease, and stroke, than those without diabetes. Management is further complicated by the multiple comorbidities that the older person with diabetes may have. In addition, older adults are at a high risk for polypharmacy, depression, cognitive impairment, urinary incontinence, injurious falls, and persistent pain from neuropathy. See **Table 11-2** for long-term complications of T2DM.

The treatment and management of older adults with

hemoglobin A1C (glycoslated hemoglobin) Glucose–hemoglobin complex that lasts the life of the red blood cell (90 to 120 days). It is a laboratory test used to assess average glucose levels over three months and does not fluctuate as does blood tests in daily testing.

BOX 11-2   Diagnostic Criteria for Diabetes

1. Symptoms of diabetes (increased thirst, urination, weight loss) AND a casual plasma glucose of 200 mg/dL. Casual is defined as any time of day without regard to time since last meal.

   AND/OR

2. Fasting blood glucose of greater than 126 mg/dL. *Fasting* is defined as no caloric intake for at least 8 hours.

   AND/OR

3. Two-hour plasma glucose of greater than 200 mg/dL during an oral glucose-tolerance test. The test should be performed as described by the World Health Organization, using a glucose load containing the equivalent of 75-gram anhydrous glucose dissolved in water.

Source: Data from American Diabetes Association. Standards of medical care in diabetes—2006. *Diabetes Care.* 2006 Jan;29 Suppl 1:S4–42; Reuben D, Herr K, Pacala J, et al. *Geriatrics at Your Fingertips, 2009.* 11th ed. New York: American Geriatric Society; 2009.

TABLE 11-2 Long-Term Complications of Type 2 Diabetes Mellitus

Complication	Pathological Change
Heart and blood vessels	Coronary artery disease; myocardial infarction; stroke; atherosclerosis; high blood pressure; diminished blood flow to feet with risk of infection, leading to potential for amputation.
Neuropathy	Damage to capillaries that nourish nerves, especially in lower extremities, resulting in numbness, tingling, and loss of sensation.
Gastroparesis	Nausea, vomiting, diarrhea, constipation (vagal nerve damage affecting the GI system).
Nephropathy	Kidney filtration system damage leading to kidney failure.
Retinopathy	Damage to blood vessels in retina leading to blindness; increased risk of cataracts and glaucoma.
Osteoporosis	Diminished bone density, leading to osteoporosis and increasing risk for fracture.
Dementia	Increased risk for Alzheimer's disease.
Infection	Skin and mouth infections, especially fungal infections, more common.
Poor healing	Diminished capability to heal cuts, sores, and wounds, and to recover from surgery.

Source: Data from Mayo Clinic Staff. Type 2 diabetes. June 13, 2009. Available at: http://www.mayoclinic.com/health/type-2-diabetes/DS00585/. Accessed July 6, 2009.

diabetes must be customized to account for individual differences. Some older diabetics have been diagnosed for years, others are recently diagnosed, and still others are not diagnosed until complications have developed after years of undiagnosed illness. In addition, some older adults with diabetes are frail, whereas others are relatively robust. The American Diabetes Association recommends that older adults who are expected to live at least ten years and who are active mentally, cognitively, and physically, and are willing to participate in the management of their illness be provided the goals and treatments afforded younger persons with diabetes. However, those older adults at risk for heart attack and stroke probably should not be aggressively managed to levels of HbA1C of less than 6%. Intensive intervention has been linked with 22% higher relative risk of death compared to maintaining the level at 7% to 7.9%

Diabetes Management

Management of individuals with any of the risk factors for diabetes includes a major effort at assisting the older adult to make lifestyle changes. This therapy has become more aggressive in recent years for the healthy older adult as well. The goals of diabetes management in the fragile or institutionalized older adult often are not managed as aggressively as those for other individuals. A balance between tight glucose control, management of comorbidities, and quality of life must be determined by the individual and the health care team.

For older adults in reasonably good health, the goal is a hemoglobin A1C of less than 7%. However, for frail older adults with a life expectancy of less than five years and others in whom the risks of intensive glycemic control appear to outweigh the benefits, a less stringent target, such as 8%, is appropriate. The goal for fasting plasma glucose is 80 to 120 mg/dL. The goal for the two-hour postprandial glucose test is less than 180 mg/dL. Other goals include a blood pressure lower than 130/80 mm Hg; low density lipoproteins (LDL) less than 100 mg/dL; and triglycerides less than 150 mg/dL and HDL greater than 40 for men and greater than 50 for women. Other components of the standard of care include the use of statins to prevent macrovascular problems, nutrition therapy and physical activity, monitoring of urinary microalbumin, an annual flu shot, an annual eye exam, regular foot exams at each health professional visit, aspirin therapy, and a pneumococcal vaccine every five to ten years.

It is essential that older adults with diabetes mellitus be managed by collaborative health care teams that include, but are not limited to, physicians, nurse practitioners, physician's assistants, nurses, dietitians, pharmacists, diabetes counselors/teachers, and mental health professionals with expertise and a special interest in diabetes. Because T2DM is a complex metabolic problem, it is imperative that all members of the team assume an active role in assisting the older adult.

Engaging the older adult in self-management is key to managing T2DM. The approach must be holistic; that is, the individual's age; physical, mental, and emotional strengths and weaknesses; cultural factors; and the presence of complications of diabetes or other chronic illnesses all must be considered. Lifestyle changes require the cooperation of the individual as well as a carefully constructed individual plan of care.

Diet and exercise are very important for all people with diabetes, regardless of the metabolic problem causing the diabetes. For type 1 diabetics, taking insulin is life-saving. The management of older adults with T2DM often requires the addition of oral antihyperglycemics as beta cell function decreases and fails. Most older adults will require insulin therapy in late stages of the disease. Many older diabetics require medications, such as ACE inhibitors or ARBs or aspirin (150 mg/day to 325 mg/day), for the management of cholesterol, hypertension, blood glucose, lipids, or other comorbidities.

Diet

Diet is a significant part of the treatment plan for the older adult with T2DM. A registered dietitian is a valuable member of the collaborative health care team who can help the older adult to plan a balanced food plan that meets his or her metabolic needs. Older adults with early detected diabetes who are able to alter their lifestyles by eating healthy, losing weight, and exercising regularly often can delay or prevent complications from T2DM.

Studies by the CDC have shown that people with prediabetes can successfully prevent or delay diabetes onset by losing 5% to 7% of their body weight. This is best done by participating in 30 minutes or more of physical activity most days of the week and following a low-calorie, low-fat diet that is rich in whole grains, fruits, and vegetables.

Metabolic syndrome is more common among those who consume a lot of meat, fried food, and diet soda. The Western dietary pattern of high intake of refined grains, processed meats, fried foods, and red meats increases the risk of metabolic syndrome. In particular, hot dogs, hamburgers, and processed meats are each associated with highest risk for metabolic syndrome. High intake of dairy and

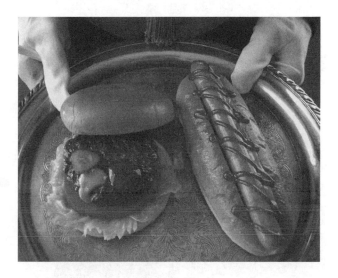

diet soda are also implicated. Sweetened beverages such as juices or sweet sodas have not been found to be associated with the syndrome.

Dietary goals for individuals with diabetes mellitus are to attain optimal metabolic outcomes, including those for blood glucose, A1C, cholesterol, and triglycerides. It is also important to maintain a healthy blood pressure and body weight. Diet is used to prevent and treat diabetes complications while assisting the individual to meet nutritional needs based on cultural and lifestyle preferences. Carbohydrates should provide 45% to 65% of the daily caloric intake for all diabetics. Low-carbohydrate diets that restrict total carbohydrates to fewer than 120 g per day are not recommended. Proteins should represent 15–20% of total daily calories; fiber, 25–50 g/day is recommended as it aids digestion and metabolism of carbohydrates. Total dietary fat less than 30% and saturated fats less than 10% and less than 7% if the LDL is greater than 100. Individuals with type 1 diabetes will need to plan carefully to fully regulate insulin administration and dietary and energy expenditures.

The focus of a diabetic diet is to manage glycemic control. A healthy diet is a good diabetic diet that the entire family can eat and enjoy. Caloric requirements must be balanced with energy expenditure. The diabetic food pyramid suggested by the American Diabetes Association consists of six major food groups (**Figure 11-2**). At the bottom of the pyramid are grains, breads, and other starches. The second tier is vegetables and fruits, followed by the milk and meat, meat substitutes, and other proteins. The top of the pyramid is fats, oils, and sweets. The diabetic food pyramid is slightly different than the USDA Food Guide Pyramid. The pyramid provided by the American Diabetic Association (ADA) classifies foods according to carbohydrate and protein content rather than their food grouping. For example,

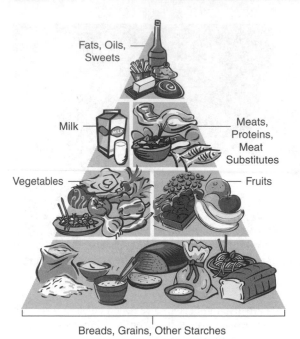

Fats, Oils, Sweets

Milk

Meats, Proteins, Meat Substitutes

Vegetables

Fruits

Breads, Grains, Other Starches

FIGURE 11-2 Food Pyramid for Diabetics

Source: Adapted from American Diabetes Association. Diabetes Food Pyramid. Available at: http://www.diabetes.org/food-nutrition-lifestyle/nutrition/meal-planning/diabetes-food-pyramid.jsp. Accessed July 6, 2009.

in the ADA pyramid potatoes and other starchy vegetables are in the grains, beans, and starchy vegetables group instead of the vegetable group.

Portion size is very important for the diabetic individual, and the ADA pyramid identifies the portion size for each food group. It also identifies the recommended servings for each group.

For older adults who wish to take an active role in planning their meals, www.MyPyramid.gov features a calculator that can be used to plan a diet based on age and activity level. This pyramid uses vertical groupings of six major food groups: grains, vegetables, fruits, oils, milk, and meat and beans (**Figure 11-3**). To the side of the pyramid are guidelines that emphasize the importance of exercise to a healthy lifestyle. The width of the food group bands indicates the amount of each food group the individual should select. A newer pyramid is the Modified MyPyramid for Older Adults (**Figure 11-4**). The flag at the top is a reminder that older people may need to take supplements of calcium, vitamin D, and vitamin B12 in addition to that which is taken from food. The Modified MyPyramid for Older Adults also indicates that packaged fruits and vegetables—for example, frozen vegetables, canned fruits, and dried fruits—can be reasonable alternatives to fresh fruits and vegeta-

bles. It also demonstrates the importance of various types of exercise that may be appropriate for the older adult.

For older adults who are overweight, a moderate reduction in calories of 500 to 1,000 per day plus a moderate exercise program will result in slow, progressive weight loss. At a minimum, women seeking to lose weight must have a diet of at least 1,000 to 1,200 Kcal a day; men need at least 1,200 to 1,600 Kcal a day. Nonnutritive sweeteners may be used by diabetic patients in moderation.

Older diabetic adults can consume alcohol in moderation (one drink or less per day for women and two or less per day for adult men). One drink is a 12-ounce beer, a 5-ounce glass of wine, or 1.5 ounces of distilled spirits. Research has demonstrated that red wine is helpful in preventing heart disease.

To reduce the incidence of vascular complications, the amount of saturated fat should be less than 7% of the total calories. Foods high in monounsaturated fats such as nuts; avocados; and olive, canola, and peanut oils are good for all people with diabetes.

Protein is restricted when there is evidence of the complication of chronic kidney disease. The recommended dietary allowance of protein is 0.8 g per kilogram of body weight per day for the older adult without kidney disease. However, proteins are restricted for older adults with both diabetes and kidney disease. For example, a 200-pound man with diabetes and kidney disease would only be allowed 72 g of protein per day (200/2.2 = 90.9 kg × .8 = 72 g). As a result of this restriction, it will take a lot of patience and persistence on the part of the older adult and the dietitian assisting in the planning of meals. Patient education is very important if the older adult is to manage his or her diet to meet nutritional and metabolic needs.

Exercise

Exercise programs must be individualized for the person with diabetes by the collaborative team. Prior to beginning an exercise program, it is always wise for the older adult to have a thorough physical examination, including a good cardiac evaluation, if warranted. The older adult should begin with a very modest amount of activity and gradually increase the duration and frequency to 30 to 45 minutes of moderate aerobic activity three to five days each week to a goal of at least 150 minutes each week. Collaborative care is very helpful; the team should enlist the evaluation of a physical therapist to help plan the activity program for older adults who may have physical limitations as a result of comorbidities such as heart disease and osteoarthritis.

Exercise is valuable because it helps reduce insulin resistance, which then results in lower blood glucose levels. For older adults who are taking insulin as part of their medication regimen, it is important that exercise be performed consistently. For some older adults, it may be help-

Anatomy of MyPyramid

One size doesn't fit all

USDA's new MyPyramid symbolizes a personalized approach to healthy eating and physical activity. The symbol has been designed to be simple. It has been developed to remind consumers to make healthy food choices and to be active every day. The different parts of the symbol are described below.

Activity
Activity is represented by the steps and the person climbing them, as a reminder of the importance of daily physical activity.

Moderation
Moderation is represented by the narrowing of each food group from bottom to top. The wider base stands for foods with little or no solid fats or added sugars. These should be selected more often. The narrower top area stands for foods containing more added sugars and solid fats. The more active you are, the more of these foods can fit into your diet.

Personalization
Personalization is shown by the person on the steps, the slogan, and the URL. Find the kinds and amounts of food to eat each day at MyPyramid.gov.

Proportionality
Proportionality is shown by the different widths of the food group bands. The widths suggest how much food a person should choose from each group. The widths are just a general guide, not exact proportions. Check the Web site for how much is right for you.

Variety
Variety is symbolized by the 6 color bands representing the 5 food groups of the Pyramid and oils. This illustrates that foods from all groups are needed each day for good health.

Gradual Improvement
Gradual improvement is encouraged by the slogan. It suggests that individuals can benefit from taking small steps to improve their diet and lifestyle each day.

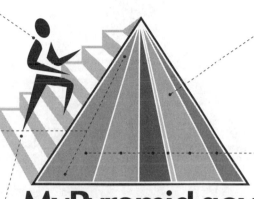

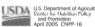

U.S. Department of Agriculture
Center for Nutrition Policy
and Promotion
April 2005 CNPP-16

USDA is an equal opportunity provider and employer.

GRAINS   VEGETABLES   FRUITS   OILS   MILK   MEAT & BEANS

FIGURE 11-3 MyPyramid

www.mypyramid.gov

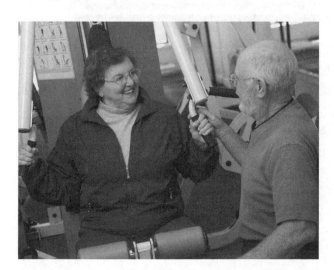

ful to monitor blood glucose both before and after exercise to avoid **hypoglycemia**.

Medical Management

Individuals with type 1 diabetes manage their blood glucose with insulin, because they are unable to secrete insulin due to damage to the beta cells. Many older adults with T2DM are maintained on insulin with or without other medications. Insulin resistance is progressive and insulin is often required in the older adult with diabetes.

Insulin is administered by injection. Insulin may be administered by either subcutaneous injection by using a specialized insulin syringe or the newer insulin pumps

hypoglycemia Abnormally low concentration of glucose in the blood; any blood glucose value lower than 40 to 50 mg/dL.

Modified MyPyramid for Older Adults

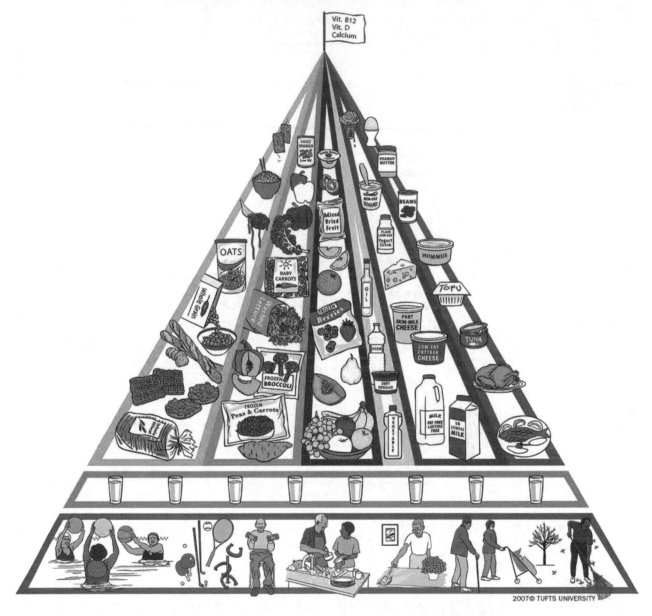

FIGURE 11-4 Modified MyPyramid for Older Adults

Source: Copyright 2007 Tufts University. Reprinted with permission from Lichenstein AH, Rasmussen H, Yu WW, Epstein SR, Russel RM. Modified MyPyramid for Older Adults. *J Nutr.* 2008;138:78–82.

that provide a continuous infusion of insulin based on blood sugar levels. A nasally inhaled insulin product had been developed that reduced or eliminated the need for injected insulin; however, long term side effects proved to be severe enough for it to be removed from the market.

Older adults with T2DM who are unable to maintain their blood glucose levels within normal limits through diet and exercise are often prescribed oral medications (**Table 11-3**). When oral medications are ineffective, insulin therapy may be prescribed. In fact, recently basal insulin (e.g., glargine)

TABLE 11-3 Commonly Prescribed Medications for Diabetes Mellitus

Medication	Trade Name	Route of Administration	Action/Information
Insulins:		Subcutaneous injection	
basal (long-acting)			
Insulin glargine	Lantus		Insulin replacement; lasts 24 hours; do not mix with other insulins; may be pain at injection site.
Insulin isophane	Humulin Novolin		Prepared mixed with regular insulin in doses: 70/30, 75/25, or 50/50; lasts 24 hours; do not add other insulins.
Non-insulin Agents:		Subcutaneous injection	
exenatide	Byetta		Incretin mimetic; adjunct to insulin, not substitution; CrCl should be greater than 30 mL/min; causes GI upset, hypoglycemia, and dizziness.
pramlintide	Symlin		Synthetic analogue of amylin; adjunct to insulin; causes GI upset, hypoglycemia; allergy.
Biguanide:		Oral	
metformin	Glucophage, GlucophageXR, Glumetza		Antihyperglycemic; Increases binding of insulin to its receptor. Potentiating insulin action. Does not increase insulin secretion. Decreases hepatic glucose; do not use in very old patients unless CrCl is greater than 50 mL/min; avoid with Cr greater than 1.5 mg/dL in men and greater than 1.4 mg/dL in women; causes weight loss.
Sulfonylureas:		Oral	
Glimepiride	Amaryl		Stimulates pancreatic beta cells to secrete insulin, decreases liver glycogenolysis and gluconeogenesis, and increases cellular sensitivity to insulin in body issues. Should not be used with rapid or very rapid-acting insulins.
Glipizide	Glucotrol		
Glyburide	Glucotrol XL DiaBeta, Glynase, Micronase		
Meglitinides:		Oral	
nateglinide	Starlix		Stimulates pancreatic beta cells to secrete insulin. Give 30 minutes before meals.
repaglinide	Prandin		
Alpha-glucosidase inhibitors:		Oral	
acarbose	Precose		Decreases glucose absorption from the GI tract. GI adverse effects common; do not use with Cr greater than 2 mg/dL. Monitor LFTs.
miglitrol	Glyset		Decreases glucose absorption from the GI tract. GI adverse effects common; do not use with Cr greater than 2 mg/dL.
Thiazolidinedione:		Oral	
Pioglitazone	Actos		Enhances insulin sensitivity. Decreases hepatic glucose output and increases insulin-dependent muscle glucose uptake in skeletal muscle and adipose tissue. Monitor LFTs.
Rosiglitazone	Avandia		

(continues)

TABLE 11-3 Commonly Prescribed Medications for Diabetes Mellitus (*Continued*)

Medication	Trade Name	Route of Administration	Action/Information
DPP-4 enzyme inhibitor:		Oral	Enhances endogenous incretins; interacts with sulfonylureas; can cause severe allergic reactions (e.g., Stevens–Johnson syndrome, anaphylaxis).
Sitagliptin	Januvia		

Source: Data from Wilson B, Shannon M, Shields K, Stang C. *Nurse's Drug Guide 2007.* Upper Saddle River, NJ: Prentice Hall; 2007; Reuben D, Herr K, Pacala J, et al. *Geriatrics at Your Fingertips, 2009.* 11th ed. New York: American Geriatric Society; 2009; *Nurse Practitioner Prescribing Reference, Spring 2009.* New York: Haymarket Media; 2009.

Cr = creatinine; CrCl = creatinine clearance; LFTs = liver function tests

Note: This list is not exhaustive

has become an early treatment according to the American Diabetes Association new treatment algorithm 2009. Insulin also has the advantage of quickly reducing blood glucose levels and can be given during periods when the individual cannot eat or drink. Insulin has drug interactions (e.g., cannot mix long-acting insulin with quick-onset insulin; potentiated by alicylates, alcohol, sulfa drugs, some ACE inhibitors; other effects with corticosteroids, thiazides, niacin, phenothiazines, B-blockers, clonidine, and lithium salts) and unless one has hypersensitivity to insulin, they are considered relatively safe for older adults. The disadvantages of insulin therapy for the management of type 1 and 2 diabetes is that it must be injected; it can result in weight gain, especially in women; and it can cause hypoglycemia if diet, exercise, and metabolic changes occur without changes in the insulin therapy (see **Box 11-3**).

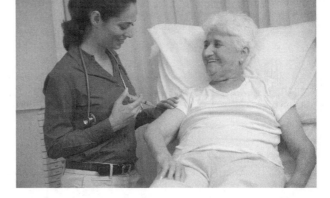

Two newer drugs, non-insulin injectables are used as adjunctive therapy for diabetes. Exenatide (Byetta©) is an incretin mimetic and pramlintide. Symlin© is an amylin analogue/amylinomimetic. Amylin is a hormone secreted by the beta cells of the pancreas and reduces postprandial glucagons levels, lowering glucose. Incretins are gut hormones released during food ingestion and augment normal insulin secretion. They account for 60% of total insulin release after eating a meal (in the normal situation). They suppress glucagon in the liver and decrease glucose output. Both drugs can cause GI upset, hypoglycemia, headache, anorexia, and allergic reactions.

Oral medications have been the mainstay of early and mid-stage type 2 diabetes management. Two important classes of oral medications are sulfonylureas and biguanides. Sulfonylureas enhance the release of insulin from the beta cells in the pancreas, decrease liver glycogenolysis and gluconeogenesis, and increase cellular sensitivity to body tissues. However, they cause weight gain. Metformin, a biguanide, decreases glucose absorption from the intestines and glucose production in the liver and improves **insulin sensitivity** in the peripheral tissues. It does not increase insulin secretion; therefore, it does not cause hypoglycemia. Biguanides do not cause weight gain and are often prescribed for overweight diabetic older adults.

Meglitinides lower blood glucose levels by stimulating the beta cells of the pancreas to produce insulin. Both of these groups of medications can result in hypoglycemia.

insulin sensitivity A measure of one's risk for heart disease. The more sensitive one is, the lower the risk for heart disease. Can be used to regulate insulin dosages. Formula for measurement:

(1) weight (lbs)/4 = _____ units of insulin

(2) total daily dose of insulin (all types of insulin) = _____ units

Line 1 is the estimated need for insulin; if the actual insulin dose on line 2 is close to this number, and patient has good control, insulin sensitivity is normal. If line 2 is *less* than line 1 and control is good, insulin sensitivity is excellent. If line 2 is much *greater* than line 1, the patient is probably getting too much insulin and may have insulin reactions.

Thiazolidinediones reduce blood glucose levels by lowering insulin resistance. They resensitize the body to its own insulin and decrease insulin resistance in the periphery and liver, thus enhancing the body's ability to process glucose. This classification of medications also has an effect on lipid metabolism. These drugs cause weight gain and also enhance fluid retention.

Alpha-glucosidase inhibitors delay the digestion and absorption of carbohydrates in the small intestine. This results in a smaller increase in blood glucose levels after food is ingested. These inhibitors are used as an adjunct to diet. Because they do not alter insulin secretion, they do not result in hypoglycemia. This class of drugs does not cause weight gain, but it is associated with GI complaints. In addition, many of these drugs are expensive.

Because insulin, the sulfonylureas, and the meglitinides stimulate insulin production, it is possible that the pancreas may secrete more insulin than is needed for the older adult's metabolic needs. Changes in activity, diet, or illness may result in the beta cells producing more insulin than can be metabolized, resulting in hypoglycemia. When the blood glucose level falls below 60 to 70 ml/dl the older adult should reverse the symptoms of hypoglycemia by ingesting 10 to 15 g of carbohydrates. Foods that can increase blood glucose in the event of hypoglycemia include:

- Glucose tablets (three to four)
- One serving of glucose gel (an amount equal to 15 g of carbohydrate)
- Fruit juice (4 oz) of any type
- Regular soft drink (not diet; 4 oz)
- Milk (8 oz)
- Hard candy (five or six pieces)
- Sugar or honey (1 tablespoon)

Note that the effects from eating these foods do not last long, so the older adult should recheck his or her blood glucose every 15 minutes until the capillary blood glucose level is about 70 on a self-monitoring device. The management of type 2 diabetes requires that older adults and significant others be educated on the signs and symptoms of hypoglycemia, know how to use a capillary glucose monitor, and be knowledgeable of the treatments that should be instituted. Everyone in the older adult's household must know where the emergency foods are kept to raise the capillary blood glucose level. They should also be aware of the signs and symptoms of hypoglycemia: tremor, anxiety, sweating, hunger and craving for sweets, palpitations, blurred vision, confusion, headache, dizziness, cold hands and feet, and less common but very serious, loss of consciousness.

A Summary of Diabetes Mellitus

Type 1 and type 2 diabetes are complex metabolic disorders. Most older adults have type 2 diabetes. The disease is chronic and progressive and requires a collaborative approach for successful management. The older adult with diabetes must maintain blood glucose levels in a normal range and prevent or control the complications that result from the metabolic changes associated with diabetes. The four keys to successful management are diet, exercise, medications, and self-care strategies. Ongoing research may change how we manage this disease in the near future. See **Boxes 11-4** and **11-5** for goals and recommendations for care of the older adult with diabetes.

> **BOX 11-5   Energy Balance, Overweight, and Obesity Recommendations**

- Modest weight loss will improve insulin resistance.
- Modify diet to low-carbohydrate or low-fat calorie-restricted diet for up to one year.
- On low-carbohydrate diet, monitor lipid profiles, renal function, and protein intake in those with nephropathy; adjust hypoglycemic therapy as necessary.
- Physical exercise and behavior modification are helpful in weight loss programs.
- Bariatric surgery for those with BMI greater than 35 or prescription of weight loss medications can be considered with physician discussion.

Source: Data from American Diabetes Association. Standards of medical care in diabetes—2008. *Diabetes Care.* 2008 Jan;31 Suppl 1:S12–54.

The Endocrine System

The endocrine glands include the pituitary, thyroid, parathyroid, pineal, thymus, **adrenal glands**, gonads (ovaries and testes), and pancreas. This section discusses the thyroid, parathyroid, and adrenal glands and the pancreas (**Figure 11-5**).

The endocrine system, through the hormones it produces and/or regulates, has far-reaching effects on the body. The pituitary gland, the "master gland," produces

adrenal glands   Two organs located close to the upper pole of each kidney. Each gland has two separate parts: a cortex and a medulla. The cortex produces the mineralocorticoid aldosterone, estrogen, androgens, and glucocorticoids. The medulla secretes epinephrine and norepinephrine.

trophic hormones   Hormones secreted to provide for survival of various cells.

pituitary (anterior and posterior)   The anterior part of the pituitary gland produces and secretes peptide hormones that regulate stress, growth, and reproduction. The posterior pituitary secretes antidiuretic hormone (ADH), also known as vasopressin, and oxytocin. Oxytocin causes contractions in childbirth. ADH controls blood plasma osmolality. It acts to increase the permeability of renal collecting ducts. ADH secretion is increased by changes in intravascular volume.

hormones that reach target glands, which in turn produce more hormones. Other factors in the body also influence some of these regulatory mechanisms. For example, ADH (antidiuretic hormone), which is produced by the posterior pituitary, influences the body's sodium balance in conjunction with the kidneys.

Pituitary Gland and Hypothalamus

The hypothalamus, although not an endocrine gland, is discussed here because it plays a major role in the function of the endocrine system. The hypothalamus and the pituitary gland make up the hypothalamic–pituitary axis, which increase or decrease inhibitory/stimulating/**trophic hormones**.

The hypothalamus is located at the base of the brain and is connected to the **anterior pituitary** (located in the sella turcica) by portal hypophysial blood vessels and to the **posterior pituitary** by the hypothalamohypophysial nerve tract.

The neurons in the hypothalamus synthesize ADH and oxytocin, which are sent to the posterior pituitary by the hypothalamohypophysial nerve tract and stored and secreted in the posterior pituitary. The hypothalamus also synthesizes releasing and inhibitory hormones that are sent to the anterior pituitary and control the trophic hormones. The trophic hormones include thyrotropin-releasing hormone (TRH), which stimulates the release of thyroid-stimulating hormone (TSH); growth-hormone-releasing factor (GRF), which stimulates release of growth hormone (GH); gonadotrophic-releasing hormone (GnRH), important to women premenarche; prolactin-inhibitor factor (PIF), another premenarche need; and substance P, which inhibits synthesis and release of adrenocorticotropic hormone (ACTH).

Hormones of the posterior pituitary include ADH and oxytocin, which causes uterine contractions in childbirth. ADH in involved in the control of plasma osmolality and water absorption. It also inhibits the increase of calcium and decrease of potassium.

Other hormones of the neuroendocrine system include those produced by the hypothalamus that reduce or increase appetite. Appetite-reducing hormones include alpha-melanocyte-stimulating hormone and cocaine-amphetamine-regulated transcript. Appetite-stimulating hormones include neuropeptide Y and agouti related protein. Leptin, a hormone produced by fat cells, has a major role in regulating food intake. Leptin inhibits the release of agouti related protein. The hypothalamus also influences hormones produced in the gastrointestinal system. Grehlin, produced by the stomach, rises prior to meals and with starvation. Levels fall after feeding. These hormones are the focus of much research in hopes of learning more about the causes of obesity. In practical terms, the hypothalamus is involved in the regulation of hunger and satiety, respiration, body temperature, water balance, and the many body functions mentioned above.

Thyroid Glands

Thyroid diseases increase with aging. The aging **thyroid gland** develops both micro- and macronodules as well as fibrous tissue and lymphocytes. There is a reduction in follicle size and colloid. The thyroid may become smaller. The resting metabolic rate (RMR) diminishes with age. Men have a higher RMR than women.

The amount of thyroxine (T4) secreted decreases, but its half-life increases. The amount of T4 and free T4 remain constant. T3 (triiodothyronine) is produced in greater quantities, and free T3 levels remain constant until very old age. TSH levels do not change with age.

Medications commonly taken by older patients can decrease the level of free T4 with lower or normal T3 and normal TSH (phenytoin, carbamazepine, phenobarbital, rifampin), increase free T4 and T3 with lower TSH (aspirin, phenylbutazone, heparin); or cause decreased or normal free T4 and T3 with lowered TSH (corticosteroids, amiodarone, dopamine therapy).

The Thyroid Gland and Its Dysfunctions

The two most common conditions affecting the thyroid gland are **hypothyroidism** and **hyperthyroidism** (**Figure 11-6**). The incidence of hypothyroidism increases with age. Approximately 0.5% to 5% of older adults over the age of 60 have hypothyroidism and 5% to 10% have subclinical hypothyroidism. Hyperthyroidism presents more commonly as toxic nodular goiters.

Hypothyroidism
Hypothyroidism results from a decrease in thyroid gland function. Diagnostic tests show increased TSH, which is a

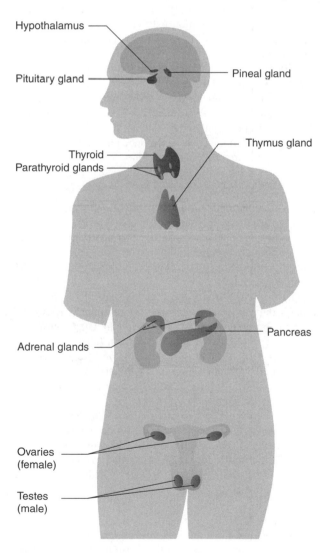

Hypothalamus

Pituitary gland — Pineal gland

Thymus gland

Thyroid
Parathyroid glands

Pancreas

Adrenal glands

Ovaries
(female)

Testes
(male)

FIGURE 11-5 Endocrine Glands

Source: National Institutes of Health, 2007.

thyroid gland Composed of two lobes that lie on either side of the trachea behind the thyroid cartilage, it is not visible but is palpated on swallowing. Thyroid cells secrete polypeptides such as calcitonin and somatostatin. Thyroid hormone secretion (TH) occurs in a feedback loop with other endocrine glands, principally the anterior pituitary and hypothalamus. Thyroid-stimulating hormone (TSH) increases iodide uptake and increases synthesis and release of prostaglandins. It helps regulate somatostatin, dopamine, and catecholamines, nutritional state, the body's response to extreme cold, and steroid levels. It regulates protein, fat, and carbohydrate catabolism in all cells. It regulates the metabolic rate of all cells. It regulates body heat production, acts as an insulin antagonist, and maintains growth hormone secretion, to name just a few of its activities.

hypothyroidism Insufficient production of thyroid hormone. Fairly common disorder; incidence is higher in older adults. Iodine deficiency can increase the risk. Early symptoms include poor muscle tone, fatigue, cold intolerance, depression, constipation, muscle cramps, arthritis, goiter, brittle fingernails and hair, dry itchy skin, and weight gain. Late symptoms include dry puffy skin, loss of hair in outer one-third of eyebrows, slow speech with hoarse voice, and low body temperature.

hyperthyroidism
Overproduction and release of thyroid hormones. May result in heart palpitations and atrial fibrillation. Symptoms include tremors, nervousness, anxiety, weight loss, and diarrhea. There may be intolerance to heat and hair loss. It is very serious and may result in death if not diagnosed and treated.

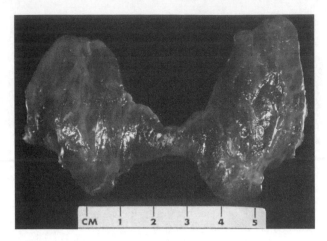

FIGURE 11-6 Thyroid Gland

Source: Reproduced from *An Introduction to Human Disease.* 7th ed. Photo courtesy of Leonard V. Crowley, M.D., Century College.

response to low levels of T3 and T4. The main causes of hypothyroidism are

- Chronic autoimmune inflammation of the gland
- Complications following thyroid surgery
- Complications following the use of radioactive iodine for hyperthyroidism
- Thyroid gland incompletely developed
- Drugs, such as lithium, propylthiouracil, carbimazole, amiodarone, and large amounts of iodine in cough syrups

Hypothyroidism often presents atypically in older adults. Common signs and symptoms that can be confused with other problems include diminished skin turgor, dry skin (common in older adults), slowed mentation, weakness, constipation, anemia, **hyponatremia**, arthritis, paresthesias, and gait disturbances. Reflexes and slowed speech also may occur. Symptoms are slow to develop and are often mistakenly identified and attributed to other morbidities or aging. Hypothyroidism is recognized in the clinical examination in only 10% to 20% of cases. Concomitant disease conditions, nutritional problems, and other endocrine problems can delay the diagnosis of hypothyroidism.

The common nutritional problem with hypothyroidism, particularly in the older patient, is hypercholesterolemia. The health care provider needs to be aware of an increase in cholesterol. The treatment of hypothyroidism will reduce the hy-

hyponatremia Abnormally low sodium concentrations in the blood due to excessive excretion of sodium (by the kidney), prolonged vomiting, or diarrhea.

percholesterolemia. Additional deficits of thyroid hormones lead to nutritional problems of hyponatremia and anemia.

Myxedema coma, a very serious effect of hypothyroidism, can occur when another concomitant nonthyroid illness occurs in the older adult with mild hypothyroidism.

Treatment

Hypothyroidism is corrected with low-dose replacement of T4, with slow increases in dose. If the older adult has cardiac problems, the dose is started even lower, but still should be given. The T4 dose will be higher for older adults who are severely hypothyroid. Laboratory work, which should be conducted at least annually, will confirm normalization. The dose will be lower in aged adults, because thyroid hormone requirements diminish with age. However, overreplacement results in osteopenia and exacerbation of heart disease.

With normalization of the hypothyroid state, elevated lipoproteins resolve. This reduces the risk of atherosclerosis. However, those who have suffered diminished cognitive function may not return to their previous functional state. Referral for specialist review is usually only necessary if there is myocardial ischemia, the need for amiodarone therapy or lithium, or evidence of pituitary disease.

Hyperthyroidism

Hyperthyroidism is defined as an increase in the function of the thyroid gland. It occurs in 0.5% to 2.3% of older adults. Serum thyroxine (T4) and serum triiodothyronine (T3) or both are elevated, with low levels of TSH (thyrotropin). Subclinical hyperthyroidism labs show elevated TSH with low T4 and T3.

Thyrotoxicosis is not the same as hyperthyroidism, although the terms are often used synonymously. *Hyperthyroidism* is the result of an overactive gland. *Thyrotoxicosis* is a very severe form of hyperthyroidism (also called "thyroid storm") that refers to the clinical pathological effects of unbound hormones. Secondary hyperthyroidism refers to causes from pituitary adenomas, thyroiditis, iodine-induced hyperthyroiditis, and others.

The most common hyperthyroid state in older adults is Grave's disease. Grave's disease is a syndrome triad of ophthalmopathy, diffusely enlarged thyroid gland, and dermopathy. Toxic multinodular goiter and autonomously functioning adenomas are more common in older rather than younger adults.

Epidemiology

Hyperthyroidism occurs more often in women than men. The median age at diagnosis in the United Kingdom is 58. In some parts of the world with low iodine availability, the disorder is not uncommon; for example, in Denmark, the incidence is 9.7%. Thyrotoxicosis occurs mainly in younger female adults, but more than 25% of cases occur in adults 60 years and older. In the United States, most cases (85% to 95%) are caused by Grave's disease.

The clinical presentation of hyperthyroidism is vague, nonspecific symptoms with elevated T3 and T4 tests and low TSH. Elevated production of T3 and T4 increases metabolism. Problems noted in the eyes include irritation; dryness; protruding, even bulbous, eyes in some Grave's disease cases; and difficulty closing the eyelids.

Common manifestations of hyperthyroidism in the older adult include irritability, weight loss, depression, agitation, edema, lethargy, dementia, and confusion. Angina may occur or may worsen. Paradoxically, in the older person with hyperthyroidism a lack of appetite occurs more frequently than an increase. Ophthalmopathy may be absent. Common findings (60%) include congestive cardiac failure and refractory atrial fibrillation. Uncommon findings include nervousness, increased diaphoresis, increased appetite, and increased bowel movements. See **Box 11-6** for general manifestations of hyperthyroidism. A low TSH is associated with three times the risk of developing atrial fibrillation within 10 years, and hyperthyroidism is present in 13% to 30% of older adults with atrial fibrillation.

Medications and certain foods can cause hyperthyroidism (e.g., amiodarone, iodine, kelp, contrast media, alpha-interferon, interleukin-2) or hypothyroidism (e.g., lithium, amiodarone, iodine, aminoglutethamide, alpha-interferon, interleukin-2) by affecting the thyroid gland. Grave's disease can also be caused or triggered by autoimmune disease resulting in goitrous or atrophic thyroiditis, subtotal thyroidectomy, smoking, stress, environment, viruses, and hereditary factors.

Apathetic hyperthyroidism is defined as hyperthyroidism but with few typical symptoms. It is almost exclusively seen in frail older adults. The clinical presentation of apathetic hyperthyroidism includes depression, inactivity, lethargy, weight loss, muscle weakness, and/or cardiac symptoms. If apathetic hyperthyroidism is not treated, the patient is likely to succumb to other problems. If treated, he or she will lose wrinkles, become more active, and lose the depression.

Nutritional problems associated with hyperthyroidism are hyponatremia, worsening of glucose tolerance, mild hyperglycemia, and anemia. Another problem that may occur if not treated is osteoporosis.

Treatment

Treatment of hyperthyroidism is directed at the underlying cause. Treatment includes a thionamide (methimazole, carbimazole, or propylthiouracil) and a beta-blocking drug. Thionamide treatment has a 50% recurrence rate in Graves' disease and is ineffective in toxic nodular goiter, so defini-

> ## BOX 11-6 General Manifestations of Hyperthyroidism at Any Age, But Not as Common in Older Adults
>
> - Nervousness, restlessness
> - Trembling hands
> - Rapid heartbeat
> - Feelings of excessive warmth and intolerance of heat
> - Hot, sweaty skin
> - Weight loss despite increased appetite
> - Severe general tiredness
> - Muscle pains and muscle tiredness
> - Frequent loose stools
> - Disturbances of menstruation

tive treatment is needed in most older patients. After an euthyroid state is reached (usually one to six months of a thionamide, with monthly serum T4 checks), administration of radioiodine or surgery can be undertaken. Surgery is usually reserved for older patients with a large goiter or ophthalmopathy.

Nodular Goiter and Thyroid Cancer in the Older Adult

Thyroid nodules are common in adults older than age 70 (90% of women older than 70; 60% of men 80 and older). Age does not increase differentiated thyroid cancer, but a rare anaplastic carcinoma involving the gland has been found only in people over age 65. The treatment of choice may be surgery, external radiation, and chemotherapy.

Parathyroid Glands and Calcium Metabolism

The **parathyroid glands** are four tiny glands located behind the thyroid gland that secrete the parathyroid hormone. This hormone is responsible for withdrawing calcium from the bone and maintaining serum calcium levels. The release of parathyroid hormone increases 30% between the ages of 30 and 80. With advancing age, the balance between bone

parathyroid glands Two to six glands located behind the thyroid gland that produce parathyroid hormone (PTH), which regulates calcium. PTH acts directly on bone and kidneys. If greatly stimulated (by low magnesium levels or phosphate), it causes breakdown and resorption of bone. If chronic stimulation occurs, bone remodeling occurs in which bone is broken down and re-formed.

resorption and bone formation lessens so that there is a decrease in bone mass, increasing the risk of osteoporosis.

Calcitonin, secreted by the thyroid gland, inhibits the release of calcium from the osteoclasts in the bone when serum calcium levels are too high. Vitamin D facilitates calcium absorption. Calcitriol is the active form of vitamin D and promotes absorption of calcium in the gastrointestinal tract (**Figure 11-7**).

Hyperparathyroidism

Hyperparathyroidism is a relatively common disorder. It is more common in women, particularly postmenopausal women, than in men. It affects approximately 2 of 1,000 women. The condition is primarily the result of gland hyperplasia. A single benign parathyroid adenoma is the most frequent underlying disease. However, malignancy is as common a cause as the benign form. It is often mild and asymptomatic and detected by a routine serum calcium laboratory report. Symptoms of related abnormalities include hypertension, muscular weakness, irritability, mild GI disturbances, renal colic, bone cysts, impaired renal function with polyuria, and diminished bone mass.

Hypercalciuria and nephrolithiasis can occur and also be asymptomatic. Even if the calcium abnormalities are reversed, renal impairment may progress. With nephrocalcinosis, the damage is irreversible.

Severe **hypercalcemia** is common and dangerous in older adults. It may result from malignancy, especially breast cancer and multiple myeloma, or from primary hyperparathyroidism that was formerly in a mild state. This change may be caused by a concomitant illness causing dehydration.

Signs and symptoms of hypercalcemia include elevated calcium levels, decreased phosphorus levels, elevated or high normal serum parathormone (PTH), osteopenia, generalized weakness, fractures, depression, mild cognitive impairment, fatigue, lack of energy, increased thirst, and polyuria. Other diagnostic measures that may be helpful are blood pressure, serum calcium and creatinine, creatinine clearance, 24-hour urine calcium, abdominal films, and bone densitometry. A BUN and creatinine should be obtained, because secondary hyperparathyroidism may occur in renal insufficiency.

Rapid onset of hypercalcemia accompanied by anemia, weight loss, and hypoalbuminemia is suggestive of malignancy. Chest X-ray and thyroid tests and serum protein electrophoresis should be done in addition to other tests to confirm or deny malignancy.

Hyperparathyroidism may be treated through surgery or pharmacological treatment. Older adults with hyperparathyroidism should avoid thiazide diuretics, dehydration, and immobilization. Treatment with medications is recommended for those who cannot tolerate surgery. Acute hypercalcemia is treated with volume replacement with IV saline and diuresis with a loop diuretic, such as furosemide, followed by intravenous biphosphonate pamidronate in doses or 60 to 90 mg or intravenous mithramycin of 25 µg/kg of body weight. Chronic hypercalcemia is treated with oral or intravenous biphosphonates. Bisphosphonates will decrease bone pain in elders with pathologic fractures of bone.

Hypocalcemia

Hypocalcemia is a decrease in serum calcium to less than 7 mg/dL. The causes are varied, but the most common ones are inadequate intake of dairy products, with decreased albumin, and decreased vitamin D intake or activation. Impaired vitamin D activation is due partially to decreased exposure to sunlight and vitamin D synthesis by the skin. Age-related decreases in hepatic and renal function lead to lower amounts of 25-hydroxycholecalciferol and 1.25-dihydroxycholecalciferol.

Drugs may reduce body stores of calcium by increasing the elimination of calcium (e.g., loop diuretics are calciuric) or reducing its absorption (e.g., anticonvulsants stimulate hydroxylation pathways that produce metabolites of vitamin D that are less effective at absorbing calcium from the GI tract).

The symptoms of hypocalcemia are frequently confused with other comorbid conditions of the older patient. Severe hypocalcemia causes tetany and is a medical emergency. Tetany is characterized by paresthesias of the mouth, lips, and tongue and muscle spasms of the hands, feet, and face. Cardiac arrhythmias and heart block may occur.

Mild hypocalcemia can be asymptomatic or have CNS signs. There may be a mimicking of depression, dementia, or psychosis. When chronic, hypocalcemia causes cataracts and calcification of the basal ganglia.

Laboratory tests often show that when calcium is low, serum phosphate is high. However, hypocalcemia can occur with hypophosphatemia in those with vitamin D deficiency and in those with magnesium and phosphate depletion.

Hypocalcemia is treated with calcitriol (1,25-dihydroxyvitamin D3) and oral calcium supplements (1 to 2 g per day of elemental calcium). These will rapidly increase the serum calcium concentration in those who have been hypocalcemic for more than one day. Calcitriol is given in divided doses because it has a short half-life. Correcting the hypomagnesiemia is also helpful in treating other deficiencies, such as calcium, potassium, and phosphate deficiencies.

calcitonin A hormone secreted by the thyroid gland in response to elevated blood calcium. It stimulates calcium deposition in bone and calcium excretion by the kidneys, thus reducing blood calcium.

hypercalcemia Abnormally high concentrations of calcium in the blood.

hypocalcemia A deficiency of calcium in the blood.

VITAMIN D: FROM SOURCE TO DESTINATION

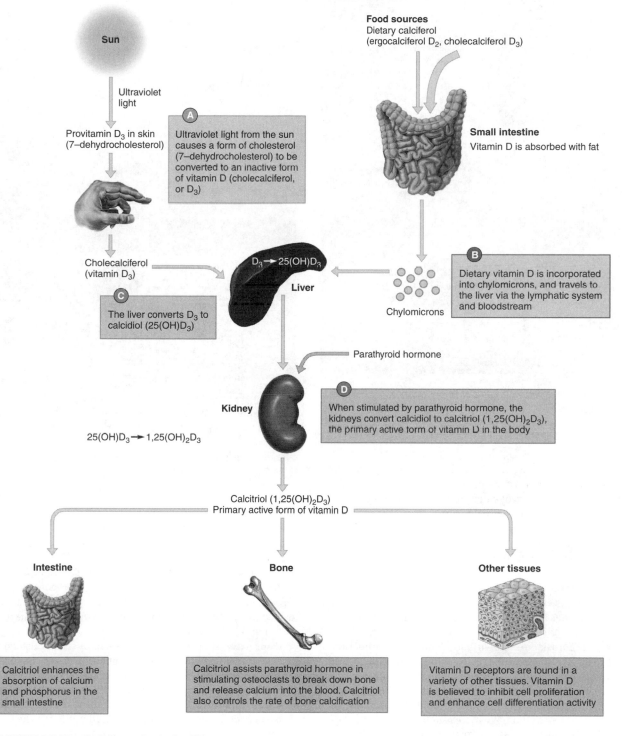

FIGURE 11-7 Vitamin D Absorption in the GI Tract

Source: Insel P, Turner RE, Ross D. *Nutrition.* 3rd ed. Sudbury, MA: Jones & Bartlett; 2007. Reproduced with permission.

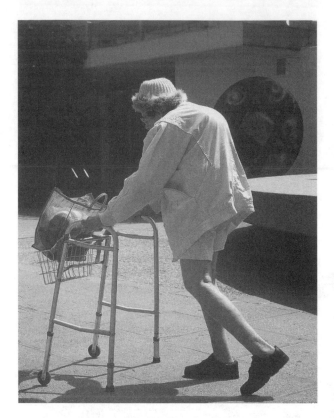

FIGURE 11-8 Visible Symptoms of Osteoporosis Due to Collapsed Vertebrae

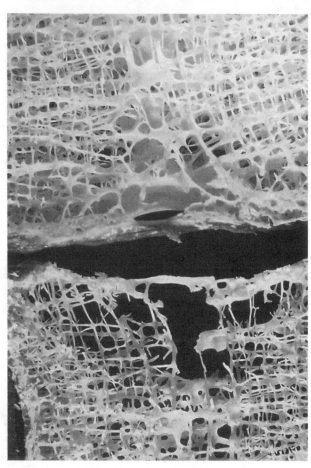

FIGURE 11-9 Normal and Abnormal Bone in Osteoporosis

Thiazide diuretic can be used to increase phosphate excretion and decrease calcium excretion. Aluminum hydroxide gel or large doses of calcium carbonate binds phosphate in the intestine and reduces its absorption.

Rarely, an IV infusion of calcium is used to treat tetany on an urgent basis. In this situation, 20% calcium gluconate is given over 5 to 10 minutes.

Osteoporosis

Osteoporosis is a common, preventable, and treatable disorder of older men and women. In women, osteoporosis often begins during menopause (**Figure 11-8**). Risk factors for osteoporosis are known and identifiable. Evaluation of bone mineral density is available to all older adults in the United States. The U.S. Preventive Services Task Force recommends using dual energy x-ray absorptiometry (DEXA) scans to screen all women 65 years and older and to screen women 60 to 64 who have increased fracture risk.

Postmenopausal osteoporosis is characterized by low bone mass, micro-architectural deterioration of bone, fragile bone, and heightened susceptibility to fracture (**Figure 11-9**). The World Health Organization (WHO) criteria for osteoporosis is a DEXA scan T-score at or below −2.5. Osteopenia (low bone mass) is a T score of −1.0 to −2.5. A normal T-score is −1.0 and higher. Nearly 8 million women in the United States meet the criteria for osteoporosis. The DEXA scan is the tool best able to diagnose osteopenia and osteoporosis. It is advised by many that older adults have a baseline DEXA scan by age 50.

Those groups most at risk for osteoporosis and osteopenia (low bone mass) are White women (one in every five) and Asian women older than 50 years. Following these high risk groups are Hispanic women, then African American women with the least of the four. Unfortunately, osteopenia and osteoporosis often are not diagnosed until after the first fracture occurs. Further, osteoporosis occurs frequently in men (20% of cases are in men), but its diagnosis is often missed.

Risk Factors/Prevention

The process of osteoporosis begins in early life, with peak bone mass occurring during an adult's 20s and 30s. Osteoporosis can be prevented by ensuring adequate calcium and vitamin D intake and making sure to receive enough sunlight. In addition, weight-bearing exercises can help to prevent osteoporosis. In some cases, hormone-replacement therapy may be used, because many studies have confirmed that osteoporosis is highest after menopause.

Estrogen loss in postmenopausal women is partially responsible for osteopenia and osteoporosis. See **Box 11-7** for other risk factors. Similarly, androgen loss in older men causes bone loss. More than 40% of men in their 60s and 80% of men in their 80s have very low levels of testosterone. Men lose their bone mass more slowly than women do because they have higher bone mass. By age 90, 17% of men have had a hip fracture compared to 37% of women.

Calcium and phosphate concentrations, which are maintained by the endocrine system, bear heavily on skeletal homeostasis. Dysfunction of this system can ultimately cause bone deterioration. Hormones commonly associated with osteoporosis include parathyroid hormone, cortisol, thyroid hormone, and growth hormone.

Treatment

The universally recommended vitamin D intake is 1200 IU per day of vitamin D3. Vitamin D levels should be obtained routinely even in younger men and women, as many levels are lower than predicted just based on a good diet. Further, Blacks need more than six times the UV radiation than do Whites. In Boston, 73% of older Blacks were found to have low vitamin D. Vitamin D insufficiency is very prevalent and has been associated with increased risk of DM I and II; breast, colon, and prostate cancers; hip and nonvertebral fractures; and osteoporosis. Supplementation with vitamin D is associated with fewer falls, and a 7% lower risk of death. Vitamin D3 is the form of vitamin D that best supports bone health. It is manufactured in the skin following direct exposure to sunlight. It is also called cholecalciferol. To a lesser extent, vitamin D3 also can be obtained from fortified milk, egg yolks, saltwater fish, liver, and supplements. As mentioned earlier, those at risk for osteoporosis should participate in weight-bearing exercise on a daily basis. They should also limit alcohol consumption and smoking.

Recommendations for calcium intake are 1,200 mg/day in men and women 31 to older than age 50. Calcium carbonate is least expensive but calcium citrate should be used for those on PPIs or who have achlorhydria. Granular forms are available for those with difficulty swallowing. See **Table 11-4** for calcium-containing foods.

In a 15-year follow up of subjects in the Framingham study, it was found that consumption of Vitamin C at sufficiently high levels was associated with nearly a 50%

BOX 11-7   Risk and Contributing Factors for Osteoporosis

Genetic	Family history of fracture, white race, older age, female sex
Build	Small stature, fair, pale-skinned, thin build (body weight <127 lb; BMI <21)
Metabolic	Early menopause, late menarche, nulliparity, obesity, low weight
Dietary	Low dietary calcium and vitamin D, low endogenous magnesium, excess vitamin A, aluminum (in antacids), excessive protein and low protein, excessive sodium/salt intake, high caffeine intake, anorexia, malabsorption
Lifestyle	Sedentary, smoker, alcohol consumption to excess, immobilization, little physical activity, falling
Disease	Rheumatoid arthritis, systemic lupus, renal insufficiency, spinal cord injury, bone marrow disorders such as thalassemia and myeloma, homocystinuria, hyperparathyroidism, thyrotoxicosis, GI surgery, inflammatory bowel disease, gastric bypass, malabsorption, pancreatic disease, primary biliary cirrhosis, ankylosing spondylitis, epilepsy, idiopathic scoliosis, prior fracture as an adult, congestive heart failure, depression, arrhythmias, malnutrition
Drugs	Corticosteroids, loop diuretics (furosemide), dilantin, methotrexate, thyroid, heparin, cyclosporine, retinoids, narcotics

Source: Data from McCance K. Huether S. *Pathophysiology.* 5th ed. Philadelphia: Elsevier Mosby; 2006; National Osteoporosis Foundation. National Osteoporosis Foundation releases new clinical recommendations for low bone mass and osteoporosis incorporating absolute fracture risk. 2008. Available at: http://www.nof.org/prevention/calciumandvitaminD.htm. Accessed March 10, 2008.

---

decrease in risk of hip and nonvertebral osteoporotic fractures. Those with the highest intake of Vitamin C, via both diet and supplement (median of 305 mg/day), had the best results. Interestingly, the increased intake did not affect bone mineral density (BMD).

Older adults at risk for osteoporosis should receive treatment. All postmenopausal women who have had a hip or vertebral fracture and all postmenopausal women with

TABLE 11-4 High-Calcium Foods

Food	Serving	Calcium per Serving (mg)
Milk	1 cup	290–300
Powdered milk	1 tsp	50
Yogurt	1 cup	240–400
Cottage cheese	1/2 cup	80–100
Ice cream	1/2 cup	90–100
Parmesan cheese	1 tbs	70
American cheese	1 oz/1 slice	165–200
Swiss cheese	l oz/1 slice	250–270
Sardines in oil & bones	3 oz	370
Orange juice with calcium	1 cup	300
Canned salmon with bones	3 oz	170–210
Broccoli	1 cup	160–180
Turnip greens	1/2 cup, cooked	100–125
Kale	1/2 cup, cooked	90–100
Cornbread	2-1/2" square	80–90
Egg	1 medium	55

Source: Data from American Geriatric Society. *Geriatrics Review Syllabus.* 6th ed. New York: American Geriatric Society; 2006.

bone mineral density values consistent with osteopenia and osteoporosis should receive treatment. Postmenopausal women (and men) with a T-score ranging from –2.0 to –2.5 *plus* one of the following risk factors for fracture—thinness, history of fragility fracture (other than skull, ankle, finger, toe) since menopause, and history of hip fracture in a parent—should receive treatment. Note that patients often do not link a fragility fracture with having osteoporosis. Most do not even know that the diagnosis of osteoporosis places them at risk for fracture. It is important to inform the older adult with osteoporosis of the risk for fractures.

Medications

A number of medications are available for the management of osteoporosis. SERMS (selective estrogen receptor modulators, e.g., Evista©) have the positive effects of estrogen but minimize its negative effects, such as those on the breast and endometrium. Other options are intranasal calcitonin (e.g., Miacalcin, Fortical) and oral sodium fluoride. The oral bisphosphonates, alendronate, ibandronate, and risedronate, are effective in reducing hip and vertebral fractures, especially in those who need to take glucocorticoid steroids for other health problems. The newer drug, teriparatide, a parathormone and anabolic agent, is given by subcutaneous injection daily to men and women at high risk for fractures. Side effects of this drug are dizziness, nausea, headache, and leg cramps. It can be given for one year at which point it must then be discontinued and bisphonates given. It should not be used in older adults with Paget's disease.

The drug ibandronate is given IV 3 mg every 3 months for 4 doses. Zoledronic acid is given IV 5 mg/year for 3 doses. Both reduce fractures.

A number of trace elements affect skeletal tissues; these include fluoride, magnesium, zinc, iodine, aluminum, copper, boron, iron, and manganese. Their exact involvement in maintaining bone health is not currently known, but they do enhance bone mass and bone turnover; help to regulate secretion of calcitonin, inhibit osteoclastic function; as well as other important functions.

Fractures carry a high morbidity and mortality rate. In one study by Bliuc, Nguyen, Milch, and colleagues, half the low-trauma fractures incurred in women and in men were followed by death. Subsequent fracture increases the mortality rate.

Paget's Disease

Paget's disease occurs in 1.3 of every 100 adults aged 45 to 74. It affects men more than women and is more common in aged individuals and those of Northern European background. It is sometimes hereditary.

With Paget's disease, increased bone remodeling occurs in localized areas, changing the bone's architecture and causing deformity and increasing the bone's tendency to fracture (**Figure 11-10**). It is usually asymptomatic. If symptomatic, pain occurs in the affected bones or from secondary osteoarthritic changes in the hips, knees, and vertebrae. It is usually found by x-ray after an unexplained elevation of the alkaline phosphatase.

The bones most commonly affected by Paget's disease are the skull, pelvis, spine, femur, and tibia. Bone deformities usually occur in the long bones of the legs, resulting in bowed legs. However, deformities can also occur in the skull, which will enlarge. The spine can be involved, causing serious curvature. The bones become very fragile (see **Figure 11-11**).

Occasionally, the disease transforms to a malignant state of osteosarcoma. Treatment is usually unnecessary for the asymptomatic disease, although there may be concern for hearing loss when the skull is involved. Nerve root and spinal cord compression can occur with vertebral involvement, and hip fracture can occur when the femoral neck is affected. The bisphosphonate risedronate is used to suppress accelerated bone turnover. Patients may be followed with bone-specific serum alkaline phosphatase or serum osteocalcin.

Adrenal Glands

The two adrenal glands are located retroperitoneally and close to the upper pole of each kidney. Each gland has an inner medulla and an outer cortex. They secrete glucocorticoids, mineralocorticoids, androgens, and estrogens. Aldosterone is the primary glucocorticoid; it conserves sodium by increasing the activity of the sodium pump of the epithelial cells.

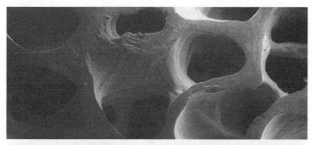

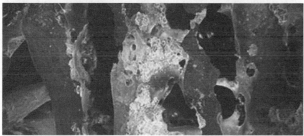

FIGURE 11-10 Paget's Disease: Normal and Abnormal Bone

Source: NIH SeniorHealth, 2007.

Water Metabolism

Water is essential to life. The body reacts to the need for water through increased thirst, increased fluid intake, and increased fluid output. Thirst perception is diminished in older adults; this can cause decreased fluid intake. Older adults also have a decreased ability to concentrate urine.

Edema, the collection of excessive fluid in interstitial compartments, may occur secondary to hypothyroidism, congestive heart failure, protein deficiency, and renal conditions. Water intoxication is excessive amounts of water throughout the body from oral or intravenous overload or hormones. Aldosterone secreted by the adrenal glands retains sodium, which in turn retains water. The antidiuretic hormone (ADH) is secreted from the posterior pituitary when there is increased osmolality of the blood. Inappropriate secretion of ADH is excessive ADH that causes hyponatremia (also known as dilutional hyponatremia).

Diseases of the Adrenal Cortex

The metabolic clearance rate of cortisol decreases with age; however, the secretion of cortisol decreases with age, thus basal serum cortisol levels do not change with increasing age. Basal levels of cortisone also remain constant. Basal adrenocorticotrophic (ACTH) levels are unchanged or slightly increased in the older patient.

Older adults are predisposed to volume depletion and free water excess. Many factors are involved in this age-related change, including alterations in ADH secretion, the osmoreceptor and baroreceptor systems, urine capability, renal hormone responsiveness, and thirst sensation.

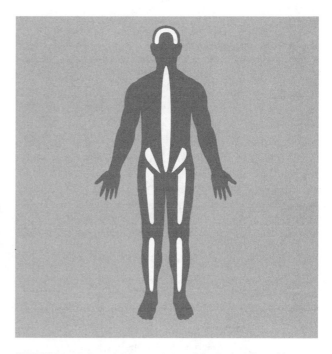

FIGURE 11-11 Paget's Disease: Areas of the Body Affected by Disease

Source: NIH SeniorHealth, 2007.

ADH secretion tends to be excessive in aged individuals. Many of the illnesses that affect older adults, such as renal insufficiency and heart failure, and the use of diuretics may cause the development of hyponatremia. Some of the medications that initiate the syndrome of inappropriate antidiuretic hormone (SIADH) are the SSRIs and Venlafaxine (for depression), tricyclic antidepressants, sulfonylureas (for diabetes), carbamazepine (for seizures), NSAIDs, and barbiturates.

Adrenal Insufficiency: Addison's Disease

Adrenal insufficiency, also called Addison's disease, is a decrease in cortisol secretion. In older adults, adrenal insufficiency is most often caused by failure of the adrenal gland rather than the pituitary gland. It can occur at any age, but the age of onset is primarily between the ages of 30 and 50.

Adrenal insufficiency can be caused by autoimmune disorders, tumors, or infection. It can also be caused by suppression of the adrenal gland by external corticoid use or by stress from trauma, surgery, hemorrhage, or infection.

Symptoms of adrenal insufficiency include abdominal pain, weakness and fatigue, nausea and vomiting, low blood pressure, hyperkalemia, hyponatremia, hyperpigmentation (skin darkening), irritability, depression, dehydration, and decreased or absent pubic hair and axiliary hair (**Figure 11-12**).

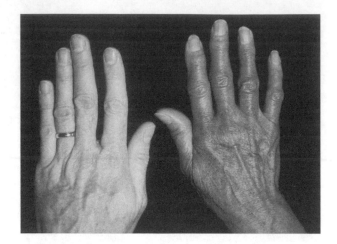

FIGURE 11-12 Hand of a Patient with Addison's Disease

Source: Reproduced from *An Introduction to Human Disease.* 7th ed. Photo courtesy of Leonard V. Crowley, M.D., Century College.

Disease onset may be sudden, resulting in Addisonian crisis, or acute adrenal failure (which also occurs if one stops taking steroid medications abruptly). Signs and symptoms of crisis are pain in the lower back, abdomen, or legs; severe vomiting and diarrhea leading to dehydration; low blood pressure with fainting; low blood sugar; elevated

potassium; and loss of consciousness. Diagnostic tests will show hyponatremia, hypoglycemia, hyperkalemia, elevated BUN and creatinine, and elevated plasma ACTH.

Disease management focuses on finding and treating the cause, if possible, and replacing the mineralcorticoids and glucocorticoids. Hydrocortisone is the drug of choice. Fludrocortisone [Florinef (c)] is added to increase salt and potassium retention. If an autoimmune disorder is present, comorbidities such as diabetes mellitus, pernicious anemia, and hypothyroidism should be investigated. Nutritional deficits of low sodium, low fluid volume, and low glucose levels must be compensated through treatment. Potassium levels must be watched and treated, if excessive. All patients with this disorder should carry a medical alert card and bracelet at all times and keep medications and syringes available in the event of an emergency.

Cushing's Syndrome

Exposure to excessive amounts of cortisol for a prolonged period of time results in Cushing's syndrome. The most common cause of Cushing's in the older adult is exogenous corticoids. The signs and symptoms of Cushing's may be difficult to identify, but central obesity, a fatty hump between the shoulders, thinning arms and legs, purple stretch marks on the skin, and a round moon face are common (**Figure 11-13**). Thin, transparent skin, bruising, muscle atrophy, and weakness occur, but these may be associated

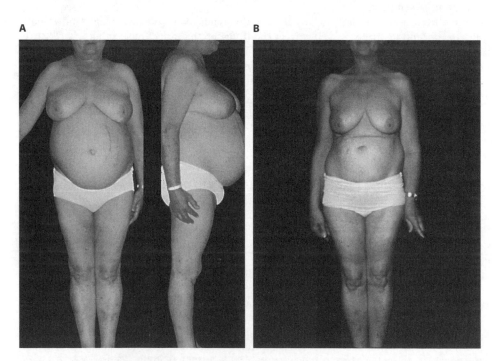

FIGURE 11-13 Older Woman with Cushing's Syndrome

Source: Reproduced from *An Introduction to Human Disease.* 7th ed. Photos courtesy of Leonard V. Crowley, M.D., Century College.

with other conditions. Other signs are slow healing or infection of cuts, wounds from insect bites; depression, anxiety, and irritability; acne; erectile dysfunction; and facial flushing. It can also result in hypertension, bone mass loss, kidney stones, unusual infections, and diabetes mellitus.

The usual cause, as stated previously, is extended use of a steroid medication to manage some illness, such as rheumatoid arthritis or asthma. Other causes, mostly endogenous ones, are difficult to diagnose.

Treatment involves eliminating the excess cortisol by reducing the use of steroids, although they cannot be stopped abruptly. If untreated, Cushing's will eventually lead to death.

Conclusion

In conjunction with the nervous system, the endocrine system synthesizes and regulates hormones that send messages throughout body. In this chapter, we examined some of the most common endocrine diseases in older adults. One of these, diabetes mellitus, is becoming more common as our society becomes more obese. We have examined the main areas of the endocrine system that affect the older adult and have described how nutrition affects it. The hypothalamic–pituitary axis is one of the most important parts of the endocrine system, because it releases and inhibits hormone release to maintain homeostasis. We examined the pituitary gland and its hormones and how they affect plasma osmolality. The thyroid gland and parathyroids regulate the body's metabolic rate, calcium metabolism, and protein, fat, and carbohydrate catabolism. Nutrition plays a very important role in the management of the disorders discussed in this chapter.

Activities Related to This Chapter

1. Review the key terms and concepts introduced in this chapter.
2. Go online and visit www.diabetes.org for the latest in treatments for diabetes mellitus in individuals of all ages.
3. Plan a diet and exercise program for a senior with T2DM.
4. Define the key terms and concepts in this chapter for a colleague and for a lay person.
5. Go online and search for endocrine-related topics.
6. Discuss the issues in this chapter with persons with specific endocrine diagnoses.
7. Relate the manifestations of the disease conditions discussed with the normal aging modifications.

Case Study

Marie is an 86-year-old widow who lives independently. She exercises and eats a healthy diet to maintain her slim, attractive figure. She is active in her church and other social activities. At a regular medical office visit with routine random laboratory studies, Marie's blood sugar was found to be 200, her triglycerides were 190, her total cholesterol 280, and her high density lipoproteins were 55. Her blood pressure was 150/74 mm Hg.

Questions

1. Which of these lab results are abnormal? What are the desirable levels?
2. Is her blood pressure high or low? What blood pressure is desirable?
3. What dietary advice would you provide to Mary?
4. What are your management/treatment goals for Mary?

REFERENCES

American Diabetes Association. Standards of medical care in diabetes—2006. *Diabetes Care.* 2006;29:S4–S42.

American Diabetes Association. Standards of Medical Care in Diabetes—2008. *Diabetes Care.* 2008;31:S12–S54.

American Diabetes Association. Using the diabetes food pyramid. Available at: www.diabetes.org/nutrition-and-recipes/nutrition/foodpyramid.jsp. Accessed May 25, 2007.

American Dietetic Association. Distribution of body fat appears independently associated with the metabolic syndrome. Available at: www.eatright.org/cps/rde/xchg/ada/hs.xsl/nutrition_1115_ENU_HTML.htm. Accessed February 12, 2008.

American Dietetic Association. Metabolic syndrome: what is it and what are the symptoms? Available at: www.eatright.org/cps/rde/xchg/ada/hs.xsl/home_4505_ENU_HTML.htm. Accessed February 12, 2008.

American Geriatric Society. *Geriatric Review Syllabus.* 6th ed. New York: American Geriatric Society; 2006.

American Geriatric Society. *Geriatric Nursing Review Syllabus.* 2nd ed. New York: American Geriatric Society; 2007.

Bedlack R. The management of diabetic neuropathy and glycemic control in long-term facilities. *Clinical Geriatrics and Annals of Long-Term Care.* 2009;17(1:S1):1-16.

Benedict C, Hallschmid M, Hatke A, Schultes B, Fehm HL, et al. Intranasal insulin improves memory in humans. *Psychoneuroendocrinology.* 2004;29(10):1326–1334.

Bliuc D, Nguyen ND, Milch V, Nguyen T, Eisman J, Center J. Mortality risk associated with low-trauma osteoporotic fracture and subsequent fracture in men and women. *JAMA.* 2009 Feb 4;301(5):513-521.

Boehm CM, Smith S. Altering the course: screening for prediabetes. *ADVANCE for Nurse Practitioners.* 2007;15(11):43–46.

Boschert S. Diabetes found in one-third of residents. *Caring for the Ages.* 2008;9(1):23.

Boyle PJ, Stolar MW. Demystifying type 2 diabetes management. *Clinician Reviews.* August 2008 (S).

British Medical Journal Clinical Evidence Handbook, Summer 2007. London: BMJ Publishing; 2007.

Centers for Disease Control and Prevention (CDC). Prevalence of diagnosed diabetes by age, 1980–2006. 2008. Available at: www.cdc.gov/Diabetes/statistics/prev/national/figbyage.htm. Accessed May 1, 2009.

Chernoff R. *Geriatric Nutrition.* Sudbury, MA: Jones & Bartlett; 2006.

del Prato S, Horton E, Nesto R. We have the evidence, we need to act to improve diabetes care. *Int J Clin Prac.* 2007;61(s157):9–15.

Desai SP. *Clinicians Guide to Laboratory Medicine.* 3rd ed. Cleveland, OH: Lexi-Comp; 2004.

Diabetes Educational Forum. Medical nutrition therapy. 2006. Available at: www.caringfordiabetes.com/Treatment-and-Prevention/Type1/Treatment_Type1.cfm. Accessed May 1, 2009.

Dudek S. *Nutrition Essentials for Nursing Practice.* 5th ed. Philadelphia: Lippincott; 2006.

Dunphy L, Brown J. *The Art and Science of Advanced Practice Nursing.* Philadelphia: F.A. Davis and Company; 2001.

Ebersole P, Hess P, Luggen A. *Toward Healthy Aging.* Philadelphia: Mosby; 2004.

Ebersole P, Hess P, Touhy T, Jett K. *Gerontological Nursing and Healthy Aging.* 2nd ed. St. Louis: Elsevier Mosby; 2005.

Eliopoulos C. *Gerontological Nursing.* 6th ed. Philadelphia: Lippincott Williams & Wilkins; 2005.

Evans J. Fractures halved with Vitamin C. *Caring for the Ages.* Jan 2009;10(1):9.

Ford E, Giles W, Dietz W. (2002). Prevalence of the metabolic syndrome among U.S. adults: findings from the third National Health and Nutrition Examination Survey. *JAMA.* 2002;287:356–359.

Gaede P, Lund-Andersen H, Parving H, Pedersen O. Effect of a multifactorial intervention on mortality in type 2 diabetes. *New Engl J Med.* 2003;358(6):580–591.

Gerstein HC, Miller ME, Byington R, Goff D, Bigger JT, Buse JB, et al. Effects of intensive glucose lowering in type 2 diabetes. *N Engl J Med.* 2008;358(24):2545-2559.

Giangregorio L, Papaioannou A, Thabane L, DeBeer J, Cranney A, et al. Do patients perceive a link between a fragility fracture and osteoporosis? *BMC Musculoskeletal Disorders.* 2008;9:38.

Goldstein B, Gomis R, Lee H, Leiter L. Type 2 diabetes—treat early, treat intensively. *Int J Clin Prac.* 2007;61(s157):16–21.

Insel P, Turner RE, Ross D. *Discovering Nutrition.* 2nd ed. Boston: Jones & Bartlett; 2004.

Insel P, Turner RE, Ross D. *Nutrition.* 3rd ed. Boston: Jones & Bartlett; 2007.

Janiszewski PM, Janssen I, Ross R. Does waist circumference predict diabetes and cardiovascular disease beyond commonly evaluated cardiometabolic risk factors? *Diabetes Care.* 2007;30(12):3105–3109

The John A. Hartford Foundation Consortium for Geriatrics in Residency Training. Tools for Geriatric Care. Stanford University Geriatric Education Resource Center; 2003.

Joy SV. Incretin mimetics in clinical practice. Pri-Med Updates, September 29–30, 2006, Cincinnati, Ohio.

Landefeld C, et al. *Current Geriatric Diagnosis and Treatment.* Chicago: Lange Medical Books/McGraw-Hill; 2004.

Leahy J. Insulin: the basics. Pri-Med Updates, September 29–30, 2006, Cincinnati, Ohio.

Lewiecki EM. Denosumab for the treatment of postmenopausal osteoporosis. *Future Medicine.* Jan 2009;5(1):15-22.

Lidow IA, Rawlings NL. Postmenopausal osteoporosis. *ADVANCE for Nurse Practitioners.* 2005;13(9):41–46.

Lutz C, Przytulski K. *Nutrition and Diet Therapy: Evidence-Based Applications.* Philadelphia: F. A. Davis and Company; 2006.

Mangione C, Brown A, Sarkisian C, et al. Guidelines for improving the care of the older person with diabetes mellitus. *J Am Geriatric Soc.* 2003;51:S265–S280.

Mayo Clinic. Addison's disease. 2006. Available at: www.mayoclinic.com/print/addison-disease/DS00361/METHOD = print&DSECTIO. Accessed March 25, 2008.

Mayo Clinic. Cushing's syndrome. 2006. Available at: www.mayoclinic.com/print/cushings-syndrome/DS00470/METHOD = print&DSECT. Accessed March 25, 2008.

Mayo Clinic. Paget's disease. 2006. Available at: www.mayoclinic.com/print/pagets-disease/. Accessed March 25, 2008.

McCance K, Huether S. *Pathophysiology: The Biologic Basis for Disease in Adults and Children.* Philadelphia: C.V. Mosby and Company; 2002.

McKenry L, Salerna E. *Mosby's Pharmacology in Nursing.* 21st ed. St Louis: Mosby; 2003.

McKoy J. Diabetes mellitus and the elderly: a review of the 2003 California Health Care Foundation (CHF)/American Geriatrics Society (AGS) guidelines. 2003. Available at: www.medscape.com/viewarticle/459093. Accessed May 27, 2003.

Merck Manual of Geriatrics. Calcium metabolism. 2008. Available at: www.merck.com/mkgr/CVMHighLight?file = /mkgr/mmg/sec8/ch58/ch58b.jsp%3 Fre. Accessed March 24, 2008.

Murray R, Zentner J. *Health Assessment Promotion Strategies Through the Life Span.* McGraw-Hill, Columbus, OH; 2000.

Nathan DM, Buse JB, Davidson MB, Ferrannini E, Holman RR, et al. Medical management of hyperglycemia in type 2 diabetes: a consensus algorithm for the initiation and adjustment of therapy: a consensus statement of the American Diabetes Association and the European Association for the Study of Diabetes. *Diabetes Care.* 2009 Jan;32(1): 193–203.

National Diabetes Information Clearing House. Hypoglycemia. Available at: http://diabetes.niddk.nih.gov/dm/pubs/hypoglycemia/index.htm. Accessed May 29, 2006.

National Osteoporosis Foundation. National Osteoporosis Foundation's updated recommendations for calcium and vitamin D intake. 2007. Available at: www.nof.org/professionals/NOF_Clinicians_Guide. Accessed March 10, 2008.

National Osteoporosis Foundation. National Osteoporosis Foundation releases new clinical recommendations for low bone mass and osteoporosis incorporating absolute fracture risk. 2008. Available at: www.nof.org/prevention/calciumandvitaminD.htm. Accessed March 10, 2008.

Palomer X, Gonzalez-Clemente J, Blanco-Vaca F, Mauricio D. Role of vitamin D in the pathogenesis of type 2 diabetes mellitus. *Diab Obes Metab.* 2008;10(3):185–197.

Reger M, Watson G, Frey W II, Baker L, Cholerton B, Keeling M, et al. Effects of intranasal insulin on cognition in memory-impaired older adults: modulation by APOE genotype. *Neurobiol Aging.* 2006;27(3):451–458.

Reger M, Watson G, Green P, Wilkinson C, Baker L, et al. Intranasal insulin improves cognition and modulates B-amyloid in early AD. *Neurol.* 2008;70:440–448.

Schneider DL, Barrett-Connor EL, Morton DJ (1994). Thyroid hormone use and bone mineral density in elderly women. Effects of estrogen. *JAMA.* 1994;271(16):1245–1249.

Sierra-Johnson J, Johnson B, Allison T, Bailey K, Schwartz G, Turner S. Correspondence between the Adult Treatment Panel III criteria for metabolic syndrome and insulin resistance. *Diabetes Care.* 2006;29(3):668–672.

Stoneking K. Initiating basal insulin therapy in patients with type 2 diabetes mellitus. *Am J Health-System Pharm.* 2005;62(5):510–518.

Stroup J, Kane M, Abu-Baker AM. Teriparatide in the treatment of osteoporosis. *Am J Health-System Pharm.* 2008;65(6):532–539.

Svec F. Challenges of type 2 diabetes: addressing glycemic targets and the incretin effect. Pri-Med Updates, September 29–30, 2006, Cincinnati, Ohio.

Swartz M. *Textbook of Physical Diagnosis History and Examination.* 4th ed. Philadelphia: W.B. Saunders; 2002.

Sweet M, Sweet J, Jeremiah M, Galazka S. Diagnosis and treatment of osteoporosis. *Am Fam Physician.* 2009 Feb 1;79(3):193-200.

Thyroid.org. Thyroid disease in the older patient. Available at: www.thyroid.org/patients/brochures/ThyroidDisorderOlder_broch.pdf. Accessed May 23, 2006.

Tufts University. Modified food pyramid for older adults, 2007. Available at: http://nutrition.tufts.edu/docs/pdf/modifiedmypyramid.pdf. Accessed May 27, 2007.

Uphold C, Graham M. *Clinical Guidelines in Family Practice.* 4th ed. Gainesville, FL: Barmarrae Books; 2003.

U.S. Department of Agriculture. My Pyramid plan. Available at www.mypyramid.gov. Accessed May 27, 2006.

Wein H. The role of diet in metabolic syndrome. National Institutes of Health Research Matters. February 25, 2008. Available at: www.nih.gov/news/research_matters/ february2008/02252008junkfood.htm. Accessed March 5, 2008.

Yaggi H, Araujo A, McKinlay J. Sleep duration as a risk factor for the development of type 2 diabetes. *Diabetes Care.* 2006;29(3):657–661.

Cancer and Nutrition in Older Adults

Ann Schmidt Luggen, PhD, GNP

CHAPTER OBJECTIVES   Upon completion of this chapter, the reader will be able to:

1. Describe the relationship between nutrition and cancer
2. State the status of current research on the relationship between antioxidants and cancer
3. Identify how ethnicity and race are associated with different cancers
4. Discuss the role of nutrition in cancer risk
5. Provide examples of the relationships among poverty, diet, and cancer
6. State the most common cancers of older adults
7. Describe the role of nutrition in cancer management

KEY TERMS AND CONCEPTS

Alpha-tocopheral

Beta-carotene

Cachexia

Heterocyclic amines

Isoflavones

Omega-3 fatty acids

Palliative care

Postmenopausal

Selenium

Epidemiology

Age is a major risk factor in cancer incidence. However, nutrition, exercise, other lifestyle factors, and environmental exposures have been implicated in cancer causation or increased risk. Heredity explains much of our cancer risk, and, as many as 50% to 75% of cancer deaths in the United States are caused by personal choices and behaviors such as smoking, physical inactivity, and poor diet.

The lifetime risk of developing cancer in the United States is one out of every two men and one of every three women. Although anyone can develop cancer, about 76% of cancers occur in people aged 55 and older. The most common cancers in older adults are those affecting the prostate, breast, lung and bronchus, colon, and rectum (**Table 12-1**).

Survival

Death rates from those cancers common in older adults have been declining in the United States, which indicates that more older adults are living with cancer. Nearly 65% of Americans with cancer now live longer than five years (**Table 12-2**). Increased longevity has meaningful implications for care. Globally, cancer incidence is increasing and is surpassing heart disease as the number one cause of death. Cancer is expected to double by 2010 and triple by 2030.

Prevention

In recent years, researchers have implicated some nutrition problems as increasing an individual's risk for developing cancer. One important nutrition problem is overweight and

TABLE 12-1 Probability of Developing Invasive Cancers by Older Age (70+) and Sex

Cancer Site	Men	Women
All	1:3	1:4
Prostate	1:8	—
Breast	—	1:16
Lung and bronchus	1:18	1:21
Colon and rectum	1:22	1:24

Source: Data from American Cancer Society. *Cancer Facts and Figures 2009.* Atlanta: American Cancer Society; 2009.

TABLE 12-2 Five-Year Survival Rates for Cancers of Older Adults (All Stages)

Cancer	Survival rate %
Prostate	99.0%
Breast	89
Lung and bronchus	16
Colon	65
Pancreas	5

Source: Data from American Cancer Society. *Cancer Facts and Figures 2009.* Atlanta: American Cancer Society; 2009.

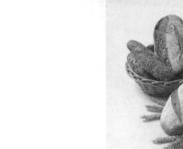

obesity. Some of the cancers that have increased risk due to excess body weight include: breast (in **postmenopausal** women), colorectal, esophageal, liver, gallbladder, pancreatic, kidney, uterine, and advanced prostate cancer. However, there is more need for research in this area.

Fruit and Vegetable Consumption

Limited fruit and vegetable consumption is a cancer risk. People who consume a diet rich in fruits and vegetables have a lower risk for cancers of the mouth, pharynx, larynx, esophagus, stomach, and lung. Some evidence suggests that this diet also might lower a person's risk for colon, pancreatic, and prostate cancer.

A diet high in plant foods helps reduce caloric intake and may help in weight control. Intake of fruits and vegetables has remained stable since 1993. In 2003–2004, the average American consumed 2.6 cups of fruits and vegetables per day. African Americans consumed slightly less than this average; Hispanics slightly more. Fruit consumption is highest among the youngest and oldest population groups. Both fruit and vegetable consumption increases with age, education, and income. See **Box 12-1**.

Healthy People 2010 suggests a minimum of five daily servings of fruits and

postmenopausal After the female menopause, after cessation of menses.

vegetables (two fruits, three vegetables [one to three dark-green/orange]). The 2005 Dietary Guidelines for Americans recommends higher intakes. Fruits and vegetables could replace the "empty calories" in many American's diets. Empty calories include those from sugars, such as honey and syrup, that are added to foods; soft drinks; and solid fats, such as butter and sour cream.

Access to nutrient-dense foods can be problematic for low-income populations, especially those in urban areas. A study that examined the relationship between food store access and household fruit and vegetable use among participants in the U.S. Food Stamp Program found that easy access to supermarket shopping was associated with increased purchase of fruits. Distance from home to the store was inversely associated with fruit use. A similar pattern was seen for vegetable purchase, but it was not statistically significant.

◗ BOX 12-1 American Cancer Society Nutrition Guidelines

Eat a variety of healthy foods with an emphasis on plant sources.

Eat five or more servings of a variety of vegetables and fruits every day:

- Have vegetables and fruits at each meal and for snacks.
- Eat a variety of the vegetables: dark green, orange, legumes, starchy vegetables.
- Limit snack potato and other chips, French fries, and other fried vegetables.
- Choose juices that are 100% juice.

Eat whole grains rather than refined (processed) grains and sugars. One-half of grain intake should be whole grains.

- Eat whole-grain cereals, breads, pastas, and rice.
- Limit consumption of refined carbohydrates such as pastries, soft drinks, and sweetened cereals.

Limit consumption of red meats, especially those high in fat, and processed meats.

- Choose poultry, fish, and beans rather than beef, pork, and lamb.
- When eating meats, choose lean cuts and small portions.
- Prepare meats by oven broiling, baking, or poaching, rather than frying or charcoal broiling.

Consume 3 cups a day of fat free or low fat milk or equivalent milk products.

Limit exposure to the aflatoxins in foods. Aflatoxins can be found in peanuts, tree nuts (pecans, walnuts, etc.), corn, wheat, and oil seeds (such as cottonseed oil).

Limit or avoid salt and salt-preserved foods.

- Avoid Chinese-style fermented salted fish.
- Avoid preserved meats.

Avoid very hot (thermally/temperature) drinks, for example, hot coffee or tea. Avoid foods that are very hot in temperature.

Choose foods to help maintain a healthy weight.

- When eating out of the home, choose foods that are low in fat, calories, and sugars.
- Eat small portions of high-calorie foods. The terms "low fat" and "fat free" do not mean "low calorie." Low-fat cakes and cookies are often high in calories.
- Substitute low-calorie foods, such as vegetables and fruits, for high-caloric foods, such as French fries, pizza, ice cream, doughnuts, and other sweets.

Maintain a healthy weight throughout life.

- Stay or become physically active.
- Balance calorie intake with physical activity.
- When drinking alcohol, limit consumption to one drink/day for women and two drinks/day for men.

Source: Data from American Cancer Society. *Cancer Facts and Figures 2009.* Atlanta: American Cancer Society; 2009.

Many fruits and vegetables contain **isoflavones** (also called phytoestrogens or phytochemicals). In studies by Lampe and colleagues and Fink and colleagues, isoflavone consumption has been found to be inversely associated with breast cancer and with fibrocystic breast conditions. More recent research finds that there is no association between flavonoid-rich foods and cancers.

The combination of tomato and broccoli has been found to enhance antitumor activity in prostate adenocarcinomas. Research has found that the benefits from the combination of these two vegetables is greater than either one alone. This information reinforces national recommendations for a diet consisting of five to ten servings of fruits and vegetables daily.

A study by Chao in 2007 of the association between beer, wine, and liquors and lung cancer found that in men consumption of one beer per day was associated with increased risk for lung cancer, but the same was not true of women. There was an inverse relationship between wine consumption (one or more glass per day) and lung cancer risk for men and women. Liquor consumption increased the risk of lung cancer in men, but not women. Further research examining the consumption of alcoholic beverages is needed.

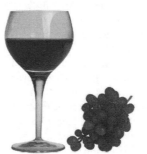

Isoflavones Plant chemicals that include genistein and daidzein and may have positive effects against cancer and heart disease. Also called *phytoestrogens*.

Weight

Increased weight, as mentioned earlier, is a risk factor for a number of cancers that are common in older adults (see Chapter 14 on weight problems of older adults). For example, a number of studies have suggested that obesity increases the risk of colorectal cancer by 30% to 60%, such as the study by Moghaddam and colleagues. Further, in the United States, overweight and obesity contribute from 14% to 20% of all cancer-related deaths. They increase the risk for cancer of the breast in postmenopausal women, colon, endometrium, kidney, and adenocarcinoma of the esophagus. There is evidence that obesity increases the risk for cancer of the pancreas, gallbladder, thyroid, ovary, cervix, myeloma, Hodgkin lymphoma, and the aggressive type of prostate cancer.

Ovarian cancer, most common in women older than 55, has no screening recommendations from the major relevant professional organizations. Further, when it is diagnosed, the cancer is in its late stages. However, subtle signs and symptoms are often present to the listening health professional: abdominal or pelvic pain, bloating, increase in abdominal size, difficulty eating or feeling full quickly (occurring more than 12 times in a month), urinary frequency or urgency. The presence of these factors is sensitive and specific.

Some tips for preventing overweight and obesity include walking daily; limiting food portions; eating more plant-based foods; choosing lean meats and poultry without skin; eating low-fat dairy products; reducing the use of butter, mayonnaise, and sweets; cooking by broiling or steaming rather than frying; limiting high-calorie snacks; starting activities that help relieve stress; and meeting with a registered dietitian for guidance.

Low-Fat Diet

Additional research by the WHI suggests that women who consume a low-fat diet may have a decreased risk of invasive ovarian cancer. Ovarian cancer is the seventh most common cancer in women and the fifth leading cause of cancer death. During the more than eight years of the WHI Dietary Study's Intervention phase, there were fewer new cases of ovarian cancer among the dietary change participants than among the "usual diet" participants. Though it can take years to see the effect of a preventive intervention on cancer risk, after four years researchers saw a 40% risk reduction among the low-fat diet participants.

WHI researchers have also examined the relationship between low fat intake and breast cancer incidence. A low-fat diet was not found to have a statistically significant impact on the development of breast cancer. However, a low-fat diet did reduce blood estradiol (estrogen) by 15%, and estrogen has been demonstrated to be a risk factor for breast cancer. In another arm of the WHI study, women who had a prior hysterectomy and took estrogen did not have a higher incidence of breast cancer than those who did not take estrogen. Women who stop taking estrogen and progesterone have a marked decrease in risk for breast cancer.

A low-fat diet did not reduce the risk of colorectal cancer in the WHI participants. The researchers concluded that a low-fat diet that includes vegetables and grains does not reduce the risk for colorectal cancer, but it did cause a diminution of polyps, which often become cancerous over time.

Trans-Fatty Acids

A number of studies, such as that by Chavarro et al., have suggested a positive association between markers of trans-fatty acid (TFA) intake and prostate cancer. However, in a study of nearly 15,000 healthy men researchers found no association between TFA and aggressive prostate cancer. However, blood levels of trans isomers of oleic and linoleic acids were found to be associated with increased risk of nonaggressive prostate tumors. Many or most prostate cancers fall into this category and can be determined by use of the prostate-specific antigen (PSA) screen in clinical practice.

Eating foods high in saturated fats, such as red and processed meats, may be a risk factor for cancer of the small intestine. This conclusion by the National Cancer Institute included 500,000 men and women who provided eating habits for 8 years. This type of cancer has been increasing in recent years.

Cholesterol-Lowering Drugs

Statins are the most commonly used drug class to lower cholesterol in the United States. A study of more than 55,000 men in the Cancer Prevention Study II Nutrition Cohort found that use of statins for five or more years was not associated with overall prostate cancer incidence. However, it was associated with a significant reduction in the risk of advanced prostate cancer.

A study from the National Cancer Institute studied a population of veterans, believing that earlier studies examined young men who were not likely to develop cancers. In this study, there was a statistically significant benefit in that older men taking statins had a decreased risk of developing cancer of any type.

Folate and Cobalamin

Studies of folate and cobalamin and their association with gastric cancer risk have shown inconsistent results. The European Prospective Investigation into Cancer and Nutrition study found no relationship between folate and gastric cancer. However, it did find that higher cobalamin levels reduced the risk of gastric cancer. Researchers postulate that low cobalamin levels are related to atrophic gastritis. Up to 30% of older adults have atrophic gastritis, which decreases the bioavailability of cobalamin (vitamin B12). For these older adults, dietary supplements and fortified foods are important.

However, a recent finding from the Women's Health Initiative found that taking multivitamin supplements did not diminish either the risk of any cancer, nor the risk of death from cancers.

Fiber

High-fiber diets continue to be recommended for prevention of colon cancer despite the lack of any evidence in clinical research trials since the theory was first proposed in the early 1970s. Two recent prospective trials—the Wheat Bran Fiber Trial and the Polyp Prevention Trial were conducted with follow-up colonoscopies two to four years after being assigned to the fiber diet or placebo. Separately, the two trials found no positive effects for fiber in the diet. Together, with pooled data, high-fiber diets were found to be moderately protective against recurrent adenomas (the polyps) in men, but not in women. It was especially protective in men who had very high fiber diets.

Omega-3 Fatty Acids

Early research on animals suggested that **omega-3 fatty acids** reduce the incidence, growth rate, and proliferation of a number of cancers. At this stage of research, however, it is not clear that the lower incidence in cancers might be due to omega-6 fatty acid intake. Multiple research studies examined the relationship between omega-3 fatty acid intake and cancer and found that omega-3 fatty acids decreased the risk of cancer. Just as many studies found an increased risk of cancer. Not enough evidence exists to suggest a significant association between omega-3 fatty acids and cancer incidence. Further, the evidence does not support the use of omega-3 fatty acid supplements as a cancer-prevention measure. Further study is needed in this area. It is known that excess omega-6 fatty acid intake relative to omega-3 promotes some cancers such as breast and prostate.

Carotenes

Carotenes are a type of antioxidant. Oxidative damage is higher in older adults, so theoretically, antioxidants would be helpful in counteracting this. Antioxidants are linked to lower mortality in older adults, including mortality from cancer and heart disease. In one study by Key et al., researchers found that consumption of beta-carotene and alpha-carotene, together, were directly associated with a lower risk of cancer (**Box 12-2**). However, the lead author of the study noted that carotenes may need to be taken with other antioxidants to have this protective effect. An important supposition by the researchers is that **beta-carotene** may act as both an oxidant and an antioxidant when consumed in high doses.

The relationship between beta-carotene and other antioxidants and cancer has been the topic of a great deal

of research. Five large-scale clinical trials published in the 1990s reached differing conclusions about the effect of antioxidants on cancer risk in different population groups. The AHRQ (Agency for Healthcare Research and Quality) summarized evidence from randomized controlled trials of vitamins for cancer prevention. Beta-carotene supplementation was found to increase the incidence of cancer in smokers, but not in nonsmokers—an important finding. However,

---

BOX 12-2 Vitamin A/Carotene

Ingested vitamin A is a "preformed" version that is converted by the body into the vitamin A. Retinol is the preformed version of vitamin A that is found in foods from animals, for example, eggs, milk, and liver. It is easily converted to vitamin A. Beta carotene is the preformed version of vitamin A in foods from plants, but only a small amount of ingested beta carotene is converted to vitamin A.

Research suggests that too much retinol is linked to weak bones and hip fractures, already a serious problem of older adults. The increase in risk begins at about 1,500 µg/day. Many of the vitamin supplements taken in older adults contain retinol, beta carotene, or both. Some vitamin manufacturers have replaced the retinol in vitamin supplements with beta carotene after publication of this research.

Plasma carotenoids, retinol, and tocopherols have been implicated as risk factors for prostate cancer. However, the European Prospective Investigation into Cancer and Nutrition Study has found no association with prostate cancer risk.

Beta carotene is the best way of obtaining vitamin A. Foods rich in this preformed version of vitamin A include leafy, dark green vegetables, such as kale and spinach, and in orange-colored foods, such as pumpkin, squash, apricots, and cantaloupe.

Source: Key TJ et al. Plasma carotenoids, retinol and tocopherols and the risk of prostate cancer in the European Prospective Investigation into Cancer and Nutrition study. *Am J Clin Nutr.* 2007 Sep; 86(3): 672–681.

---

omega-3 fatty acids Any polyunsaturated fatty acid in which the first double bond starting from the methyl (CH_3) end of the molecule lies between the third and fourth carbon atoms.

beta-carotene Yellow carotenoid in vegetables and fruits that contain vitamin A.

this study examined beta-carotene levels that were considerably higher than average dietary intake.

The report also summarized a study by Ritenbaugh et al., who examined the use of beta-carotene plus retinol as prevention for lung cancer. After four years, there were statistically significant *increases* in lung cancer. In another study comparing retinol with beta-carotene for prevention of lung cancer, the incidence of lung cancer was not any lower in the retinol group. In the Vitamins and Lifestyle (VITAL) study, long-term use of individual B-carotene, retinol, and lutein supplements were linked to increased lung cancer risk.

The Chinese Cancer Prevention Study looked at beta-carotene, vitamin E (**alpha-tocopherol**, which is found in almonds, wheat germ, safflower, corn and soybean oils, broccoli, and mangos), **selenium** (a mineral micronutrient containing antioxidant enzymes found in rice and wheat), and development of cancer in healthy Chinese men and women who are at high risk for gastric cancers. This study found that all three of these nutrients significantly reduced the incidence of gastric cancer and all cancers.

A Finnish study found that lung cancer rates in Finnish male smokers *increased* significantly with beta-carotene, but were not affected by vitamin E. A second study, the CARET (Beta-Carotene and Retinol Efficacy Trial) examined beta-carotene and retinol (vitamin A; retinol is vitamin A1; vitamin A2 is 3,4-didehydroretinol; and vitamin A3 is 3-hydroxy-retinol). Foods rich in vitamin A include sweet potatoes, carrots, milk, egg yolks, mozzarella cheese, and liver. The CARET study found a possible increase in lung cancer with these antioxidants.

A second Chinese study, this one by Kamangar and colleagues, examined the effect of supplementation with four different combinations of vitamins and minerals in the prevention of lung cancer in nearly 30,000 healthy adults. The study lasted 5.25 years, but subjects were followed for 10 years. No differences in lung cancer death rates were found for any combination of the supplements tested (retinol and zinc, riboflavin and niacin, ascorbic acid and molybdenum, B-carotene and alpha-tocopherol and selenium) versus placebo.

In the United States, the Physician's Health Study (PHS) found no change in cancer incidence associated with beta-carotene and aspirin in male physicians. There was no impact of beta-carotene on lung cancer incidence in an average-risk population with a low prevalence of smokers.

The Women's Health Study (WHS) found no benefit (or harm) for lung cancer prevention from beta-carotene supplementation

alpha-tocopheral A potent form of vitamin E found in germ oils or via synthesis.

selenium A member of the family of antioxidant enzymes. Prevents membrane damage. Also involved in the metabolism of iodine and thyroid hormone.

This arm of the WHS was discontinued due to the lack of benefit of beta-carotene and the possibility of adverse effects.

Vitamin D

Epidemiological research on geographic location as a risk factor for prostate cancer suggests that decreased production of vitamin D increases prostate cancer risk. Both in vitro and in vivo studies (in test tubes or cultures versus in real-life animal or human clinical studies) show that the active form of vitamin D (1a,25-dihydroxyvitamin D3) inhibits the proliferation of cancer cells in the prostate. Data from the NHANES III study has found that vitamin D levels in men have been falling in recent years.

A recent study by Autier, et al. in 2007 found that taking ordinary doses of vitamin D supplements decreased mortality in prostate cancer patients. Interestingly, a study by Oregon Health and Science University found that men from Norway who were diagnosed in summer and/or autumn months, when vitamin D production is highest, were more likely to survive prostate cancer. Men diagnosed in summer and fall had a 20% lower risk of dying from prostate cancer within three years of diagnosis. The research suggests that high-dose activated vitamin D (calcitriol) combined with chemotherapy may increases survival in men with prostate cancer.

A study that included the Nurses' Health Study (NHS), the Health Professionals Follow-Up Study (HPFS), and the Physicians' Health Study (PHS), found that there was an inverse association of vitamin D and colorectal cancer in the NHS and HPFS cohorts. In the NHS, there was a 30% risk reduction for breast cancer. In all men and women there was a lower risk for pancreatic cancer. The study did not find any role for vitamin D in middle-aged or elderly men for prostate cancer risk. Further, the study revealed that poor vitamin D status in African-Americans contributed to higher incidence and mortality from malignancies.

Aspirin and Vitamin E

The WHI's major trial of nearly 40,000 women 45 years and older also examined the impact of low-dose aspirin (100 mg/day) and vitamin E (600 IU) to determine if they were protective against cancer (and cardiovascular disease). Aspirin was not found to be protective for cancer breast, colorectal, and other site-specific cancers. They did find that it was somewhat protective against lung cancer, but believe that further study needs to be conducted on this dose and higher doses. Vitamin E supplements were not found to be protective against cancer (or cardiovascular disease).

Another study testing aspirin in women, this one by van Dyke, et al., found that use of adult-strength aspirin resulted in a significant reduction in the risk of lung cancer (non-small-cell lung cancer) in White women aged 55 to 64 years. In women aged 65 to 74 years, baby aspirin and NSAIDs (nonsteroidal anti-inflammatory drugs, such as ibuprofen) use was associated with a significant reduction in risk. It should be noted, however, that NSAIDs carry a significant risk of GI bleeding in older adults when used on a regular basis.

A report from the American Cancer Society states that aspirin and other anti-inflammatory drugs have been found to be protective against colon cancer. Hormones such as estrogen and progestin were also found to be protective, but none of these are recommended for prevention because they all have adverse effects as well.

A review from the SELECT (Selenium and Vitamin E Cancer Prevention Trial) Study showed that selenium and vitamin E supplements, together or alone, did not prevent prostate cancer. There was a small increased trend in prostate cancer in men older than 50 in those taking only vitamin E.

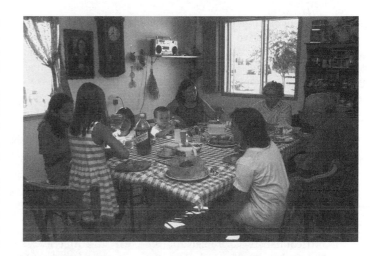

Multivitamin Use

People of every age take multivitamins, and many believe that more is better. A cohort of the WHI who followed subjects for nearly eight years showed convincing evidence that multivitamin use has little or no influence on risk for common cancers or total mortality in postmenopausal women.

Coffee

A study of more than 80,000 women in the Nurses' Health Study (NHS) looked at the relationship between coffee consumption and ovarian cancer. The researchers found an inverse relationship between caffeine intake and ovarian cancer risk (that is, higher amounts of coffee reduced risk of ovarian cancer). The study also examined alcohol consumption. The findings indicated that alcohol consumption was not related to the risk for ovarian cancer.

Meat Mutagens

Meats cooked at high temperatures, such as with grilling or pan-frying, have long been thought to be a source of carcinogens. Cooking meat at high temperatures causes the formation of **heterocyclic amines (HCAs)**, which are carcinogens found in cooked muscle meats, such as those from beef, pork, fowl, and fish.

One study by Koutros and colleagues found that meats that were well done or very well done were associated with increased risk for prostate cancer. A similar study by Stolzenberg-Solomon and colleagues examined more than 500,000 subjects, and looked for an association between meats cooked at high temperatures and pancreatic cancer. The researchers found that red meat intake, and particularly meat cooked at high temperatures, may play a role in the development of pancreatic cancer in men, but not women.

A study from the National Cancer Institute's Division of Cancer Epidemiology and Genetics reports a link between stomach cancer and the consumption of medium-well-done and well-done meats. The incidence of stomach cancer was three times greater among those who ate medium-well and well-done meats compared to those who ate rare or medium-rare meats. The researchers also found that those who eat beef four or more times per week had more than twice the risk of stomach cancer compared to those who ate meat less frequently. A number of other studies have found an increased risk for colorectal, pancreatic, and breast cancer with high intake of well-done, fried, or barbequed meats.

Researchers have determined that carcinogens are not a problem with meats from fast-food restaurants, because the cooking time is slow. However, it is a much more significant problem in home cooking and in non-fast-food restaurants.

Coffee has been found to be protective against some breast cancers. Drinking two to three cups per day can either reduce the total risk of developing certain types of breast cancer or slow the onset. The onset of cancer was delayed until older age and these cancers are more benign and easily treated than those in younger women.

Ethnicity, Culture, and Cancers

American and Alaskan Natives

The federal government recognizes over 100 Native American tribes, each with its own culture. American and Alaskan natives are among the poorest population groups in the United States. Native Americans speak 217 native languages, and most of these languages do not have a word for "cancer."

Cancer rates among Native Americans and Alaskan Natives have been increasing in the past 20 years, and cancer is the second leading

heterocyclic amines
Carcinogens found in cooked muscle meats such as those from beef, pork, fowl, and fish.

cause of death in those over the age of 45. However, the diversity of Native Americans and Alaskan Natives makes generalizations difficult. The incidence and mortality from kidney and renal pelvis cancers are higher than any other group. Liver and bile duct cancers are higher (as is mortality) in women than any group except for Asian Americans and Pacific Islanders. Mortality (but not incidence) from uterine cervix cancer is higher in women except for African American women. The Northern Plains tribes have a greater incidence of lung, cervical, breast, and prostate cancers; and the Southwestern tribes have mainly stomach and gallbladder cancers. However, in those residing in Indian Health Service (IHS) Contract Health Service Delivery Areas, cancer mortality rates during 2001 to 2005 were stable. Data for trends of cancer is not available at this time.

Health care is problematic for the Native Americans. This group is second only to Hispanics in lacking health insurance. Fewer than 90 physicians are available for every 100,000 Native Americans (the national average is 229 physicians per 100,000 people). Native American women with breast cancer are likely to receive their first cancer-directed surgery more than six months after diagnosis.

African Americans

There are more than 35 million African Americans, comprising 13% of the U.S. population. Most African Americans live in the southern United States (55%); 19% live in the Northeast; 18% live in the Midwest; and 8% in the West. The term *African American* is applied to very diverse peoples, including those from the West Indies, other Caribbean areas, Nigeria, Ethiopia, and South Africa.

Cancer is the second leading cause of death in African Americans. Of all cultural and ethnic groups, the incidence and mortality from cancer is highest in African American men. African American women are second in incidence only to White women and their mortality is highest of all women groups. One problem in this population is that cancers are diagnosed in later stages, often after metastasis, than it is in other groups.

Lung cancer accounts for the most cancer deaths in African American men. African American women are second only to White women. The incidence and deaths from prostate cancer are higher than any group. Colorectal cancers rank third in African American men and women and are higher than any group. Cancer survival is lower compared to Whites in the United States. Kidney cancer is highest in African American men and deaths from stomach cancer is highest in men and second highest in African American women, after Asian Americans and Pacific Islanders.

Obesity has been a problem among African American women for decades. In the 1960s, approximately 42% of African American women were overweight, jumping to 64% in the late 1990s.

Recent data shows that African American youth are less likely to eat fruits and vegetables and more likely to eat high-fat foods compared to White youths. Nearly 31% of African Americans have incomes below the poverty level.

Asian Americans

Asian Americans are also a very diverse people and include Asian Indian, Korean, Pakistani, Vietnamese, Japanese, Filipino, Chinese, Malayan, Thai, and many more ethnic groups and cultures. In the United States, the majority of Asian Americans are Chinese (23.8%), followed by Filipinos (20.4%), Japanese (12.3%), Asian Indian (11.8%), Korean (11.6%), and Vietnamese (8.9%).

Cancer is the number one cause of death of Asian American women. Many Asian American women do not have or seek access to the health care system. Some use herbal remedies to manage illness. For example, 22% of Chinese women with breast cancer use herbal remedies. Cervical cancer is a problem among Asian American women, and it is the most common cancer in Vietnamese women in the United States. Many have never had, nor heard of, the Pap smear test.

Liver cancer in Asian Americans is more than twice as high as in Whites. It is more common in men and women in this group than any other ethnic, cultural, or racial group. The mortality from liver cancer is also higher than any group. Vietnamese men have the highest rate of liver cancer of all racial and ethnic groups. Korean men have the highest rate of stomach cancers of all groups, and five times that of Whites. Asian Americans (men and women) have the highest incidence of stomach cancer of any group; mortality is highest in women and second highest in men after African American men.

The poverty rate among Asian Americans is much higher than the national average. In 1990, 64% of Hmong people, 43% of Cambodians, and 35% of Laotians lived in poverty, compared to the U.S. poverty rate of 20%. As a consequence, they have had no or little access to medical services.

Native Hawaiians and Pacific Islanders

Native Hawaiians and Pacific Islanders comprise a very small percentage of the U.S. population (0.1%). They are very diverse, with many groups having different languages and histories. Most live in California and Hawaii. Native Hawaiians are 19% of Hawaii's population (fewer than 5,000). The income of Hawaiian Americans and Pacific Islanders is 27% below the national average. They are underserved in terms of access to health care and social services.

In Hawaii, Native Hawaiians have the second highest incidence of cancers and of cancer-related mortality compared to all other groups. The cancer mortality rate for Hawaiian Native women is 2.6 times higher than the general state population. The incidence of breast cancer in this group is second among all U.S. women and it has the third highest death rate from breast cancer. They have the highest incidence of and death from endometrial cancer than any other group of women in the United States. Cancer-related mortality rates for this group have increased 123% for all cancers from 1976 to 1990, especially colon cancer (134%), liver (135%), lung (293%), breast (158%), and uterine (313%).

In Hawaiian men, mortality rates have increased 62% for all cancers from 1976 to 1990. Most of the increases have been in colon (228%), rectal (117%), pancreatic (83%), lung (74%), and prostate (117%).

Pacific Islanders have significant health-related high-risk behaviors. Smoking, high alcohol intake, and obesity are problems. Diets are high in calories, cholesterol, saturated fats, and salt. American Samoan men who live in Hawaii are similar in incidence of cancers to Native Hawaiian men. Samoan women differ from other groups in that the most common site-specific cancers are the breast, uterus, blood, cervix, and thyroid.

Seventh-Day Adventists

The Seventh-day Adventist church is a Protestant religious group. Seventh-day Adventists in the United States, which include a large number of African Americans, are known to have a very low incidence of cancer. Church members' vegetarian dietary habits (including a high soy intake, comparable to that used in China), the absence of alcohol and tobacco use, and their willingness to participate in research helps researchers delineate more clearly the association of diet and cancer.

In 2005, the General Council of Seventh-Day Adventist Nutrition Council adopted the U.S. Department of Agriculture's Pyramid for Vegetarian Diet. It allows no fish, fowl, or meat, but accepts three egg yolks per week. Dieters abstain from tobacco, alcohol, coffee, tea, and other caffeinated beverages. It advocates nine servings of fruits and vegetables and six or more servings of whole grain combinations, cereals, and legumes.

Common Cancers and Dietary Recommendations

The following four sections are briefs on cancers most common in older adults and specific dietary and lifestyle recommendations for reducing the risk of these cancers. Many of these guidelines are similar to recommendations for reducing heart disease and other chronic problems of older adults. In general, limited fruit and vegetable consumption is a cancer risk. People who consume diets rich in fruits and vegetables have a lower risk for cancers of the mouth, pharynx, larynx, esophagus, stomach, lung, and perhaps colon, pancreas, and prostate.

Among older adults, increased weight and obesity can significantly increase the risk of certain cancers, including those of the breast, colon, rectum, esophagus, liver, gallbladder, pancreas, kidney, uterus, and prostate. A study at Harvard, the Nurses' Health Study, and the Health Professionals Follow-up Study are evaluating the impact of changes in eating patterns and diet quality over time on the risk of breast cancer and colorectal cancer.

The probability of one developing a cancer is great. Men have a one in two chance to develop a cancer in their lifetime. Women have one in three chances. The most probable cancer to develop in men is prostate cancer, and a man has a one in six chance. Women have a one in eight chance to develop breast cancer. Those are the most common cancers and these and other cancers are most likely to develop at age 70 or older.

Prostate Cancer

Prostate cancer is the most diagnosed cancer in men. More than 65% of cases of prostate cancer occur in men older than 65 years. African American men and Jamaican men of African descent have the highest incidence of prostate cancer in the world. It is rare in Asia and South America and common in North America and northwestern Europe.

Risk factors for prostate cancer include age (older), race (African American), geographic area (northern, non-sun areas), and family history of the disease. Some data suggests that obesity is actually a protective factor.

Experts recommend limiting the intake of red meat and full-fat dairy products and eating at least five servings of fruits and vegetables daily. It is not clear which specific fruits and vegetables are the most beneficial; more clinical research is needed in this area. However, some research suggests that diets high in tomatoes, dried peas, and beans may lower prostate cancer risk. At present, vitamin D is not recommended for protection against prostate cancer.

The early stages of prostate cancer are usually asymptomatic. Diagnosis has increased because of the PSA test, which measures prostate-specific antigen, a protein made in the prostate.

Breast Cancer

Since the advent of mammography in the 1980s, more breast cancers have been diagnosed earlier and treated longer. Although it is the second highest cause of cancer deaths in women after lung cancer, mortality rates are declining. Age is a major risk factor (43% of cases occur in older women) as is a lengthy menstrual history, overweight or obesity after menopause, use of oral contraceptives and postmenopausal hormone therapy, nulliparity, lack of physical activity, and drinking alcohol to excess. Older women who smoke or have smoked for many years appear to be at very high risk for breast cancer.

A disparity of incidence and mortality is present between African American women and White women. The incidence of breast cancer is highest in White women of all ethnic and cultural groups, followed by African American women. However, African American women have a mortality rate that is the highest of all groups; it is nearly double other groups, with the exception of White women. African American women are less likely to have screening mammograms and are more likely to have breast cancer diagnosed at later stages. However, there is little difference in time of diagnosis among African American and White women who receive regular mammograms.

Survival is 88% at five years and 80% at ten years. Mortality from breast cancer increases with age in both African American and White women. However, African American women are more likely to die from breast cancer at an earlier age than White women. This disparity is thought to be due to differing responses to new medical interventions or differential access to them. Being overweight adversely affects survival for postmenopausal women.

Treatment for breast cancer may include lumpectomy (local tumor removal) or mastectomy (surgical removal of the breast). Women may have radiation therapy, chemotherapy, and/or hormone therapy; often two or more of these methods are used.

Women at risk for breast cancer should exercise at least four hours each week as part of their effort toward weight control. Further, because of a diminished metabolic rate and limited exercise in many older adults, limiting food intake is recommended.

High folate intake has been linked to lower risk of breast cancer (and colon cancer). Enriched cereal grains are fortified with folic acid (the synthetic form of natural folate; folic acid is absorbed twice as readily as folate). The average intake of folate in the United States is 200 mcg. A cancer protective dose would be 400 mcg or greater. Many over-the-counter dosages are 400 mcg.

Literature has demonstrated the importance of limiting alcohol intake to no more than one drink, and preferably less, per day. A study reported at the American Society of Clinical Oncology (ASCO) meeting in 2005 revealed that the relationship of alcohol to breast cancer occurred in postmenopausal (older) women, but not premenopausal women. Further, even very modest amounts of alcohol in older women demonstrated an association, especially in estrogen-receptor + and progesterone + breast cancers. However, a prospective study by Baglietto, et al., in Australia of more than 17,000 women aged 40 to 69 years over a 13-year period examining the relationship of folate on alcohol and breast cancer found that an adequate dietary intake of folate (200 mcg/day) could protect against the known increased risk of breast cancer with alcohol consumption. One caveat is that it has been clearly demonstrated that moderate alcohol intake is useful in management of heart disease. Heart disease is the number one cause of mortality; therefore, drinking alcohol must be weighed carefully

Lung and Bronchus Cancers

The incidence of lung and bronchus cancers is declining. There had been a significant increase in women, but this has now stabilized and is decreasing. However, lung cancer is still the leading cause of cancer deaths (30% in men and 26% in women). Estimates of new lung cancer cases in 2009 are 15% of all cancers for men, and 14% of all cancers for women. This is less than 25% for new prostate cases and 27% of new breast cancers.

Symptoms of lung and bronchus cancers are persistent cough, sputum with blood streaks, chest pain, voice change, and recurrent pneumonias or bronchitis. It is well known that cigarette smoking is the most important risk factor, closely followed by exposure to secondhand smoke. Tuberculosis is also a risk factor, as are numerous occupational environmental exposures, such as air pollution, radon, asbestos, and benzene. There is a genetic susceptibility, but in these cases lung cancer usually occurs in younger persons.

No early detection method is currently readily available. Treatment includes surgery, radiation therapy, chemotherapy, and biological therapies. If the tumor is localized, surgery is the treatment of choice. If it has metastasized, treatment involves chemotherapy and/or radiation. Some patients have long remissions; the one-year survival rate is 42% and the five-year survival rate is 15%.

Diets high in phytochemicals have been shown to decrease the risk of lung and bronchus cancers. One study by Schabath et al., that examined the relationship between dietary intake of phytochemicals and the risk of lung cancer found benefits, even in smokers, although the benefits were less in former smokers. Foods high in phytochemicals include soy, spinach, carrots, and broccoli.

Researchers have found a statistically significant joint effect between hormone therapy use and phytochemical intake in women. High intake of lignans enterolactone and enterodiol and the use of hormone therapy were associated with a 50% reduction in the risk of lung cancer. However, women appear to benefit from phytochemicals from food sources only. In men, decreased risk was associated with phytosterols (24%) and isoflavones (44%).

It is recommended that smokers try to stop smoking. The American Cancer Society recommends eating at least five servings of fruits and vegetables every day.

Colon and Rectum

Colon and rectum cancers are the second most common causes of cancer deaths in men ages 40–59 and 60–79. They are the third most common causes in men aged 80 or older, after lung and prostate cancers. In women, they are the third most common causes of cancer death in those ages 40–59 and 60–79, after breast and lung cancers. They are the second most common causes in women 80 and older, after lung cancer. Nine percent of all cancer deaths are from colorectal cancers. Because of increased screening for polyps, there has been a decline in incidence and deaths from these cancers. The primary risk factor for colorectal cancers is age—90% of people diagnosed are older than 50 years. The risk grows with a family history of this cancer and/or polyps. Other risk factors include obesity; smoking; heavy alcohol use; physical inactivity; diets high in saturated fats and red meat and processed meat; and inadequate intake of fruits and vegetables. Men and women who are overweight are more likely to develop and die from colorectal cancer. Risk factors identified in the National Health Interview Study were age (older than 50), smoking, and race (White). A report from the American College of Gastroenterology states that those with diabetes are three times more likely to develop colorectal cancers than nondiabetics.

Surgery is the most common treatment for colorectal cancers and may be curative. Often, chemotherapy alone or in combination with radiotherapy is given before or after surgery to those older adults who have cancer that has metastasized (spread). The one-year survival rate is 83%, the five-year survival rate is 64%, and ten-year survival rate is 58%.

Experts recommend increasing physical activity, avoiding obesity, limiting red meat consumption, and increasing fruit and vegetable intake. The new MyPyramid for Older Adults recommends that older adults eat leaner meats in an effort to prevent colorectal cancer. The American Cancer Society recommends the inclusion of sufficient dietary fiber in all adults, but research is inconclusive about its protective effect in this cancer. The EPIC (European Prospective Investigation into Cancer and Nutrition) study has found that high fiber intake and fish consumption are protective for colorectal cancers. No other nutrients have been associated at this time, and the study is continuing.

The WHI examined the effects of a low-fat diet on risk of colorectal cancer in postmenopausal women. The researchers concluded that the low-fat dietary intervention did not reduce the risk of most colon cancers in postmenopausal women; however, it did reduce the risk of ovarian cancer in this age group.

The Modified MyPyramid for Older Adults suggests that older adults consume low-fat and nonfat dairy products in order to obtain sufficient calcium and vitamin D. Some evidence suggests that dairy products can provide a protective effect in people with colon and breast cancers. A study from the National Cancer Institute pooled data from ten studies from five countries that followed 500,000 people. Milk and calcium intake was inversely related to colorectal cancer—that is, higher milk intake equaled lower incidence of colorectal cancer (**Table 12-3**). Calcium intake was also inversely related to colorectal cancer.

Cancer Treatments

Whether the intent is to cure or to provide palliative care, older adults provide a considerable challenge. Cancers in older adults are different from cancers in younger adults. Breast cancer, for example, is usually less aggressive in older adults. However, the toxic effects of cancer treatments are worse in older adults and they occur at lower doses than in younger adults.

Many therapies for the treatment of cancer are aggressive, and the patient may require aggressive nutrition management. Prior to cancer therapy, the health care team will discuss a treatment plan with the patient. The plan may include surgery, radiation therapy, chemotherapy, hormone therapy, or biologic immunotherapy, or a combination of these. Each of these therapies is discussed later in this section.

Dietary counseling is part of the treatment plan, and the patient should meet with a registered dietitian, if at all possible. Early assessment prior to therapy is imperative. Good nutrition before, during, and after therapy can make an important difference in the patient's life. The older adult will be much more able to cope with some of the more difficult therapies and side effects if nutrition is good. The patient should know that in therapy, the plan is to kill cancer cells, but that some healthy cells may be damaged as well.

No therapy will be without side effects that affect eating and nutrition. Some side effects of cancer therapies include loss of appetite, weight changes, sore mouth, dry mouth, dental and gum problems, change in smell and taste, nausea and vomiting, diarrhea, lactose intolerance, constipation, fatigue, and depression. A useful tool to keep track of

TABLE 12-3 Potential Anticancer Activity of Milk Components

Cancer	Whey Protein Concentrate	Lactoferrin and Lactoperoxiddase	Conjugated Linoleic Acid	Bovine Serum Albumin	Peptide
Colon	+	+	+	+	+
Breast	+	−	+	+	+

Source: Data from Ohio State University. Available at: http://www.fst.ohio-state.edu/People/HARPER/Functional-foods/Potential%20 Anti-Cancer. Accessed March 5, 2006.

▶ **BOX 12-3   Monitoring Side Effects**

Name: _____

Week of: _____

Type of treatment: _____

Date of treatment: _____

Type of treatment: _____

Date of treatment: _____

Weight: _____ lbs (measured once/week)

Make a check next to any side effect listed below that you experienced in the week. Next to each one checked, indicate on a scale of 1 to 3 how severe the side effect was for you. 1–mild; 2–moderate; 3–severe.

Side Effect	M	Tu	W	Th	F	Sa	Sun
Sore/dry mouth							
Nausea							
Vomiting							
Constipation							
Diarrhea							
Fatigue							
Other:							

For any other questions or concerns, use the space below to write.

Source: Adapted from National Cancer Institute. Eating hints for cancer patients: before, during, and after treatment. Available at: http://www.cancer.gov/cancertopics/eatinghints/allpages. Accessed January 20, 2008.

side effects is provided in **Box 12-3**. Some of these will be discussed further under symptom management.

Surgery

Sixty percent of patients with cancer will undergo a cancer-related surgical procedure. If malnourished, the patient is at high risk for postoperative morbidity and mortality. Macronutrient and micronutrient deficiencies should be corrected prior to surgery, if time permits. This may require oral supplements or even enteral or parenteral nutritional support. Immediately after surgery, the patient's diet is usually restricted to clear liquids. As the patient recovers, more food types are allowed in progression (**Box 12-4**).

After surgery, the body needs extra calories and protein for wound healing and recovery. The patient may be unable to eat a normal diet due to surgery-related side effects, including pain and fatigue. This is a good time to eat small, frequent meals and snacks, especially those that are low in fat and easy to digest. Encourage the patient to sip water or juice in small amounts throughout the day to prevent dehydration; at least eight 8-oz glasses each day is needed.

Depending on the surgical site, there may be a number of side effects, including taste changes, dry mouth, loss of appetite, and fatigue. The patient may experience fat intolerance, feelings of fullness, indigestion, heartburn,

▶ BOX 12-4 Post-Surgery Diet Progression

Step 1:
Clear liquids
Weak tea
Juices, strained
Clear, fat-free broth
Sports drinks
Gelatin, plain
Clear carbonated drinks
Bouillon
Fruit ices
Popsicles
Strained lemonade
Consommé
Vegetable broth, strained
Water

Step 2: Easy-to-digest foods
All foods in step 1
Plain crackers, chicken, turkey
Plain milkshakes
All juices
Instant hot cereal
White breads
Soft baked custard
Plain puddings
Fruit nectar
Fruits and vegetables: canned and
　peeled
Angel food cake
Lean beef, fish, skinned chicken,
　turkey
Smooth ice cream

Cream soups, strained
Refined cereals
Milk of all types
Ice milk
Pasteurized eggnog
Frozen yogurt
Fruits and vegetables: canned and
　peeled

Step 3: Regular diet allowed,
　but avoid
Gassy foods: beans, melons,
　cruciferous vegetables, milk and
　milk products
High-fat, greasy, deep-fat fried foods
Large meals

Source: Data from American Cancer Society. Surgery. Available at: http://www.cancer.org/docroot/MBC/content/MBC_6_2X_When_You_Have_Cancer_Surgery.asp?sitearea=MBC. Accessed July 13, 2009.

milk intolerance, diarrhea, gas, cramping, constipation, and bloating.

There is considerable controversy whether the very old (those older than 85) should have surgery. Many state that older adults recover as well as young adults. Age 70 used to be the cutoff point for any surgery; this has changed. The biggest problem for very old adults is the lack of reserve; they do not tolerate complications. Because many older people with cancer are not healthy, surgery may not be a choice.

Chemotherapy

Unlike surgery and radiation therapy, chemotherapy is a systemic therapy, meaning it affects the entire body. Chemotherapy has more side effects than other cancer therapies, although it is important to remember that patients may receive all three treatments—surgery, radiation, and chemotherapy. Sometimes side effects are minimal; however, many people experience nausea and vomiting, anorexia, taste changes, early satiety, mucositis and esophagitis, fatigue, constipation, and diarrhea. Poor nutrition during therapy can affect the patient's ability to stay on treatment schedules. High-calorie and high-protein liquid supplements in between meals may help maintain adequate nutrient and caloric intake.

Sometimes it is advisable to pack a small nutritious meal to take before treatment. Often this helps in avoiding nausea. Fried foods are to be avoided. Small, frequent meals are to be encouraged. Drinking plenty of fluids is essential. Specialists suggest that patients avoid their favorite foods prior to chemotherapy so that they don't begin to make an association between the food and nausea.

If the older adult is having trouble with fatigue, meal delivery can often be arranged. The American Cancer Society has a toll-free number (1-800-ACS-2345) and a website at www.cancer.org for suggestions of resources within a particular community.

Radiation Therapy

Good nutrition is very important during radiation therapy (RT). RT affects healthy tissues as well as diseased tissues. Side effects depend on the area that is irradiated and the volume of radiation. Side effects are usually acute and begin the second or third week of therapy. They diminish two or three weeks after therapy is completed; however, some side effects are chronic and continue indefinitely. The gastrointestinal tract is most susceptible to nutrition-related radiation side effects. Radiation to the head and neck, lungs, esophagus, cervix, uterus, colon, rectum, and pancreas can affect the gastrointestinal tract.

RT side effects may include painful swallowing, xerostomia, mucositis, stricture of the upper esophagus, enteritis, diarrhea, nausea and vomiting, and malabsorption of nutrients. Nutritional counseling and dietary modification have been demonstrated to be efficacious. Patients may need artificial saliva and oral comfort via hard candies and popsicles.

Immunotherapy

Monoclonal antibodies (MAb) are the widely used form of cancer immunotherapy at this time. These antibodies are made in the laboratory as opposed to those made in one's own immune system. It is considered passive immunotherapy. MAbs are presently in clinical trials for people with almost every type of cancer. As researchers find more cancer-associated antigens, they are able to make MAbs against these cancers. Some presently in use include Herceptin for breast cancer; Campath for chronic lymphocytic leukemia; Erbitux for colorectal and some lung and breast cancers; and Avastin for colorectal, some lung cancers, and advanced breast cancer. MAbs may cause many side effects, such as nausea and vomiting, diarrhea, chills, weakness, headache, low blood pressure, rashes, and fever. Side effects of interferon immunotherapy are similar but include anorexia and fatigue. Interleukin-2 therapy can cause weight gain or the need for nutrition support.

Side Effects of Therapy: Nutrition and Symptom Management

No therapy is without side effects that affect eating and nutrition. To help patients cope with these side effects and meet their dietary needs, advise them to eat when they are hungry, rather than at set mealtimes, or when they feel best, often in the morning when rested. They should also eat their favorite foods, dine with family and friends, and, if possible, have others prepare their foods. Usually a waiver from dietary restrictions is granted for religious holidays or special events. Attractive foods look better and taste better, so add garnishes such as lemon wedge, orange slices, cherry tomatoes, parsley.

The patient should be encouraged to eat small, frequent meals and snacks throughout the day. Maintaining hydration is very important, and, with the exception of anorexia treatment, the older cancer patient should carry a water bottle and drink eight to ten cups of fluid daily.

The patient may not feel up to grocery shopping, but the pantry and refrigerator need to remain well stocked. Encourage the patient to ask family or friends to help with shopping. Foods requiring little preparation and dinners frozen in advance in meal-sized portions are useful.

Protein-Calorie Malnutrition

The most common nutrition diagnosis associated with cancer is protein-calorie malnutrition (PCM). With some

TABLE 12-4 Signs and Symptoms of Malnutrition

Protein Malnutrition	Protein-Calorie Malnutrition
Marked hypoalbuminemia	Weight loss
Anemia	Diminished basal metabolism
Edema	Depletion of subcutaneous fat and tissue
Muscle atrophy	Poor turgor
Delayed wound healing	Bradycardia
Impaired immunocompetence	Hypothermia

Source: Data from RxKinetics. Section 1—Malnutrition. Available at: http://www.rxkinetics.com/tpntutorial/1_2.html. Accessed January 20, 2008.

cancers, the older adult may be unable to digest certain foods. Metabolic abnormalities may occur, such as glucose intolerance, insulin resistance, anemia, an increase in lipolysis, an increase in whole-body protein turnover with marked hypoalbuminemia, muscle atrophy, delayed wound healing, and impaired immunocompetence. See **Table 12-4** for a more complete list of signs and symptoms of malnutrition. If left untreated, PCM can lead to progressive wasting, weakness, debilitation, and death.

The Immunocompromised Patient

Both cancer and cancer therapy can weaken the body's immune system by affecting the blood cells that protect against disease and bacteria. **Box 12-5** contains a list of specific foods to avoid that may contain infection-causing organisms in older patients. See **Box 12-6** for food-handling considerations.

Anorexia

Anorexia, the loss of appetite or the desire to eat, is a common problem of older adults with cancer. It is present in 15% to 25% of all cancer patients at diagnosis and occurs as a side effect of many therapies. In widespread cancer, metastasis, it occurs in nearly 100% of patients. Depression, a common accompaniment to a cancer diagnosis, often causes anorexia. The following advice should be offered to the patient suffering from anorexia:

- Eat small, frequent, high-calorie meals every two hours
- Add extra protein and calories to food
- Eat one-third of daily protein and calories at breakfast
- Snack between meals and at bedtime
- Limit liquids with meals, because they may be filling and limit the desire for high-calorie foods; drink 30 to 60 minutes before or after meals
- Provide foods that appeal to the sense of smell
- Be creative with foods (vary color and texture)
- If permitted, have a small amount of wine or beer before meals, because these may stimulate the appetite

BOX 12-5   Foods to Avoid when Immunocompromised

- Cold smoked fish (salmon), lox, and pickled fish
- Herbal preparations and nutrient supplements
- Nuts in the shell, unroasted nuts
- Salads from a delicatessen
- Commercial salsas in the refrigerated case
- Raw grain products
- Cold brewed tea made with warm or cold water
- Unrefrigerated cream-filled pastries (those stored at room temperature)
- Meats and cold cuts from the delicatessen
- Cured hard salami in a natural wrap
- Unpasteurized milk and milk products, including cheese and yogurt
- Cheeses with molds: blue, Roquefort, gorgonzola, sharp cheddar, brie, camembert, feta, farmers' cheese
- Stilton cheese containing chili pepper or other uncooked vegetables

- Fresh salad dressings that contain aged cheeses (blue, Roquefort) or raw eggs
- Unwashed raw vegetables and fruits and those with visible mold
- All raw vegetable sprouts (e.g., alfalfa, mung beans)
- Unpasteurized commercial fruit and vegetable juices
- Raw or non-heat-treated honey or honey in the comb
- All miso-based products (e.g., tempeh, and mate tea)
- Any outdated products, moldy products
- Unpasteurized beer
- Raw, uncooked brewer's yeast
- Well water, unless tested yearly and found safe; if severely immunocompromised, no well water unless tested daily; use bottled, distilled, or boiled water
- Filtration devices are not safe unless the water is chlorinated

Source: Data from American Cancer Society. People with Weak Immune Systems. Available at: http://www.cancer.org/docroot/MBC/content/MBC_6_2X_Impact_of_Altered_Immune_Function.asp?sitearea=MBC. Accessed July 13, 2009.

- Provide frequent mouth care to decrease aftertastes
- Avoid foods that do not smell good to you
- Provide a pleasant ambience with meals (soft music, candles)

Recommended foods include cheese and crackers, muffins, puddings, milkshakes, yogurt, ice cream, peanut butter, cream cheese, deviled ham, canned fruit in heavy syrup, nuts, cottage cheese, and chocolate milk.

Cachexia

Cachexia is a wasting syndrome characterized by weakness and progressive weight loss, fat loss, and muscle wasting. It is often an immediate cause of death in many patients with cancer. The cause is probably multifactorial—metastasis, tumor factors, and metabolic abnormalities. The cause is not well understood. Medications used to treat cachexia include progestational agents, such as megestrol acetate and medroxyprogesterone; glucocorticoids; antiemetics; antihistamines; the antidepressant mirtazipine; and omega-3 fatty acids. Pancreatic enzymes are used for those with pancreatic cancer. Some therapeutic interventions may inhibit tumor-induced catabolic activity and increase lean body mass. These interventions include branched-chain amino

acids such as leucine, isoleucine, and valine; cannabinoids; melatonin; and thalidomide. Thalidomide has been found to be very effective in advanced pancreatic cancers at 200 mg per day. More studies are being conducted to determine its effect in other cancers.

Fatigue

The fatigue resulting from cancer therapy can be a serious obstacle to good nutrition management if the patient is too tired to fix snacks and meals. Encourage the patient to take rest breaks from work and take several naps per day rather than long rests. Regular short walks will also help to alleviate fatigue.

Consider the following when attempting to manage fatigue:

- Dehydration makes fatigue worse, so fluids are essential.
- If weight loss is a problem, the fluids should have calories.
- Avoid sugary foods; these can cause an energy

cachexia Loss of weight and muscle mass, often due to loss of appetite. One may be cachectic without stopping eating; frequently indicates a medical problem, often cancer.

> ### BOX 12-6   Food Handling Tips for Immunocompromised Patients

- Refrigerate foods at or less than 40°F.
- Wash hands with warm soapy water before and after food preparation and eating.
- Keep hot foods hot (more than 140°F.) and cold foods cold (less than 40°F).
- Wash fruits and vegetables under running water before peeling/cutting. Do not use soap, detergents, or chlorine bleach solutions.
- Rinse leafy vegetable leaves individually under running water; do not use commercial produce rinses.
- Rinse packaged salads and slaws, even if it states it is prewashed.
- Clean rough skin and rinds with a scrubber.
- Thaw meat, fish, and poultry in microwave or in refrigerator in a dish to catch drips. Do not thaw at room temperature.
- Use defrosted foods immediately and do not refreeze.
- Put perishable foods in refrigerator within two hours of use.

- Egg, cream, and mayonnaise dishes should be refrigerated within one hour of use.
- Do not buy produce that has been precut at the grocery store.
- Wash canned food lids with soap and water before opening.
- Use two different utensils for stirring and then tasting.
- Use a clean knife for cutting each different food.
- When grilling, use a clean plate for the grilled item after cooking.
- Cook eggs until whites are hard and yolks thickened.
- Throw away eggs with cracked shells.
- Boil tofu five to ten minutes before using.
- Throw out foods that look or smell strange.
- Cook meats until juices run clear and are no longer pink.
- Meats are cooked to 160°F; poultry 180°F.
- Cook hot dogs and lunch meats to steaming (165°F).
- Do not eat uncooked eggs, such as in cookie dough.

Source: Data from American Cancer Society. People with Weak Immune Systems. Available at: http://www.cancer.org/docroot/MBC/content/MBC_6_2X_Impact_of_Altered_Immune_Function.asp?sitearea=MBC. Accessed July 13, 2009.

"boost" that leaves one more tired after the boost is over.

- To maintain healthy blood glucose levels, eat protein, fat, and/or fiber at each snack.
- Meet basic calorie needs.
- Consider a multivitamin supplement with just 100% of the RDA of each nutrient.
- Do not take large amounts of vitamins and minerals without first consulting a physician, nurse, or registered dietitian.
- Avoid stress.

Weakness and Falls

Weakness, which can lead to falls, is a very common side effect of cancer therapy and cancer. Many older adults are already at risk of falling from general fatigue, weakness, age-related loss of priopriception, osteoarthritis of the hip or knees, and many other causes. One study by Bischoff-Ferrari and colleagues found that vitamin D (cholecalciferol) may reduce the risk of falls if it is started early and used over a long period of time (see Chapter 4). The research protocol used 700 IU of cholecalciferol plus 500 mg of calci-

um citrate malate per day in the study subjects. In ambulatory older women, falls were reduced by 46%; in less active women falls were reduced by 65%. However, these findings did not hold true for older men. Another study by Prince and colleagues found that older adults with vitamin D insufficiency who are at risk for falls and who live in sunny climates benefited from ergocalciferol (vitamin D2) supplementation in addition to calcium citrate (1000 IU/day).

Vitamin D production is diminished in older adults. Further, consistent use of sunscreens will decrease the synthesis of vitamin D. Older adults who live in northern latitudes are especially at risk for vitamin D deficiency. Sixty percent of women in hospitals in Boston were found to be deficient in the vitamin. Because of this, it is recommended that older adults increase their vitamin D intake. Some experts suggest 1,000 IU/day of vitamin D, higher than the currently recommended 600 IU/day. Because vitamin D is not found naturally in many foods, it is important for older adults to take a multivitamin (400 IU) every day. Milk is fortified to 100 IU per cup; however, this is known to vary considerably. It is advisable to take calcium supplements that include vitamin D, which should add another 400 to

500 mg of calcium and 200 to 400 IU of vitamin D. Foods high in vitamin D include fortified milk; oily fish, such as salmon; egg yolks; and butter.

Altered Taste

Taste perception is often altered as a result of therapy. Patients with cancer may develop an aversion to meat, leading to protein deficiencies. When meats do not taste "right," advise the patient to substitute poultry, fish, eggs, and cheese for red meat. Also, suggest that the patient eat other high-protein foods, such as beans, peas, cheeses, custards, egg dishes, eggnog, instant breakfast drinks, macaroni and cheese, milkshakes, nuts, peanut butter, pudding, and yogurt. Also, suggest marinating the meat or eating meat in combination with other foods, such as chili, lasagna, spaghetti sauce, stews, or soups. The patient could add sauces and seasonings and try spicy or smoked meats such as ham, sausage, cold cuts. Meats might be more palatable when eaten with something sweet, such as jelly, applesauce, or cranberry sauce. Another idea is to eat meat when it is cold or at room temperature, such as cottage cheese plates; macaroni salad with shrimp, tuna, egg, ham, or chicken salad; luncheon meat sandwiches; or cold salmon. Note, however, that these foods should not be at room temperature for more than 60 minutes to avoid food poisoning.

If the patient is experiencing a bitter or metallic taste, suggest that the patient use plastic utensils, suck lemon drops or mints, check with dentist to determine if there are dental problems, and check with physician or nurse to see if any medications could cause odd tastes. To avoid bad aftertastes, the patient should drink tasty liquids, eat mints or hard candies, or chew gum.

To give food more flavor, add bacon bits; chopped green peppers; chopped onions; ham, nuts; cheeses, especially sharp cheddar; barbecue sauce; extracts and flavorings; ketchup; meat marinades; mustards; salad dressings; soy sauce; spices and herbs; teriyaki sauce; vinegar; or wine.

To sweeten food, use brown sugar, maple syrup, honey, cinnamon, dates, or raisins rather than white sugar. When foods taste too sweet, add salt or lemon juice, yogurt, buttermilk, fresh fruit, instant coffee powder, or extra milk. Dilute fruit juices, milk, buttermilk, lemonade, ginger ale, and sports drinks, such as Gatorade or PowerAde.

If foods taste salty, have the patient or care giver check product labels for sodium content and avoid seasonings that contain salt.

Xerostomia (Dry Mouth)

Management of xerostomia can include the following advice to the patient:

- Brush four or more times a day; avoid commercial mouthwashes, especially those with alcohol content.

- Brush and rinse dentures after each meal.
- Keep water available to moisten the mouth.
- Drink eight to ten cups of liquid per day.
- Avoid liquids and foods with high sugar content.
- Consume sweet or tart foods and beverages that stimulate saliva.
- Drink fruit nectar rather than juices.
- Use a straw to drink liquids.
- Suck on sugarless candy or gum, especially lemon drops.
- Avoid alcoholic and acidic beverages.
- Avoid tobacco.
- Limit caffeine-containing drinks/foods, such as coffee, tea, colas, and chocolate.
- Eat soft, moist foods that are cool or at room temperature.
- Use a blender to process fruits and vegetables, soft-cooked chicken and fish, popsicles, and slushies.
- Avoid foods that stick to the mouth, such as peanut butter, bananas, cookies, cakes, pies, dry breads, rolls, pasta, rice, pretzels, chips, cereals, dry meats, and poultry.
- Use a cool-mist humidifier to moisten room air especially at night (keep it clean to avoid bacterial spread).
- If salivary glands have been removed or damaged by radiation, use saliva substitutes and nutritional supplements, such as liquid meal replacements.

Mucositis and Stomatitis

The following can be used to manage mucositis and stomatitis:

- Eat soft foods that are easy to chew and swallow: bananas, applesauce, peaches, pears, apricot nectars, watermelon, cottage cheese, mashed potatoes, macaroni and cheese, custard, puddings, gelatin, milkshakes, soft pies, sherbets, scrambled eggs, oatmeal or other cooked or cold cereals, pureed or mashed vegetables, tuna noodle casserole, creamed soups, and pureed meats.
- Avoid irritating foods such as citrus fruits, spicy foods, foods with vinegar, and rough, coarse foods, such as crackers, crusty breads, toast, granola, or raw vegetables.
- Avoid irritating beverages, such as tomato juice, caffeinated beverages, and alcohol.
- Use a straw to drink liquids.
- Eat foods cold or at room temperature.
- Practice good oral hygiene.
- Increase fluid intake by adding sauces, gravy, or broths to foods.
- Numb the mouth with ice chips or ice pops.

Dysphagia

Management of dysphagia centers on having the patient puree or thicken food or liquids in a food processor to a consistency that is easy to swallow. Baby rice cereal makes very thick products. Soften cakes, cookies, or sandwiches by saturating them with gelatin (1 tablespoon unflavored gelatin in 2 cups liquid until dissolved). Liquids can be thickened with tapioca, flour, or cornstarch (these thickeners should be cooked before consuming). The following are some additional tips for managing dysphagia:

- Meet with a speech therapist.
- Call a physician or nurse if you choke when eating; call immediately if fever occurs (it may indicate aspiration pneumonia).
- Drink six to eight cups of thickened fluid per day.
- Use liquid supplements if unable to eat enough food to meet caloric requirements.
- Use pureed vegetables in soups.

The following foods are generally well tolerated by those with dysphagia: thickened milk; yogurt without fruit; cottage cheese; sour cream; pureed meat, poultry, and fish; casseroles; scrambled eggs; thick broth and soup; Cream of Wheat and cream of rice; pureed fruits and vegetables without seeds or skin; mashed potatoes; thickened juice and nectars; milkshakes; custards; pudding; syrup; honey. If these foods are well-tolerated, a mechanical soft thick-liquid diet may be appropriate. Such a diet includes milk, yogurt, cheeses, all eggs, ground meats, fish, sandwiches with spread or ground meat, soft breads, graham crackers, cookies, soft cold cereal in milk, pancakes, waffles, rice, bananas, canned fruit, well-cooked or pureed vegetables, soft desserts, and soft cakes.

Nausea and Vomiting
The following are tips for managing nausea and vomiting:

- Sip clear liquids frequently to avoid dehydration.
- If vomiting, rinse mouth, and continue to drink or sip clear liquids such as apple, grape, or cranberry juice; frozen flavored ices; flat soda; or broth.
- Eat dry foods such as crackers, toast, and bread sticks during the day.
- Sit up or keep head raised for one hour after eating.
- Eat bland, soft easy-to-digest foods, not heavy meals; avoid greasy, sweet, fried, and spicy foods.
- Eat away from odors; eat foods with little odor.
- Eat in a cool, rather than a warm, room.
- Rinse out mouth before and after eating with a baking soda and salt mouthwash (1 quart water, 3/4 tsp salt, 1 tsp baking soda).
- Suck on hard candies such as lemon drops and peppermints if there is a bad taste in the mouth.
- On chemotherapy treatment days, eat easy-to-digest foods such as Cream of Wheat and chicken noodle soup with saltine crackers.
- Ask a physician or nurse about antinausea medications.

Diarrhea
The following are some tips for managing diarrhea:

- Drink room-temperature fluids throughout the day.
- Drink one cup of liquid after each loose bowel movement.
- Limit milk products to two cups per day; yogurt and buttermilk are good alternatives.
- Avoid foods that can cause gas, such as sodas, legumes, lentils, cruciferous vegetables, and gum.
- Avoid sugar-free gum and candies made with sugar alcohols (sorbitol, mannitol, or xylitol).
- Avoid high-fiber foods such as nuts, seeds, whole grains, dried fruits, raw fruits and vegetables, shredded wheat, coconut, popcorn, granola, and wild rice.
- Avoid pears, melons, chocolate, licorice, pickles, and hot sauces.
- Eat small frequent meals and snacks.
- Eat high-sodium foods such as broths, soups, sports drinks, crackers, and pretzels.
- Drink high-potassium liquids and foods such as fruit juices and nectars, sports drinks, potatoes without skin, and bananas.
- Eat foods high in soluble fibers such as applesauce, bananas, canned peaches and pears, oatmeal, and white rice.

Constipation
The following are some tips for managing constipation:

- Eat high-fiber foods regularly, but add them to the diet slowly. The following are some high-fiber foods: bran cereals, popcorn, brown rice, whole wheat bread and pasta, wheat bran, kidney beans, navy beans, nuts, carrots, brussels sprouts, potato with skin, banana, apple with peel, blueberries, pear with skin, prunes, oranges, raisins, and strawberries.
- Drink eight to ten cups of fluid daily, including water, prune juice, warm juices, decaffeinated teas, and lemonade.
- Try to eat at the same times each day.
- Try to have a bowel movement at the same time each day.
- Use laxatives only if directed by a physician or nurse.
- Contact a physician or nurse if no bowel movement for three days or more.
- If constipation is an ongoing problem, establish a bowel plan using Senekot, Colace, Metamucil, or other preparation with psyllium fiber.
- Limit gas-causing drinks and foods: dried beans and peas, string beans, turnip greens, milk, mushrooms, fried foods, cucumbers, pickles, peppers, broccoli, cabbage, melons, beer, eggs, corn, onions, collards, asparagus, avocado, nuts, sauerkraut, cauliflower, spinach, raw apples and juice, fatty foods, fish, sweet potatoes, spicy foods, lentils, and pastries.

- Limit chewing gum, talking while eating, chewing with mouth open, and using straws.
- Exercise.

Advanced Cancers

Near the end of life, patients often have no appetite and lose weight rapidly. Usually this is caused by the cancer and is not in the patient's control. Even if the older adult understands the importance of eating and wants to eat, it is difficult to force oneself to eat.

The American Cancer Society offers the following suggestions for nutrition in advanced cancers:

- Make the most of days when it feels good to eat.
- Keep nutritious foods and drinks handy so they are there when appetite is present.
- Eat small, frequent snacks.
- Eat high-protein, high-calorie foods.
- Avoid food odors caused by food preparation.
- Eat favorite foods.
- Don't force eating.
- Try to maintain present weight.
- Drink sufficient fluids so that bowels function regularly.
- Eat with others at a table when possible.

A number of appetite stimulants may be effective in managing weight loss, anorexia, and cachexia in older adults with advanced cancer. Other agents, for example, megestrol acetate (MA), have sometimes been found to be useful. In those with digestive tract cancers, certain targeted nutritional strategies, such as digestive enzymes or elemental diets, may be useful.

In the final days of life, the body cannot use the food or fluid, and continuing them can increase discomfort. Food should not be a source of stress between the patient and the family or caretakers. Usually, care at this time includes treatment of dry mouth and thirst and helping the older adult's family understand and cope with feelings about stopping nutrition.

Methods of Nutrient Delivery

Methods of nutrition care include the oral route (preferred); total parenteral nutrition, although there is little evidence of improved outcomes in those with advanced cancer with this route; nasogastric tube; and percutaneous endoscopic gastrostomy tube.

Nasogastric Tubes

Nasogastric tubes (NG) are used for short periods of time, such as prior to surgery or for a few days postoperatively. The tube may be used during radiation therapy if the upper airway is not painful. They usually are not used during chemotherapy because the oral cavity can be quite painful from side effects. The NG tube is a cost-effective management of nutrition. Except for GI surgery, enteral therapy is preferred because it continues to use the gut; has fewer complications, such as infection and organ malfunction; and is easy to administer.

Percutaneous Endoscopic Gastrostomy Tubes

The malnourished older adult with cancer often is fitted with a percutaneous endoscopic gastrostomy (PEG) tube. With a PEG tube, the patient is able to eat and drink what he or she prefers and does not need to focus on maintaining adequate nutrition. They are usually used for long-term enteral feedings (more than two weeks). The risk of aspiration is lower with PEG tubes because there is less of a chance for migration of the large tube up into the esophagus, compared to NG tubes.

It is better to provide nutrition through the PEG tube via the bolus method, rather than by long-term infusion, because it resembles normal eating. Boluses can be administered three to six times a day over 10 to 15 minutes. However, this feeding should only be delivered into the stomach, not the duodenum or jejunum.

Note that there is not sufficient evidence that function, nutrition, or subjective health is improved with the use of the PEG tube. The PEG tube should probably not be used when the overall health prognosis is not conducive to aggressive nutrition therapy.

Parenteral Nutrition

Parenteral nutrition is initiated in those patients with a nonfunctioning gut or those with profound nausea. It is indicated in patients who are unable to use the oral or enteral routes. Contraindications are a functioning gut, a poor prognosis, and the need for nutritional support for fewer than five days.

Parenteral nutrition can be delivered via a central venous catheter or a peripheral venous catheter in a large vein such as the subclavian. High blood flow is essential. The peripheral line is a PICC line (peripherally inserted central catheter) used for long-term support and inserted into the superior or inferior vena cava.

A number of organizations advise against routine use of parenteral nutrition in cancer patients.

Palliative Care

Incurable and advanced-staged cancers are best managed with **palliative care** to maintain comfort and quality of life as long as the older adult lives. Pain, confusion, and shortness of breath are common symptoms at this time. Nutrition at end of life is less a primary care issue and more about comfort care. Nutrition and hydration are considered medical interventions that can be stopped.

Family members of the older patient may be at odds

palliative care Care given not to cure, but rather to help the patient live better with the disease while dying.

with the hospice or end-of-life needs of cancer patients. They often will be in a "do everything" mode of thinking. This involves very careful discussions, even if the older adult has made a living will, because the needs of the family members are often different from the plans of the patient from an earlier time in the cancer management. It is prudent to begin discussion with the family as early after diagnosis as possible so that they may understand and adjust to the downhill trajectory of the older adult with this disease.

Where the patient will die has become problematic. Priorities for enabling the older adult with cancer to die at home are family support and good home-based care. When the patient becomes very weak and has limited function and mobility, it becomes essential for there to be live-in relatives (more than just an older adult spouse) and/or caregivers. The patient's preference may be to die at home, or, fearing lack of care, to die in the hospital or nursing home facility.

At the end of life, it is advisable not to force eating and drinking. Instead, offer ice chips, soft drinks, juices, popsicles, or whatever may be of interest (nutritional or not). Avoid carbonated beverages and gas-producing foods. Apply petrolatum to dry lips and moisture to dry tongues and mucous membranes.

Conclusion

The goal of nutrition therapy for the older adult with cancer is to provide optimal nutritional status to prevent or reverse nutrient deficiencies, preserve lean body mass, better tolerate therapy, minimize nutrition-related side effects and complications, maintain strength and energy, protect immune function, decrease the risk of infection, aid in healing and recovery, and maximize quality of life.

Activities Related to This Chapter

1. Give examples of the key terms that you defined in this chapter.

2. Go to the American Cancer Society website and locate statistics on some of the most common cancers of older adults. How are the statistics changing? Are people living longer with cancer?

3. Select a cancer common to older adults and plan a nutritional care program throughout the spectrum of life of the disease in the older person.

Case Study

Mrs. D, a 77-year-old widow, was recently diagnosed with lung cancer after a prolonged period of bronchitis with chronic cough. She had never smoked, although her husband smoked two packs a day for most of their married life. Mrs. D has two children, a son and daughter, and four grandchildren; however, all live out of state. When told of the diagnosis, each adult child came for a week to visit with their mother and meet with physicians. Mrs. D did not wish to move from her home to live with either family member.

After her son and daughter left, Mrs. D became progressively depressed and her appetite diminished considerably. She had not been a large woman prior to this time. The oncologists determined that radiation would be the best course for Mrs. D and a courtesy car took her to and from appointments. After several weeks, her throat became very sore and other than cool drinks, she ate very little. Her radiation oncology nurse noted considerable weight loss and referred Mrs. D to the registered dietitian.

Questions

1. Based on this case study, what is your nutrition plan?
2. What do you know about the progress of this cancer?
3. What are the effects of radiation to this area?
4. If Mrs. D's prognosis is good, what diet plan will you recommend?
5. If Mrs. D's prognosis is poor, what diet plan will you recommend?

REFERENCES

American Cancer Society. *Cancer Facts and Figures 2009*. Atlanta: American Cancer Society; 2009.

American Cancer Society. Chemotherapy. May 2006. Available at: www.cancer.org/docroot/MBC/content/MBC_6_2X_When_You_Have_Chemotherapy. Accessed January 21, 2008.

American Cancer Society. People with weak immune systems. May 2006. Available at: www.cancer.org/docroot/MBC/content/MBC_6_2X_Impact_of_Altered_Immune_. Accessed January 21, 2008.

American Cancer Society. Preparing yourself for cancer treatment. May 2006. Available at: www.cancer.org/docroot/MBC/content/MBC_6_2X_Preparing_Yourself_for_Cancer. Accessed January 21, 2008.

American Cancer Society. Radiation therapy. May 2006. Available at: www.cancer.org/docroot/MBC/content/MBC_6_2X_When_You_Have_Radiation_T. Accessed January 21, 2008.

American Cancer Society. Surgery. May 2006. Available at: www.cancer.org/docroot/MBC/content/MBC_6_2X_When_You_Have_Cancer_Surg. Accessed January 21, 2008.

American Cancer Society. Unwanted weight gain. 2006. Available at: www.cancer.org/docroot/MBC/content/MBC_6_2X_Unwanted_Weight_Gain.asp?si. Accessed January 21, 2008.

American Cancer Society. The complete guide—nutrition and physical activity. 2006. Available at: www.cancer.org. Accessed January 28, 2008.

American Cancer Society. Coping with physical and emotional changes: dry mouth or thick saliva. 2006. Available at: www.cancer.org/docroot/MBC/content/MBC_6_2X_Dry_Mouth_or_Thick_Saliva.asp?sitearea = MBC. Accessed January 2, 2008.

Autier P, Gandini S. Vitamin D supplementation and total mortality: a meta-analysis of randomized controlled trials. *Arch Intern Med.* 2007;167(16):1730–1737.

Baglietto L, English D, Gertig D, Hopper J, Giles G. Does dietary folate intake modify effect of alcohol consumption on breast cancer risk? Prospective cohort study. *BMJ.* 2005;331 (7520):807.

Beer T. Vitamin D, taxotere combination extends the lives of men with advanced prostate cancer. Oregon Health & Science University Cancer Institute News & Information: November 2, 2005. Available at: www.ohsu.edu/ohsuedu/newspub/releases/110205taxotere.cfm. Accessed Mary 4, 2006.

Beresford S, Johnson K, Ritenbaugh C, Lasser N, Snetselaar L, Black H, et al. Low-fat dietary pattern and risk of colorectal cancer. *JAMA.* 2006;295(6):643–654.

Bischoff-Ferrari H, Orav E, Dawson-Hughes B. Effect of cholecalciferol plus calcium on falling in ambulatory older men and women. *Arch Int Med.* 2006;166(4):424–430.

Buijsse B, Feskens E, Schlettwein-Gsell D, Ferry M, Kok F, Kromhout D, et al. Plasma carotene and a-tocopherol in relation to 10-y all-cause and cause-specific mortality in European elderly: the Survey in Europe on Nutrition and the Elderly, a Concerted Action (SENECA). *Am J Clin Nutr.* 2005;82(4):879–886.

Callahan C, Haag, K, Weinberger M, Tierney W, Buchanan N, Stump T, et al. Outcomes of percutaneous endoscopic gastrostomy among older adults in a community setting. *JAGS.* 2000;48:1048–1054.

Canene-Adams K, Lindshield B, Wang S, Jeffery E, Clinton S, Erdman Jr. J. Combinations of tomato and broccoli enhance antitumor activity in Dunning R3327-H prostate adenocarcinomas. *Cancer Res.* 2007;67:836–843.

Chao C. Associations between beer, wine, and liquor consumption and lung cancer risk: a meta-analysis. *Cancer Epidemiol Biomarkers Prev.* 2007;16(11):2436 2447.

Chavarro J, Stampfer M, Campos H, Kurth T, et al. A prospective study of trans-fatty acid levels in blood and risk of prostate cancer. *Cancer Epidemiol Biomarkers Prev.* 2008;17(1):95–101.

Cho E, Smith-Warner A, Spiegelman D, Beeson W, van den Brandt P, Colditz G, et al. Dairy foods, calcium, and colorectal cancer: a pooled analysis of 10 cohort studies. *J Natl Cancer Inst.* 2004;96(13):1015–1022.

Clarke-Pearson DL. Clinical practice. Screening for ovarian cancer. *N Engl J Med.* 2009 Jul 9;361(2):170–177.

Dudek SG. *Nutrition Essentials for Nursing Practice.* 5th ed. Philadelphia: Lippincott; 2006.

Farwell W, Scranton R, Lawler E, Lew R, Brophy M, et al. The association between statins and cancer incidence in a veteran's population. *J Nat Cancer Inst.* 2008;100(2):134–139.

Feskanich D, Singh V, Willett W, Colditz G. Vitamin A intake and hip fractures among postmenopausal women. *JAMA.* 2002;287(1):47–54.

Fink B, Steck S, Wolff M, Britton J, et al. Dietary flavonoid intake and breast cancer survival among women on Long Island. *Cancer Epidemiol Biomarkers Prev.* 2007;16(11):2285–2292.

Fraser GE. Seventh-day Adventist Cohort Study: cancer epidemiology in Adventists—a low risk group. May 30, 2006. Available at: http://epi.grants.cancer.gov/ResPort/Adventist.html. Accessed January 28, 2008.

Gomes, B. What's needed for terminally ill patients to die at home? *BMJ.* 2006;332:515–521.

Gonzalez C. The European Prospective Investigation into Cancer and Nutrition (EPIC). *Pub Health Nutr.* 2006;9(1):124–126.

Harvard Medical School. Vitamins: the quest for just the right amount. *Harvard Health Letter.* 2004;29(8):4–5.

Hess P. End-of-life issues. In P Ebersole, P Hess, A Luggen (eds.). *Toward Healthy Aging.* 6th ed. St. Louis: Mosby; 2004.

Hodges D. ACG: Study confirms three-fold greater risk of colorectal cancer among diabetics. March 4, 2006. *Medical Post.* Available at: www.medicalpost.com/mpcontent/article.jsp?content=20051127_200543_4100. Accessed January 28, 2009.

Hu FB. Dietary patterns, diet quality and cancer risk. Ongoing study: RO1, CA095589, 5/1/03–4/30/07. http://researchportfolio.cancer.gov/cgi-bin/abstract.pl?SID=491846&Project ID=84497. Accessed March 2, 2006.

Insel P, Turner RE, Ross D. *Nutrition.* 3rd ed. Boston: Jones & Bartlett; 2008.

Intercultural Cancer Culture. American Indians/Alaskan Natives and cancer. Available at: http://iccnetwork.org.

Intercultural Cancer Culture. African Americans and cancer. Available at: http://iccnetwork.org/cancerfacts/ICC-CFS1.pdf. Accessed February 1, 2009.

Intercultural Cancer Culture. Asian Americans and cancer. Available at: http://iccnetwork.org/cancerfacts/ICC-CFS3.pdf. Accessed February 1, 2009.

Intercultural Cancer Culture. Native Hawaiians/Pacific Islanders and cancer. Available at: http://iccnetwork.org/cancerfacts/ICC-CFS5.pdf. Accessed February 1, 2009.

Jacobs E, Lanza E, Alberts D. Fiber, sex, and colorectal adenoma: results of a pooled analysis. *Am J Clin Nutr.* 2006;83:343–349.

Jacobs E, Rodriguez C, Bain E, Wang, Y et al. Cholesterol-lowering drugs and advanced prostate cancer incidence in a large U.S. cohort. *Cancer Epidemiol Biomarkers Prev.* 2007;16(11):2213–2217.

Jatoi I, Anderson W, Rao S, Devesa S. Breast cancer trends among black and white women in the United States. *J Clin Onc.* 2005;23(31):7836–7841.

Kamangar F, Qiao Y, Binbing Y, Sun X, Abnet C, et al. Lung cancer chemoprevention: a randomized double-blind trial in Linxian, China. *Cancer Epidemiol Biomarkers Prev.* 2006;15:1562–1564.

Koutros S, Cross A, Sandler D, Hoppin J, et al. Meat and meat mutagens and risk of prostate cancer in the Agricultural Health Study. *Cancer Epidemiol Biomarkers Prev.* 2008;17(1):80–87.

Landefeld CS, Doyle C, Kushi L, Byers T, Courneya K, Demark-Wahnefried W, Grant B, et al. Nutrition and physical activity during and after cancer treatment: An American Cancer Society Guide for informed choices. *CA Cancer J Clin.* 2006;56:323–353.

LaMonica V. Weigel S, Weigel N. Vitamin D and prostate cancer. *Exper Biol and Med.* 2004;229:277–284.

Lampe J, Nishino Y, Ray R, Wu, C, Li W, et al. Plasma isoflavones and fibrocystic breast conditions and breast cancer among women in Shanghai, China. *Cancer Epidemiol Biomarkers Prev.* 2007;16(12):2579–2586.

Lee IM, Cook N, Manson J, et al. Beta-carotene supplementation and incidence of cancer and cardiovascular disease: the Women's Health Study. *J Natl Cancer Inst.* 1999;91:2102–2106.

Looker AC, Pfeiffer CM, Lacher DA, Schleicher RL, Picciano MF, et al. Serum 25-hydroxyvitamin D status of the US population: 1988-1994 compared with 2000-2004. *Am J Clin Nutr.* 2008 Dec;88(6):1519–1527.

Luggen AS. Unhealthy alcohol intake among older adults. *Geriatrics & Aging.* 2007;10(6):347–360.

MacLean C, Newberry S, Mojica W, Khanna P, Issa A, Suttorp M, et al. Effects of omega-3 fatty acids on cancer risk. *JAMA.* 2006;295(4):403–415.

Mayo Clinic. Cancer: No appetite? How to get the nutrition you need. 2006. Available at: http://www.mayoclinic.com/health/cancer/HQ01134. Accessed January 21, 2008.

McCarthy E, Burns R, Coughlin S, Freund K, Rice J, Marwill S, et al. Mammography use helps to explain differences in breast cancer stage at diagnosis between older black and white women. *Annals of Int Med.* 1998;128(9):729–736.

Moghaddam AA, Woodward M, Huxley R. Obesity and risk of colorectal cancer: a meta-analysis of 31 studies with 70,000 events. *Cancer Epidem Biomarkers Prev.* 2007;16(12):2533–2547.

Mortimer JE, McElhaney J. Cancers in the geriatric population. Current geriatric diagnosis & treatment. In Landefeld CS, Pamer R, Johnson MA, Johnston C et al, Eds. Current geriatric diagnosis. McGraw Hill Professional, 2004.pp 305–313.

National Cancer Institute. Nutrition in cancer care: health profession version. Available at: www.cancer.gov/cancertopics/pdq/supportivecare/nutrition/healthprofessional. Accessed February 1, 2009.

National Cancer Institute. Antioxidants and cancer fact sheet. Available at: www.cancer.gov/cancertopics/factsheet/antioxidantsprevention. Accessed February 1, 2009.

National Cancer Institute. Cancer trends progress report—2007 update. Available at: http://progressreport.cancer.gov/doc.asp?pid=1&did=2007&mid=vcol&chid=71. Accessed January 18, 2008.

National Cancer Institute. Heterocyclic amines in cooked meats. Available at: www.cancer.gov/cancertopics/factsheet/Risk/heterocyclic-amines/print? Accessed February 1, 2009.

National Cancer Institute. Nutrition in cancer care. 2007. Available at: www.cancer.gov/cancertopics/pdq/

supportivecare/nutrition/HealthProfessional/4.cdr. Accessed January 29, 2008.

Oncology Nutrition Dietetic Practice Group. *The Clinical Guide to Oncology Nutrition*. 2nd ed. Chicago: American Dietetic Association; 2006.

Oregon Health and Science University. OHSU Cancer Institute. Norwegian researchers find that prostate cancer survival affected by seasons. September 27, 2007. Available at: www.ohsu.edu/ohsuedu/newspub/releases/092707prostate.cfm. Accessed January 27, 2008.

Palmer RM, Johnson MA, Johnston CB, Lyons WL (eds.). *Current Geriatric Diagnosis and Treatment*. New York: Lange; 2004.

Prentice R, Caan B, Chlebowski R, Patterson R, Kuller L, Ockene J, et al. Low-fat dietary pattern and risk of invasive breast cancer: the Women's' Health Initiative Randomized Controlled Dietary Modification Trial. *JAMA*. 2006;295(6):629–642.

Prince R, Austin N, Devine A, Dick I, Bruce D, Zhu K. Effects of ergocalciferol added to calcium on the risk of falls in elderly high-risk women. *Arch Intern Med*. 2008;168(1):103–108.

Ritenbaugh C, Streit K, Helfand M. Agency for Healthcare Research and Quality (AHRQ). Routine vitamin supplementation to prevent cancer: summary of evidence from randomized controlled trials. 2003. Available at: www.ahrq.gov/clinic/3rduspstf/vitamins/vitasum.htm. Accessed January 23, 2008.

Rock C, Flatt S, Natarajan L, Thomson C, Bardwell W, Newman V, et al. Plasma carotenoids and recurrence-free survival in women with a history of breast cancer. *J Clin Onc*. 2005; 23(27):6631–6638.

Rose D, Richards R. Food store access and household fruit and vegetable use among participants in the US Food Stamp Program. *Pub Health Nutr*. 2004;7(8):1081–1088.

Schabath MB, Hernandez L, Wu X, Pillow P, Spitz M. Dietary phytoestrogens and lung cancer risk. *JAMA*. 2005;294(12):1493–1504.

Schild S, Stella P, Brooks B, Mandrekar S, Bonner J, McGinnis W, et al. Results of combined-modality therapy for limited-stage small cell lung carcinoma in the elderly. *Cancer*. 2005;103(11):2349–2354.

Seventh-Day Adventist Dietetic Association. A position statement on the vegetarian diet. Available at: http://www.sdada.org/position.htm. Accessed July 14, 2009.

Steiner M, Price D, Israeli R, Mitchell J. Higher prostate cancer incidence in nonobese patients than in obese patients in a study in men with high-grade prostatic intraepithelial neoplasia. ASCO Meeting, 2005, abstract no. 26.

Stolzenberg-Solomon R, Cross A, Silverman D, Schairer C, et al. Meat and meat mutagen intake and pancreatic cancer risk in the NIH-AARP Cohort. *Cancer Epidemiol Biomarkers Prev*. 2007;16(12):2664–2675.

Tufts University. Modified pyramid for older adults, 2007. Available at: http://nutrition.tufts.edu/docs/pdf/releases/ModifiedMyPyramid.pdf. Accessed December 25, 2007.

Tworoger S, Gertig D, Gates M, Hecht J, Hankinson S. Caffeine, alcohol, smoking and the risk of incident epithelial ovarian cancer. *Cancer*. 2008;112(5):1169–1177.

van Dyke A, Cote M, Prysakl G, Claeys G, Wenzlaff A, Schwartz A. Regular adult aspirin use decreases risk of non-small cell lung cancer among women. *Cancer Epidemiol Biomarkers Prev*. 2008;17(1):148–157.

Vollset S, Igland J, Jenab M, Fredriksen A, Meyer K, et al. The association of gastric cancer risk with plasma folate, cobalamin and methylenetetrahydrofolate reductase polymorphisms in the European Prospective Investigation into Cancer and Nutrition. *Cancer Epidemiol Biomarkers Prev*. 2007;16(11):2416–2424.

Women's Health Initiative. Low-fat dietary pattern and cancer. October 9, 2007. Available at: http://www.whi.org. Accessed January 23, 2008.

Women's Health Initiative. Low-fat dietary pattern and risk of breast cancer, colorectal cancer and cardiovascular disease: the Women's Health Initiative (WHI) Randomized Controlled dietary Modification Trial. February 2006. Available at: http://www.whi.org/findings/dm/dm.php. Accessed January 23, 2008.

World Health Organization. Diet, nutrition, and the prevention of chronic diseases. WHO technical report, series 19, (2003). Geneva, Switzerland.

Yates M, Kwak M, Egner P, Groopman J, Bodreddigari S, Sutter T, et al. Potent protection against aflatoxin-induced tumorigenesis through induction of Nrf2-regulated pathways by the triterpenoid 1-[2-cyano-3,12-dioxooleana-1,9(11)-dien-28-Oyl] imidazole. *Cancer Res*. 2006;66(4):2488–2394.

CHAPTER 13

Neurological Changes Affecting Nutrition in Older Adults

Ann Schmidt Luggen, PhD, GNP

CHAPTER OBJECTIVES   Upon completion of this chapter the student will be able to:

1. Describe age-related changes of the brain and nervous system
2. Describe the sequelae of stroke and the role of good nutrition in its management
3. List some of the common neurological problems affecting older adults and how they affect nutrition
4. Explain how postpolio syndrome can affect nutrition
5. List strategies to help an older adult with dementia eat a meal

KEY TERMS AND CONCEPTS

Alzheimer's disease

Anorexins

Amyloid

Apraxia

Hypothalamus

Neurofibrillary tangles and plaques

Parageusia

Parkinson's disease

Parosmia

Polypharmacy

Selective serotonin-reuptake inhibitors (SSRIs)

The central nervous system (CNS) is remarkably complex. It enables people to interact with their environment, regulate their activities, and have consciousness. The CNS drives the organs in the body and transmits messages, both via chemicals and electrical current. It is "control by committee". Many changes in the brain occur with normal aging, and brain disorders are more common in older adults. Many of the neurological disorders in the aged affect diet and nutrition. Nearly all of them will affect nutritional status through loss of cognition, apathy, weakness, fatigue, or hormonal dysfunction.

The most common brain disorders in this group are mood disorders, such as depression and anxiety; **Alzheimer's disease**; Lewy body dementia; seizure disorders; Parkinson's disease; brain tumors; vascular dementias; strokes; trauma from falls; delirium; acute confusional states, such as those from drug side effects or from multiple drug use; hypothyroid dementia; Pick disease; myasthenia gravis; brain tumors; neuropathies; Huntington disease; and others. Some neurological disorders are caused by nutritional deficiencies, for example, vitamin B12 dementia; thiamine deficiency; niacin deficiency causing acute confusional states; vitamin B6 deficiency causing neuropathies; and folic acid

> **Alzheimer's disease** Progressive and fatal neurological disorder occurring primarily in older adults. Characterized by problems with memory, physical function, and behavior. It is the most common form of dementia.

and biotin deficiencies associated with depression. Some begin in middle adulthood and continue into later years. Some begin de novo in old age.

The brain plays an essential role in the decision to eat or not eat through integration of multiple hormonal and neural signals. The regulation of hunger and satiety occurs in the **hypothalamus**, which also regulates such important functions as respiration, body temperature, and water balance. The hypothalamus is also an important emotion center and controls molecules that make one feel happy or unhappy, both of which may affect the desire to eat or not to eat.

The taste, aroma, and texture of food are enjoyed through the parietal lobes of the brain. In the frontal part of these lobes are primary sensory areas that receive information about temperature and taste, as well as touch and movement.

Visual information plays a role in the decision to eat or not to eat. The occipital lobes at the back of the brain process images from the eyes and link the information with images stored in memory. The processing of all this information occurs in the cerebral cortex ("gray matter"), which is approximately one-half-inch thick covering over the cerebrum and cerebellum. Any injury to the brain that affects any of these areas can affect the desire or interest in eating. Approximately 50 million people in America (one in five) suffer damage to the brain and nervous system. Most of the damage occurs in older adults.

Appetite and Anorexia

Diminished appetite and/or anorexia in the older adult can result from a number of causes. The consequence of diminished appetite and anorexia is, of course, malnutrition. This can have severe consequences on quality of life, morbidity, and mortality. It is almost a universal symptom of those with serious and life-threatening illness. See Chapter 12 on cancer and appetite for supplemental information on this topic. See Chapter 20 for nutritional support for the older adult.

Physical Causes of Anorexia

Morely (1986) described the "anorexia of aging," suggesting that diminished nutrient intake in older adults is a result of diminished metabolic rate and decreased energy output. He also noted that inadequate food intake often may be due to compromised socioeconomic situations, depression, and/or dementia. Functional dependency can contribute to a slow, sustained weight loss.

Endocrine changes with aging also affect the appetite. Testosterone, leptin, cytokines, and cholecystokinin are involved in some of these changes. Other **anorexins** that act to suppress appetite include insulin, corticotropin-releasing hormone (CRF), and urocortin (a CRF satiety-signaling hormone).

With the diminution of the senses of smell and taste with aging, interest in food often diminishes. Diminution occurs because of loss of sensory neurons, loss of fungiform papillae of the tongue, and loss of cells in the olfactory bulbs.

Parageusia, an abnormal unpleasant taste, may occur in older adults and is common in those receiving chemotherapy for cancers. Nutrient deficiencies can also cause change in taste, as can many chronic illnesses and brain injury. (See Chapter 6 for more on this topic.) A number of medications can change the taste of foods and diminish interest in eating.

A simple questionnaire can be used to assess appetite. Questionnaires can be used with older adults living in the community and in hospitals, as well as those living in long-term care facilities. One good tool is the Simplified Nutritional Appetite Questionnaire (SNAQ). Another is the Council on Nutrition Appetite Questionnaire (CNAQ). These tools can be used to predict weight loss in these populations. Another nutrition assessment tool is the Mini Nutritional Assessment, which is used to identify older adults at risk of malnutrition.

If the older adult is at the end of life, actively dying, and does not want to eat, he or she should not be forced to eat. The use of ice chips, popsicles, moist compresses, or artificial saliva is useful in people with dry mouth. Lemon glycerine swabs are not used, because they irritate cracked mucosa. The drugs megestrol acetate and corticosteroids cause weight gain (mainly fat) and can improve quality of life of older adults with anorexia, but they do not prolong life.

Chronic mental health problems are often disabling. Common problems, including Huntington's chorea, dementias, oral health problems, antidepressants causing dry mouth, and depression, all contribute to lack of appetite/anorexia. Many of these disabilities cause difficulty in shopping, cooking, and eating.

Strategies

Social support is essential in managing the patient with lack of appetite/anorexia. It is often useful to collaborate with a registered dietician, home nursing caregiver, social workers, and family and friends. Consult with a pharmacist about medications that may be part of the anorexia problem. See that false teeth are clean and available. Advise the patient to avoid alcohol and tobacco, spicy food, and dry mouth. Water should be kept available for frequent sipping. Improve oral intake by providing meals of interest to the older adults via Meals on Wheels and family or neighbor

---

hypothalamus Link between the central nervous system and the endocrine system. Synthesizes and secretes neurohormones. Responsible for regulation of body temperature, hunger, thirst, and anger.

anorexins Anything causing anorexia (loss of appetite).

parageusia Unpleasant, abnormal taste of a food; often a metallic taste; may be caused by some medications.

support. Keep small nutritional snacks handy in the refrigerator or near the older adult. Keep areas clean from bad odors, such as those from bedpans and urinals. Caregivers should be encouraged to sit with the older adult or provide companionship during meals.

Cancer Cachexia and Anorexia

Cachexia is a complex metabolic wasting syndrome associated with anorexia with progressive unintentional weight loss, and depletion of host reserves of adipose tissue, skeletal muscle, and essential amino acids. The patient may be eating adequate calories and protein but is unable to absorb the nutrients because of the disease state. If the older adult loses more than 5% of premorbid weight in a six-month period, cachexia should be suspected.

The cause of cachexia is unknown, but it frequently occurs with cancers and can be a cause of considerable morbidity and mortality in older adults with cancer and in those undergoing chemotherapy. Cancer-related cachexia is associated with 20% to 40% of cancer deaths. Those with gastrointestinal cancers in the upper tract, lung cancers, and pancreatic cancers are especially likely to suffer significant weight loss. See Chapter 12 for care of the older adult with cancer.

Unfortunately, good nutrition, nutritional supplements, and dietary counseling do not always make a difference with cachexia. With anorexia, which is present in 15% to 25% of all cancers and is a side effect of cancer therapy, early satiety is a problem. If good nutrition can be obtained, malnutrition can be avoided because nutrition stores can be maintained.

A number of therapies of potential benefit are available for those with anorexia/cachexia. Some of these include the use of androgens/anabolic agents; cysteine and other amino acids; omega-3 fatty acids, especially eicosapentaenoic acid (EPA); progestational hormones; cardiovascular drugs, such as statins and ACE-inhibitors; some of the macrolide antibiotics; and creatine.

Depression in Older Adults

Depression is very common in older adults in the community and is even more common in hospitals and other institutional settings. It affects at least 50% of the patients in long-term care facilities. Depression is a mental disorder; it is not a normal part of aging. Depression is often a component of other mental disorders as well as a significant problem alone. In 2005 and 2006, 81.9% of adults older than 50 had received treatment for depression. In comparison, 70.3% of adults 35 to 49 and 64% of those adults 26 to 34 had been treated in the prior year. Depression is often a life-long disability.

It has been estimated that 65% to 70% of older adults in nursing facilities have significant mental disorders. Of adults with dementia, 30% to 40% have behavioral and psychiatric symptoms.

Malnutrition is prevalent in hospitalized older adults. An examination of older adults in hospitals found that only 18% were well nourished. Fifty-eight percent were at risk of malnutrition and 24% were malnourished. Those who had dementia or were cognitively impaired were significantly lower in frequency of good nutrition and higher in frequency of malnutrition.

In assisted living facilities, depression has long gone unrecognized, and therefore untreated, in older adults. Some older adults have suffered a lifelong depression. Others develop depression in response to losses of children, spouses, financial independence, and health (especially sight and hearing losses). These losses may manifest as vague clinical complaints, especially gastrointestinal complaints; isolation; attempts to gain attention; poor appetite; weight loss or weight gain; fatigue; depressed mood; insomnia; hypersomnia; loss of concentration; functional impairment; and loss of interest and pleasure. Because eating is often a pleasant activity, the sign of both of these—poor appetite and loss of interest and pleasure—may be synergetic in weight loss. **Parosmia**, abnormal sense of smell, can occur with severe depression.

Risk factors for depression include prior episodes of depression; a family history of depression; alcohol or other substance abuses; female gender; stresses, such as loss of spouse or child, divorce, retirement, trauma, physical or emotional abuse; perceived loss of social support; chronic illnesses and disability; and polypharmacy.

Suicide is a consideration in older adults with depression, especially in men aged 85 and older. Older adults have the highest incidence of suicide in the United States. The health care practitioner should ask if the older adult has considered suicide; sometimes it seems to the person that this is the only way out of a situation that seems hopeless. Social isolation is an important risk factor for suicide, as is a prior suicide attempt.

Some of the major causes of new onset of depression or worsening of a lifelong depression include cancer diagnosis, worsening health status, current alcohol abuse or other substance abuse, dementia, Parkinson's disease, stroke, arthritis, hip fracture, heart attack, chronic pulmonary disease, and functional disability. One must have an index of suspicion for depression when these disorders occur. The Geriatric Depression Scale is a useful tool to use during assessment. See **Box 13-1** for the short form.

Other systemic and metabolic disorders may have a depression component. Depression may be a prodrome of dementia, such as Alzheimer's disease (AD).

parosmia Distorted sense of smell; the person smells something unpleasant rather than the normal smell.

Other disorders with a depression component include infections, diabetes, obesity, cancers, anemias, hypothyroidism, and hyperthyroidism.

Some evidence suggests that functional deficiencies of omega-3 highly unsaturated fatty acids (HUFA), which have become relatively deficient in modern diets, may also be causative. Folate deficiency may be causative for onset of depression; however, it also reduces symptoms of depression in some individuals. Depressive symptoms are the most common neuropsychiatric manifestation of folate deficiency. The laboratory levels may be low or borderline.

Medications often have a depressive effect. Medications that have been linked with depression include steroids, narcotics, sedatives/hypnotics/antihypertensives, histamine-2 antagonists, beta blockers, antipsychotics, immunosuppressive agents, and cytotoxic agents.

Anxiety is a common mood disorder problem in the aged and is often linked with depression. Significant concurrent anxiety symptoms are found in two-thirds of older adults with depression. Concomitant anxiety and depression constitute a more severe illness and increase the probability of suicide.

Pain is often accompanied by depression. Pain and depression together are a vicious cycle that requires interruption. Enhance social supports and physical functioning. Identify strengths and capabilities.

Treatment

Treatment of depression with medication is usually successful. Treatment with **selective serotonin reuptake inhibitors (SSRIs)** has been found to diminish the number of suicides in older adults with both minor and major depression. SSRIs used as a first-line therapy for treatment of depression in older adults include citaloram, fluoxetine, and paroxetine. If it is a recurrent depression, the older adult should probably be maintained on a medication indefinitely. If it is a new depression, treatment should continue for six to nine months and medication slowly reduced and stopped and the patient reevaluated. The depression screening can be performed by a geriatric psychiatrist, the patient's primary care physician, or a nurse practitioner.

Side effects of SSRIs include somnolence, nausea, xerostomia, diaphoresis, anxiety, anorexia, diarrhea, and dyspepsia. Alcohol and nutraceuticals such as valerian, St. John's wort, SAMe, kava kava, and gotu kola should be avoided because they increase central nervous system depression.

Note that about 25% to 30% of patients with depression actually have bipolar illness with a component of mania or hypomania (fewer "high" symptoms). With bipolar illness, SSRIs may actually precipitate mania.

selective serotonin reuptake inhibitors (SSRIs) A class of antidepressants used to treat depression and anxiety disorders.

> **BOX 13·1   Geriatric Depression Scale, Short Version**
>
> - Are you basically satisfied with your life?
> - Do you often get bored?
> - Do you often feel helpless
> - Do you prefer to stay home rather than go out and do new things?
> - Do you feel pretty worthless the way you are now?
>
> *Source:* Data from Stanford University, Aging Clinical Research Center. Geriatric depression scale. Available at: http://www.stanford.edu/~yesavage/GDS.html. Accessed July 13, 2009.

In this instance, different medications are used. Lithium is the standard therapy for bipolar illness, although it is less effective in older adults. An anticonvulsant, such as valproate, and an atypical antipsychotic, such as quetiapine, are sometimes used together and have fewer side effects than lithium.

Many of the SSRIs also are useful in managing anxiety with depression. In addition, venlafaxine, a SNRI (serotonin-norepinephrine reuptake inhibitor), is another first-line drug in treatment for anxiety. Benzodiazepines should be used on a short-term basis to alleviate severe anxiety, although this class of drug is known to contribute to falls.

Psychotherapy is an important component in the treatment of depression. Medication plus psychotherapy has more benefit than either alone. Therapy may be done by a geriatric psychiatrist, geriatric nurse practitioner (GNP), geriatric psychiatric NP, social worker, psychologist, or other counselor. An assessment tool should be used to monitor the success, or lack of success, of therapy. Severe major depression is treated with electroshock therapy.

Treatment of depression in the older adult should also include frequent monitoring and promotion of good nutrition, elimination, sleep and rest, and physical comfort. Assess internal and external influences on hunger and appetite. Stress and mood can influence appetite just as do digestive functioning, metabolic influences, social situations, and even time of day. Depression is known as a treatable cause of weight loss. If the depression is caused by a nutritional deficiency, this should be managed.

Isolation

Isolation can contribute to depression. Living alone often results in the inability to meet dietary needs. People who have lost their spouses often lose their appetites, are lonely, and lose interest in cooking. They may eat very little and eat only one or two meals every day. Widowers often have never cooked meals and continue living alone without cooked meals. A well-balanced diet may not occur to this man; even those who do know how to cook often do not take the time to prepare adequate meals. Widows lose their appetites, are lonely, and lose interest in cooking. They may eat very little and eat one or two meals every day. Difficulty walking, lack of transportation, and similar problems may limit access to stores and shopping. Health problems may restrict cooking ability. These factors may affect the older adult's ability to maintain adequate nutrition. Lack of social supports worsens this situation. Widows lose their appetites, are lonely, and lose interest in cooking. They may eat very little and eat one or two meals every day.

Long-Term Care

Older adults who reside in long-term care facilities frequently are required to "eat what is served." In many instances, it is either a diet that is restricted for medical necessity or due to cost-saving measures by the facility. Medical nutrition therapy must balance medical needs and individual desires to maintain quality of life. The position of the ADA is that through liberalization of the diet prescription, superior quality of life and nutritional status may occur. Each patient should have an individualized nutrition intervention plan. An unpalatable diet or one that is personally unacceptable to the older adult leads to poor nutrition and fluid intake, weight loss, undernutrition, and negative health status. Be-

cause of the ADA's stance, long-term care facilities are developing person-centered or resident-centered care whereby the residents are involved in decision making about menus, schedules, and dining location. This enhances the desire to eat, the enjoyment of the food, and diminishes the risk for weight loss, undernutrition, and poor hydration.

Alzheimer's Disease and Other Dementias and Nutrition

The specific cause of Alzheimer's disease (AD) and most dementias remains unknown. However, people with AD have a large number of **neurofibrillary tangles and plaques** that form around a core of **amyloid**, which deposits in cerebral arteries (**Figures 13-1**). Dementias are not common in middle-aged or younger adults. Interestingly, there is substantially less AD neuropathology in older adults who have been treated with antihypertensive medications, suggesting a salutary effect of these drugs against AD neuropathology.

Researchers have found neurotransmitter defects in AD patients, prompting research in medications to treat AD. Commonly used medications include done-

neurofibrillary tangles and plaques Tangles are protein aggregates found in the neurons in Alzheimer's disease. Beta amyloid plaques are proteins found around the neurons in Alzheimer's disease. Together, they destroy neurons in the brain.

amyloid Insoluble proteins that aggregate abnormally. They are associated with a number of diseases, including Alzheimer's disease.

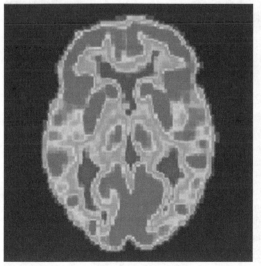
A.

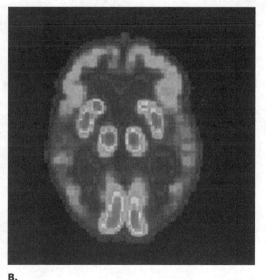
B.

FIGURE 13-1 Alzheimer's Disease Shown in PET Scans: (a) Normal Brain (b) Brain in Alzheimer's.

Source: Courtesy of the Alzheimer's Disease Education and Referral Center, a service of the National Institute on Aging

BOX 13-2 Drugs for Alzheimer's Disease and Side Effects

Drug	Problem Effects
Donepezil	Bradycardia (slow heart rate), diarrhea, nausea, vomiting, bladder outlet obstruction, headache, anorexia, weight loss, fecal incontinence, GI bleeding, frequent urination, muscle cramps. Avoid St. John's wort—decreases drug levels.
Galantamine	Nausea, vomiting, diarrhea, bradycardia, dizziness, anorexia, weight loss, abdominal pain, dyspepsia, flatulence, anemia. Avoid alcohol and St. John's wort.
Rivastigmine	Nausea, vomiting, diarrhea, anorexia, abdominal pain, dizziness, headache, fatigue, insomnia, dyspepsia, constipation. Avoid cigarettes, alcohol.
Memantine	Allergic reaction with hives, cough, shortness of breath, or rash; nausea, vomiting, diarrhea, constipation, anorexia, weight loss, tachycardia, edema of hands and feet. Avoid cigarettes.

Source: Data from Neighborcare. *Geriatric Drug Therapy Handbook, 2004–2005.* Hudson, OH: Lexi-Comp; 2004; Martignoni ME, Kunze P, Friess H. Cancer Cachexia. Molecular Cancer. 2003;2:36. Available at: http://www.molecular-cancer.com/content/2/1/36. Accessed August 2, 2006.

pezil, galantamine, rivastigmine, and memantine. See **Box 13-2** for side effects of some of these drugs. It should be noted that many psychiatrists and clinicians are treating AD with a combination of drugs. This decreases symptoms more than a single drug alone.

In 2007, nearly 47% of all nursing home residents had a diagnosis of AD. In assisted living, 45% to 67% have AD or another dementia. It is the fifth leading cause of death in adults 65 and older. Further, when adults with AD are hospitalized with a fractured hip or pneumonia, more than half die within six months compared with only 15% of those cognitively intact.

Vascular dementia is caused by atherosclerotic disease in small vessels in the brain. It does not cause the major symptoms of stroke, as with atherosclerosis of the larger vessels. The damage caused to the small vessels results in multiple infarcts and strokes in small areas, the incidence of which increases over time. With each small stroke, the symptoms of vascular dementia worsen. This stepping-stone-like change is diagnostic for vascular dementia. In one study by Vernooij and colleagues, researchers found that the prevalence of "microbleeds" in the cerebrum is quite high, occurring in approximately 18% of adults aged 60 to 69 and 38% and higher in those older than age 80. Many of these microbleeds were caused by hypertension and atherosclerosis. Those with more cardiovascular risk factors were found to have microbleeds in some areas of the brain. Microbleeds in other areas of the brain were caused by cerebral amyloid angiopathy.

Weight loss is a major concern for older adults with AD and other dementias in the later stages of illness. The stages of AD with signs and symptoms are presented in **Box 13-3**.

BOX 13-3 Stages of Alzheimer's Disease

Stage	Years After Diagnosis	Clinical Findings
I	1 to 3	Memory loss, especially recent memory, diminished visual-spatial skills, anomia (inability to retrieve words), irritability, apathy, depression
II	2 to 10	Severely impaired memory, spatial disorientation, fluent aphasia (impaired language), **apraxia** (inability to carry out motor activities despite intact motor function), indifference, apathy, agitation, wandering, pacing, screaming, cursing, repeating words and phrases, moaning, attention-seeking behaviors, sexual advances (verbal or physical), sleep disturbances, delusions, paranoia, hallucinations (visual and auditory), loss of judgment
III	8 to 12	Very deteriorated intellectual function, memory loss for old memories deteriorates so that only childhood memories remain, limb rigidity with difficulty moving, flexion posture, urinary and fecal incontinence, seizures

Source: Data from McCance K, Huether S. *Pathophysiology.* 5th ed. Philadelphia: Elsevier Mosby; 2006; Kempler D. Neurocognitive Disorders in Aging. Thousand Oaks, CA: Sage; 2005.

BOX 13-4 Management of Alzheimer's Disease and Other Dementias

- Use teamwork whenever possible; care is exhausting and often causes depression in the primary caregiver.
- Promote function and allow older adult to do what he or she is able to do.
- Use a preventive approach; put away unsafe items that may be consumed.
- Look for other safety issues; taking away the car keys is one of the most difficult tasks.
- Obtain identification bracelet or anklet in event that patient gets lost or wanders.
- Use humor with patient and self when possible to maintain joy in life.
- Keep patient at home as long as is possible; institutionalization often causes regression, increase in symptoms.
- Be cognizant of other chronic or acute health problems.
- Continue with glasses and hearing aids; loss of such aids can cause isolation.
- Try to prevent or reduce behavioral disturbances of older adult with dementia.
- Use medications as prescribed when possible; sometimes with paranoia, the older adult will refuse pills—try things like giving it with a favorite drink or food even if the drink is not healthy (like a cola).
- Use daycare when it is available so that caregivers can have a break.

- Use reminiscence to access retained memories.
- Avoid trialing herbals/nutraceuticals that have false claims for cure.
- Initiate activities to avoid apathy.
- Manage depression.
- Help orient to time, place, person. Introduce yourself every meeting time.
- Help family understand that they may need to introduce themselves to the patient.
- Recognize sleep disorders; often, night becomes day; obtain medical help.
- Continue with healthy exercising; patient might be able to use stationary bicycle or walk in the garden.
- Facilitate socialization, such as through dining or daycare.
- Anticipate problems with hospitalization and institutionalization, work to minimize; try to obtain specialized services such as those found in Alzheimer's units.
- Plan respite care for caregivers.
- Provide support groups for patients in first stage of illness.
- Get home care services when possible.
- Work with others to plan advanced directives, ethical decision making, health care proxies. Make sure family members are aware of disease progression so that they can plan palliative care and avoid inappropriate life support.

Source: Kempler D. *Neurocognitive Disorders in Aging*. Thousand Oaks, CA: Sage; 2005.

Weight loss may be caused by increased energy output in pacing and wandering; increased incidence of infections; inadequate food intake; loss of the ability to self-feed; as well as from depression and forgetfulness.

Management

Strategies for dealing with malnutrition and weight loss are found in many areas of the book. Strategies that are particularly useful for older adults with dementias are presented in **Box 13-4**. One of the most important strategies is establishing a routine so that failure to remember times or places does not cause anxiety and agitation. Another tool is the use of memory aids, such as large clocks, large dials on telephones, photographs of patient and family members from long ago (often the patient does not know children or spouse at this time, but does recall who they are with a photo when they were young or when first married).

Strategies for good nutrition include continuing to serve well-balanced meals and drinks that the patient likes and has always eaten. Consuming sufficient fluids is an ongoing challenge, because the patient may be unaware of thirst due to sensory losses. Alcohol and caffeine should be avoided. The patient should be given plenty of time to eat a meal. In addition, it is useful to make

apraxia Speech disorder whereby the person is unable to say what he or she wishes to say. There are two types: one occurs after a stroke in the area of the brain where speech originates, rending the patient unable to speak or unable to say what he wishes to say. The second type is caused by muscle weakness affecting the muscles used in speech.

mealtime a pleasant experience by providing music that the patient enjoys. Prompts will be necessary to initiate eating, because the older adult may not recognize why he or she is sitting at a table. Finger foods are useful after the patient is no longer able to eat with utensils. When feeding, focus on one food at a time. In late stages, pureed foods and thickened liquids may be required. The patient may also need to be fed. In some cases, tube feeding may be necessary.

The Mediterranean diet may be protective against mild cognitive impairment (MCI) which often precedes AD. Researchers have found that those who adhere to this diet have a reduced risk of developing MCI and a reduced risk of conversion to AD. Other studies have demonstrated that a simple walk every day helps keep the older adult mentally sharp. One therapy that does not work to prevent cognitive impairment is gingko biloba, a drug thought by many to be the panacea for many ills. One study by Dekosky et al. found that it was not effective in reducing dementia or the incidence of AD in older adults with normal cognition or in those with MCI.

Parkinson's Disease and Dietary Problems

Parkinson's disease (PD) is a form of Parkinsonism, a syndrome characterized by tremor, bradykinesia (slowed movements), rigidity, and postural instability. It is one of the most common neurological disorders. See **Box 13-5** for signs and symptoms of early, mid, and late stages of PD. The disease emerges primarily during middle-age and worsens dramatically with age. Many older adults with this disease become greatly disabled. Many have a concomitant dementia, frequently Lewy body dementia.

The etiology of PD remains unknown. Research suggests the incidence of PD is significantly lower in older adults who smoke and who have a higher intake of vitamin B6. The rationale is that high homocysteine levels accelerate dopaminergic cell death in PD through neurotoxic effects. Vitamin B6, folate, and vitamin B12 are cofactors in homocysteine metabolism. Dietary folate and vitamin B12 were not found to be associated with lower risk for PD.

Parkinson's Disease and Eating

Swallowing becomes more difficult with disease progression. Aspiration becomes common, and the risk for pneumonia increases. A number of techniques can be used to reduce the risk of aspiration and increase the comfort of eating a meal. The setting of the meal should be a quiet, relaxed atmosphere in which the older adult does not need to participate in the conversations at the table. Taking a breath to speak can cause aspiration of food. Lighting should be good so that all foods and consistencies can be seen. Eating when stressed or tired increases the risk for choking and aspiration.

▶ BOX 13-5 Signs and Symptoms of Parkinson's Disease by Disease Stage

Early Stage	Mid Stage	Late Stage
Fatigue	Resting tremor, "pill-rolling tremor" in fingers and thumbs, disappears in sleep	Inability to move (akinesia) or "freezing"
Malaise		Postural instability, unable to maintain balance
Personality changes	Asymmetrical tremor in body parts, head	Festinating gait (fast shuffling) forward momentum of body, propulsion
Weakness	Shaking	
Clumsiness	Sleep disorders	Dysphagia, aspiration, drooling
Incoordination	Micrographia (small writing)	Bradyphrenia (slowed thinking, cognition)
Difficulty writing	Seborrhea (oily skin and dandruff)	Dementia (20–40%), Alzheimer's disease, or vascular dementia
Pain, tension in muscles	Constipation	
	Difficulty and diminished swallowing	On-off phenomenon with medications
	Slumped forward posture	Hallucinations, psychosis (drug-induced)
	Low blood pressure	
	Dysarthria (soft, muffled, slurred speech)	
	Depression and anxiety	
	Diminished eye blinking	
	Short stepping and shuffling gait	

Source: Data from Kempler D. *Neurocognitive Disorders in Aging.* Thousand Oaks, CA: Sage; 2005; Mumenthaler M, Mattle H. *Neurology.* 4th ed. New York: Thieme; 2003.

In the nursing facility setting, it is better for those who require assistance with feeding to eat in the dining room. Those who eat in their rooms are at greater risk for unintentional weight loss. However, many older adults with PD spill food and drink during meals because of tremor and may wish to eat in isolation to avoid embarrassment. Further, it is helpful for them not to have social interactions during the meal, which distracts from careful chewing and planned swallowing.

Strategies for Eating

People suffering from PD should sit upright when eating snacks or meals or drinking fluids. When swallowing, they can tilt the head downward pointing the chin toward the chest. It may help to rest their elbows on the table with the chin resting in the palm of the hands to maintain the downward position of the head. They should remain seated for twenty to thirty minutes after the snack or meal.

Patients should be encouraged to eat four to six small meals/snacks throughout the day rather than eating the traditional three larger meals a day. Meals should be limited to 25 minutes or less. Patients should eat slowly and pause between bites of food and sips of fluids. Foods should be cut into tiny bites—one-half teaspoon or less—and served with a small spoon and sauces applied to dry foods. Other helpful measures to take when eating include using the elbow as a pivot to raise the fork or spoon from the plate to the mouth. Further, one can purchase or adapt utensils so that they are weighted for easier feeding.

When drinking, a straw may be helpful in controlling the amount of fluid taken, compared to a cup or glass. If the patient prefers a cup, both hands should be used to lift the glass or cup to the mouth. Ideally, use a plastic cup with double handles and a small opening for drinking.

The patient should avoid dry, tough, crumbly, particle foods like rice, foods with kernels or seeds, and stringy foods. Pureed, soft, or blenderized foods are easier to swallow. Liquids are often thickened to a honey or milkshake consistency. Commercial thickeners are available. If aspiration is common, it is best to avoid acidic and spicy foods, because these increase the risk of developing aspiration pneumonia.

All of these methods can be used when an older adult chokes and aspirates foods. An eating plan can be individualized and kept in a food diary so that different strategies that have been tried are known to anyone who helps care for this older adult. Consultation with a speech therapist is often useful.

Medications for Treatment of Parkinson's Disease

Surgical treatments are available for PD; however, the mainstay of management is drug therapy. A trial of levodopa can be used to diagnose early suspected PD. It will relieve symptoms that are vague and nondiagnostic. Although there is controversy as to whether to start levodopa early or late in the disease, the older adult often benefits from the drug and in many cases is able to continue with a normal lifestyle for a period of time. However, the effectiveness of levodopa decreases with extended use and as the disease worsens. The most frequently used medication therapy is a combination of carbidopa-levodopa once or twice a day or a sustained-release carbidopa-levodopa once a day. These drugs are not without side effects, including nausea and vomiting, which can be severe with considerable weight loss. See **Box 13-6** for other commonly used drugs for treatment of PD and their side effects.

Nutrition Management for Drug Side Effects

Levodopa/carbidopa has a number of drug and diet interactions that need to be considered. Alcoholic beverages should be avoided because they depress the central nervous system. High-protein diets are to be avoided because they interfere with absorption of the drug. Foods containing high amounts of vitamin B6 are to be avoided (however,

BOX 13-6 Side Effects of Drugs Used to Treat Parkinson's Disease

Drug	Side Effects
Carbidopa/Levodopa	Nausea, vomiting, hypotension, confusion, dyskinesia (involuntary movements)
Bromocriptine	Hypotension, nausea, edema, skin blotches (livido reticularis), confusion
Pergolide	Hypotension, nausea, edema, skin blotches, confusion
Pramipexole	Nausea, hypotension, sleep attacks, sedation, hallucinations
Ropinirole	Nausea, hypotension, sleep attacks, sedation
Entacapone	Hematuria (blood in urine), diarrhea
Tolcapone	Hematuria, diarrhea
Amantadine	Hypotension, nausea, edema, skin blotches, confusion
Benztropine mesylate	Anticholinergic: confusion, hallucinations, blurry vision, dry mouth, urinary retention, nausea
Selegiline	MOA oxidase inhibitor: agitation, insomnia, vivid dreams, and hallucinations

Source: Data from the National Parkinson Foundation. *Parkinson's Disease: Medications.* 2nd ed. Miami: NPF; 2003.

note that B6 has been suggested to reduce the development of PD). Herbal remedies and nutraceuticals containing more that 10 to 25 g of pyroxidine should be avoided; higher doses decrease the efficacy of levodopa/carbidopa. Kava also diminishes the effects of levodopa/carbidopa.

Patients should take levodopa/carbidopa 30 minutes before or at least one hour after mealtime. It should be taken with 4 to 8 ounces of water. A nonprotein snack—especially a light salty or sweet snack, such as pretzels or crackers—may be taken to minimize nausea. Ginger in any form is excellent for treating nausea and vomiting, which is particularly prominent when first starting levodopa/carbidopa. See **Box 13-7** for instructions on how to make ginger tea. Alternatively, crystallized ginger (available as a cooking spice or candy) can be sprinkled on food or kept handy to be nibbled as soon as queasiness begins.

Gastric emptying time is often delayed in older adults with PD. This will be exaggerated or aggravated by high-fat or high-fiber meals. A delay in gastric emptying will cause the drug to remain in the stomach for a prolonged period. The drug is designed to be absorbed in the small intestine, which is why it is best to take it 30 minutes prior to a meal.

Another component of PD is constipation. See Chapter 7 for information dealing with this topic.

The Older Patient with Stroke

Stroke is the third most common cause of death in the United States, after heart disease and cancer. In adults older than 70 years, stroke is the second highest cause of death. It is the main cause of focal neurologic dysfunction and the main cause of disability and death in older adults. Two-thirds of all strokes occur in adults older than age 65. It is less common in older women than in older men, except after age 85.

Four million people in the United States have survived a stroke and live with the aftereffects. One-third of stroke victims have only mild impairments; however, another third are moderately impaired, and another third are severely impaired.

Stroke (also called a cerebral infarction, cerebrovascular accident [CVA], or brain attack) is diagnosed based on signs and symptoms reported to the health professional by the patient or spouse or caregiver. Often the older adult has reported TIAs (transient ischemic attacks) over time, which heightens the ability to diagnose an imminent stroke and treat the underlying causes.

TIAs last less than 24 hours, although they are often only 2 to 15 minutes in duration and are reversible. In contrast, strokes are permanent, or nearly so. TIAs manifest as unilateral, bilateral, or alternating weakness; loss of coordination; and/or sensory disturbances of the face or limbs. The TIA may cause dysphasia, transient blindness of one or both eyes, gait disturbances, loss of equilibrium, diplopia (double vision), dysphagia, dysarthria (motor weakness of the mouth and speech) and dizziness.

Similarly, a stroke can have many different signs and symptoms. A stroke is caused by either an occlusion, such as from atherosclerosis or a thromboembolic event (most often), or a bleed in the brain. This causes loss of blood flow and cell death. The signs and symptoms of stroke depend on where in the brain the infarction occurs. Usually, it affects a particular region of the brain, causing focal neurological damage. Therefore, following a stroke some older adults will be paralyzed on one side or both; some will be unable to speak; and some will have sensory disturbances. Communication deficits may also occur following a stroke, including inappropriate verbal and nonverbal communication. This makes it difficult for the patient to convey his or her needs and wishes to another person, including health professionals. Other neurological changes include the loss of writing ability, aphasia (loss of the ability to produce or comprehend language), and perseveration. With aphasia, the patient's speech may be slow and halting and he or she might omit prepositions and articles, using just nouns or verbs. With perseveration, the patient uses the same term or label over and over to describe or define different objects.

Stroke Prevention

Risk factors for stroke that can be managed include hypertension (high blood pressure), heart disease, overweight and obesity, elevated homocysteine levels, dyslipidemia, smoking, lack of exercise, elevated CRP levels, and atherosclerosis. See **Figure 13-2** for the stages of atherosclerosis. Many of these risk factors are also seen in diabetes, making diabetes itself a risk factor. These risk factors can be managed with diet and exercise and medical interventions. Tight management of blood glucose may reduce the risk of stroke. Management of hypertension alone diminishes the risk for stroke by 40%. See Chapter 8 on cardiovascular disease and

---

◗ BOX 13-7 Ginger Tea for Nausea and Vomiting of Levodopa/Carbidopa

One-inch slice of ginger root.

Cover ginger root with water in a pan.

Bring to a boil and simmer 30 minutes.

Source: Data from Imke S. Parkinson's disease. More than meets the eye. *Adv Nurse Pract.* 2003 Sep;11(9): 42-54.

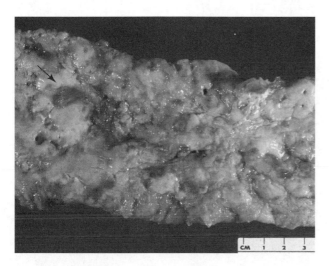

FIGURE 13-2 Stages of Atherosclerosis

Source: From *An Introduction to Human Disease.* 7th ed. Photo courtesy of Leonard V. Crowley, M.D., Century College.

Chapter 11 on endocrine problems for more information on management strategies for these risk factors.

Elevated homocysteine is associated with higher risk of cerebrovascular disease. In the HOPE 2 trial (Heart Outcomes Prevention Evaluation 2), the researchers found that lowering the homocysteine level with daily folic acid, vitamin B6, and vitamin B12 reduced the risk of stroke. However, when the subjects did have a stroke, it did not diminish the severity or disability.

Many older adults have atrial fibrillation (AF), which is an irregular heartbeat. AF can cause emboli (blood clots), which are treatable with medication. Low dose aspirin is often prescribed for older adults to reduce the development of blood clots, even in older adults without AF. Similarly, low to moderate amounts of alcohol (two or fewer drinks a day) can have a protective effect against atherosclerosis in the heart and brain. However, high intake of alcohol (more than five drinks a day) is highly correlated with stroke causation.

One new study by Jeffrey found that treatment for people with normal lipid levels with a statin drug (usually used to treat high lipid levels) had a 48% relative risk reduction for stroke. The subjects did have elevated C-reactive protein (CRP). High CRP is an inflammatory marker that may predict future stroke. Statins reduce CRP.

The Mediterranean diet is known to diminish risk for coronary heart disease. A new study by Fung, et al., has demonstrated that adherence to this diet also lowered risk for stroke in older women.

A meta-analysis of nine research studies by Arab, et al., found that people consuming more than three cups of black or green tea per day had a lower risk of stroke. The subjects had a 21% lower risk than those consuming less than one cup of tea per day.

Stroke Sequelae

Nearly 25% to 30% of those with a hemorrhagic stroke (bleed) die, and another 20% to 30% die within a month of the acute event. However, most strokes are occlusive, and a high percentage live with deficits. Initially after a stroke, a spontaneous recovery often occurs over three months, probably due to decreased swelling in the brain and return of local blood flow.

Some of the issues caregivers have in managing the patient with stroke include bladder and bowel function; cognition; other comorbid conditions; venous embolism; difficulty with communication; limb pain and dysfunction; osteoporosis; depression; and dysphagia. Even though many patients are fed nonorally, researchers in one study by Smucker found that 86% developed lower respiratory tract infections. Survivors of stroke are at increased risk for death from heart disease (35%); recurrent stroke (25%); pneumonia (15%); and pulmonary embolus (10%). This reflects the severity of the underlying illness.

Vitamin B12 Deficiency Dementia

The bioavailabilty of vitamin B12 (cobalamin) from food sources diminishes with age and there is a decline of serum B12 to low normal levels. Adults 50 years and older should eat foods fortified with vitamin B12 and take vitamin B12 supplements. However, reports indicate that 0% to 50% of older adults living in the community do not consume the recommended amount of vitamin B12 (2.4 µg/day).

Low-normal and subnormal amounts of vitamin B12 result in vague symptoms, which may not call attention to the seriousness of later signs and symptoms, which may be irreversible. Clinical signs of B12 deficiency include mood swings, infections, GI disturbances, kidney problems, and cardiac problems. Further, low levels of vitamin B12 (and folate) lead to increased levels of homocysteine, which is implicated in heart disease. Because so many older adults are found to have low levels of vitamin B12 and folate, it is reasonable to give oral doses, because 10% will be absorbed even in those without intrinsic factor (a protein made by the stomach and needed to absorb vitamin B12 in the large intestine).

Pernicious anemia (PA), the most common type of megaloblastic anemia (see Chapter 10), is diagnosed predominantly in adults older than 60 years; however, it probably is present for 20 to 30 years prior to diagnosis. This vitamin B12 deficiency is the result of chronic atrophic autoimmune gastritis, type A. This disorder was once fatal. It occurs in females more often than males and at an earlier age in African American females.

Later clinical signs and symptoms at time of diagnosis are usually severe. Signs of pernicious anemia include weakness, fatigue, and paresthesias of the feet and fingers, which cause difficulty walking. The neurological manifestations are often the result of neuron cell death. The spinal cord may be affected with loss of position and vibration senses, ataxia, and spasticity. Cognitive changes range from loss of concentration to memory loss, disorientation, and dementia. Again, this is usually not reversible. Other signs and symptoms include sallow skin and a combination of pallor and icterus. The tongue may be beefy red from atrophic glossitis. The liver can be enlarged, indicating right-sided heart failure, which is often the cause of death.

The diagnosis of pernicious anemia is made with the combination of low serum B12, normal folate, high MCV (mean corpuscular volume), high plasma iron, high ferritin, and normal total iron-binding capacity. The hemoglobin and hematocrit are low; however, blood levels are neither necessarily anemic nor megaloblastic. Some specialists may order bone marrow aspiration, gastric biopsy, and the Schilling test for urinary secretion of B12 (rarely done today). Early tests include homocysteine and methylmalonic acid serum levels, which are elevated in early pernicious anemia.

Treatment consists of replacement of cobalamin or vitamin B12. It is administered intramuscularly once a month for life. Early management is intramuscular cobalamin once a week until laboratory studies are corrected.

Postpolio Syndrome

It is uncommon during a patient assessment to ask about polio, which has been eradicated in the United States. This viral disease was devastating in the early to mid-twentieth century, causing much fear and curtailment of social activities, especially in summer months.

Polio survivors have been reporting new or renewed symptoms decades after the disease subsided. A prominent symptom described by polio survivors is profound weakness and fatigue similar to ALS (amyotrophic lateral sclerosis). These older adults have what is described as "metabolic exhaustion" and often lose their ability to function. There is no diagnostic tool for this new picture of polio.

Management is basically the conservation of energy, with frequent rest periods throughout the day. However, planned exercise is important so that there is no further decline in muscle strength.

Nutrition counseling is essential. Older adults with postpolio syndrome often have difficulty swallowing and may require softer foods and a schedule of meals at times of the day when fatigue and weakness and pain are at their lowest. Support includes community services such as food preparation and/or delivery and support group therapy. It is best if they are managed by a registered dietician who is experienced with polio survivors.

Conclusion

The brain is an immensely complex part of the body that regulates all of the organs. Neurological disorders can result in anorexia, gait disturbance, depression, dizziness, dementia, sleeplessness, psychosis, and stroke, to name just a few. With careful assessment, early diagnosis of many of these problems may occur so that treatment and prevention of further disability may allow the older adult to live with the greatest quality of life possible.

Activities Related to This Chapter

1. Discuss in a group the changes in the brain with the different neurologic problems of older adults.
2. Describe how to manage the older adult with stroke who is paralyzed on the right side of the body.
3. List ways you could assist the older patient with postpolio syndrome with diet management.
4. Meet with a patient with dementia and develop a plan of care for nutrition management.

Case Study

Mr. Collins is an 84-year-old widower who lives in an assisted-living facility. He has been fairly healthy, walks with a walker to meals, and is socially inclined. Very recently he had a stroke and is now paralyzed on the right side of his body. He is a right-handed person. Plan your nutrition support for this patient.

Questions

1. What strengths does Mr. Collins have in his favor?
2. How can you assist him in beginning to eat?
3. What kinds of foods will he start eating at this time?
4. How will you progress this regimen?
5. How will you approach his right-handedness?

REFERENCES

Alpert J, Fava M. Nutrition and depression: the role of folate. *Nutr Rev* 2003; 55(5):145–149.

Alzheimer's Association. Alzheimer's disease facts and figures 2008, part 4. *Assisted Living Consult.* 2008;4(5):22–27.

Alzheimer's Association. Alzheimer's disease facts and figures 2008, part 5. *Assisted Living Consult.* 2008;4(6):16–18.

American Geriatric Society. *Geriatric Review Syllabus, 2006.* New York: American Geriatric Society; 2006.

American Geriatric Society. *Nursing Geriatric Review Syllabus, 2007.* New York: American Geriatric Society; 2007.

American Dietetic Association. Position of the American Dietetic Association: Liberation of the diet prescription improves quality of life for older adults in long-term care. *JADA.* 2005;105(12):1955–1965.

American Family Physician. Managing cancer cachexia. 2004. Available at: www.aafp.org/afp/20040215/tips/21.html. Accessed August 2, 2006.

Arab L, Weiqing L, Elashoff D. Green and black tea consumption and risk of stroke. A meta-analysis. *Stroke.* 2009;40:1786–1792.

Chapman I. Endocrinology of anorexia of aging. *Best Pract Res Clin Endocrin Metabol.* 2004; 18(3):437–452.

Chernoff R. *Geriatric Nutrition.* 3rd ed. Sudbury, MA: Jones & Bartlett; 2006.

Dekosky S, Williamson J, Fitzpatrick A, Kronmal R, et al. Ginkgo biloba for prevention of dementia. *JAMA.* 300(19):2253–2262.

deLau LML, Koudstaal PJ, Witteman JCM, Hofman A, Breteler MMB. Dietary folate, vitamin B12, and vitamin B6 and the risk of Parkinson disease. *Neurology.* 2006;67:315–318. Ebersole P, Hess P, Touhy T, Jett K, Luggen A. *Toward Healthy Aging.* 7th ed. Philadelphia: Mosby/Elsevier; 2008.

Family Medicine. Family practice notebook: cachexia in cancer. Available at http://www.fpnotebook.com/HEM36.htm. Accessed August 2, 2006.

Fung T, Rexrode K, Mantzoros C, Manson J, et al. Mediterranean diet and incidence of and mortality from coronary heart disease and stroke in women. *Circulation.* 2009;119:1093–1100.

GeroNurseOnline. Depression. Available at: http://www.geronurseonline.org/index/cfm?section_id=35&geriatric_topic_id=15&sub_se. Accessed August 1, 2006.

Hoffman L, Schmeidler J, Lesser G, Beeri M, et al. Less Alzheimer disease neuropathy in medicated hypertensive than nonhypertensive persons. *Neurology.* 2009;72(20):1720–1726.

Imke S, Parkinson's disease, more than meets the eye. *Adv for NPs.* 2003;11(9):42–54.

Insel P, Turner RE, Ross D. *Nutrition.* 2nd ed. Sudbury, MA: Jones & Bartlett: Sudbury MA; 2004.

Jackson WC. Strategies in the treatment of bipolar disorder. Pri-Med Updates. September 29–30, 2006, Cincinnati, Ohio.

Jeffrey S. JUPITER stroke results show significant reduction in stroke risk. Report from the American Stroke Association International Stroke Conference 2009. Available at: http://www.medscape.com/viewarticle/588515/. Accessed May 27, 2009.

Kempler D. *Neurocognitive Disorders in Aging.* Thousand Oaks, CA: Sage; 2005.

Kennedy G, Katz I, Conwell Y. Prevention of suicide in older persons: lessons and limitations of evidence-based interventions. *Annals of LTC.* 2004;12(8):43–48.

Ludwig S. Oral health and careful eating and swallowing. *The Grapevine, Ohio Parkinson Foundation.* 23(4):3.

Martignoni ME, Kunze P, Friess H. Cancer cachexia. *Mol Cancer.* 2003;2:36.

McCance KL, Huether SE. *Pathophysiology.* 5th ed. Philadelphia: Elsevier/Mosby; 2006.

Morely J, Silver A, Fiatarone M, et al. Nutrition and the elderly—Grand rounds. *J Am Ger Soc.* 1986;34:823–832.

Mumenthaler M, Mattle H. *Neurology.* 4th ed. New York: Thieme; 2003.

National Cancer Institute, National Institutes of Health. Nutrition in cancer care. 2006. Available at: http://www.nci.nih.gov/cancertopics/pdq/supportivecare/nutrition/healthprofessional. Accessed August 1, 2006.

National Institute on Aging. Depression. Available at: http://www.nia.nih.gov/healthinformation/publications/depression.htm. Accessed May 21, 2008.

National Institute of Neurological Disorders and Stroke. Brain basics: know your brain. Available at: http://www.ninds.nih.gov/disorders/brain_basics/know_your_brain.htm. Accessed May 21, 2008.

National Parkinson Foundation. Parkinson's Disease: Medications. 2nd ed. Miami, FL: National Parkinson Foundation; 2003.

NeighborCare. *Geriatric Drug Therapy Handbook, 2004–2005.* Hudson, OH: LexiComp; 2004.

Orsitto G, Fulvio F, Tria D, Turi V, et al. Nutritional status in hospitalized elderly patients with mild cognitive impairment. *Clin Nutr.* 2009;28(1):100–102.

Ravindran L, Conn D, Ravindran A. Pharmacotherapy of depression in older adults. *Geriatrics & Aging.* 2005;8(8):20–27.

Reuben DB, Herr KA, Pacala JT, Pollock BG, Potter JF, Semla TP. *Geriatrics at Your Fingertips, 2007–2008.* 9th ed. New York: American Geriatric Society; 2007.

Richardson AJ. The role of omega-3 fatty acids in behaviour, cognition, and mood. *Scandinavian J Nutr.* 2003;47(2):92–98.

Saposnik G, Ray J, Sheridan P, McQueen M, et al. Homocysteine-lowering therapy and stroke risk, severity and disability. Additional findings from the HOPE 2 Trial. *Stroke.* 2009;40(4):1365–1372.

Scarmeas N, Stern Y, Mayeux R, Manly J, et al. Mediterranean diet and mild cognitive impairment. *Arch Neurol.* 2009;66(2):216–225.

Searle J. Eating and swallowing. Kansas University Medical Center. Available at: http://www.kumc.edu/hospital/huntingtons/swallowing.html. Accessed August 10, 2006.

Simmons SF, Levy-Storms L. The effect of dining location on nutritional care quality in nursing homes. *J Nutr Health Aging.* 2005;9(6):434–439.

Smeets P, deGraaf C, Stafleu A, van Osch M, Nievelstein R, van der Grond J. Effect of satiety on brain activation during chocolate tasting in men and women. *Am J Clin Nutr.* 2006;83(6):1297–1305.

Smucker WD. Stroke: recognition, management and prevention in long-term care. *Caring for the Ages*, supplement, highlights of a symposium March 8, 2008, Salt Lake City, Utah.

Stefanacci RG. How big an issue is depression in assisted living? *Assisted Living Consult.* 2008;4(4):30–40.

Truesdell DD. The efficacy of nutrition and lifestyle approaches in the treatment of depression. *Topics in Clin Nutr.* 2009;24(1):55–66.

Vernooij M, van der Lugt A, Ikram M, Wielopolski A, Niessen W, et al. Prevalence and risk factors of cerebral microbleeds. *Neurology.* 2008;70:1208–1214.

Williams G, Jiang JG, Matchar D, Samsa GP. Incidence and recurrence of total stroke. *Stroke.* 1999;30(12):2523–2528.

Wilner A. Study shows combination therapy superior for Alzheimer's disease. *CNS Senior Care.* 2008;7(4):1,14.

Wilson M, Thomas D, Rubenstein L, Chibnall J, Anderson S, Baxi A, et al. Appetite assessment: simple appetite questionnaire predicts weight loss in community-dwelling adults and nursing home residents. *Am J Clin Nutr.* 2005;82(5):1074–1081.

Weight Loss and Obesity in Older Adults

Bonnie L. Callen, RN, PhD, CPHCNS-BC and
Ann Schmidt Luggen, PhD, GNP

CHAPTER OBJECTIVES   Upon competition of this chapter, the reader will be able to:

1. Discuss the importance of weight management in older adults
2. Recognize the factors associated with weight loss in older adults
3. Describe interventions for management of undernutrition
4. Examine the importance of psychosocial factors that contribute to weight loss or obesity in older adults
5. Understand the impact of obesity in older adults
6. List some interventions the dietician or health professional can use to help with weight problems in older adults.

KEY TERMS AND CONCEPTS

BMI (body mass index)   Protein-energy malnutrition (PEM)

Malnutrition   Undernutrition

Obesity

It cannot be emphasized enough that proper nutrition is essential for maintaining health, function, and overall well-being. The term **malnutrition** covers a broad spectrum of conditions, including **undernutrition**, in which nutrients are undersupplied; overnutrition, in which food and sometimes nutrients are oversupplied (**obesity**); or specific nutrient deficiencies. The malnourished individual may, therefore, be obese, of normal weight, or thin. **Protein-energy malnutrition (PEM)** is the most common type of undernutrition in older adults and is a significant cause of weight loss.

Other nutritional problems and deficiencies include fiber, long-chain omega-3 fats, vitamin D, magnesium, calcium, folic acid, B6, B12, selenium, zinc, chromium, and iron. Correcting many of these is not an easy task because the recommended daily allowances the government has established do not clarify optimal intake. Decreases in cholesterol to less than 160 predicts mortality.

Although the reliability of clinically significant malnutrition is important when targeting and evaluating nutritional interventions, assessment of nutritional status remains a controversial issue in clinical practice. Nutritional status is

malnutrition Failure to achieve nutrient requirements, which can impair physical and/or mental health. May result from consuming too little food or a shortage or imbalance of key nutrients.

undernutrition Poor health resulting from the depletion of nutrients due to inadequate nutrient intake over time. It is most often associated with poverty, alcoholism, and certain eating disorders.

obesity BMI at or above 30 kg/m^2.

protein-energy malnutrition (PEM) A condition resulting from long-term inadequate intakes of energy and protein that can lead to wasting of body tissues and increased susceptibility to infection.

probably best detected through a combination of laboratory measures, assessment of nutrient intake, and anthropometric measurements.

Anthropometric methods of nutritional assessment are commonly used in the community setting to describe nutritional health. These methods are simple, inexpensive, and fairly reliable. Undernutrition, or a lack of sufficient protein or calorie intake, is most commonly assessed using **body mass index** (**BMI**), which is the ratio of weight in kilograms to height (in meters) squared. A BMI of 21 or less is consistent with malnutrition in older adults. Nearly 25% of older adults living in the community are malnourished.

Common biochemical indicators of mild undernutrition are a serum albumin 2.8–3.5 g/dL; moderate depletion is a serum albumin of 2.1–2.7 g/dL; and severe depletion is less than 2.1 g/dL. Albumin has a half life of 15–20 days. A prealbumin is another important indicator and its half life is 1–2 days; it is useful for assessment of short-term PEM. Mild depletion is 10–15 g/dL; moderate deletion 5–10 g/dL; and severe is less than 5 g/dL. Low levels are linked to an increase in morbidity and mortality. A serum cholesterol less than 160 mg/dL (low) is indicative of insufficient calories being consumed. Total lymphocyte count of less than 1500–1800 is considered malnourished; a count of less than 1000 is severely malnourished. Some of these parameters may be abnormal in several conditions not associated with malnutrition; nonetheless, they are useful indicators of malnutrition.

Signs and symptoms of older adults who are undernourished may not change. If only protein is deficient, weight may be normal or even higher. Many older adults, however, lose their muscle mass and body fat and are clearly underweight. When severely underweight, bones protrude and temples of the head appear hollow. The skin is pale, cold, thinned, dry, and inelastic. Hair is dry and sparse. The patient feels tired, weak, sleepy, and often dizzy, and may fall. Infections are more likely and wounds less likely to heal. The older adult may not be aware of any of these changes, although family members often are. Underweight is associated with increased hospitalizations, length of time in hospital, and higher risk for mortality.

The combination of aging and undernutrition can lead to a downward spiral of poor health. It can contribute to physical illness and exacerbate existing medical conditions. Undernutrition has been positively correlated with poor functional status, increased burden of disease and disease-related complications, increased severity of disability, and diminished quality of life in older persons. Despite the high prevalence of undernutrition in the older adult population, physicians and other health-care professionals often overlook and fail to treat it.

body mass index (BMI) Ratio of weight in kilograms to height (in meters) squared.

Importance of Undernutrition and Weight Loss

Unintentional weight loss represents a cardinal symptom of frailty in the older adult. In 1859, Florence Nightingale wrote, "Thousands are annually starving in the midst of plenty." Nearly 150 years later, she might have written the same thing. Understanding the causes of frailty in older adults and managing it is a research goal of the National Institute of Aging.

Weight loss is an important predictor of early institutionalization among community-dwelling older adults. Over 90% of older adults admitted to a skilled nursing facility after hospitalization either have malnutrition or are at high risk of undernutrition. One-fourth to two-thirds of older adults in the nursing facility are malnourished. Undernutrition and weight loss are common and potentially serious problems among older residents of long-term care (LTC). The incidence of weight loss and cachexia in this population has been reported to be as high as 55% to 65%. Compared to other nursing home residents, those who have lost weight or who are underweight have worse clinical outcomes.

Due to illness prior to hospitalization, older adults may already be malnourished when they are admitted to the hospital. In the months before hospitalization, 65% of males and 69% of females have had insufficient energy intake. One study published by the Library of the National Medical Society found that 15% of older adults ate less than 1000 kcal/day and just 30% of impoverished older adults ate more than 1000 kcal/day.

It is estimated that 40% to 60% of hospitalized older patients are malnourished. When undernourished older adults are admitted to the hospital, they fare worse than their well-nourished counterparts. Nutritional deficits are likely to get worse during hospitalization, because the majority of patients are unable to eat enough to meet most of their basal protein or energy requirements. Further, the rigid diets offered in hospitals (an average of 2128 kcal) are wasted because few older adults are able to eat this. To sustain weight, 1400 kc/day are required. There is a need for quality nutritional care before, during, and after hospitalization.

Dramatic weight loss and hypoalbuminemia often follow acute hospitalization. In a study by Thomas, Zdrowski, and colleagues of 837 older patients admitted to a subacute care unit, almost one-third (29%) were malnourished and almost two-thirds (63%) were at risk of malnutrition. The Geriatric Depression Score was higher in malnourished subjects than in nutritionally at-risk subjects. A study of undernutrition and risk of mortality in older adult patients within one year of hospital discharge by Sullivan, Liu, et al. found that a BMI below 20 and weight loss in the year prior to hospital admission were strong predictors of post-discharge mortality.

Factors Contributing to Poor Nutrition

Many factors are associated with poor nutrition among the older adult population (See **Box 14-1**). These include normal physiological changes of aging, mechanical barriers, medical conditions, psychological factors, and social factors.

Physiological Changes of Aging

Some of the physiological changes of aging include changes in height and weight distribution, decreased taste and smell, and decreased appetite (see Chapter 2). These contribute to poor nutrition in older adults.

Reduction in Height and Weight Distribution

BMI is widely used as a noninvasive measure of nutritional status. BMI combines weight and height into a single number. It is a useful predictor of undernutrition, especially in community settings where laboratory markers are not available. However, BMI is influenced by normal changes with aging, such as reduction in height and changes in fat distribution. Identification of the presence of protein-energy malnutrition (or obesity) can be facilitated by determination of BMI.

Height decreases between 1 and 2 cm per decade after age 50, and even faster in people older than 85 years old. A loss of 2 or more inches in adulthood is a strong predictor of osteoporosis of the hip and risk of hip fracture. Loss of 2 to 3 inches is four times the risk for osteoporosis and 3 or more inches increases the risk ten times. In one study by Dey, the subjects were women, average age 60 and postmenopausal. The loss of estrogen dramatically increased bone loss. A European 25 year longitudinal study reported a height decrease of 4–4.9 cm in men and women between the ages of 70 and 95. The principle causes were vertebral compression, height and morphologic changes of vertebral discs, loss of muscle tone, and loss of bone mineral density. Height needs to be measured accurately for many of the tools used to assess nutrition. Often patients and families will offer the height from younger years. Further, measuring the usual way is not always possible with older frail adults. According to Collins, one accurate method is to measure knee height (KH). The formula for the older adult is: stature equals 59.01 plus (2.08 KH) for white men. For white women, stature equals 75 plus (1.91 KH) minus (0.17 [age in years]).

In men, body weight tends to peak at age 65 and then decreases in the following years. In women, maximum weight is reached at age 75. In both genders, mean BMI decreases after the 70s. An important cause of weight loss during aging is the reduction in muscle mass, called sarcopenia, which occurs with aging. Still another change with aging is the progressive increase of adipose tissue in the trunk and abdomen, while subcutaneous fat decreases, especially in the limbs. Because body fat in the abdominal cavity in-

creases with aging, BMI becomes a poorer indicator of both overall and central fatness in older adults.

Caloric requirement decreases with aging. However, required nutrients do not diminish. The Harris Benedict equation is useful for determination of caloric need and includes height, weight, age, activity level, and stress level. This tool can be seen at www.bmi-calculator.net/bmr-calculator/harris-benedict-equation/.

BOX 14-1 Conditions Associated with Undernutrition

1. Physiological Conditions of Aging
   a. Alterations in taste and smell
   b. Loss of appetite/anorexia

2. Mechanical Barriers
   a. Poor oral health status/dentition
   b. Poor eyesight
   c. Poor motor coordination
   d. Slow eating pace
   e. Therapeutic or mechanically altered diet
   f. Dysphagia

3. Medical Conditions Leading to Increased Energy Requirements
   a. Cancer
   b. Infections
   c. COPD
   d. Wounds, burns, fractures

4. Medical Conditions Leading to Interferences with Eating
   a. Congestive heart failure
   b. Malabsorption syndrome
   c. Diabetic gastroparesis
   d. Cholelithiasis

5. Psychological Conditions
   a. Depression
   b. Dementia
   c. Paranoia

6. Social Factors
   b. Poverty
   c. Isolation
   d. Ethnicity/preferences

Source: Data from Thomas DR. Are older people starving to death in a world of plenty? *Nestle Nutr Workshop Ser Clin Perform Programme.* 2005;10:15-23; discussion 23-19.

Reduction in Taste and Smell

Among the normal age-related changes are diminished taste and smell (see Chapter 6). With aging, the taste sensory threshold increases and the sense of smell decreases. Individuals with a history of smoking or poor dental hygiene are more likely to experience decline in their ability to taste. This may be related to swelling and blockage of the salivary ducts. Medications and disease may also cause alterations in taste. These deficits make food less appealing and flavorful and may decrease food consumption, contributing to negative changes in eating behaviors.

Decrease in Appetite and Anorexia

A decrease in appetite with age is a major contributor to declining nutrition and subsequent weight loss in older adults. Older adults feel full with less food due to an increased satiety effect thought to be caused by nitric oxide deficiency. One consequence of this caloric decline is that when older adults develop disease processes, they are more at risk for malnutrition. A physiological anorexia of aging affects nearly all older persons with a decline in caloric intake over the lifespan. This appears to be predominantly due to altered gastric signals resulting in early satiation. Leptin levels decrease with loss of body fat, which decreases at about age 70 in women. Men have increased levels of leptin with fat loss, probably due to loss of testosterone. Further, many of the medications taken by older adults have anorexia as a major adverse effect (e.g., digoxin, phenytoin, SSRIs, calcium-channel blockers, proton-pump inhibitors, ipratropium bromide, and furosemide) or they may reduce nutrient availability in the older adult (e.g., antacids, levodopa, laxatives, metformin, salicylates, digoxin, and diuretics) (**Box 14-2**).

The older adult population does not show changes in their feelings of hunger in response to the caloric content of ingested nutrients. This means that there appears to be a decoupling of hunger and nutrient ingestion in older individuals. There is a satiety index, although it has not been tested specifically on older adults. With the index, foods are compared to white bread, which is the index food. Those with the same or higher level of satiety as white bread include ice cream, cookies, crackers, lentils, cheese, eggs, baked beans, fish, beef, oatmeal, oranges, French fries, pastas, rice, boiled potatoes (highest), and whole grain bread. Many of these foods contain fewer nutrients than we would hope to see in a healthy diet.

Anorexia may be associated with illness, drugs, dementia, or mood disorders. Depression is commonly associated with anorexia.

Polypharmacy is prevalent in older adults and is one of the strongest indicators of malnutrition. Many drugs are associated with anorexia (see **Box 14-2**).

BOX 14-2 Medications that Produce Anorexia

Generic Name	Brand Name
Amblodipine	Norvasc
Aspirin	
Cholecystamine	Questran
Ciprofloxacin	Cipro
Conjugated equine estrogen	Premarin
Digoxin	Lanoxin
Enalapril	Vasotec
Famotidine	Pepcid
Fentanyl	Duragesic
Fluoxetine	Prozac
Furosemide	Lasix
Hydralazine	Apresoline
Levothyroxine	Synthroid
Nifedipine	Procardia
Nizatidine	Axid
Omeporazole	Prilosec
Paroxitine	Paxil
Phenytoin	Dilantin
Potassium replacement	K-Dur
Propoxyphene/Acetaminophen	Darvocet, Propacet
Quinidine	Quinadine Duratabs
Ranitidine	Zantac
Resperidine	Risperidal
Sertraline	Zoloft
Theophylline	
Vitamin A	
Warfarin	Coumadin

Source: Data from Endoy MP. Anorexia among older adults. *The American Journal of Nurse Practitioners.* 2005;9(5), 31-38.

Mechanical Barriers Contributing to Poor Nutrition

Poor oral health may contribute to malnutrition. Tooth or mouth pain or poor-fitting dentures may make a person avoid crisp foods such as fresh fruits and vegetables that have high nutrient content. Food consistency and the unpalatability of some special diets may result in reduced intake.

Physical activity may become more difficult with declining mobility, failing eyesight, or fear of falling. Declining mobility makes it more difficult to shop for and prepare food. Pain from arthritis may make it more difficult to prepare fresh fruits and vegetables and other foods. Older adults with arthritis become less mobile. Dependence on others for assistance in eating may reduce intake if meals are hurried for older adults who eat slowly. This is especially a problem in understaffed nursing facilities.

Therapeutic diets have been shown to be associated with weight loss. Special restrictive diets for cholesterol, salt, or sugar reduction often reduce intake without significantly helping the individual's clinical status. Some older adults excessively restrict their food intake based on studies showing a link between caloric restriction and longevity in animals, leading to malnutrition. Others try to limit their diet in an effort to lower their cholesterol. A recent 2-year study by Sacks, et al. has demonstrated what we already knew: a decrease in calories equals a decrease in weight, just as an increase in calories leads to an increase in weight.

Unrecognized feeding problems and failure to provide proper feeding techniques for those with dysphagia may cause weight loss. This occurs in older adults with stroke and disorders such as Parkinson's disease.

Medical Conditions Contributing to Poor Nutrition

Many diseases are associated with protein-energy malnutrition or are worsened by malnutrition. Increased metabolic requirements may be precipitated by fever, infection, or the presence of chronic skin wounds. One study by Guo, et al. of older patients with hip fractures and slow wound-healing evaluated tools and measures to identify those at risk for delayed healing.

Although acute illness is characterized by a spontaneous decrease in food intake, healing increases the need for nutrients. Cancer, in particular, is a cause of weight loss in some older adults. Undernutrition in these patients impacts survival. People with COPD have an increased resting metabolic rate, but a decrease in their physical activity. They become hypoxic while eating because of a lack of oxygen needed to maintain the therapeutic energy of eating. This leads to food avoidance and severe anorexia and weight loss. Gallstones can present with early satiation, leading to declining nutrition. Hepatic congestion decreases albumin production and loss of protein from the gut. Uncontrolled diabetes is also associated with weight loss due to changes in metabolism and the speed at which food moves through the digestive tract. GERD (gastroesophageal reflux disease), peptic ulcers, constipation, diarrhea, and irritable bowel disease can all contribute to poor nutrition. Arthritis, gout, and other musculoskeletal disorders contributing to immobility are other medical and mechanical problems that contribute to poor nutrition. In the instance of a person with Parkinson's disease the metabolism is higher, caus-

ing weight loss, just as the intake is less, enhancing the problem. Additional medical conditions that are associated with protein-energy malnutrition include anemia, pressure ulcers, sarcopenia, bone loss and hip fractures, declining immune function, impaired immune response to vaccinations, infections, and cognitive impairment.

In addition, chronic disease can result in difficulties with the mechanical requirements of eating. In long-term care facilities, nearly 50% of all residents are unable to eat independently. The intake of many residents is less than 1000 kcal/day. As a result, 5% to 59% of adults in long term care are at significantly higher risk for death than those adults who are overweight.

Psychological Factors Contributing to Poor Nutritional Status

Depression is one of the most common reversible causes of weight loss (or weight gain) in the older population. Older women report more depressive symptoms than men. Common situations such as institutionalization, widowhood, loneliness, sense of abandonment, feeling useless, and isolation, may lead to depression, which in turn, leads to either weight loss or obesity. A major contributor to depression in older adults is the high rate of illness and disability. Depression is common in patients with cancer, and 80% of all cancers occur in persons older than 60 years. A diagnosis of failure to thrive has also been closely correlated with depression in older adults.

Reports of the prevalence of depression in the older adult population vary widely across settings. One report found 8% to 16% of community-dwelling older adults to be depressed. Other reports have found that depression affects 10% to 22% of those in long-term care and 36% to 46% of older hospitalized patients. In Greece, 35.8% of a sample of 682 seniors aged 60 and older met the Geriatric Depression Scale-4 criteria for depression.

Nearly one-third of older adults with weight loss have depression. The relationship between age and depression has been reported to be U-shaped. A study of 1,408 U.S. adults participating in the 1996 General Social Survey showed that depression decreased in young adulthood into midlife and then increased among the oldest-old. This upturn was associated with less education, lower sense of control, and widowhood.

Sometimes older adults are offered a glass of wine or sherry to enhance appetite. However, excessive alcohol intake may interfere with appropriate nutrition. Further, abuse of alcohol by older adults is little known in the medical community.

Dementia often results in skipping meals due to forgetfulness. In late dementia, weight loss becomes a considerable concern. The older adult is unaware of the need to eat, unaware of hunger, and often uses excessive energy pacing and wandering. Older adults with dementia may also develop apraxia of swallowing.

Malnutrition is prevalent in hospitalized older adults with mild cognitive impairment (MCI). Malnutrition leads to cognitive deficits. In a study by Orsitto and colleagues of older adults with dementia including some with MCI, 18% of the subjects were found to be well; 58% were at risk for malnutrition; and 24% were malnourished. Compared with those who had normal cognition, patients with MCI and dementia less frequently were well and more frequently were at increased risk for malnutrition.

Social Factors Associated With Undernutrition

Many older adults are women who have outlived their husbands, the household breadwinners, and are left to live on Social Security and enter poverty status. With income inelasticity, food is an item in the budget that may have the most potential for reduction. Further, despite the fact that a diet high in fruits and vegetables has been associated with a decreased risk of some cancers, reduced morbidity and mortality from heart disease, and enhanced weight management, older adults living in poverty may have insufficient funds to purchase food, especially nutrient-dense foods. In a sample of 908 homebound older adults, those who were food insecure were 70% more likely than other older adults to report unintentional weight change over the previous six months. About 16% of older adults in the community consume less than 1000 kcal each day.

A study by Yeh et al. that surveyed a number of different ethnic groups found that cost, an obesogenic environment, early home food environment, and limited access to fresh produce all contributed to inadequate consumption of fruits and vegetables. The participants were aware of the government guidelines to promote consumption.

Although most older adults consume less than the recommended dietary allowances for multiple nutrients, food-insecure older adults have significantly lower intakes of energy, protein, carbohydrates, saturated fats, niacin, vitamins B6 and B12, magnesium, iron, and zinc. Data from the Third National Health and Nutrition Examination Survey (NHANES III) and the Nutrition Survey of the Elderly in New York State (1994) found that food-insecure older adults were 2.33 times more likely to report fair/poor health status and had higher nutritional risk. According to a study by the Department of Agriculture's Continuing Survey of Food Intakes by Individuals (CSHF), nutritional intake differs between persons of low and high socioeconomic status (SES).

Social isolation adversely affects food intake among older adults. Reliance on family or neighbors to shop for food can have a negative impact on availability of fresh foods. Loneliness in older persons has also been shown to be related to malnutrition. Women aged 65 and older are more likely than men (41% of women vs. 17% of men) to live alone, and a higher proportion of older adults living alone skip meals.

Loneliness may also diminish the desire to prepare and eat balanced meals. The result may be snacking throughout the day. Women eat more (by 13%) when men are present. Both men and women eat more (by 23%) with family present. Meals eaten in a group tend to be up to 44% larger than meals eaten alone and they include larger amounts of carbohydrates, fats, proteins, and alcohol. One study by Suda and colleagues found that older adults receiving Meals on Wheels will eat more if the person delivering the meals stays while the older adult eats.

Rural older adults have been found to be particularly vulnerable to nutritional inadequacies. Contributing factors include social and geographic isolation, limited access to transportation, and limited availability of nutrition-related services.

Culture also plays a role in nutrition through food preferences and choices. Older adults are more likely to eat foods that are familiar and that they enjoy.

Consequences of Weight Loss in the Older Adult

Weight loss in older adults often leads to death. Weight loss suggests a loss of lean body mass. Both intentional and unintentional weight loss may follow the development of disease; this can pose considerable risk for decreased survival, especially when initial body weight is low. Nutritional deficiencies and weight loss can also predispose older adults to increased risk and worse outcomes for community-acquired pneumonia. The incidence of eating disability in the long term care facility is high; nearly 50% of all residents are unable to eat independently.

Weight loss has been shown to be associated with bone loss and hip fractures. In one study by Ensrud and colleagues, older men with weight loss had higher rates of hip bone loss. The researchers postulate that the hip bone loss may be related to a decline in mechanical load on the weight-bearing skeleton, which may alter bone remodeling; the production of lower levels of endogenous estrogen in adipose tissue and muscle; reduced calcium and nutrient intake; or subclinical illness.

Finally, many medications used with older adults can cause anorexia, nausea, increased energy metabolism, or malabsorption, resulting in weight loss. Numerous causes of weight loss are reversible (**Box 14-3**). Further, there are drugs and medications that can be used to manage undernutrition. Among these are steroids and hormones. One study by Chapman et al. examined the use of testosterone and nutritional support, alone and in combination. The results demonstrated that the combined treatment decreased

BOX 14-3   Reversible Causes of Weight Loss—the MEALS ON WHEELS Mnemonic

Medications

Emotional (depression)

Alcoholism, elder abuse, anorexia, tartive

Late life paranoia

Swallowing disorders

Oral problems

Nosocomial infections, no money, poverty

Wandering and other dementia related behaviors

Hyperthyroidism, hypoadrenalism, hypoglycemia, hypercalcemia

Enteral problems (gluten enteropathy, pancreatic insufficiency)

Eating problems

Low salt, low cholesterol diet

Stones (gallstones), shopping problems

Source: Data from Morley JE. Pathophysiology of weight loss in older persons. *Nestle Nutr Workshop Ser Clin Perform Programme.* 2005;10:167-172; discussion 131-137, 172-168.

hospitalizations and decreased the length of stay when hospitalized in this vulnerable group.

Another study by Vanderkroft et al. examined nutritional care in hospitalization of older adults. The conclusion was that practice in hospitals needed to support supplementation to minimize nutrition problems. Alternative diets need to be developed for those at high risk.

Interventions

It is vital that declining nutrition be recognized early enough for effective interventions that increase caloric intake. Some possible interventions include:

- Detection and treatment of depression to improve quality of life.
- Providing a pleasant mealtime in a social environment.
- Providing a well-lighted, unhurried mealtime environment.
- Provision of nutrient-dense food choices.
- Identification of dysphagia and swallowing disorders and referrals for further evaluations for altered food consistency and assistance with feeding.

- Older persons eat more in the morning, a shift that is more pronounced after the development of dementia. Older people, especially those with dementia, should increase their food intake at breakfast.
- Mealtime assistance should be provided as needed
- Flavor amplifiers may improve the palatability of food, and enhancers have been shown to reverse weight loss. Appetite enhancers for nursing home residents have been found to be effective in increasing appetite.
- If appetite is small, make meals more appetizing by providing different flavors, textures, temperatures, and colors. Tastes and smells can be enhanced with spices.
- Physical activity such as walking before a meal may help stimulate appetite.
- A review of medications may help identify drugs that affect taste and appetite, or cause nausea.
- High-energy protein oral supplements between meals have been found to be the most common means of increasing daily energy intake.
- If funds are limited, food stamps, Meals on Wheels, and organizations such as churches may assist in providing needed nutrition.
- Treat dental problems so that dentures fit properly to make eating easier.
- Consult with a dietitian so that the family and patient know which foods help an undernourished person and which foods do not.
- Discuss drugs to stimulate appetite and promote weight gain with a primary care physician or nurse if all other efforts are ineffective.
- Consider other methods of feeding such as tubes or intravenous.
- These common nutrient deficiencies can be treated by eating or taking the following:

Folate: fortified breads, pastas, and cereals; raw leafy green vegetables; citrus fruits; supplements

Vitamin B12: monthly B12 injection or supplements

Vitamin C: foods rich in vitamin C or supplements. Foods richest in vitamin C are kakadu plum, camu camu, rose hips, acerola, seabuckthorn, jujube, Indian gooseberry, baobab, black currant, red pepper, parsley, guava, kiwi fruit, broccoli, red currant, and brussel sprouts

Vitamin D: milk fortified with vitamin D; supplements; sunlight

Calcium: milk and dairy products; fortified orange juice, or soy, or rice milk; green leafy vegetables; almonds; supplements

Magnesium: leafy vegetables, nuts, and seeds; wheat and oat bran; whole grains, soy products; seafood; supplements

Phosphorus: large quantities of milk, supplements

Fiber: fruits, vegetables, whole grains, legumes, nuts

Long-chain-omega-3 fats: cold-water/small-mouth fish; mussels; oysters; fish-oil supplement

Selenium, Zinc, Chromium, Iron: supplements

The older adult and caretakers should be provided with nutritional education and with helpful hints for healthy eating. The older adult should be encouraged to:

- Have a piece of fruit with every meal or as a snack.
- Eat two portions of vegetables or salad with many meals.
- Have bread with meals or sandwiches, using mainly whole grain breads.
- Eat a large bowl of breakfast cereal daily.
- High-carbohydrate foods (e.g., rice, pasts, and potatoes) should take up about one-third of the plate at main meals.
- Eat fish two or three times each week, particularly fatty fish such as sardines, mackerel, herring, and salmon.
- Have a half pint of skim/2% milk or low-fat yogurt daily; use reduced fat spreads and cheese.
- If eating is difficult, chop food finely, mash, or blend it. Sources of protein in this situation are eggs, cheese, yogurt, beans, or peanut butter. Egg protein is the standard of quality for measuring protein quality because of their essential amino acid profile and high digestibility.
- Undernourished older adults should limit alcohol consumption to one drink each day.
- Do not add table salt to food and eat fewer salty foods.
- Restrict intake of cakes, cookies, sweets, and ice cream.

Obesity

People who have too much body fat may be overweight or obese. Some people believe that being overweight or obese means being too well nourished. However, overweight or obese people may not consume enough of the nutrients needed for good health, making them undernourished. The prevalence of obesity, defined as a BMI of 30 kg/m2 or greater, continues to increase for both men and women in all age groups. Further, middle aged and older adults are more likely to be obese than those in any other age group. BMI is age-dependent and does not account for body fat distribution. However, it should be recognized that as much as 30 pounds over ideal weight is healthier than ideal weight. It is protective from mortality. A goal might be a BMI greater than 25 but less than 30.

The National Health and Nutrition Examination Survey 1999–2000 found that 38.1% of men and 42.5% of women between 60 and 69 years of age were obese. The corresponding figures are 28.9% of men and 31% of women between the ages of 70 and 79 years. For those older than 80 years, the prevalence of obesity declines precipitously.

Older adults 70–79 who are obese have the greatest risk of being disabled, even though they do not have an increased risk of death.

In the past two decades, the problem of increasing obesity has become a major public health concern in the United States. Projections for obesity in older adults in the United States have been estimated for 2010. The estimated prevalence of obesity in adults 60 and older increases from 32% in 2000 to 37.4% in 2010. The number of obese older adults increases from 14.6 million in 2000 to 20.9 million in 2010. The prevalence of normal weight adults 60 and older decreases from 30.6% in 2000 to 26.7% in 2010.

Obesity has had disease status since 1986. In the United States, it is estimated that between 280,000 and 325,000 deaths a year are attributable to obesity, making it second only to smoking as a preventable cause of death. Obesity is associated with greater health care use and costs, particularly pharmaceutical and laboratory costs. Further, the higher the BMI in older adults, the greater the number of health-related problems, especially mobility and the ability to do everyday tasks. Only severe obesity increases the risk of death.

There are differences in obesity by race and gender. The prevalence of BMI greater than 30 is higher in women than men. There is a relatively high BMI status among older adult minority group members. Among women, the incidence of obesity and overweight are highest among African American women. In this population, more than half of women aged 40 and older are obese and more are overweight.

Physiological Changes

At the population level, some researchers have found that the prevalence of obesity and increase in body fat peaks at age 40 in men and at age 50 in women. There is a loss of lean tissue, but intraabdominal and intramuscular fat increase with age. Visceral body fat also increases with age.

Fat is stored as excess calories which is protective in illness when great weight loss may occur. Excess fat is protective from injuries and falls and helps to maintain core body temperature in vulnerable adults who are likely to become hypothermic. Excess accumulation causes medical complications; a high waist to hip ratio is associated with high risk for hypertension, type 2 diabetes, coronary artery disease, and premature death. Women usually have a lower waist to hip ratio than men. These effects of obesity, negative and positive, on health have been shown to persist well into later life.

Overeating, diminishing physical activity, and resting metabolic rates increase obesity in older adults. Older men decrease their activity levels by 20% compared to younger men. Women decrease activity levels 13%. Women's metabolic rates do not change very much because they continue to do much of the household work all their lives.

Sarcopenic obesity (SO) is a new term used to describe the loss of muscle mass relative to the increase in fat in older adults. This phenomenon is caused by peptides produced by adipose tissue. Obesity and SO may potentiate each other with maximum effects on disability marked as well as increased mortality.

The following factors contribute to obesity in old age:

1. **Inactivity**. This is the major cause of obesity in older adults. The increase of chronic diseases causing disability in older adults causes reduced motor function and, consequently, a reduction in energy expenditure. Physical inactivity is considered one of the main causes of obesity. In 2005–2006, 22% of adults 65 and older reported engaging in regular leisure time physical activity. The percentage of those engaging in regular activity was lower at older ages, ranging from 26% in adults 65–74 and 10% among adults 85 and older. Men over 65 are more likely to exercise than women of that age. Older non-Hispanic White people report higher levels of physical activity (23%) than non-Hispanic Blacks (16%) or Hispanics (14%).

2. **Reduced hormone levels**. With aging, growth hormone and testosterone decrease. This causes diminution of muscle and increase in body fat. Since muscle burns more calories than fat, this change contributes to weight gain.

3. **Poor nutrition.** Older adults tend to choose less expensive foods because of economic problems or low socioeconomic status. They may choose foods that are usually rich in added sugars, but poor in proteins. This is called the "empty calorie syndrome." If older adults choose convenience or restaurant foods, even if they are eaten in small amounts, they often contain high amounts of calories which results in weight gain. People also may eat poorly if they are lonely, bored, depressed, or under stress.

4. **Other**. Drugs used to treat common medical and psychiatric disorders cause weight gain. Some of these are antidepressants, insulin, and steroids. Hypothyroid disorders may cause weight gain because calories are used slowly due to a diminished metabolic rate. Nicotine in tobacco decreases appetite and increases the metabolic rate, but stopping smoking often results in weight gain because the metabolic rate slows and the body burns fewer calories. Further, those who smoke may remain thin but fat accumulates in the waist and abdomen. This increases the risk for health problems even if they remain in a normal weight range.

Problems Associated with Obesity

There is a clear association between obesity and disability. The obese are more likely to become and remain disabled, with decreases in functioning in old age. One study by Lang and colleagues found that obesity was more strongly related to morbidity and disability than to mortality. High body fatness is predictive of mobility loss. Women have higher rates of functional limitation within all BMI categories than do men and the BMI value at which risk increases is lower for women than for men. In a longitudinal study of 7,132 community-dwelling adults aged 70 and older followed for four years by Reynolds, Saito, and Crimmins, obese women at aged 80 had a 27% likelihood of becoming disabled; for nonobese women, the figure was 18%.

Being overweight or obese makes one more likely to experience the onset of functional impairment across various domains including lower body mobility and activities of daily living (ADLs). Older adults who gain more than 5% of their BMI are more likely to experience the onset of lower body mobility impairment. Higher BMI is associated significantly with poorer upper and lower body function, and has a negative impact on both ADLs and IADLs (independent activities of daily living). Mid-life obesity has been associated with a twofold increase in the odds of ADL limitations later in life. Among U.S. older adults in the community, the prevalence of significant pain in the head, neck, and shoulders, back, legs, and feet, and abdomen and pelvis occurs with obesity.

Other Consequences of Obesity

Obesity is associated with numerous diseases and problems. These include coronary heart disease, stroke, type 2 diabetes, hypertension, osteoarthritis, dyslipidemia, gallbladder disease, sleep disturbances and sleep apnea, some cancers, pain, depression, fatty liver disease, metabolic syndrome, and increased risk of death. The risk of developing diabetes is 2.9 times greater for people ages 10 to 75 years old who are overweight relative to those who are not overweight. Studies have linked being overweight with depression, discrimination, social stigmatization, eating disorders, poor self-image, and reduced quality of life.

Twenty percent of adults have metabolic syndrome and it increases with aging. The syndrome consists of abdominal obesity, impaired glucose metabolism, dyslipidemia, and hypertension (see chapter 11). Metabolic syndrome increases the risk for diabetes and cardiovascular diseases. The prevalence of this disorder is due to significant overweight and obesity in older adults.

Increasing weight increases the likelihood of osteoarthritis (OA) in the knees. There is an overall 45% risk that Americans will develop OA in their knees by age 85. These odds increase with increased weight gain so that the odds are 60% among obese men and women. History of knee injury increases rise significantly. Severe OA of the knee often requires major surgery for correction.

Depression is associated with both weight loss and obesity. Factors associated with depression and obesity included younger age, female gender, lower education, functional impairment, and diabetes.

Being overweight but not obese did not have a significant impact on health-related quality of life (HRQOL) in a sample of 1326 community-dwelling adults (mean age 72) in one study by Groessl et al. However, obese older adults tended to have a lower HRQOL than those who were overweight or of normal BMI. The lower quality of well-being score associated with obesity translated into millions of quality adjusted life years lost each year.

Some interesting reports in the literature indicate that obesity does have some favorable aspects in addition to being protective for falls and mortality in older adults. One study from the Nutrition Research Newsletter found that older women who were obese had increased muscle strength compared to those who were not obese.

Another study by Compher and colleagues demonstrated that obesity decreased the risk for pressure ulcer in older adults. Those who were most obese had the lowest risk for pressure ulcers.

Still another study by Dahl et al. has demonstrated that increased BMIs may be protective against dementia in women. Those older women with higher BMIs had less dementia than those with lower BMIs. This did not hold true for older overweight or obese men.

To Lose or Not to Lose Weight

The most effective interventions for weight loss in older people utilize nutrition education, diet, exercise counseling, and behavioral strategies. However, there has been considerable controversy over recommendations of weight loss for obese older adults. A small study of 18 subjects by Jensen and colleagues demonstrated that it is feasible for self-selected obese older women to achieve moderate weight loss and to increase physical activity, resulting in short-term improvements in laboratory values, physical performance, self-reported function, vitality, and life-quality outcomes. Another researcher demonstrated that treatment-induced weight loss among mildly to moderately overweight persons improves health-related quality of life (HRQOL) with at least some of the benefits maintained at one-year follow-up, regardless of whether the weight loss was maintained. A study of overweight individuals by Schneider et al. compared those who were sedentary with those given an exercise regimen. Those individuals who had a negative mood became more negative with the exercise regimen and consumed more energy intake than those who were sedentary and without the exercise plan. Further, frequent weight fluctuations may have negative consequences, such as a higher risk of all-cause and cardiovascular disease mortality. Therefore, health care providers should promote a commitment to help individuals maintain weight loss and avoid weight fluctuations.

Health care providers can encourage obese older adults to increase their level of exercise in pleasant ways that can be sustained over time, such as walking with a friend in the mall or exercising to a videotape. Reducing calories by eliminating between-meal snacks or foods with empty calories should also be encouraged.

Unfortunately, several studies, such as those by Edelstein and colleagues and Latner and colleagues, have found that healthcare providers are biased against obese individuals and therefore, may not be as helpful as they might be. The bias against obese individuals was found to be greater than bias against homosexuality in medical settings as well as interpersonal, employment, and educational settings. Among dietitians, there is a strong to moderate preference for thin people compared to "fat" people. Registered dietitians were found to be less tolerant of obesity than those among the general population (2.5 million subjects). Clearly, this has implications for the education of dietitians for improving tolerance with overweight patients.

Losing Weight

The Tufts pyramid for older adults provides nutrition guidelines for older adults. The addition of more exercise will help the obese older adult lose weight. There are many different diets that are popular from time to time and are found in the popular press. The Mediterranean diet seems to be the best all around for improving health, because it allows greater flexibility, is easy to adapt to various cultures, and has been proven to lower lipid levels and reduce mortality due to heart disease. It should be put into practice for use over the long term. This will reduce weight and then keep the weight off. The only problem with this or any healthy diet is that it can be too expensive for many older adults with a low income.

Counseling by a dietitian is a good way to help older adults find a daily diet that works for him or her. Diet diaries are helpful for weight loss. One report by Clinical Advisor found that diaries doubled the weight loss. In that reported study in which nearly 80% were obese older Americans, those who tracked everything they ate and drank every day for 20 weeks lost 6.2–9.5 pounds. The mean weight loss was 12.8 pounds and 69% of subjects lost more than 8.8 pounds. Those who did not keep a record lost 3.5–4.25 pounds. Of additional importance, African American women in the study lost an average of 9 pounds and the men lost about 12 pounds. Because African Americans have a higher risk for diabetes and cardiovascular disease aggravated by increased weight, this weight loss is highly significant because it reduces that risk.

Telephone counseling by dietitians also is effective for weight loss. A large study by Digenio et al. of obese patients taking silbutramine measured percent of body weight loss at the 6 months endpoint. There were five interventions: high-frequency face-to-face counseling; low frequency face-to-face counseling; high frequency telephone counseling; high frequency email counseling; or no dietitian contact. The high frequency face-to-face and telephone counseling had similar mean weight loss of nearly 9%, which was significantly higher than low frequency face-to-face or email or no dietitian contact. This appears to be a meaningful way to produce lifestyle changes in patients. Silbutramine, the drug used in the study, is an antiobesity drug; a serotonin and noradrenaline reuptake inhibitor. These drugs were provided by physicians in the study. There are many weight-loss drugs that are not approved by the FDA. The FDA recently released a warning about drugs that have pharmaceutical agents that put patients at risk. Some of these are marketed as dietary supplements and claim to be natural or contain only herbal ingredients. The drugs sometimes contain prescription drugs that greatly exceed safe doses. Silbutramine is in some of these marketed drugs and can cause hypertension, seizures, palpitations, heart attack, and stroke. Another ingredient, rimonabant, is found in the marketed drugs and was not approved by the FDA for use in the United States. It is used in Europe and increases the risk for depression and suicide and has resulted in deaths. Health care providers should always ask patients what other medications they are taking, including herbals, to help provide correct information and avoid these kinds of problems. Further information can be obtained at www.fda.gov/cder/consumerinfo/Weight-loss-products.htm.

Conclusion

Because obesity and diabetes are rapidly growing problems in this country and others, research will continue to examine diets in terms of composition as it pertains to immediate weight loss as well as weight loss management and prevention of obesity. Exercise should be an integral part of any research about diet therapy in those with undernutrition as well as in obese individuals.

Activities Related to This Chapter

1. Find a BMI calculator (many are available online), calculate your BMI, and determine your weight category. The government website for the new pyramid also has a BMI calculator.
2. Visit the CDC website and examine obesity trends in the United States over the past two decades. Go to http://www.cdc.gov/nccdphp/dnpa/obesity/trend/maps/index.htm.
3. Lead a group discussion on the leading cause of weight loss in the older adult population.

4. Name two normal physiological factors of aging that may impact nutrition.
5. Identify some of the psychological conditions that are associated with undernutrition.
6. List some of the reversible causes of weight loss.
7. Identify some of the mechanical barriers associated with undernutrition.
8. Describe interventions that may reverse undernutrition.
9. List some of the common diseases associated with obesity in the older adult population.
10. Name some of the diseases associated with protein-energy malnutrition in the older adult population.
11. What are the relationships between overweight and mortality among older adults?
12. What are the relationships between obesity and mortality among older adults?

Case Study

Katherine, 66, has been diagnosed with bipolar disorder. She is taking several medications, and in the three years since she started them she has gained over 100 pounds. She is 5′2″ and is inactive. She is a teacher and twice divorced. She has one son, who lives out of state, and a daughter and grandson, who live nearby. She has recently had an outpatient procedure that ties off part of the stomach so that she feels full after only a small meal. She does, however, eat much of a full meal and does not cut out sweets, having always had a sweet tooth. Since she has gained all the weight she has been told that she has a heart problem. How can you help her?

Questions

1. What is Katherine's most important problem?
2. How does one motivate someone like Katherine?
3. Clearly, she cares about her problem or she wouldn't have had the surgery, but she has not instituted any lifestyle changes. Does she need medication to control her appetite?
4. What will you do first? What is your beginning plan with Katherine?

REFERENCES

Andersen, RE, Crespo CJ, Bartlett SJ, Bathon JM, Fontaine KR. Relationship between body weight gain and significant knee, hip, and back pain in older Americans. *Obes Res.* 2003;11(10):1159–1162.

Apovian CM, Frey CM, Wood GC, Rogers JZ, Still CD, Jensen GL. Body mass index and physical function in older women. *Obes Res.* 2002;10(8):740–747.

American Geriatric Society. *Geriatric Nursing Review Syllabus.* 2nd ed. New York: American Geriatric Society; 2007.

Arterburn D, Crane P, Sullivan S. The coming epidemic of obesity in elderly Americans. *J Am Geriatr Soc.* 2004;52(11):1907–1912.

Beers MH (ed.) *Merck Manual of Geriatrics.* 3rd ed. 2000–2009. Available at: http://www.merck.com/mkgr/mmg/home.jsp. Accessed May 28, 2009.

Blanc-Besson C, Fonck M, Rainfray M, et al. Undernutrition in elderly patients with cancer. *Crit Rev Oncol Hematolog.* 2008;67(3):243–254.

Blazer DG, Moody-Ayers S, Craft-Morgan J, Burchett B. Depression in diabetes and obesity: Racial/ethnic/gender issues in older adults. *J Psychosom Res.* 2002;53(4):913–916.

Burger S, et al. Malnutrition and dehydration in nursing homes: issues in prevention and treatment, 2000. Available at: http://www.cmwf.org/programs/elders/burger_mal_386.asp. Accessed July 24, 2004.

Centers for Disease Control and Prevention. Overweight and obesity: Obesity trends: U.S. Obesity trends 1985–2003. Available at: http://www.cdc.gov/nccdphp/dnpa/obesity/trend/maps/. Accessed September 23, 2005.

Chapman J, Visvanathan R, Hammond A, Morley J, et al. Effect of testosterone and a nutritional supplement, alone and in combination on hospital admission in undernourished older men and women. *Am J Clin Nutr.* 2009;89(3):880–889.

Chen CC, Schilling LS, Lyder CH. A concept analysis of malnutrition in the elderly. *J Adv Nurs.* 2001;36(1):131–142.

Clinical Advisor. Diet diaries double weight loss. 2008. Available at: http://www.clinicaladvisor.com/Diet-diaries-double-weight-loss/article/119338/. Accessed May 29, 2009.

Clinical Advisor. Weight gains boost odds for arthritic knees. 2008. Available at: http://www.clinicaladvisor.com/Weight-gains-boost-odds-for-arthritic-knees/article/120670/. Accessed May 29, 2009.

Collins N. Measuring height and weight. *Adv Skin Wound Care.* 2002;15(2):91–92.

Compher C, Kinasian B, Ratsliffe S. Obesity reduces the risk of pressure ulcers in elderly hospitalized patients. *Journal of Gerentology.* 2007;62A(11):1310–1312.

Consada P, Ravasco P, Camillo M. Rigid diets offered in hospitals. *J Nutr Health Aging.* 2009;13(2):158–164.

Crotty M, Miller M, Giles L, Daniels L, Bannerman E, Whitehead C, et al. Australian longitudinal study of ageing: Prospective evaluation of anthropometric indices in terms of four-year mortality in community-living older adults. *J Nutr Health Aging.* 2002;6(1):20–23.

Dahl A, Lopproven M, Isaoho R, Berg S, et al. Overweight and obesity in old age are not associated with greater dementia risk. *J Am Geriatr Soc.* 2009;56(12):2261–2266.

Davis MA, Murphy SP, Neuhaus JM, Gee L, Quiroga SS. Living arrangements affect dietary quality for U.S. adults aged 50 years and older: NHANES III 1988–1994. *J Nutr.* 2000;130(9):2256–2264.

de Castro JM, Stroebele N. Food intake in the real world: implications for nutrition and aging. *Clin Geriatric Med.* 2002;18(4):685–697.

de Groot CP, Enzi G, Matthys C, Moreiras O, Roszkowski W, Schroll M. Ten-year changes in anthropometric characteristics of elderly Europeans. *J Nutr Health Aging.* 2002;6(1):4–8.

Defay R, Delcourt C, Ranvier M, Lacroux A, Papoz L. Relationships between physical activity, obesity and diabetes mellitus in a French elderly population: The POLA study. Pathologies oculaires liees a l' age. *Int J Obes Relat Metab Disord.* 2001;25(4):512–518.

Dey D, Rothenberg E, Sudh V, et al. Height and body weight in the elderly. A 25 year longitudinal study. *Europ J Clin Nutr.* 1999;53(12):905–914.

Dey DK, Lissner L. Obesity in 70-year-old subjects as a risk factor for 15-year coronary heart disease incidence. *Obes Res.* 2003;11(7):817–827.

Diaz VA, Mainous AG III, Everett CJ. The association between weight fluctuation and mortality: results from a population-based cohort study. *J Comm Health* 2005;30(3):153–165.

Digenio A, Mancuso J, Gerber R, Dvorak R. Comparison of methods for delivering a lifestyle modification program for obese patients: a randomized trial. *Ann Intern Med.* 2009;150(4):255–262.

DiMaria-Ghalili RA, Amella E. Nutrition in older adults. *Am J Nurs.* 2005;105(3):40–50.

Droyvold WB, Lund Nilsen TI, Lydersen S, Midthjell K, Nilsson PM, Nilsson JA, et al. Weight change and mortality: The Nord-Trondelag health study. *J Intern Med.* 2005;257(4):338–345.

Duffy E. Malnutrition in older adults. *Adv for NPs.* 2008;16(9):28–34.

Edelstein S, Silva N, Mancini L. Obesity bias among dietitians by using the Fat People–Thin People Implicit Association Test. *Topics in Clin Nutr.* 2009;24(1):67–72.

Endoy MP. Anorexia among older adults. *Am J Nurse Pract.* 2005;9(5):31–38.

Ensrud KE, Ewing SK, Stone KL, Cauley JA, Bowman PJ, Cummings SR. Intentional and unintentional weight loss increase bone loss and hip fracture risk in older women. *J Am Geriatric Soc.* 2003;51(12):1740–1747.

Ensrud KE, Fullman RL, Barrett-Connor E, Cauley JA, Stefanick ML, Fink HA, et al. Voluntary weight reduction in older men increases hip bone loss: the osteoporotic fractures in men study. *J Clin Endocrinol Metab.* 2005;90(4);1998–2004.

Federal Interagency Forum on Aging-Related Statistics. 2008 Older Americans: Key indicators of well-being. Available at: http://www.agingstats.gov/Agingstatsdotnet/Main_Site/Data/Data_2008.aspx. Accessed May 29, 2009.

Ferraro KF, Thorpe RJ Jr, Wilkinson JA. The life course of severe obesity: does childhood overweight matter? *J Gerontol B Psychol Sci.* 2003;58(2):S110–S119.

Flegal KM. Estimating the impact of obesity. *Soz Praventivmed.* 2005;50(2):73–74.

Flegal KM, Carroll MD, Ogden CL, Johnson CL. Prevalence and trends in obesity among us adults, 1999–2000. *JAMA.* 2002;288(14):1723–1727.

Fontaine KR, Barofsky I. Obesity and health-related quality of life. *Obes Rev.* 2001;2(3):173–182.

Fontaine KR, Barofsky I, Bartlett SJ, Franckowiak SC, Andersen RE. Weight loss and health-related quality of life: Results at 1-year follow-up. *Eat Behav.* 2004;5(1):85–88.

Fontaine KR, Redden DT, Wang C, Westfall AO, Allison DB. Years of life lost due to obesity. *JAMA.* 2003;289(2):187–193.

Fried LP, Tangen CM, Walston J, Newman AB, Hirsch C, Gottdiener J, et al. Frailty in older adults: evidence for a phenotype. *J Gerontol A Biol Sci Med Sci.* 2001;56(3):M146–M156.

Friedmann JM, Elasy T, Jensen GL. The relationship between body mass index and self-reported functional limitation among older adults: a gender difference. *J Am Geriatr Soc.* 2001;49(4):398–403.

Gillick M. Pinning down frailty. *J Gerontol A Biol Sci Med Sci.* 2001;56(3):M134–M135.

Groessl EJ, Kaplan RM, Barrett-Connor E, Ganiats TG. Body mass index and quality of well-being in a community of older adults. *Am J Prev Med.* 2004;26(2):126–129.

Guo J, Yang H, Qian H, Huang L, et al. The effects of different nutrition measurements on delayed wound healing after hip fracture in the elderly. *J Surg Res.* 2008 Oct 16. [Epub ahead of print].

Guthrie JF, Lin BH. Overview of the diets of lower- and higher-income elderly and their food assistance options. *J Nutr Ed Behav.* 2002;34(suppl 1):S31–S41.

Heiat A, Vaccarino V, Krumholz HM. An evidence-based assessment of federal guidelines for overweight and obesity as they apply to elderly persons. *Arch Intern Med.* 2001;161(9):1194–1203.

Himes CL. Obesity, disease, and functional limitation in later life. *Demography.* 2000;37(1):73–82.

Holmes S. Nutritional screening and older adults. *Nurs Stand.* 2000;15(2):42–44.

Huang KC, Lee MS, Lee SD, Chang YH, Lin YC, Tu SH, et al. Obesity in the elderly and its relationship with cardiovascular risk factors in Taiwan. *Obes Res.* 2005;13(1):170–178.

Inelmen EM, Sergi G, Coin A, Miotto F, Peruzza S, Enzi G. Can obesity be a risk factor in elderly people? *Obes Rev.* 2003;4(3):147–155.

Jenkins KR. Body-weight change and physical functioning among young old adults. *J Aging Health.* 2004;16(2):248–266.

Jenkins KR. Obesity's effects on the onset of functional impairment among older adults. *Gerontologist.* 2004;44(2):206–216.

Jenkins KR, Fultz NH, Fonda SJ, Wray LA. Patterns of body weight in middle-aged and older Americans, by gender and race, 1993–2000. *Soz Praventivmed.* 2003;48(4):257–268.

Jensen GL, Roy MA, Buchanan AE, Berg MB. Weight loss intervention for obese older women: Improvements in performance and function. *Obes Res.* 2004;12(11):1814–1820.

Kenchaiah S, Evans JC, Levy D, Wilson PW, Benjamin EJ, Larson MG, et al. Obesity and the risk of heart failure. *N Engl J Med.* 2002;347(5):305–313.

Lang I, Llewellyn D, Alexander K, Melzer D. Obesity, physical function and mortality in older adults. *J Am Geriatr Soc.* 2008;56(8):474–478.

Latner J, O'Brien K, Durso L, Brinkman L, et al. Weighing obesity stigma: the relative strength of different forms of bias. *Int J Obes.* 2008;32(7):1145–1152.

Layman D, Rodriguez N. Egg protein as a source of power, strength, and energy. *Nutrition Today.* 2009;44(1):43–48.

Lechleitner M. Obesity and metabolic syndrome in the elderly. *Gerentology.* 2008;54(5):253–259.

Ledikwe JH, Smiciklas-Wright H, Mitchell DC, Jensen GL, Friedmann JM, Still CD. Nutritional risk assessment and obesity in rural older adults: a sex difference. *Am J Clin Nutr.* 2003;77(3):551–558.

Lee IM, Blair SN, Allison DB, Folsom AR, Harris TB, Manson JE, et al. Epidemiologic data on the relationships of caloric intake, energy balance, and weight gain over the life span with longevity and morbidity. *J Gerontol A Biol Sci Med Sci.* 2001:56(spec. no 1):7–19.

Lee JS, Frongillo EA Jr. Nutritional and health consequences are associated with food insecurity among U.S. Elderly persons. *J Nutr.* 2001;131(5):1503–1509.

Library of the National Medical Society. Undernutrition in the elderly. 2008. Available at: http://www.medical-library.org/journals3a/undernutrition_elderly.htm. Accessed May 28, 2009.

Liu L, Bopp MM, Roberson PK, Sullivan DH. 2002. Under-nutrition and risk of mortality in elderly patients within 1 year of hospital discharge. *J Gerontol A Biol Sci Med Sci.* 57(11);M741–M746.

Loeb M, High K. The effect of malnutrition on risk and outcome of community-acquired pneumonia. *Respir Care Clin N Am.* 2005;11(1):99–108.

Luggen AS, Bernstein M, Touhy T. Nutritional needs. In P Ebersole, P Hess, et al. (eds.) *Toward Healthy Aging.* 7th ed. St. Louis; Mosby; 2008

Masley S. Correcting common nutritional deficiencies. *The Clinical Advisor.* 2008;pp. 60–66.

Mathey MF, Siebelink E, de Graaf C, Van Staveren WA. Flavor enhancement of food improves dietary intake and nutritional status of elderly nursing home residents. *J Gerontol A Biol Sci Med Sci* 2001,56(4):M200–M205.

McCarthy L, Bigal M, Katz M, Derby C, et al. Chronic pain and obesity in elderly people: results from the Einstein aging study. *J Am Geriatr Soc.* 2009;57(1):115–119.

Merck Manual of Health & Aging. Undernutrition. n.d. Available at: http://www.merck.com/pubs/mmanual_ha/sec3/ch17/ch17b.html. Accessed May 28, 2009.

Morley JE. Anorexia and weight loss in older persons. *J Gerontol A Biol Sci Med Sci.* 2003;58(2):131–137.

Morley JE. Pathophysiology of weight loss in older persons. *Nestle Nutr Workshop Series Clin Perform Programme* 2005;10:167–172.

National Institute of Aging, National Institutes of Health. Research goal A: improve our understanding of healthy aging and disease and disability among older adults. 2008. Available at: www.nia.nih.gov/AboutNIA/Strategic Directions/goal_a_.com. Accessed February 2, 2009.

National Institute of Diabetes and Digestive and Kidney Diseases, National Institutes of Health. Excess fat around waist may increase death risk for women. Available at: http://www.nih.gov/news/health/apr2008/niddk-07.htm. Accessed April 13, 2008.

Nightingale F. *Notes on Nursing.* Philadelphia: J. B. Lippincott; 1992.

Nutrition Research Newsletter. Is muscle strength related to obesity in elderly women? 2004. Available at: http://findarticles.com/p/articles/mi_m0887/is_5_23/ai_n6076503/. Accessed May 29, 2009.

Ogden CL, Carroll MD, Flegal KM. Epidemiologic trends in overweight and obesity. *Endocrinol Metab Clin North Am.* 2003;32(4);741–760, vii.

Orsitto G, Fielrio F, Tria D, Venezia A, et al. Nutritional status in hospitalized elderly patients with mild cognitive impairment. *Clin Nutr.* 2009;28(1):100–102.

Parashos IA, Stamouli S, Rogakou E, Theodotou R, Nikas I, Mougias A. Recognition of depressive symptoms in the elderly: What can help the patient and the doctor. *Depress Anxiety.* 2002;15(3):111–116.

Payette H, Coulombe C, Boutier V, Gray-Donald K. Nutrition risk factors for institutionalization in a free-living functionally dependent elderly population. *J Clin Epidemiol.* 2000;53(6):579–587.

Peeters A, Bonneux L, Nusselder WJ, De Laet C, Barendregt JJ. Adult obesity and the burden of disability throughout life. *Obes Res.* 2004;12(7):1145–1151.

Pirlich M, Lochs H. Nutrition in the elderly. *Best Pract Res Clin Gastroenterol.* 2001;15(6):869–884.

Raj A. Depression in the elderly. Tailoring medical therapy to their special needs. *Postgrad Med.* 2004;115(6);26–28, 37–42.

Reynolds S L, Saito Y, Crimmins EM. The impact of obesity on active life expectancy in older American men and women. *Gerontologist.* 2005;45(4):438–444.

Russell A, Remington P, Rumm P, Haase R. Increasing prevalence of overweight among Wisconsin adults, 1989–1998. *WMJ.* 2000;99(3):53–56.

Sacks F, Bray G, Carey V, et al. Comparisons of weight loss diets with different compositions of fat, protein and carbohydrates. *N Engl J Med.* 2009;360:859–873.

Schieman S, Van Gundy K, Taylor J. Status, role, and resource explanations for age patterns in psychological distress. *J Health Soc Behav.* 2001;42(1):80–96.

Schneider K, Spring B, Pagoto S. Exercise and energy intake in overweight sedentary individuals. *Eat Behav.* 2009;10(1):29–35.

Senior Health. Screening height loss. 2004. Available at: http://seniorhealth.about.com/cs/osteoporosis/qt/height_osteopor.htm. Accessed May 28, 2009.

Sharkey JR. Nutrition risk screening: the interrelationship of food insecurity, food intake, and unintentional weight change among homebound elders. *J Nutr Elderly.* 2004;24(1):19–34.

Suda Y, Marske CE, Flaherty JH, Zdrodowski K, and Morley JE. Examining the effect of intervention to nutritional problems of the elderly living in an inner city area: a pilot project. *J Nutr Health Aging.* 2001;5(2):118–123.

Sullivan DH, Bopp MM, Roberson PK. Protein-energy undernutrition and life-threatening complications among the hospitalized elderly. *J Gen Intern Med.* 2002;17(12):923–932.

Sullivan DH, Liu L, Roberson PK, Bopp MM, Rees JC. Body weight change and mortality in a cohort of elderly patients recently discharged from the hospital. *J Am Geriatr Soc.* 2004;52(10):1696–1701.

Tariman JD. Obesity in men. Exercise as a weight loss intervention. *Adv NP.* 2008;16(2):26–27.

Teresi J, Abrams R, Holmes D, Ramirez M, Eimicke J. Prevalence of depression and depression recognition in nursing homes. *Soc Psychiatry Psychiatr Epidemiol.* 2001;36(12):613–620.

Thomas DR. Are older people starving to death in a world of plenty? *Nestle Nutritional Workshop Series Clin Perform Programme.* 2005;10:15–23.

Thomas DR, Zdrowski CD, Wilson MM, Conright KC, Lewis C, Tariq S, et al. Malnutrition in subacute care. *Am J Clin Nutr.* 2002;75(2):308–313.

Torgerson JS, Lindroos AK, Naslund I, Peltonen M. Gallstones, gallbladder disease, and pancreatitis: cross-sectional and 2-year data from the Swedish obese subjects (SOS) and SOS reference studies. *Am J Gastroenterol.* 2003;98(5):1032–1041.

Turcato E, Bosello O, Di Francesco V, Harris TB, Zoico E. Bissoli I., et al. Waist circumference and abdominal sagittal diameter as surrogates of body fat distribution in the elderly: their relation with cardiovascular risk factors. *Int J Obes Relat Metab Disord.* 2000;24(8):1005–1010.

U.S. Food and Drug Administration. FDA expands warning to consumers about tainted weight loss pills. Available at: http://www.fda.gov/bbs/topics/NEWS/2008/NEW01933.html. Accessed May 29, 2009.

Vanderkroft D, Collins C, Fitzgerald M, Lewis S, et al. Minimising undernutrition in the older inpatient. *Int J Evid-Based Health Care.* 2007;5(2):110–181.

Visscher TL, Rissanen A, Seidell JC, Heliovaara M, Knekt P, Reunanen A, et al. Obesity and unhealthy life-years in adult Finns: an empirical approach. *Arch Intern Med.* 2004;164(13):1413–1420.

Wedick NM, Barrett-Connor E, Knoke JD, Wingard DL. The relationship between weight loss and all-cause mortality in older men and women with and without diabetes mellitus: the Rancho Bernardo study. *J Am Geriatric Soc.* 2002;50(11):1810–1815.

Weill Medical College of Cornell University. Food and fitness advisor. The satiety index, p. 8. June 2006.

Wolf AM. Economic outcomes of the obese patient. *Obes Res.* 2002;10(suppl 1):58S–62S.

Yamashita BD, Sullivan DH, Morley JE, Johnson LE, Barber A, Olson JS, et al. The gain (geriatric anorexia nutrition) registry: the impact of appetite and weight on mortality in a long-term care population. *J Nutr Health Aging.* 2002;6(4):275–281.

Yeh M, Ickes S, Lowenstein L, Shuval K, Ammerman A, et al. Understanding barriers and facilitators of fruit and vegetable consumption among a diverse multi-ethnic population in the USA. *Health Promotion Int.* 2008;23(1):42–51.

Young KW, Binns MA, Greenwood CE. Meal delivery practices do not meet needs of Alzheimer patients with increased cognitive and behavioral difficulties in a long-term care facility. *J Gerontol A Biol Sci Med Sci.* 2001;56(10):M656–M661.

Young KW, Greenwood CE. Shift in diurnal feeding patterns in nursing home residents with Alzheimer's disease. *J Gerontol A Biol Sci Med Sci.* 2001;56(11):M700–M706.

Zamboni M, Mazzali G, Fantin F, et al. Sarcopenic obesity: a new category of obesity in the elderly. *Nutr Metab Cardiovasc Dis.* 2008;18(5):388–395.

Zicarelli KR. Weight loss for patients with metabolic syndrome. *Adv NP.* 2008;16(3):59–62.

Zuliani G, Romagnoni F, Volpato S, Soattin L, Leoci V, Bollini MC, et al. Nutritional parameters, body composition, and progression of disability in older disabled residents living in nursing homes. *J Gerontol A Biol Sci Med Sci.* 2001;56(4):M212–M216.

Alcohol Use in Older Adults

Ann Schmidt Luggen, PhD, GNP and
Mary B. Neiheisel, BSN, MSN, EDD, CNS, APRN-FNP, FAANP

CHAPTER 15

CHAPTER OBJECTIVES   Upon competition of this chapter, the reader will be able to:

1. Discuss age-related changes that make older adults more susceptible to alcohol's damaging effects
2. Describe the benefits of alcohol intake
3. Relate the different systems affected by high alcohol intake
4. Discuss some of the pharmacologic and nonpharmacologic methods of management of high alcohol intake in older adults
5. State one strategy that the student health professional can use with an older adult with high alcohol intake

KEY TERMS AND CONCEPTS

Bone mineral density (BMD)   Gamma aminobutyric acid (GABA)

Cirrhosis   Glutamate

Dementia   Hepatitis

Dopamine   Macrocytosis

Alcohol is both a tonic and a poison. The "French paradox" has been recognized for over 200 years. The French diet is high in butter, cheese, and alcohol, especially red wine. Yet, the French have a lower incidence of cardiac problems compared with people in other European countries where wine consumption is not as high. Researchers think that it might be the red wine that makes the difference. Studies have found that cardiovascular benefits occur when red wine is consumed with the meal. Alcoholic beverages, especially wines, contain substances that appear to prevent blood clots, having antithrombotic activity; relax blood vessel walls; and prevent the oxidation of low-density lipoproteins (LDLs), the "bad" cholesterol that causes plaques in arteries. Alcoholic beverages raise high-density lipoproteins (HDLs), which protect against heart disease. Wine offers greater benefits than do beers or spirits.

As just discussed, alcohol, in the right amounts, may be good for you. However, it is the amount that is of concern. Alcohol is known to be good for the heart and the circulatory system. It is also thought to be protective against diabetes and gallstones. However, *heavy* drinking is a major cause of preventable death. Excessive alcohol consumption can damage the heart, liver, stomach, brain, breasts, and cognition. Associations have been found with breast and colorectal cancers. *Moderate* drinking increases sex steroid hormone levels and may interfere with folate metabolism. In addition, heavy drinking leads to falls; motor vehicle accidents; accidents with potentially dangerous equipment, such as cutting knives; and argumentative behavior that may cause dangerous interactions or fights with others.

Alcohol and Alcohol Use Defined

There is a lack of consensus regarding what constitutes light versus moderate versus heavy alcohol use. When the health benefits outweigh the risks, it can be considered moderate drinking. The prevailing thought today is that one to two drinks a day for men and one drink a day for women older than age 65 is moderate drinking. In the United States, one drink of alcohol is defined as 12 ounces (oz.) of beer, 5 oz of wine, or 1 1/2 oz of spirits (e.g., whiskey). Each drink contains 12 to 14 grams of alcohol. Beer, wine, and liquor have different alcohol levels. Beer may be 5% to 6% alcohol; wine, 8% to 14%; and hard liquors, 35% to 45%. A liquor that is 35% liquor is said to be 70 proof; 45% is 90 proof.

Alcohol eludes classification in terms of nutrition. It provides energy—7 Kcal/gram—when metabolized; therefore, it is a food. But alcohol is not a nutrient. Beer and wine do contain unfermented carbohydrates and traces of protein, but no mineral substances. A serving a beer contains 1.8 mg niacin, which is 10% of the daily value.

Alcohol is not stored in the body. It acts like a drug, producing euphoria as well as a depressive effect. It is addictive for some people, and it is characterized by tolerance (needing more and more to get the same effect), dependence, and withdrawal symptoms.

Epidemiology

No major population studies have been done to determine the number of older adults consuming or abusing alcohol. However, 14 million Americans (7.4% of the population) meet the standard criteria for alcohol abuse/alcoholism (**Figure 15-1**). About 50% of adults older than age 65 report the use of alcohol occasionally. Further, there are geographic differences in alcohol consumption in older adults. In East Boston, 70% of older adults report drinking alcohol in the past year. Of these, 8.4% report drinking two or more drinks per day. Contrast this with the rural Midwest, where just 46% report drinking in the past year and 5.4% report drinking two or more drinks per day. In American primary care settings, 4% to 10% of older adults are diagnosed with alcoholism. Ten to 15% of older patients drink heavily but are not considered alcoholics. One study by Brody found that 10% to 15% of older patients seeking medical attention have an alcohol-related problem. In the hospital setting, 10% to 21% of older adults and 3% to 49% of nursing home patients are diagnosed as alcoholic.

One estimate from a research study in England by the Institute of Alcohol Studies concluded that 5% to 12% of men in their 60s have alcohol problems. Another study in England found that 17% of men drank excessively. A survey in 1994 in the United Kingdom found that of those aged 65 and older, 17% of men and 7% of women exceeded rec-

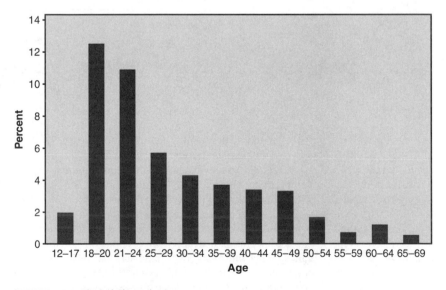

FIGURE 15-1 Alcohol Abuser by Age

Source: National Institute on Alcohol Abuse and Alcoholism of the National Institutes of Health, 2008.

ommendations for moderate drinking. Only a small number of these ever receive treatment.

Additional research suggests that alcohol use/abuse is the twelfth leading cause of death. In the 65- to 74-year age group, chronic liver disease and **cirrhosis** cause more deaths than Alzheimer's or Parkinson's disease. Hepatitis has increased to 35% of older alcoholics and cirrhosis is present in 20%. Cirrhosis causes death in 50% of older adults within one year of diagnosis, but only 7% in patients under 60 years old.

Alcohol dependence is one of the top three psychiatric disorders in the United States. In one study of suicides in older adults reported by Seniors in Sobriety, alcohol abuse occurred in 35% of men and 18% of women.

Two national surveys, one in 1984 and one in 1990 by Midanik and Clark, reported relevant data with regard to alcohol use/abuse in older adults. In the 1984 study, 59% of men aged 60 and older were current "drinkers." In 1990, this number increased to 66%. This trend does not hold for older women. In 1984, 49% were current drinkers; in 1990, only 37% were drinkers.

Table 15-1 shows data from a study of men who reported having four or more drinks on any single day in the past 30 days by ethnicity. The same data for women shows a very different situation. In all racial/ethnic groups, nearly all women deny having four or more drinks a day over a 30-day period. In the 56 and older group, fewer than 10% consume four drinks a day; in the 61 years and older group, 5% to 8%; and in the 66 and older age group, 0% to 2% admit to four or more drinks a day over the past 30 days.

Although limited data is available on the drinking patterns of older adults, there *is* data to suggest that drinking is a problem. Injuries and deaths in alcohol-related accidents demonstrate the need for concern. In 1994, 11% of drivers aged 65 to 74 years who were in fatal crashes tested positive for alcohol. U.S. statistics show that deaths rose 7% in drivers 75 years and older. A person's risk of auto crash increases at age 55 and by age 80 the risk exceeds that of young beginning drivers. Further, accidents involving an overturned vehicle increase the likelihood of fatality by 220% in older men but only 154% in younger men. In older women, the likelihood of fatality in these accidents increased 523% compared to only 113% in young women. Alcohol has been shown to be a causative factor in fatalities in middle-aged women but is not statistically significant in older women. However, alcohol intake may have an indirect effect in terms of speed and not wearing a safety belt. One study by Higgins, Wright, and Wrenn of the prevalence of alcohol or drug use in older adults admitted to an emergency room found that 14% had a positive alcohol screen. Twenty-one percent of older men had a positive screen. Only one-half were able to be discharged to home.

Gender

Men are twice as likely as women to drink excessively. Women who live with a spouse who drinks excessively are more likely to drink heavily. Older women, in general, drink less than young women. Women who are unemployed or work part time drink more than those who are employed full time. Heavy drinking may occur following a medical illness or psychiatric illness. Being single, separated or divorced, or socially isolated are risk factors for alcoholism in older age groups.

Women are more vulnerable than men to the physical and medical consequences of alcohol use. They develop cirrhosis, cardiomyopathy, and neuropathy more rapidly than do men.

In 1985, a national interview study by the Harvard School of Public Health found that moderate drinkers were more likely than nondrinkers or heavy drinkers to be at a healthy weight, to sleep 7 to 9 hours each night, and to exercise regularly. Many other confounding variables were examined, and it seems clear that there are some benefits to moderate alcohol consumption. In two other national studies (the Nurses' Health Study and the Health Professional's Follow-Up Study), the prevalence of gallstones and type 2 diabetes were lower in moderate drinkers than nondrinkers.

Alcoholism Theories

A number of theories attempt to explain why some people succumb to alcoholism. The biogenetic model proposes that there are genetic risk factors for alcoholism. The sociocultural model suggests that external factors such as poverty, parental values, and behavior can lead to alcoholism. The learning theory/behavior model postulates that alcoholism is

TABLE 15-1 Percent of Men Reporting Four or More Drinks in One Day in the Past 30 Days

Age Group	Hispanic	Black	White
56–60	33%	19%	18%
61–65	30	16	19
66+	20	12	8

Source: Data from Jackson J, Williams D, Gomberg E. A life course perspective on aging and alcohol use and abuse among African Americans. In: Gomberg E, Hegedus A, Zucker R, eds. *Alcohol Problems and Aging.* NIH Pub. 98-4163. Bethesda, MD: NIAAA; 1998

cirrhosis Severe, life-threatening problem related to alcohol abuse (usually). Leads to end-stage liver disease, jaundice, esophageal varices with bleeding, ascites (abdominal fluid), coma, and death.

a learned behavior through social interactions, stress, or pain. The psychological-psychodynamic model suggests that an underlying psychopathology, such as depression, power-seeking behavior, or a dependency conflict predisposes an individual to alcohol abuse.

Genetics

A number of studies, such as those by Schuckit and Dick, confirm that there is a genetic component to alcoholism. Strong evidence suggests that a high correlation between first-degree relatives' risk of alcohol dependence largely results from shared genetic risk factors, rather than from purely environmental mechanisms. Studies on adoptees conducted since the 1970s have demonstrated that alcoholism risk is correlated with the alcoholism histories of the adoptees' biological parents rather than their adoptive parents. One study found that sons of male alcoholics are three to four times more likely to be alcoholics whether or not they were reared by biologic or adoptive parents. An estimated 20% to 25% of sons and brothers of alcoholics become alcoholics, and 5% of the daughters and sisters. Most researchers believe the influences of both genes and environment combine to determine alcoholism risk.

Age-Related Changes Affecting Alcohol Intake

Age-related physical changes may make older adults less tolerant of alcohol. The body water to fat ratio decreases, which means there is diminished alcohol dilution. Hepatic blood flow is decreased, enhancing liver damage. Liver enzymes diminish in efficiency, decreasing alcohol metabolism so that alcohol will have a more rapid effect on the brain. There is increased permeability of the blood-brain barrier, allowing more alcohol to enter the brain. This affects the neurotransmitters and acts as a central nervous system depressant.

Nutritional Intake

Energy requirements usually decrease over later adult years due to diminished physical activity and decreased BMR (basal metabolic rate), which is associated with diminished muscle mass. A gradual reduction in caloric intake is recommended starting at age 40 to 50 years. Alcoholic beverages add many calories without a nutritional benefit. Between the ages of 20 and 80 years, mean caloric intake decreases by 1,000 to 1,200 calories in men, and 600 and 800 calories in women. Older adults' nutritional patterns change; they consume a great proportion of calories in carbohydrates and fewer in fats. Protein intake is relatively

dementia Progressive decline of cognitive function that occurs most often in very old adults. There is loss of memory, attention, and problem solving abilities. There are many types of dementia, the most common being Alzheimer's disease.

stable. Nutritional deficiencies occur if calories are reduced but higher quality nutritional intake does not occur.

Risk Factors

Risk factors for nutritional problems in older adults are great because of the number of age-related changes and the chronic health problems that occur and increase with increasing age. Some of these include loss of teeth or missing teeth; recent weight loss; psychiatric diagnoses such as depression and **dementia**; living alone; number of medications especially diuretics and antidepressants, and declining functional status. The Institute of Alcohol Studies and others report physical changes in elderly people making them less tolerant of alcohol. The body water to fat ratio decreases leading to less water so that there is diminished alcohol dilution. Hepatic blood flow is decreased enhancing liver damage. Liver enzymes diminish in efficiency decreasing the alcohol metabolism. There are benefits and risks of moderate drinking over one's lifetime. Risks exceed benefits until middle age, when cardiovascular disease is an increasing cause of morbidity and mortality. See **Box 15-1** for risks and benefits of alcohol consumption with aging.

Alcohol, Physiology, and Pathophysiology

Ethanol is the active ingredient in alcoholic beverages. Alcohol absorption begins in the mouth and esophagus. Small

> **BOX 15-1   Risks and Benefits of Alcohol with Aging**
>
> - **Person with liver disease, recovering alcoholic:** Moderate drinking offers little benefit, has potential risks.
> - **Person taking one or more medications that interacts with alcohol:** moderate drinking offers little benefit, has potential risks.
> - 60-year-old man: Daily drink protects from heart disease (if not prone to alcoholism).
> - 60-year old woman: Risk-assessment is difficult. Women fear breast cancer more than heart disease, but more women die of heart disease (ten times more) than breast cancer. Alcohol benefits heart disease, but contributes to breast cancer.
>
> *Source:* Data from Harvard School of Public Health. Men with high blood pressure who drink moderate amounts of alcohol may have a lower risk of heart attack. January 1, 2007. Available at: http://www.hsph.harvard.edu/news/press-releases/2007-releases/press01012007.html. Accessed March 1, 2007.

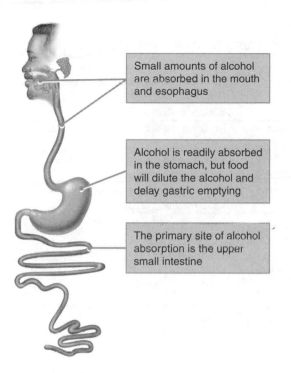

Small amounts of alcohol are absorbed in the mouth and esophagus

Alcohol is readily absorbed in the stomach, but food will dilute the alcohol and delay gastric emptying

The primary site of alcohol absorption is the upper small intestine

FIGURE 15-2 Alcohol Absorption

Source: Insel P, Turner RE, Ross D. *Nutrition.* 3rd ed. Sudbury, MA: Jones & Bartlett; 2007, p. 306. Reproduced with permission.

amounts enter the bloodstream. Some alcohol is absorbed in the stomach, but the primary site of absorption is the upper small intestine (**Figure 15-2**). It is then metabolized in the liver.

Drinking on an empty stomach causes the alcohol to rush into the bloodstream. If food is eaten prior to drinking, alcohol absorption is delayed and oxidizing enzymes are able to break down the alcohol. Food dilutes the contents of the stomach, decreasing the concentration of alcohol and the rate of absorption.

Most alcohol and enzyme products travel to the liver via the portal vein where alcohol metabolism occurs. Metabolism results in energy production, and by metabolizing it quickly, protects the body from alcohol's damaging effects and the even more damaging metabolite acetaldehyde.

A single bout of heavy drinking can cause fat to accumulate in the liver. Fatty liver is the first stage of liver destruction in alcoholism. Those adults with genes favoring a strong immune response are at most risk of alcohol liver disease.

Alcohol has a more serious damaging effect in women compared to men, and it takes less alcohol to cause damage. Heavy drinking often occurs in older women following a medical or psychiatric illness. Women suffer the consequences of high alcohol intake more rapidly than do men. They experience the problems of cirrhosis, cardiomyopathy, and peripheral neuropathy more quickly than men.

Alcohol stimulates appetite—not to be ignored in elders; it improves digestion, and is relaxing. However, alcohol is addictive. Physical dependence occurs and tolerance occurs—that is, it takes gradually more and more alcohol to obtain the same relaxed or desired effect from alcohol over time.

The Brain and Nervous System

Alcohol diffuses readily into the brain from the circulating blood. Memory impairments can result after just a few drinks. If large quantities of alcohol are taken on an empty stomach, a "blackout" can occur. In this situation, the whole event may be lost to memory.

The craving for alcohol is mediated by dopaminergic pathways in the brain. Alcohol facilitates **dopamine** transmission by decreasing the activity of **GABA** (gamma-aminobutyric acid) receptors.

Alcohol consumption causes a number of changes in the brain's normal activity. Sleep can be disrupted even with moderate intake of alcohol; the amount of quality rapid eye movement (REM) sleep is reduced. Even moderate alcohol intake can result in poor judgment, euphoria, loss of inhibition, somnolence, respiratory suppression, and stupor. Excessive amounts of alcohol can cause a person to enter a coma. If one drinks heavily over a long period of time, brain deficits occur that persist after sobriety occurs and is maintained. Further, chronic alcoholism produces and/or is concomitant with many mental disorders. Usually, malnutrition is a factor in these, even if the diet appears to be sufficient. However, older adults who drink heavily are particularly susceptible to decline in cognitive and physical functioning. The number of drinks consumed is a risk factor for falls and accidents.

There has been much research on the association of alcohol misuse and depression. One study by Fergusson and colleagues found that alcohol misuse leads to an increase in major depression, which is already a problem for many older adults.

Withdrawal from alcohol causes a number of symptoms in the brain and nervous system, even if the withdrawal is brief, for example, having drinks with lunch and then not having a drink until late evening. Withdrawal symptoms include hangovers; tremors; and if the withdrawal is

dopamine A hormone and neurotransmitter in the brain. It is also in a medication used to treat Parkinson's disease.

gamma aminobutyric acid (GABA) Main inhibitory neurotransmitter in central nervous system. Regulates excitation of neurons. Implicated in such disorders as anxiety, epilepsy, and addiction.

prolonged, hallucinations, partial or generalized seizures, and delirium tremens (DTs).

A complication of alcohol-induced liver disease is hepatic encephalopathy (brain disease). This is caused by the inability of the liver to detoxify wastes.

Vitamin and Nutrient Deficiencies

Excessive alcohol intake decreases the absorption of vitamins and minerals, causing overt nutritional deficiencies. Deficiencies of thiamine, folate, pyridoxine niacin, and vitamin A are common among alcohol abusers. **Table 15-2** summarizes some of the more common nutritional deficiencies associated with chronic alcohol use. See **Figure 15-3** for information on alcohol and malnutrition. These nutritional deficiencies are not difficult to identify, but they are difficult to correct. Poor diet is common in many older adults and is common in heavy drinkers, but less common in women who drink to excess. Other risk factors for nutritional deficiencies are male sex, poverty, homelessness, and lack of cooking facilities. Loneliness, isolation, depression, anxiety, and chronic pain are additional risk factors. Lack of appetite is a common characteristic of those with alcoholism.

Thiamine

In Western countries, the most frequent cause of thiamine deficiency is alcohol misuse. Impairment of the brain and neurological system is the result. There is the risk of Wernicke-Korsakoff (WN) syndrome with thiamine deficiency. WN is an encephalopathy that causes vision impairment, ataxia, memory loss, confusion, and death if not treated. Thiamine deficiency is also called beriberi.

Folic Acid

Folic acid, a form of folate, is needed to decrease homocysteine in the body (**Box 15-2**). Homocysteine, a byproduct of protein metabolism, is involved in atherosclerosis, the accumulation of cholesterol plaques in the walls of arteries. These plaques contribute to heart attacks and to strokes. Alcohol blocks the absorption of folic acid and inactivates folic acid in the blood and tissues, thus increasing the risk of atherosclerosis.

Chronic alcohol abuse may result in **macrocytosis** (enlarged red blood cells often seen in folate and B12 deficiency). Laboratory studies of folate and B12 should be checked periodically in the older adult.

In the Nurses' Health Study, women who drank more than one drink per day and had high levels of folic acid were 90% less likely to develop breast cancer than those with low levels of folic acid. One study suggests

macrocytosis Enlarged red blood cells. Seen in certain anemias, vitamin B12 deficiency, and alcohol abuse.

TABLE 15-2 Alcohol-Caused Nutritional Deficiencies

Nutrient	Consequences
Calories	Weight loss, protein loss, anemia
Protein	Poor healing, hypoalbuminemia, loss of protein-binding of drugs
Fat	Inability to absorb vitamins A, D, E, K
Vitamin A	Dry skin and eyes, night blindness, visual sensitivity to light (photophobia)
Vitamin B1, thiamine	Anorexia, neuropathy, muscle weakness, dementia, heart disease
B2, riboflavin	Chelitis, glossitis, blepharitis, conjunctivitis, visual sensitivity to light
B3, niacin	Depression, dementia, diarrhea, dermatitis, stomatitis
B9, folate	Macrocytic anemia, high homocysteine levels
Magnesium	Disorientation, irritability of nervous system, heart arrhythmias

Source: Data from Miller CA. *Nursing for Wellness in Older Adults.* 4th ed. Philadelphia: Lippincott; 2004.

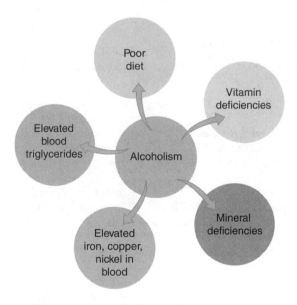

FIGURE 15-3 Alcohol and Malnutrition

Source: Insel P, Turner RE, Ross D. *Nutrition.* 3rd ed. Sudbury, MA: Jones & Bartlett; 2007, p. 319. Reproduced with permission.

that 600 μg of folic acid will counter the effect of moderate alcohol consumption on the risk of breast cancer.

Hormones

In this same study, it is reported that women who take unopposed estrogen have a 23% higher chance for breast

> ### ► BOX 15-2 Folic Acid
>
> Folate is essential for DNA synthesis.
>
> Folate is essential for amino acid metabolism.
>
> Folate is essential for cell division.
>
> Folate is essential for red blood cell maturation.
>
> Folate may stave off dementia in older adults.
>
> *Source:* Data from Insel P, Turner RE, Ross D. *Nutrition.* 3rd ed. Sudbury, MA: Jones & Bartlett; 2007; Collingwood J. Folic acid supplements could prevent dementia. January 24, 2007. Available at: http://psychcentral.com/lib/2007/folic-acid-supplements-could-prevent-dementia/. Accessed July 15, 2008.

cancer; in estrogen plus progesterone there is a 67% increased risk when taken for more than 10 years. Compared to never drinking alcohol, drinking one drink per day increases risk for breast cancer up to age 70 by 7%.

Liver

Cirrhosis of the liver is the twelfth leading cause of death in the United States and the fiftieth cause of mortality in those of late middle age. Excessive use of alcohol causes inflammation of the liver, which is known as alcoholic **hepatitis**. Many alcoholics have excess iron accumulation in the liver that may contribute to the development of alcoholic liver disease. Elevated liver enzymes are found in 18% of older alcoholics. In heavy drinkers, the serum GGT, AST, ALT, ferritin, and albumin are all higher than in moderate drinkers or than in those who abstain. The biomarkers are higher in moderate drinkers compared to abstainers. Severe liver disease from long-term alcohol use is life threatening.

Alcoholic liver disease progresses in three phases. Patients may have one or more of these at one time:

1. Fatty liver—reversible with abstinence
2. Alcoholic hepatitis—liver inflammation
3. Cirrhosis—scarring of the liver

Cirrhosis, or scarring of the liver, is potentially fatal. Cirrhosis increases the incidence of cancer of the liver, and women are more vulnerable to liver cancer than are men. Those with hepatitis and cirrhosis have a high death rate, greater than 60%, in four years, with the majority of deaths occurring within 12 months of diagnosis. Oddly, many people who are heavy drinkers do not develop liver disease.

Changes in nutrition are associated with the development and progression of alcohol-induced liver disease. The degree of malnutrition correlates with the development of serious liver complications such as ascites (fluid retention), encephalopathy (brain injury causing abnormal mental functioning), and impaired renal (kidney) function.

Malnutrition is correlated with mortality. Researchers have found an inverse relationship between calorie intake and mortality. In one study by Mendenhall and colleagues, participants who consumed 3,000 calories/day had high survival rates, but 80% of those who consumed fewer than 1,000 calories/day died. Heavy consumption of alcohol is associated with severe anorexia. However, obesity is a risk factor for alcoholic liver disease.

Recent studies by Klatsky, et al. have shown that coffee intake is inversely related to the risk of alcoholic cirrhosis. Those who drink more coffee and who have excessive intake of alcohol are less likely to develop cirrhotic livers. Aspartate aminotransferase and alanine aminotransferase levels are low in those who drink coffee compared to those who do not. This finding does not hold true for tea drinkers.

Supplemental iron intake exacerbates alcohol-induced liver injury. Alcohol actually increases the iron content in hepatocytes (liver cells). Iron seems to play a role in scarring of the liver—the last stage of liver disease.

Esophageal Cancer

Drinking alcohol is a risk factor for esophageal cancer. The risk is much higher if the person also smokes. A new report shows that those who have flushing in the face when drinking alcohol have a much higher risk for developing esophageal cancer than those who do not. The flushing is accompanied by tachycardia and nausea. The reaction is due to an inherited lack of the enzyme aldehyde dehydrogenase2 (ALDH2). This is most common in Japanese, Chinese, and Korean people. One may be ALDH2 deficient or may completely lack the enzyme. Even if one is a moderate drinker, the risk is high. There is no risk to non-drinkers. Esophageal cancer is one of the deadliest cancers. The five-year survival rate in the U.S. is 15.6%.

Stomach

Alcohol use decreases the amount of the stomach enzyme alcohol dehydrogenase, which breaks down alcohol. Gastritis is more common in heavy drinkers. Deficiencies of certain vitamins such as thiamine, folate, pyridoxine, niacin, and vitamin A are common occurrences. Alcohol intake causes gastrointestinal bleeding, a serious problem. The bleeding is caused by varices that occur in the portal vein of the liver and in the varices in the esophagus and stomach.

Pancreas

There is a moderately increased risk of pancreatic

> **hepatitis** Inflammation of the liver. It has many causes, however, in this chapter, it is associated with alcohol abuse.

cancer in heavy drinkers. This holds true especially for consumption of liquor (as opposed to beer or wine).

Heart

Damage to the heart muscle, cardiomyopathy, may occur with chronic alcohol abuse. Genetics plays a role in the development of cardiomyopathy in those who consume excessive alcohol. Alcohol dehydrogenase metabolizes alcohol. A variant, alcohol dehydrogenase type 3 (ADH3), may have two effects: it will either cause the body to break down alcohol quickly or it will cause it to metabolize it more slowly. If a person has two copies of the gene for slow-acting metabolism, they are at low risk for cardiac disease. Moderate consumers with two copies of the gene for the quick breakdown of alcohol have a higher risk for cardiac disease because the alcohol does not have the time to beneficially affect clotting factors nor create more HDL. Further, blood pressure is elevated with chronic high alcohol intake (hypertension), which may lead to strokes.

Older adults are at particular risk for alcohol-related cardiac problems. They metabolize the alcohol more slowly, thus it stays in the body longer. Health conditions that are prevalent in older adults such as hypertension, stroke, and neurodegeneration and the medications used to treat them put older adults at higher risk for interactions and exacerbations.

Overuse of alcohol is associated with increased body weight, elevation of triglycerides, increase in systolic blood pressure, and impaired left ventricular function. Alcohol also appears to have a direct cardiotoxic effect on the myocardium (heart muscle). Dysrhythmias may cause dizziness, syncope (faint), and even death.

Musculoskeletal

Chronic alcohol use may cause the development of myopathy, resulting in more frequent falls and fractures. Osteoporosis is common in the older person, and when combined with alcohol use the risk of unsteadiness, falls, and hip fractures increases. Of interest, moderate drinking appears to be beneficial for bone in men and postmenopausal women. Intake of more than two drinks of liquor a day was associated with low BMD. Hip and spine BMD were significantly greater in older women consuming more than 2 drinks a day of total alcohol or wine.

Immune System

Alcohol abusers are often immunocompromised and have more infections and poorer outcomes. Alcohol compounds the problem of immunocompromise in older adults because of age-related changes to the immune system that occur in older adults with increasing age (see Chapter 2).

Cancers

Excessive alcohol intake has been linked to several cancers. Cancers of the mouth, throat, esophagus, colon, and breast have been found to be associated with long-term alcohol consumption. Two or more drinks a day increase the lifetime risk of breast cancer from 12 in 100 in nondrinkers to 14 to 15 in 100 in drinkers. The risk of developing a cancer increases with every drink taken. Specific cancer risks that increase with increased consumption in women are breast, rectum and liver. Women who also smoked had a greater increased risk of cancer of the oral cavity and pharynx, esophagus, and larynx. Further, if a woman has had breast cancer in one breast and smokes and drinks, there is a high risk for cancer in the other breast.

Sleep

Although alcohol acts as a sedative and calming drug and may induce sleep, the quality of sleep is fragmented. It increases the number of times one awakens during the night, especially the later half of sleep as alcohol wears off. Older adults are at particular risk for alcohol-related sleep disorders because they have higher levels of alcohol in the blood and brain. Alcohol at bedtime also leads to unsteadiness in walking and potential injury when getting out of bed during the night.

Drug and Alcohol Interactions

Alcohol interacts with many of the over-the-counter drugs and medications commonly taken by older adults, including selective serotonin reuptake inhibitors (SSRIs) prescribed for depression and or anxiety; painkillers; sedatives; and anticonvulsants. Some specific drugs include Prozac, Zoloft, Paxil, Luvox, Serzone, and the diet pills Fen-Phen and Redux. Further, the drugs appear to cause a compulsion to drink alcohol when one tries to abstain from drinking.

Alcohol increases the potential hepatotoxicity (liver toxicity) of certain drugs, including acetaminophen (Tylenol). Heptatotoxicity is characterized by liver necrosis. Symptoms include nausea, vomiting, diaphoresis, confusion, and possibly jaundice (yellow-coloring in the skin and sclerae from increased bilirubin), and coma. Because acetaminophen is contained in many drugs, it is easy to take too much. Older adults should not take more than 4 grams (4,000 milligrams) (and some say much less than this) per day. Each Tylenol Extra-Strength capsule is 500 mg of acetaminophen. A person taking two tablets four times a day would be at the 4,000-mg limit. In an older adult who consumes alcohol, the acetaminophen dose should be reduced.

Diuretics, such as thiazides or furosemide, used to treat hypertension, heart failure, and peripheral edema, in combination with alcohol may cause hypokalemia (low potassium) and severe muscle damage, including the heart

BOX 15-3 Drug–Alcohol Interactions

Alprazolam	Morphine sulfate
Aripiprazole	Phenobarbital
Buproprion	Phenytoin
Carbamazepine	Quietapine
Ceftrioxone	Risperidone
Chlorpropamide	Selective serotonin-reuptake inhibitors (SSRIs)
Codeine	
Desipramine	Tolbutamine
Fentanyl	Trazadone
Lamotrigine	Venlafaxine
Lorazepam	Verapamil

Source: Lexidrug, 2004.

BOX 15-4 CAGE Screening Tool

1. Have you ever felt that you should cut down?
2. Have people annoyed you by criticizing your drinking?
3. Have you ever felt guilty about your drinking?
4. Have you ever had a drink first thing in the morning to steady your nerves or get rid of a hangover?

Source: National Institute on Alcohol Abuse and Alcoholism. *The Physician's Guide to Helping Patients with Alcohol Problems.* NIH Publication No. 95-3769.

muscle. This is called hypokalemic myopathy. A list of the drugs that cause physiological reactions with alcohol and that are commonly prescribed to older adults is found in **Box 15-3**. Some side effects, such as flushing, are more of an embarrassment than a physical problem. However, others, such as verapamil, may increase the effect of alcohol by 30% and cause a prolonged alcohol effect.

Screening for Alcohol Dependence

A number of tools are available to screen for alcohol abuse that can be used when conducting patient nutrition assessments. The most common one used in practice is CAGE—an acronym for **c**ut down, **a**nnoyed, **g**uilty, **e**ye-opener (**Box 15-4**). If the patient answers "yes" to one of these questions, closer examination may reveal a problem. The CAGE questionnaire has been found to identify 60% to 70% of those who are alcohol dependent.

However, even if the older adult answers "no" to all questions, he or she may be drinking heavily. Another, more detailed, tool is the ten-item Alcohol Use Disorders Identification Test (AUDIT) available from the NIAAA (National Institute of Alcohol Abuse and Alcoholism). The AUDIT is shown in **Appendix 15-1** and is more indicative of problem drinking than the CAGE. The AUDIT can be administered as a paper-and-pencil test, but the CAGE should be administered face to face. On the AUDIT, a score of eight or more for men and four or more for women indicates problem drinking.

There exists both a Michigan Alcoholism Screening Test (MAST) and a version specific to older adults, the Michigan

Alcoholism Screening Test-Geriatric Version (MAST-G). A score of two or more indicates a problem with alcohol. The National Institute on Alcohol Abuse and Alcoholism recommends asking the following three questions:

- On average, how many days per week do you drink alcohol?
- On a typical day when you drink, how many drinks do you have?
- What is the maximum number of drinks you had on any given occasion in the past month?

Sometimes if the older adult denies a problem or the health professional is unsure of the extent of the problem it is possible to obtain information from the family or the spouse. The important thing is to screen.

Positive Effects of Alcohol in Older Adults

Alcohol stimulates appetite, and this effect should not be ignored in older adults. It also improves digestion and promotes relaxation. Moderate consumption can provide other benefits as well. The NIAAA completed an extensive review of current scientific knowledge of the health risks and potential benefits of moderate alcohol consumption. The key findings are shown in **Box 15-5**.

Bone Mineral Density

Research suggests that moderate alcohol intake in older women results in higher **bone mineral density (BMD)**. In a twin study, women who drank more than eight drinks per week had higher bone density at the hip and

bone mineral density (BMD) Measured by a DEXA scan. Measures minerals in bone. The higher the bone mineral content, the less likely one is to fracture a bone. Used in diagnosis of osteoporosis, a common problem of older adults.

lumbar spine compared to their twins who drank minimal amounts of alcohol. Confirming other studies, those women who smoked had lower bone mineral density.

Cardiovascular Benefits

A number of studies, such as that by the *Havard Heart Letter*, have shown that men who have one or two drinks per day are less likely to die of cardiovascular problems. One major study, the Physicians' Health Study, found that physicians who drank one or two drinks a day were 44% less likely to die of heart attack or stroke and less likely to develop heart failure with hypertension. The researchers believe that alcohol increases HDL cholesterol, decreasing the risk of cardiovascular disease. Further, alcohol, like aspirin, decreases the tendency of platelets to clump, suppressing the formation of blood clots that may cause stroke or heart attack. However, as interesting as these studies are, they are not proof that alcohol reduces heart disease. It certainly may be that those who drink one to two drinks per day may also be healthier, exercise more, and have better nutrition. More studies are needed to confirm these findings.

In the Physicians' Health Study, researchers examined the relationship of alcohol consumption and renal dysfunction. The conclusion was that alcohol consumption is inversely correlated with renal dysfunction, thus a beneficial effect with moderate drinking.

Dementia

Little research has been conducted on the relationship between alcohol intake and the incidence of dementia in older adults in the U.S. A number of European studies have dem-

onstrated lowered risk of dementia with moderate alcohol intake. One study at the University of Bari in Italy evaluated the incidence of mild cognitive impairment in nearly 1,500 unimpaired adults aged 65 to 84. The researchers found that those adults with mild cognitive impairment who were moderate drinkers (fewer than one drink a day for women or two drinks a day for men) had a lower rate of progression to dementia than those who abstained from alcohol. Higher levels of drinking (more than one drink a day) did not increase progression to dementia compared to the abstainers, who did progress.

One U.S. study, the Washington Heights Inwood-Columbia Aging Project, followed the alcohol intake of 980 community-dwelling older adults aged 65 and older without dementia. After four years of follow-up, the researchers found that consumption of up to three servings of wine daily was associated with a significantly lower risk of dementia and Alzheimer's disease (AD) in older adults who do not have the APOEe-4 allele (the APOEe-4 allele is associated with development of AD). Those older adults who had light to moderate intake (one to two glasses a day) of wine also had a lower risk of developing dementia, although this was not statistically significant. A rationale for this finding is that alcohol intake is related to diminution of cerebrovascular disease (CVD) risk, and dementia is frequently caused by CVD. Further, there is ongoing research on prevention of dementia with antioxidant vitamins, and alcohol has an antioxidant effect.

However, the Washington Heights Inwood-Columbia Aging Project study found that beer and liquor did not have the same positive effect that wine did. This confirms, according to the authors, the findings from several European studies. The authors state that no prescription should be made from this study; further research with larger samples is needed. Further, it is known that heavy alcohol intake causes dementia.

There is increasing evidence that moderate intake of alcohol improves cognitive function, psychological well-being, and quality of life in elderly people. One report found that there was evidence to support that limited alcohol intake in earlier adult life may be protective against dementia in later life.

Recommendations

Whether to consume alcohol for medicinal purposes is a balancing act. If the older adult is physically active, of normal weight, and a nonsmoker; has healthy diet; and does not have a family history of heart disease, moderate alcohol intake is not likely to hurt. If the middle-aged or older adult does not drink, it is not usually beneficial to start. Similar benefits can accrue from exercise and a healthier diet.

If there is no history of alcoholism and the older adult is at moderate to high risk for heart disease, a daily alcoholic beverage may reduce the risk. If the older adult has low HDL that is unresponsive to diet and exercise, moderate drinking also may be beneficial. An older woman who has no family history of alcoholism and is at moderate to high risk for heart disease must balance the benefits of a daily drink with the small increase in risk of breast cancer. If she has a history or family history of alcohol abuse, it is wise not to start.

Management of Alcohol Dependence

Older adults tend to drink less than other age groups (see **Figure 15-1**). However, national research suggests that to-day older adults drink more than previous older generations. Because people are living longer, drinking will last longer into the lifespan, thus drinking by older adults may become a national health issue.

Vitamins

The easiest course of management when dealing with the older adult with an alcohol abuse problem is prescribing a 400 mg folic acid and/or a multivitamin/multimineral supplement every day. Alcohol blocks absorption of folic acid, which is needed to lower homocysteine. Alcohol also lowers the body's magnesium, which is needed for the electrical activity of the heart. Older adults with alcohol problems should be prescribed 1 mg of magnesium each day.

Medications

Drug trials of medications used to treat alcoholism indicate that they are not as effective in older adults as compared to younger and middle-aged adults. In the recent past, two drugs were used to manage alcohol dependence: disulfiram and naltrexone. Disulfiram has been available since the 1940s and acts as an aversive agent. If the patient takes the drug, then drinks alcohol, aversive symptoms occur. These include, flushing, headache, nausea, and vomiting. Naltrexone was approved by the FDA in 1994. The mechanism of action is unknown; however, the drug reduces the craving properties of alcohol. Recently, the FDA approved an injectable naltrexone, Vivitrol, given once a month in the buttocks. It is thought to block neurotransmitters in the brain and reduce alcohol craving.

The FDA (Federal Drug Administration) has approved acamprosate (Campral®) for the treatment of alcoholism. This drug works by stabilizing the **glutamate** system in the brain. The glutamate system is strongly affected by chronic alcohol use. Acamprosate speeds the process to "normalcy" and allows abstinence. The drug has been used in Europe for 15 years to prevent relapse in alcoholics.

Another drug, topiramate, reduces dependence on the "rewarding" effects of alcohol. It works by enhancing GABA function and decreasing glutamate activity. This is an "off-label" use of topiramate, which is an anticonvulsant. De-pakote, another anticonvulsant, is also used "off-label" to reduce cravings for alcohol.

Nonpharmacologic Intervention: Therapy and Education

Research suggests that treatment is effective in managing alcohol use/abuse in older individuals. In fact, older adults tend to respond better to treatment especially when it is conducted in a group of people their own age.

Psychiatric therapies have moved from "talk" therapy, such as cognitive-behavioral therapy, to medications for many conditions. However, behavioral therapy is still used for the treatment of alcohol dependence, partly because very few successful medications are available. A health care professional can facilitate one-on-one counseling or group therapy, including (1) cognitive-behavioral therapy; (2) group and family therapies; or (3) self-help groups.

Alcoholics Anonymous (AA) offers a model of helpful, positive partnering with another older adult who has been through the same situation and understands how difficult it is to stop or slow down the intake of alcohol. Few older adults wish to attend regular AA meetings, because most of the people are young to middle-aged, but several AA chapters have developed programs targeted at older adults. The health professional can help the older adult identify these and all other resources, including telephone numbers for help when it is needed.

The health care professional can teach the use of healthy coping strategies. The health care professional should find out what has worked successfully for the person in the past and emphasize the usefulness of this strategy. One example of a successful strategy is positive self-talk ("I can do it!"). The health care professional can plan with the patient, set goals, and review the goals periodically. When helping the older adult with alcoholism, it is essential not to judge or criticize failures.

The health care professional should note the patient's reading level in the patient's charts so that other health professionals know the educational level required to work with the patient. The chart should include documentation that the patient has been told of the physiological dangers of drinking too much as well as the dangers of drinking and driving and of combining alcohol with prescription and over-the-counter medications.

Conclusion

As with all preventable medical disorders, the prevention of alcoholism begins with early teaching of the dangers of alcohol abuse, early recognition of risk factors for alcohol abuse, and

> **glutamate (glutamic acid)**
> Excitatory neurotransmitter. Excitotoxicity is associated with stroke, amyotrophic lateral sclerosis, and other disorders.

early interventions. Alcoholism is a real problem in the older adult that can lead to social, functional, economic, psychological, and physiological consequences. It is imperative that health care providers be alert to the possible diagnosis and always include questions related to drinking frequency in the nutritional assessment. The use of tools such as the MAST-G can be helpful, especially in the early interview with the older patient. Health care providers and significant others must remain nonjudgmental, caring, and prompt with interventions.

Activities Related to This Chapter

1. Define the key terms in this chapter.
2. Visit the website of the National Institute of Alcohol Abuse and Alcoholism (*www.niaaa.nih.gov*).

Case Study

Helen is age 76 and retired. She lives at home with her husband, a distinguished retired English professor. They have no children, but they do have an active social life and many friends. Unknown to anyone but her husband, Helen drinks two bottles of wine every day. Recently, she has felt very weak and has been unable to go walking with friends, as she is accustomed to doing.

She went to her primary care physician. He performed tests but did not find anything wrong with her. He did not ask her about alcohol intake. He referred her to a neurologist. She eventually saw many physicians, none of whom asked about alcohol intake. One day, Helen was sick with a gastrointestinal virus and had vomiting and diarrhea for two days and was unable to keep down any foods or liquids. She went into delirium tremens and was taken to the hospital by the EMTs and then to the intensive care unit, where she stayed for ten days. She eventually went to a nursing facility for three weeks until she "dried out" completely. Now she is home again. She has begun to drink again, occasionally.

Questions

1. Why didn't anyone ask her about alcohol intake?
2. What information might the health professionals have gotten if they had asked?
3. What do you assume her nutritional status to be at this time?
4. How will you manage her?
5. What should be her treatment plan?

REFERENCES

Alatalo P, Koivisto H, Puukka K, et al. Biomarkers of liver status in heavy drinkers, moderate drinkers and abstainers. *Alcohol and Alcoholism.* 2009;44(2):199–203.

Alcohol and Seniors. Dangers of acetaminophen use and drinking. Available at: http://www.agingincanada.ca/dangers_of_acetaminophen.htm. Accessed June 1, 2009.

Allen N et al, Million women study shows even moderate alcohol consumption associated with increased cancer risk. *JNCI J Natl Cancer Inst.* 2009;101:296–305.

American Society of Addiction Medicine (ASAM). FDA approves acamprosate for the treatment of alcoholism. Available at: http://www.asam.org/news/FDA%20APPROVES%20ACAMPROSATE%202004.htm. Accessed November 24, 2004.

American Society of Addiction Medicine (ASAM). NIAAA publishes report on moderate alcohol use. Available at: http://www.asam.org/ews/NIAAA%2MODERATE%20ALCOHOL%20USE%202004.htm. Accessed November 3, 2004.

Bagnardi V, Blangiardo M, LaVecchia C, et al. Alcohol consumption and the risk of cancer. *Alc Res & Health.* 25(4):263–270.

Beers M, Berkow R. Diabetes mellitus. In *The Merck Manual of Geriatrics.* Whitehouse Station, NJ: Merck and Company, Inc.; 2000–2007.

Bogh-Sorensen L, Biltoft-Jensen A, Groth MV, Matthiessen J, Fagt S, Hels O. Association between alcohol intake and diet quality. Ugeskr Laeger. 2009;171(9):695–699.

Brody JA. Aging and alcohol abuse. *J Am Geriatric Soc.* 1982; 30:123–126.

Brody JE. Global Action on Aging. Hidden plague of alcohol abuse by the elderly. April 2, 2002. Available at: http://www.globalaging.org/health/world/hiddenalcohol.htm. Accessed June 1, 2009.

Brooks P, Enoch MA, Goldman D, et al. The alcohol flushing response: an unrecognized risk factor for esophageal cancer from alcohol consumption. *PLoS Med.* 2009;6(3):e50.

Buddy T. Genetics and alcohol liver disease: strong immune response a factor. July 1, 2006. Available at: http://alcoholism.about.com/cs/liver/a/aa001116a.htm. Accessed June 1, 2009.

Burke MM, Laramie J. *Primary Care of the Older Adult: Multidisciplinary Approach.* Philadelphia: Mosby; 2004.

Carlen P, McAndrews M, et al. Alcohol-related dementia in the institutionalized elderly. *Alcohol Clin Exp Res.* 1994;18(6):1330–1334.

Centers for Disease Control (CDC). Healthy aging health statistics/research, 2007. Available at http://www.cdc.gov.agingstats.htm. Accessed March 3, 2007.

Chedid A, Mendenhall C, Gartside P, French S, Chen T, Rabin L. Prognostic factors in alcoholic liver disease.

VA Cooperative Study Group. *Am J Gastroenterology.* 1991;86(2):210–216.

Colditz G, Rosner B. Cumulative risk of breast cancer to 70 years according to risk factor status data from the Nurses Health Study. *Am J Epidem.* 152(10):950–964.

Dar K. Alcohol use disorders in elderly people: fact or fiction? *Adv in Psychiatric Treatment.* 2006;12:173–181.

Dick DM, Agrawal A. National Institute on Alcohol Abuse and Alcoholism. The genetics of alcohol and other drug dependence. 2008. Available at: http://pubs.niaaa.nih.gov/publications/arh312/111-118.htm. Accessed June 1, 2009.

Djousse L, Gaziano J. Alcohol consumption and heart failure in hypertensive US male physicians. *Am J Cardiol.* 2008;102(5):593–597.

Dufour M, Stinson F, Caces M. Trends in cirrhosis morbidity and mortality: United States, 1979–1988. *Semin Liver Dis.* 1993;13(2):109–125.

Fergusson D, Boden J, Horwood LJ. Tests of causal links between alcohol abuse or dependence and major depression. *Arch Gen Psychiatry.* 2009;66(3):260–266.

Gaziano J, Gaziano T, Glynn R, et al. Light-to-moderate alcohol consumption and mortality in the Physicians' Health Study enrollment cohort. *J Am Coll Cardiol.* 2000;35(1):96–105.

Goldman D. Alcohol abuse: Best practice of medicine. April 10, 2002. Available at: http://merck.micromed.conf/index.asp?page = bhg/tables&articles-id = BHGO1PSO3&table. Accessed October 24, 2005.

Harvard Heart Letter. Benefits from moderate drinking extended? July 2004. Available at: http://www.health.harvard.edu. Accessed October 12, 2005.

Harvard Mental Health Letter. Brief treatment for problem drinkers. 2004;21(2):4–6.

Harvard School of Public Health (HSPH). Alcohol. Available at: http://www.hsph.harvard.edu/nutritionsource/alcohol.html. Accessed March 12, 2007.

Harvard School of Public Health (HSPH). Men with high blood pressure who drink moderate amounts of alcohol may have a lower risk of heart attack. Press release. January 21, 2007. Available at: http://www.hsph.harvard.edu/press/releases/press01012007.html. Accessed March 1, 2007.

Harvard School of Public Health (HSPH). The Nutrition Source. Alcohol: the bottom line. 2009. Available at: http://www.hsph.harvard.edu/nutritionsource/what-should-you-eat/alcohol/index.html. Accessed June 1, 2009.

Heath AC, Phil D, and Nelson EC. Effects of the interaction between genotype and environment research into the genetic epidemiology of alcohol dependence. *Alcoholic Res*

Health. 2002. Available at: http://pubs.niaaa.nih.gov/publications/arh26-3/193-201.htm. Accessed October 1, 2005.

Higgins J, Wright S, Wrenn K. Alcohol, the elderly, and motor vehicle crashes. *Am J Emergency Med.* 1996;14(3):265–267.

Institute of Alcohol Studies. Alcohol and the elderly. n.d. Available at: http://www.ias.org.uk. Accessed March 25, 2009.

Jackson J, Williams D, Gomberg E. A life course perspective on aging and alcohol use and abuse among African Americans. In Gomberg E, Hegedus A, Zucker R, eds. *Alcohol Problems and Aging.* NIH Pub. 98-4163. Bethesda, MD: NIAAA, 1998.

Jackson V, Sesso H, Buring J, Gaziano J. Alcohol consumption and mortality in men with preexisting cerebrovascular disease. *Arch Int Med.* 2003;163(10):1189–1193.

Jiao L, Silverman D, Schairer C, et al. Alcohol use and risk of pancreatic cancer: the NIH-AARP Diet and Health Study. *Am J Epidemiol.* 2009;169(9):1043–1051.

Johnson BA. Topiramate reduces intake and craving in alcoholics who are drinking. *Alcohol Clin Exp Res.* 2004;28:1137–1144.

Johnson BA, Ait-Daoud N, Bowden C. Oral topiramate for treatment of alcohol dependence: a randomized controlled trial. *Lancet.* 2003;361(9370):1677–1685.

Klatsky A, Morton C., Udaltsova N, Friedman G. Coffee, cirrhosis, and transaminase enzymes. *Arch Int Med.* 2006;166:1190–1195.

Knight J, Bernstein L, Largent J, et al. Alcohol intake and cigarette smoking and risk of a contralateral breast cancer. *Am J Epidemiol.* 2009;169(8):962–968.

Luchsinger J, Tang M, Siddiqui M, Shea S, Mayeux R. Alcohol intake and risk of dementia. *J Am Geriatric Soc.* 2004; 52(4):540–546.

Mancinelli R, Cecanti M. Biomarkers in alcohol misuse: their role in the prevention and detection of thiamine deficiency. *Alchol Alcohol.* 2009;44(2):177–182.

Mark T. Are medications for alcoholism underutilized? An analysis of private-sector and Medicaid. *Drug Benefit Trends.* 2004;16(3):154–158.

Mayo Clinic. Alcoholism. October 2006. Available at: http://www.mayoclinic.com/printinvoker.cfm?objectid=BA6DB211-57CE-4DB7- A3614C2B60219EB5. Accessed March 12, 2006.

MayoClinic. Alcoholism: Treatment and drugs. May 8, 2008. Available at: http://www.mayoclinic.com/health/alcoholism/DS00340/DSECTION = treatments%2Dand%2Ddrugs/. Accessed June 1, 2009.

Mendenhall C, Roselle G, Moritz T, Veterans Administration Cooperative Study Groups 119,275. Relationship of protein calorie malnutrition to alcoholic liver disease: a re-examination of data from two Veterans Admin-

istration Cooperative Studies. *Alcohol Clin Exp Res.* 1995;19(3):635–641.

Merck Manual of Geriatrics. Alcohol abuse and dependence. n.d. Available at: http://www.merck.com/mkgr/mmg/sec4/ch37/ch37a.jsp. Accessed June 1, 2009.

Midanik L, Clark W. The demographic distribution of U.S. drinking patterns in 1990: Descriptions and trends from 1984. *Am J Public Health.* 1994;84(8):1218–1222.

Miller CA. *Nursing for Wellness in Older Adults.* 4th ed. Philadelphia: Lippincott; 2004.

Mukamal K, Rimm EB. Alcohol consumption: risks and benefits. *Curr Atheroscler Rep.* 2008;10(6):536–43.

Mumenthaler M, Mattle H. *Neurology.* 4th ed. New York: Thieme; 2004.

National Highway Traffic Safety Administration. *Traffic Safety Facts, 1994.* Washington, DC: NHTSA; 1995.

National Institute of Alcoholism and Alcohol Abuse. National Institutes of Health. Alcohol alert. Alcohol research: a lifespan perspective. January 28, 2008. Available at: http://www.niaaa.nih.gov/publications/AA74/AA74.htm. Accessed May 3, 2008.

National Institute on Aging. National Institutes of Health. AgePage: Alcohol use and abuse. February 2008. Available at: http://www.nia.nih.gov/HealthInformation/Publications/alcohol.htm. Accessed May 3, 2008.

O'Connell H, Chin A et al. Alcohol use disorders in elderly people—redefining an age-old problem in old age. *BMJ.* 2003;327:664–667.

Ohtake T, Saito H, Hosoki Y, Inoue M, Miyoshi S, Suzuki Y, Fujimoto Y, Kohgo Y. Hepcidin is down-regulated in alcohol loading. *Alcoholism: Clin and Exper Research.* 2007;31(suppl 1):S2–S8.

Peters R, Peters J, Warner J, et al. Alcohol, dementia and cognitive decline in the elderly: a systematic review. *Age Ageing.* 2008;37(5):505–512.

Rigler SK. Alcoholism in the elderly. *Am Fam Physician.* 2000;61(6):10–16.

Ruitenberg A, van Swieten J, Witteman J, et al. Alcohol consumption and risk of dementia: the Rotterdam study. *Lancet.* 2002;359(9303):281–286.

Saremi A, Arora R. The cardiovascular implications of alcohol and red wine. *Am J Ther.* 2008;15(3):265–277.

Schaeffner E, Kurth T, deJong P, et al. Alcohol consumption and the risk of renal dysfunction in apparently healthy men. *Arch Intern Med.* 2005;165(9):1048–1053.

Schuckit M. An overview of genetic influences in alcoholism. *J Subst Abuse Treat.* 2009;36(1):S5–14.

Senior Journal. Elderly drivers increasingly more likely to die in auto accidents. January 5, 2007. Available at: http://seniorjournal.com/NEWS/Aging/2007/7-01-05-ElderlyDrivers.htm. Accessed June 1, 2009.

Seniors in Sobriety. Alcoholism in the senior population: an abridged resource guide. n.d. Available at: http://www.

seniorsinsobriety.org/SIS-AlcoholismintheElderly.pdf. Accessed June 1, 2009.

Solfrizzi V, D'Introno A, Colacicco A, Capurso C, Del Parigi A, Baldassarre G, et al. Alcohol consumption, mild cognitive impairment, and progression to dementia. *Neurology.* 2007;68:1790–1799.

Spector T. Moderate alcohol intake tied to increased bone mineral density: a study of female twins. *Ann of Rheum Disease.* 2005;64:309–310.

Talwalkar J, Kamath P. Influence of recent advances in medical management of clinical outcomes of cirrhosis. *Mayo Clin Proc.* 2005;80:1501–1508.

Tracy AB. International Coalition for Drug Awareness. SSRIs and alcohol. 2009. Available at: http://www.drugawareness.org/ssris-and-alcohol.html. Accessed June 1, 2009.

Tucker K, Jugdaohsingh R, Powell J, et al. Effects of beer, wine, and liquor intakes on bone mineral density in older men and women. *Am J Clin Nutr.* 2009;89(4):1188–1196.

Vieten C. Alcoholism—Is it genetic? 2005. Available at: http://www.familystudies.com/alcoholism&genetics.htm. Accessed October 1, 2005.

WebMD and The Sleep Medicine Center at the Cleveland Clinic. Drug and alcohol related sleep problems. 2009. Available at: http://www.webmd.com/sleep-disorders/drug-alcohol-related/. Accessed June 1, 2009.

Wetterliing T, Backhaus J, Junghanns K. Addiction in the elderly–an underestimated diagnosis in clinical practice? *Nervenarzt.* 2002;73(9):861–866.

Appendix 15-1

The Alcohol Use Disorders Identification Test (AUDIT)

The alcohol use disorders identification test (AUDIT) is the best test for screening because it detects hazardous drinking as well as alcohol abuse. Furthermore, it has a greater sensitivity in populations with a lower prevalence of alcoholism. One study suggested that questions 1, 2, 4, 5, and 10 were nearly as effective as the entire questionnaire. If confirmed, AUDIT would be easier to administer. Extensive information is available from the World Health Organization, which offers a PDF file for free download for the primary care provider at *http://whqlibdoc.who.int/hq/2001/WHO_MSD_MSB_01.6a.pdf.*

AUDIT Questionnaire					
Questions	**0 Points**	**1 Point**	**2 Points**	**3 Points**	**4 Points**
1. How often do you have a drink containing alcohol?	Never	Monthly or less	2–4 times a month	2–3 times a week	4 or more times a week
2. How many drinks containing alcohol do you have on a typical day when you are drinking?	1 or 2	3 or 4	5 or 6	7–9	10 or more
3. How often do you have six or more drinks on one occasion?	Never	Less than monthly	Monthly	Weekly	Daily or almost daily
4. How often during the past year have you found that you were not able to stop drinking once you had started?	Never	Less than monthly	Monthly	Weekly	Daily or almost daily
5. How often during the past year have you failed to do what was normally expected of you because of drinking?	Never	Less than monthly	Monthly	Weekly	Daily or almost daily
6. How often during the past year have you needed a first drink in the morning to get yourself going after a heavy drinking session?	Never	Less than monthly	Monthly	Weekly	Daily or almost daily
7. How often during the past year have you had a feeling of guilt or remorse after drinking?	Never	Less than monthly	Monthly	Weekly	Daily or almost daily
8. How often during the past year have you been unable to remember what happened the night before because you had been drinking?	Never	Less than monthly	Monthly	Weekly	Daily or almost daily
9. Have you or has someone else been injured as a result of your drinking?	No		Yes, but not in the past year		Yes, during the past year
10. Has a relative, friend, or a doctor or other health care worker been concerned about your drinking or suggested you cut down?	No		Yes, but not in the past year		Yes, during the past year

Score of eight or more for men and four or more for women indicates problem drinking.

Source: Courtesy of the World Health Organization.

CHAPTER 16

Nutritional Assessment for the Older Adult

Melissa Bernstein, PhD, RD, LD

• •

CHAPTER OBJECTIVES   Upon completion of this chapter, the reader will be able to:

1. Discuss the importance and objectives of nutrition screening methods
2. Identify the need for nutritional assessment
3. List and define the essential components of a nutritional assessment for an older adult, including anthropometric, biochemical, clinical, and dietary components
4. Define the key components of a dietary assessment for an older adult

KEY TERMS AND CONCEPTS

Anthropometry   Nutrition assessment

Dietary assessment   Nutrition screening

Food security   Nutritional status

• •

Every careful observer of the sick will agree in this that thousands of patients are annually starved in the midst of plent...

—Florence Nightingale, *Notes on Nursing: What It Is, and What It Is Not* (1859).

Nutritional Status

Good nutritional status is essential to adequate functioning and sense of well-being in older adults. Older adults are at nutritional risk due to numerous factors, including poor dietary intake, chronic medical conditions, and a variety of physical, economic, and social factors (**Figure 16-1**). **Nutritional status** can be determined by evaluating how diet affects the health of an individual or group of people. Assessment of nutritional status measures the processes of dietary intake, digestion, absorption, transport, storage, and metabolism, as well as the elimination of wastes from food and their metabolic products. Therefore, nutritional evaluation of older adults requires consideration of many interrelated factors that contribute simultaneously to nutritional status.

As discussed in Chapter 2, progressive aging and chronic disease lead to altered physiology and diminished functionality, which may have a negative impact on food intake, and thus on overall health status. Nutrition screening and assessment form the basis for initiating a care plan for the older adult. Detection of risk for malnutrition and

> **nutritional status** The state of a person's overall health and body as influenced by levels of nutrients and diet.

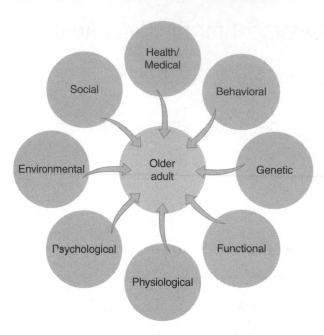

FIGURE 16-1 Nutritional Risk Factors for Older Adults

early intervention may lessen negative consequences associated with malnutrition, such as greater susceptibility to infection, longer hospital stays, and increased mortality.

Nutrition Screening

Patterns of dietary intake reflect an individual's habitual consumption of foods and beverages and can be used to assess nutritional risk. Nutrition screening is the process of identifying these risks based on food intake and food-related behaviors and circumstances. The American Dietetic Association defines **nutrition screening** as the process of identifying characteristics known to be associated with nutritional problems. The purpose of nutrition screening is to identify individuals who are at nutritional risk or who are malnourished.

The Nutrition Screening Initiative and the Mini-Nutrition Assessment are two of the most widely accepted nutrition screening tools for older adults. The Nutrition Screening Initiative (NSI) recommends that nutrition screening and intervention be provided by health care agencies and be included in the chronic disease management for our nation's aging population. The NSI also states that routine nutrition screening and intervention could contribute to health maintenance and the prevention and management of many chronic diseases, thereby leading to improved self-sufficiency, vitality, and quality of life.

nutrition screening The process of identifying factors known to be associated with nutritional problems.

Goals of Nutrition Screening

One of the major goals of effective nutrition screening is keeping older adults at home and in community-based settings by facilitating the prevention and early detection of nutrition-related complications that could contribute to medical complications and decreased ability to live independently. According to the NSI, "it is important to assess the physiologic changes associated with aging that affect nutritional status and the food intake, such as changes in taste and thirst and to be aware of the psychosocial factors that may contribute to poor intake such as poverty and isolation" when performing nutrition screening. Nutrition screening can contribute to positive health outcomes by identifying and treating nutritional risk factors early as a result of improved collaboration among all members of the health care team.

A screening process should have the following five characteristics:

1. It can be completed in any setting.
2. It facilitates the completion of early intervention goals.
3. It includes the collection of relevant data on risk factors and the interpretation of data for intervention/treatment.
4. It determines the need for a nutrition assessment.
5. It is cost-effective.

The effectiveness of a screening tool lies in its ability to identify an individual at risk so that there can be a beneficial outcome from the screening. A number of nutrition screening instruments have been developed for use with older adults (**Table 16-1**). Appropriate nutrition monitoring and intervention can then take place after screening has occurred.

Nutrition Screening Instruments

The Nutrition Screening Initiative (NSI) is a broad, multidisciplinary joint effort of the American Academy of Family Physicians, the American Dietetic Association, the National Council on Aging, and a diverse coalition of more than 25 national health, aging, and medical associations. The goal of the NSI is to promote routine nutrition screening and intervention for older adults as a cost-effective strategy to improve the health of older Americans. Both inadequate and excessive caloric and nutrient intakes, body weight, and physical activity can be identified and addressed through nutrition screening and intervention. Disease-specific nutrition screening and intervention are crucial to the management of many of the chronic diseases that affect older adults. Without proper screening and intervention, chronic conditions such as diabetes, hypertension, chronic obstructive pulmonary disease, renal disease, osteoporosis, congestive heart failure, coronary heart disease, high blood pressure, and undernutrition could lead to preventable adverse health outcomes and higher medical expenses.

TABLE 16-1 Nutrition Screening Tools

Purpose: Identify individuals at nutritional risk and provide appropriate intervention before malnutrition or related complications occur.

Tools
Nutrition Screening Initiative (NSI)
Mini Nutrition Assessment (MNA)
Nutrition Risk Index (NRI)

Scales
Subjective Global Assessment (SGA)
Nutrition Risk Assessment (NRA)
Simplified Nutrition Appetite Questionnaire (SNAQ)
Malnutrition Universal Screening Tool (MUST)
Nutrition Risk Screening (NRS 2002)

DETERMINE

The NSI focuses on identifying older Americans who are at nutritional risk and then improving their nutritional status. The DETERMINE Your Nutritional Health Checklist was developed by the NSI as a self-assessment screening tool to increase older adults' awareness of their nutritional status and to promote routine nutritional screening (**Figure 16-2**). The DETERMINE checklist is composed of ten yes/no items that are associated with nutritional health in older adults. Individuals can answer the questions themselves or with the help of a caregiver. Although the DETERMINE checklist does not evaluate nutritional status, low scores indicate low risk of poor nutritional status. An older adult with a score greater than six on the DETERMINE checklist is identified as being at high risk for malnutrition and more likely to have low nutrient intake. A higher score also indicates increased

---

The warning signs of poor nutritional health are often overlooked. Use this checklist to find out if you or someone you know is at nutritional risk.

Read the statements below. Circle the number in the yes column for those that apply to you or someone you know. For each yes answer, score the number in the box. Total your nutritional score.

	YES
I have an illness or condition that made me change the kind and/or amount of food I eat.	2
I eat fewer than two meals per day.	3
I eat few fruits or vegetables, or milk products.	2
I have three or more drinks of beer, liquor or wine almost every day.	2
I have tooth or mouth problems that make it hard for me to eat.	2
I don't always have enough money to buy the food I need.	4
I eat alone most of the time.	1
I take three or more different prescribed or over-the-counter drugs a day.	1
Without wanting to, I have lost or gained 10 pounds in the last 6 months.	2
I am not always physically able to shop, cook and/or feed myself.	2
TOTAL	

Total your nutritional score. If it's —	
0–2	**Good!** Recheck your nutritional score in 6 months.
3–5	**You are at moderate nutritional risk.** See what can be done to improve your eating habits and lifestyle. Your office on aging, senior nutrition program, senior citizens center, or health department can help. Recheck your nutritional score in 3 months.
6 or more	**You are at high nutrition risk.** Bring this checklist the next time you see your doctor, dietician or other qualified health or social service professional. Talk with them about any problems you may have. Ask for help to improve your nutritional health.

Remember that warning signs suggest risk, but do not represent diagnosis of any condition. Turn the page to learn more about the warning signs of poor nutritional health.

FIGURE 16-2 DETERMINE Your Nutritional Health

Source: Courtesy of Abbott

(Continues)

The Nutrition Checklist is based on the warning signs described below. Use the word DETERMINE to remind you of the warning signs.

Disease

Any disease, illness or chronic condition that causes you to change the way you eat, or makes it hard for you to eat, puts your nutritional health at risk. Four out of five adults have chronic diseases that are affected by diet. Confusion or memory loss that keeps getting worse is estimated to affect one out of five or more older adults. This can make it hard to remember what, when, or if you've eaten. Feeling sad or depressed, which happens to about one in eight older adults, can cause big changes in appetite, digestion, energy level, wight and well-being.

Eating Poorly

Eating too little and eating too much both lead to poor health. Eating the same foods day after day or not eating fruit, vegetables and milk products daily will also cause poor nutritional health. One in five adults skips meals daily. Only 13 percent of adults eat the minimum amount of fruits and vegetables needed. One in four older adults drinks too much alcohol. Many health problems become worse if you drink more than one or two alcoholic beverages per day.

Tooth Loss/Mouth Pain

A healthy mouth, teeth, and gums are needed to eat. Missing, loose or rotten teeth or dentures that don't fit well or cause mouth sores make it hard to eat.

Economic Hardship

As many as 40 percent of older Americans have incomes of less than $6,000 per year. Having less—or choosing to spend less—than $25 to $30 per week for food makes it very hard to get the foods you need to stay healthy.

Reduced Social Contact

One-third of all older people live alone. Being with people daily has a positive effect on morale, well-being and eating.

Multiple Medicines

Many older Americans must take medicines for health problems. Almost one half of older Americans take multiple medicines daily. Growing old may change the way we respond to drugs. The more medicines you take, the greater the chance for side effects such as increased or decreased appetite, change in taste, constipation, weakness, drowsiness, diarrhea, nausea, and others. Vitamins or minerals when taken in large doses act like drugs and can cause harm. Alert your doctor to everything you take.

Involuntary Weight Loss/Gain

Losing or gaining a lot of weight when you are not trying to do so is an important warning sign that must not be ignored. Being overweight or underweight also increases your chance of poor health.

Needs Assistance in Self Care

Although most older people are able to eat, one of every five has trouble walking, shopping, and buying and cooking food, especially as they get older.

Elder Years Above Age 80

Most older people lead full and productive lives. But as age increases, risk of frailty and health problems increase. Checking your nutritional health regularly makes good sense.

FIGURE 16-2 DETERMINE Your Nutritional Health (Continued)

risk of adverse health conditions and fair or poor perceived health status.

Based on the results of the DETERMINE checklist, level I or II screens are then used to perform a more in-depth assessment. The level I screen is designed to distinguish between those older adults who require immediate and intensive nutritional assessment by a health professional and those individuals who do not have nutritional deficits that require immediate medical care. The level II screen should be administered to those individuals who require more specific diagnostic information on nutritional status. It can be used by health care professionals to identify common medical problems, such as protein-energy malnutrition, obesity, hyperlipidemia, and osteoporosis. Following a level II screen, nutrition interventions should be implemented to prevent further declines in nutritional status and to correct any nutritional deficiencies.

Mini Nutrition Assessment

The Mini Nutrition Assessment (MNA) is another useful tool to assess nutritional risk. It is considered by many to be the "gold standard" for ambulatory older adults living in the community setting as well as those living in long-term care facilities. The MNA was designed be a quick, economical, and noninvasive method for assessing the nutritional risk of frail older persons. The MNA is useful for clinical practice because it is a well-validated tool that can be used to measure nutritional status and screen for malnutrition, to detect early risk of malnutrition, and to facilitate nutritional intervention follow up in older adults. It can also be used in the community and clinical setting by dietitians, nurses, and physicians, as well as numerous health care professionals. The MNA is commonly used for community-based individuals before they enter a nursing facility. It can also be used for screening and assessment in hospitals and long-term care facilities and for monitoring changes in nutritional status over time.

The MNA is an 18-item questionnaire composed of anthropometric measures and questions pertaining to lifestyle, medication, mobility, diet, and self-perception of health and nutrition (**Figure 16-3**). A higher score on the MNA identifies an individual with good nutritional status, whereas moderate scores (17 to 23) suggest the need for multidisciplinary geriatric intervention to alleviate risk and prevent malnutrition. A score less than 17 identifies a person with protein-energy malnutrition, which requires further assessment to quantify the severity of the malnutrition as well as to develop the appropriate nutritional intervention.

A short version of the MNA (MNA-SF) has also been developed and takes fewer than 4 minutes to complete. The MNA-SF is useful for screening older acute medical patients for malnutrition and risk of malnutrition. A positive score on the MNA-SF indicates the need to complete the full MNA. Both the MNA and MNA-SF are sensitive, specific, and accurate in identifying nutritional risk.

The MNA has been found useful in identifying the following:

- Prevalence and risk of malnutrition in community-dwelling older adults
- Prevalence of undernutrition in outpatient and home care older adults
- Prevalence of undernutrition and the risk of malnutrition in hospitalized and institutionalized older adults

One main advantage of using the MNA for assessing the nutritional status of older adults is that it does not require any biochemical tests. The MNA can also be used to distinguish between those older adults with adequate nutritional status, those at risk of malnutrition, and those with malnutrition. The MNA is also a useful tool for reassessment and for monitoring nutritional status following intervention. Changes in nutritional status are associated with changes in MNA score. Therefore, once risk for malnutrition or malnourishment has been identified, the MNA can be used as a guide for a successful nutritional intervention.

Other Nutrition Screening Methods

A number of other nutrition screening methods are available to identify nutritional risk.

The Nutrition Risk Index

The Nutrition Risk Index (NRI) focuses on mechanics of food intake, prescribed dietary restrictions, conditions that would affect food intake, and significant changes in dietary habits. The index consists of 16 questions that can be administered in a variety of settings by personnel with limited training. The higher the score, the greater the risk for poor nutritional status, poor health in general, and greater use of health care services. The NRI is helpful for identifying older adults in need of nutritional interventions and more in-depth nutrition assessment.

SCALES

SCALES is a useful tool for identifying older individuals at nutritional risk, especially protein-energy malnutrition (**Box 16-1**). It is a simple screening tool developed for use by dietitians and physicians that includes anthropometric, clinical, biochemical, as well as functional indicators of nutrition status.

Subjective Global Assessment

The Subjective Global Assessment (SGA) was originally developed for use with gastrointestinal surgery patients. The SGA includes questions about changes in weight and dietary intake, gastrointestinal disturbances, and functional capacity. The physical examination assesses subcutaneous

Nestlé Nutrition INSTITUTE

Mini Nutritional Assessment
MNA®

Last name:	First name:	Sex:	Date:

Age:	Weight, kg:	Height, cm:	I.D. Number:

Complete the screen by filling in the boxes with the appropriate numbers.
Add the numbers for the screen. If score is 11 or less, continue with the assessment to gain a Malnutrition Indicator Score.

Screening

A Has food intake declined over the past 3 months due to loss of appetite, digestive problems, chewing or swallowing difficulties?
0 = severe loss of appetite
1 = moderate loss of appetite
2 = no loss of appetite

B Weight loss during the last 3 months
0 = weight loss greater than 3 kg (6.6 lbs)
1 = does not know
2 = weight loss between 1 and 3 kg (2.2 and 6.6 lbs)
3 = no weight loss

C Mobility
0 = bed or chair bound
1 = able to get out of bed/chair but does not go out
2 = goes out

D Has suffered psychological stress or acute disease in the past 3 months
0 = yes   2 = no

E Neuropsychological problems
0 = severe dementia or depression
1 = mild dementia
2 = no psychological problems

F Body Mass Index (BMI) (weight in kg) / (height in m²)
0 = BMI less than 19
1 = BMI 19 to less than 21
2 = BMI 21 to less than 23
3 = BMI 23 or greater

Screening score (subtotal max. 14 points)
12 points or greater   Normal – not at risk – no need to complete assessment
11 points or below   Possible malnutrition – continue assessment

Assessment

G Lives independently (not in a nursing home or hospital)
0 = no   1 = yes

H Takes more than 3 prescription drugs per day
0 = yes   1 = no

I Pressure sores or skin ulcers
0 = yes   1 = no

Ref. Vellas B, Villars H, Abellan G, et al. Overview of the MNA® - Its History and Challenges. J Nut Health Aging 2006;10:456-465.
Rubenstein LZ, Harker JO, Salva A, Guigoz Y, Vellas B. Screening for Undernutrition in Geriatric Practice: Developing the Short-Form Mini Nutritional Assessment (MNA-SF). J Geront 2001;56A: M366-377.
Guigoz Y. The Mini-Nutritional Assessment (MNA®) Review of the Literature - What does it tell us? J Nutr Health Aging 2006; 10:466-487.

© Nestlé, 1994, Revision 2006. N67200 12/99 10M

For more information : www.mna-elderly.com

J How many full meals does the patient eat daily?
0 = 1 meal
1 = 2 meals
2 = 3 meals

K Selected consumption markers for protein intake
• At least one serving of dairy products (milk, cheese, yogurt) per day   yes ☐ no ☐
• Two or more servings of legumes or eggs per week   yes ☐ no ☐
• Meat, fish or poultry every day   yes ☐ no ☐
0.0 = if 0 or 1 yes
0.5 = if 2 yes
1.0 = if 3 yes

L Consumes two or more servings of fruits or vegetables per day?
0 = no   1 = yes

M How much fluid (water, juice, coffee, tea, milk…) is consumed per day?
0.0 = less than 3 cups
0.5 = 3 to 5 cups
1.0 = more than 5 cups

N Mode of feeding
0 = unable to eat without assistance
1 = self-fed with some difficulty
2 = self-fed without any problem

O Self view of nutritional status
0 = views self as being malnourished
1 = is uncertain of nutritional state
2 = views self as having no nutritional problem

P In comparison with other people of the same age, how does the patient consider his/her health status?
0.0 = not as good
0.5 = does not know
1.0 = as good
2.0 = better

Q Mid-arm circumference (MAC) in cm
0.0 = MAC less than 21
0.5 = MAC 21 to 22
1.0 = MAC 22 or greater

R Calf circumference (CC) in cm
0 = CC less than 31   1 = CC 31 or greater

Assessment (max. 16 points)

Screening score

Total Assessment (max. 30 points)

Malnutrition Indicator Score
| 17 to 23.5 points | at risk of malnutrition |
| Less than 17 points | malnourished |

FIGURE 16-3 Mini Nutrition Assessment (MNA)

Source: Vellas B, Villars H, Abellan G, et al. Overview of the MNA®–Its History and Challanges. *J. Nutr Health Aging*. 2006;10:456–465; Rubenstein LZ, Harker JO, Salva A, Guigoz Y, Vellas B. Screening for undernutrition in geriatric practice: developing the Short-Form Mini Nutritional Assessment (MNA-SF). *J Geront*. 2001; 56A:M366–377; Guigoz Y. The Mini Nutritional Assessment (MNA®) Review of the Literature–What does it tell us? *J Nutr Health Aging*. 2006;10:466–487. ®Société des Produits Nestlé S.A., Vevey, Switzerland, Trademark Owners.

fat loss, muscle wasting, and the presence of edema. The results of the physical examination and interview are then used to subjectively classify individuals as well nourished (SGA class A), mild/moderately malnourished (SGA class B), or severely malnourished (SGA class C). Although the SGA was not developed specifically for older adults, it appears to identify older adults at risk of nutrition-associated complications and death. The SGA has been used to identify nutrition-associated complications and death in nursing home residents.

Additional Assessment Tools

The Nutrition Risk Assessment (NRA) form developed by the American Dietetic Association includes strategies and interventions to guide the health care team in providing care for the nursing home resident.

Another form recently developed as an appetite-assessment tool to predict weight loss in community-dwelling adults and long-term care residents is the Simplified Nutrition Appetite Questionnaire (SNAQ). SNAQ is a short four-question tool that is clinically efficient and evaluates appetite as a distinct, singular item, which is useful for the early identification of older adults at risk for anorexia-related weight loss.

The Malnutrition Universal Screening Tool (MUST) questionnaire was developed to screen adults for risk of malnutrition. This tool, used frequently in the United Kingdom, has been found to predict mortality and length of hospital stay in acutely ill, hospitalized older adults.

Nutrition Risk Screening (NRS 2002) was developed specifically for hospitalized patients who need nutritional support and is useful in the acute care setting. NRS 2002, as well as SGA and MUST, have all been shown to accurately assess nutritional status and risk in hospitalized patients.

Nutrition Assessment

Definition and Purpose

The primary purpose of **nutrition assessment** is to interpret and expand on the data from the nutrition screening process. A comprehensive nutrition assessment defines nutritional status by using medical, nutritional, and medication histories; physical examination; anthropometric measurements; and laboratory data. A nutritional care plan is developed, implemented, and evaluated following the assessment. **Table 16-2** summarizes the nutrition assessment methods, their purpose and components, and discusses the methods in more detail.

Components of Nutritional Assessment

Once a person has been identified to be at nutritional risk, a comprehensive nutrition assessment is then used to investigate further the person's anthropometric, biochemical, clinical, dietary, psychosocial, economic, functional, mental health, and oral health status. The selection of nutritional indicators to assess nutritional status depends on several factors, including the amount of time available for the assessment, the type of personnel available, and the financial resources at hand to support the evaluation. Many risk factors and categories need to be considered during a nutritional assessment, including food and nutrient intake patterns, psychological and social factors, physical conditions and diseases/disorders, abnormal laboratory values, and medications. Each category should be used as a guide to help professionals establish if there is a history or evidence of risk factors and to determine the client's risk level. The severity of the risk factors will depend on the age and physical condition of the individual being assessed.

Nutrition assessment involves determining the health status of individuals and population groups. Measuring nutritional assessment is central to providing appropriate medical nutrition therapy (MNT) to older individuals. MNT is a two-step process of (1) assessment of nutritional status and (2) development of an individualized intervention plan.

The mnemonic ABCD can be used to remember the four primary components of nutritional assessment: *A* for *a*nthropometric measurements, *B* for *b*iochemical parameters, *C* for *c*linical assessment, and *D* for *d*ietary history.

Anthropometric measurements are used to estimate the amounts of the various body components, such as muscle fat. These methods are particularly useful in detecting protein-energy malnutrition. Anthropometric measures can generally be obtained by trained personnel with relatively inexpensive and

nutrition assessment Defines nutritional status by using medical, nutritional, and medication histories; physical examination; anthropometric measurements; and laboratory data.

TABLE 16-2 Nutrition Assessment Methods

Purpose: Provide a comprehensive evaluation of nutritional status and appropriate nutrition intervention to prevent and treat malnutrition and associated conditions.

Methods

1. Anthropometric

   Purpose: Determine and monitor changes in body weight, height, body composition, and body fat distribution. Establish protein and energy reserves and assess risk for acute and chronic diseases.

   Components:
   - Weight and height/stature
   - BMI
   - Circumference
   - Skinfolds
   - Body composition

2. Biochemical

   Purpose: Objective evaluation of nutrient intake. Determine stored and functional levels of nutrients. Determine risk and monitor changes for nutrition-related diseases.

   Components:
   - Protein status
   - Cholesterol levels
   - Vitamin and mineral status

3. Clinical

   Purpose: Obtain complete nutritional and medical history, including cognitive, physical, functional, and oral status. Determine the presence of nutritional deficiency signs and symptoms.

   Components:
   - Medical history
   - Signs and symptoms
   - Cognitive and physical function
   - Oral health
   - Medication use

4. Dietary

   Purpose: Obtain and monitor food and beverage consumption, supplement use, and food-related behaviors by individuals or groups to determine quality of the diet. Identify and evaluate dietary patterns.

   Components:
   - Food and beverage intake
   - Food security
   - Supplement use
   - Food preferences, cultural practices, beliefs, rituals
   - Dietary preferences

Source: Data from Schlenker ED. *Nutrition in Aging.* 3rd ed. Boston: McGraw Hill; 1998.

noninvasive measures. Biochemical methods are the most sensitive indicators of nutritional status; however, they are not always specific for the nutrient involved. In addition, they can be influenced by factors such as chronic disease, hydration status, and inflammation.

Biochemical assessment generally involves invasive techniques; it can be time-consuming and expensive. Nutritional inadequacies result in clinical signs that are useful in assessing nutritional status. It is important to remember, however, that many of the signs seen in the older adult may have both nutritional and non-nutritional causes. In addition to physical signs, clinical assessment also involves the evaluation of functional status, oral status, and mental and cognitive status.

Several methods are useful for the assessment of dietary intake in older adults. Each method has numerous strengths and weaknesses. It is necessary to identify the objective and the subject population before selecting a dietary assessment method. Many of these methods are valuable for identifying older people at nutritional risk and those who are in need of nutritional education and intervention.

Anthropometry

Anthropometry is the measurement of body size, weight, and proportions to assess the physiologic effects of either undernutrition or overnutrition. It can be used as part of an evaluation of the nutritional status of older persons. One of the primary objectives of nutritional anthropometry is to establish an individual's protein-energy reserve. Anthropometric measurements can be used as both indicators of an acute illness or injury or as long-term indicators of slower progressing, debilitating conditions related to loss of available energy stores (undernutrition) as well as obesity (overnutrition). In addition, anthropometric measurements can also be used to monitor the appropriateness and effectiveness of nutrition intervention. Therefore, to produce meaningful information, care should be taken to ensure that the measurements taken are accurate and reliable.

The anthropometric measures most commonly used for assessing nutritional status are body weight, height, various circumferences, and skinfold thicknesses. The major benefits of anthropometry for use in older adults are its relatively low cost and the noninvasiveness. However, the usefulness of such measures as predictors of nutritional status in older adults has been questioned due to the many physiologic changes in body size and composition that occur with normal aging. Due to the heterogeneous nature of the older adult population, comparison to reference standards based simply on age can lead to misclassification of nutritional status. Care must be used when interpreting the results of anthropometric measures. There is limited data available on older adult subjects, there is a lack of appropriate standards. In addition, physical impairments common to older adults can limit the ability to obtain adequate and

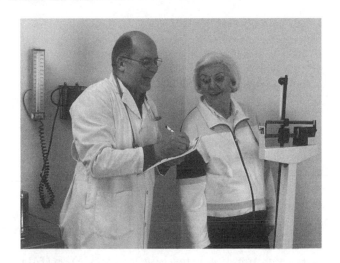

reproducible data. Therefore, anthropometric measures are best used in conjunction with clinical, laboratory, dietary, psychological, and functional data.

Weight

One of the simplest, most routinely collected measures used to monitor individuals is body weight. The measurement of body weight is used as a rough estimate of energy stores. The most accurate method for obtaining body weight is a calibrated scale. However, some older adults are unable to walk or stand; in these cases, the assessment of body weight requires the use of a calibrated wheelchair or bed scale. Accurate weights are critical for the evaluation of nutritional status; therefore, the older adult should be measured using standard procedures as much as possible to increase reliability and reproducibility. The older adult should be weighed on the same scale, wearing the same type of clothing, at the same time of day. Indicators, such as edema and hydration status, that may influence body weight should be recorded. Because changes in body weight can have a significant impact on nutritional health, achieving and maintaining a stable/usual body weight is generally a preferred standard for many older adults.

Weight Changes

Body weight tends to peak during a person's 40s and 50s, hold steady until about age 60, and then begins to decrease. Weight change has been shown to be a predictor of negative health outcomes in older adults. Monitoring weight changes allows for the early identification of problems and enables early intervention, including nutrition therapy. Care should be taken to obtain an accurate weight history. The evaluation of body weight over time will provide more clinically useful information than relative body weight. Standard procedures should be followed, and weight status should be routinely documented. When weight change does occur,

it is important to determine the degree of weight change, which correlates with health status. When possible, it is important to determine the causes of weight change so that appropriate interventions can be implemented to prevent further variances. A weight gain or loss of 10 pounds or 10% over a 6-month period requires investigation into nutritional and health status that may be related to weight change.

In addition to body weight, body composition also changes with age. Shifts in body composition are a well-known age-related change. Older adults have 10% more body fat compared to younger adults. Simultaneously, body weight and lean body mass (muscle) decline with advancing age (**Figure 16-4**).

> **anthropometry** The measurement of body size, weight, and proportions to assess the physiologic effects of undernutrition or overnutrition.

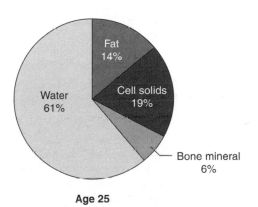

Age 25

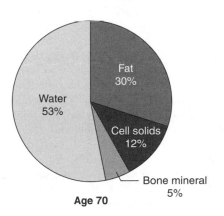

Age 70

FIGURE 16-4 Comparison of Body Composition Compartments in a Young Man Versus an Older Man

Source: Adapted from Shock NW. *Biological Aspects of Aging.* New York: Columbia University Press; 1962.

It is important to keep in mind that the measurement of body weight alone gives little insight into changes in body composition that can dramatically affect health and functional status. Additional methods for investigating body fat, as well as muscle mass, are recommended for a complete nutritional assessment.

Weight for Height

Many of the currently used indicators of appropriate body weight require the knowledge of an individual's height. Relative weight for height is the ratio of an individual's present weight to a reference weight based on the individual's height and gender. The Anthropometric Standardized Reference adapted for older adults offers recommendations for measuring the height of older adults. Once height and weight measurements have been obtained, they should be compared to standards most representative of the population being evaluated. Keep in mind that the average height–weight tables for persons aged 64 years and older may not be representative of the entire older adult population due to the limited number of subjects aged 85 and older and the fact that the subjects were predominantly White men and women. The National Health and Nutrition Examination Survey (NHANES) III, which collected data from 1988–1991 on a sample of 600 individuals ages 60 and older and equal numbers of Whites, African Americans, and Hispanics, provides more recent and comprehensive data on the older adult population.

Height

The progressive decrease in height with age due to compression of the vertebral disc space has been well documented. Because height is an important reference point for anthropometric measurements, it should be measured annually. Unfortunately, accurate measures of stature are difficult to obtain from most aged subjects because of the physical and medical changes that occur with aging. Physical limitations and chronic diseases, such as arthritis, osteoporosis, Parkinson's disease and other disorders that affect the neurological system, as well as kyphosis and scoliosis make it difficult, if not impossible, for many older adults to stand erect. This presents a major obstacle for obtaining accurate height measurements. It is not clear which is better: actual height (done as well as possible, considering the limitation) or maximal height of an individual as a young adult.

Surrogate Measures of Height

Stature of those older adults capable of standing upright should be measured with a stadiometer. If it is impossible to obtain a standing height in older adults due to physical or medical complications, recumbent length can be measured. A number of predictive stature values are considered acceptable surrogates in nutritional indices. Distance from crown to heel can be measured to determine recumbent length. Alternate methods also include arm span, total arm length, or knee height. There has been limited agreement between standing height and methods of estimating height in acutely ill older adults; therefore, it should be clearly documented that these are estimated height measurements and that they should be interpreted with caution.

Arm Span. Arm span is highly correlated with height at maturity for both men and women. Therefore, it can be used as a surrogate measure of height in an individual who is unable to be measured while standing. Arm span includes both arms and the breadth of the shoulders when the subject's arms are outstretched. Measurements can be taken from the tip of one middle finger to the tip of the other.

Total Arm Length. Problems similar to those encountered while measuring standing height can also prevent the measurement of arm span. In this case, total arm length (TAL) can be used as an alternative measure to approximate height. TAL is the distance from the tip of the right acromial process of the scapula to the end of the styloid process of the ulna of the elbow when bent at a 45-degree angle.

Knee Height. Knee height is recommended because it is an easy method for health professionals and it can be measured in either the sitting or the recumbent position. Knee height is measured as the distance from the sole of the foot at the heel to the anterior surface of the thigh with the ankle and the knee, each flexed at a 90-degree angle. Nationally representative equations to predict stature using knee height and age for racial/ethnic groups of the older adult population in the United States have also been developed from the NHANES III data. These equations should be applied when a measure of stature cannot be obtained. **Figure 16-5** shows an example of segmented measurements of an older person.

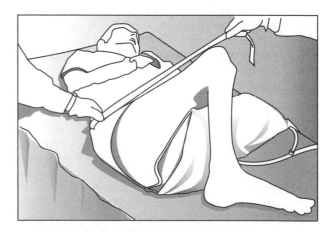

FIGURE 16-5 Segmented Measurements of an Older Adult

Source: Chernoff R. *Geriatric Nutrition.* 3rd ed. Sudbury, MA: Jones & Bartlett; 2006, p. 437. Reproduced with permission.

Body Mass Index

Once measures of weight and stature are available, body mass index (BMI) can be calculated. BMI is a useful indicator of body composition because it correlates significantly with body fatness. BMI is a weight-to-height ratio calculated as weight in kilograms divided by height in meters squared. **Box 16-2** shows how BMI is calculated. Charts for calculating BMI are widely available as are tables for the direct conversion of weight and height to BMI (**Table 16-3**).

BMI is most useful in assessing degrees of obesity; it is less informative for evaluating body fatness in people

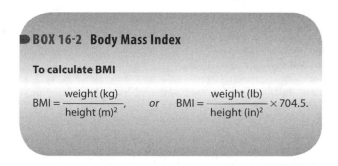

BOX 16-2 Body Mass Index

To calculate BMI

$$BMI = \frac{weight\ (kg)}{height\ (m)^2}, \quad or \quad BMI = \frac{weight\ (lb)}{height\ (in)^2} \times 704.5.$$

TABLE 16-3 Adult BMI Chart

Locate the height of interest in the left-most column and read across the row for that height to the weight of interest. Follow the column of the weight up to the top row that lists the BMI. BMI of 18.5–24.9 is the healthy weight range, BMI of 25–29.9 is the overweight range, and BMI of 30 and above is in the obese range.

BMI	19	20	21	22	23	24	25	26	27	28	29	30	31	32	33	34	35
Height							Weight in Pounds										
4'10"	91	96	100	105	110	115	119	124	129	134	138	143	148	153	158	162	167
4'11"	94	99	104	109	114	119	124	128	133	138	143	148	153	158	163	168	173
5'	97	102	107	112	118	123	128	133	138	143	148	153	158	163	158	174	179
5'1"	100	106	111	116	122	127	132	137	143	148	153	158	164	169	174	180	185
5'2"	104	109	115	120	126	131	136	142	147	153	158	164	169	175	180	186	191
5'3"	107	113	118	124	130	135	141	146	152	158	163	169	175	180	186	191	197
5'4"	110	116	122	128	134	140	145	151	157	163	169	174	180	186	192	197	204
5'5"	114	120	126	132	138	144	150	156	162	168	174	180	186	192	198	204	210
5'6"	118	124	130	136	142	148	155	161	167	173	179	186	192	198	204	210	216
5'7"	121	127	134	140	146	153	159	166	172	178	185	191	198	204	211	217	223
5'8"	125	131	138	144	151	158	164	171	177	184	190	197	203	210	216	223	230
5'9"	128	135	142	149	155	162	169	176	182	189	196	203	209	216	223	230	236
5'10"	132	139	146	153	160	167	174	181	188	195	202	209	216	222	229	236	243
5'11"	136	143	150	157	165	172	179	186	193	200	208	215	222	229	236	243	250
6'	140	147	154	162	169	177	184	191	199	206	213	221	228	235	242	250	258
6'1"	144	151	159	166	174	182	189	197	204	212	219	227	235	242	250	257	265
6'2'	148	155	163	171	179	186	194	202	210	218	225	233	241	249	256	264	272
6'3'	152	160	168	176	184	192	200	208	216	224	232	240	248	256	264	272	279
	Healthy Weight						Overweight					Obese					

Source: U.S Department of Agriculture and Health and Human Services. *Dietary Guidelines for Americans*, 6th ed. Washington DC: US Government Printing Office; 2005.

who are not obese. BMI is being included more often in the evaluation of nutritional status of older adults. The NSI includes the use of BMI and states that older individuals with a BMI of less than 24 or greater than 27 may be at risk for poor nutritional status and recommends intervention. Low BMI values are associated with decreased functional status and increased mortality in older adults. For people older than age 70, the best health status and lowest risk of mortality have been observed in those who maintain a BMI between 25 and 32, which is higher than the optimal BMI for younger people.

The appropriateness of the use of BMI in adults older than 65 has been questioned because older adults tend to "grow shorter" with age and the BMI values are based on data collected from younger people. BMI does not consider the variable height loss with age. If a person's height decreases while weight remains stable, BMI increases, which is not a true indicator of nutritional status. Any limitations associated with obtaining an accurate height in older adults will also contribute to error in determining BMI. As a result of these limitations, the use of BMI for predicting health outcomes should be interpreted cautiously.

Body Composition

Body weight is only one indication of energy stores. At times, it is desirable to evaluate the composition of these stores and the degree to which lean body mass is being preserved. Depletion of lean body mass is critical because of the role that proteins play in the body as well as the relationship between loss of lean body mass and declines in functional status and independence in older adults. *Sarcopenia* refers to the loss of lean muscle with aging. Anthropometry provides clinically applicable procedures for assessing changes in both muscle mass and adipose stores, specifically circumference, skinfold, and bioelectric impedance methods. Anthropometry, particularly skinfold and circumference measurements, are the most clinically applicable methods for evaluating changes in muscle and fat. As mentioned earlier, age-related changes in height, weight, and body composition make it difficult to interpret these measures.

Circumference Measurements

Anthropometric measures, in particular circumference and skinfold measurements, are currently the most clinically applicable methods for assessing the degree of muscle loss and adipose mass depletion in older adults. However, these measures also must be interpreted with care in older adults due to limited standardization of techniques and limited reference values for this population. Circumference measurements are becoming increasingly important in the anthropometric assessment of older adults due to their simplicity and relatively noninvasive, simple methodology.

Waist-to-Hip Ratio. One main reason to measure circumference in older adults is the association between fat distribution and health outcomes. Fat tends to shift from the extremities to the trunk, especially in women, and from subcutaneous to deep adipose tissue in both women and men. Disease risk increases when the waist-to-hip ratio is about 1.0 for men and 0.8 for women. Anthropometric measures of abdominal adiposity are associated with all-cause, coronary vascular disease, and cancer mortality independent of body mass in women. Abdominal fat accumulation appears to increase progressively with age, thus raising concern for increased heart disease risk.

Arm Circumference. As mentioned previously, the benefits of circumference measures are that they are fairly simple to obtain and require minimal equipment. Circumference measurement requires only the use of a flexible tape measure. Measurements are taken at various sites on the body, and then are compared to standards. Mid-upper-arm circumference (MAC) is a measure of both the subcutaneous fat and the muscle of the arm. A change in this measurement reflects either a change in muscle mass, a change in fat mass, or both. Monitoring MAC is useful for assessing the progress of nutrition interventions. Measurements should be compared to reference standards such as percentiles for MAC measurements, which are available for people aged 60 years and older who were examined in the first phase of NHANES III. Repeated measures can help to detect abnormal changes and monitor the effectiveness of nutrition intervention programs. However, one problem with this method is the inconsistency with regards to where the measuring tape is placed for measurement.

Calf Circumference. In addition to arm circumference, the World Health Organization recommends that calf circumference also be included as a measure of nutritional status of the older adult. Measurement of calf circumference has been recommended as a more sensitive indicator of the loss of total body muscle mass. Calf circumference is included as part of the MNA form developed for assessing nutritional status of older adults. Circumference measurements can be used alone or in combination with skinfold measurements to help evaluate nutritional status.

Skinfolds. Body density equations may not be applicable in older adults due to age-related changes in body composition. Physical changes experienced by older individuals, such as the redistribution of fat, reduction in skin elasticity, alterations in skin thickness, as well as changes in hydration and compressibility of the skin, connective, and adipose tissues will limit the reliability of skinfold measurements and the accuracy of equations used to predict total body fat. Despite this, however, skinfold measurements are

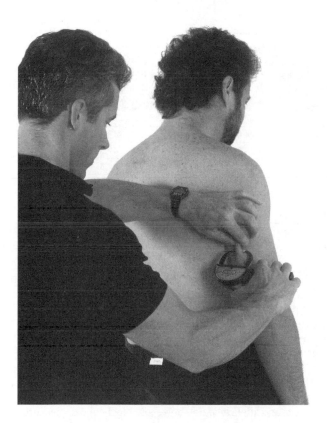

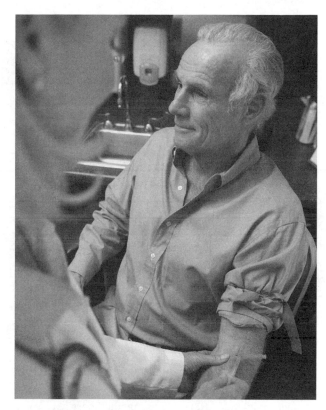

simple and noninvasive to obtain and have been shown to correlate with body fatness.

Despite this, collection of skinfold measurements from multiple sites may help improve the reliability of body fat estimation in older adults. All circumference and skinfold measurements should be taken from the same side of the body. In the older adult, skinfold measurements obtained from the trunk in men and the extremities in women may be more reliable in estimating body fat. Common sites of measurement are the triceps, biceps, subscapular, and suprailiac, and standardized methods for performing these measurements should be followed to ensure accuracy. Standardized formulas are available to predict body fat and calculate fat-free mass using one or multiple skinfold measurements.

The most common skinfold measure is the triceps skinfold (TSF). TSF can be obtained through the use of calibrated skinfold calipers, such as the Lange, Harpenden, or Holtain calipers. The calipers are used to measure a double fold of the subcutaneous fat on the back of the mid-upper arm over the triceps muscle. **Table 16-4** presents the percentile values obtained from TSF thickness of men and women ages 60 to 89. Individuals with a TSF measurement below the 5th percentile are generally considered underweight, whereas those with a measurement above the 95th percentile are considered obese. TSF measurements and the MAC,

discussed earlier, can be used to calculate arm-muscle circumference (AMC) and arm-muscle area (AMA). Both the AMC and AMA are estimates of body muscle mass.

Bioelectrical Impedance Assessment

Bioelectrical impedance analysis (BIA) has great appeal in assessing the older adult because it places little physical demands on the subject. Additional advantages of BIA is that it is a simple, quick, noninvasive, safe, relatively inexpensive, and highly reproducible method for measuring body composition. BIA determines body fatness by measuring conductivity. The body's resistance to an electric current is measured and used to calculate total body water. Lean tissue conducts a mild electrical current; fat tissue does not. Electrodes are placed on the hands and feet while an electric current is passed through the body. Fat-free mass and percent body fat are then calculated using age-appropriate equations. It is important to ensure that subjects are adequately hydrated, otherwise errors in estimating fat mass can occur.

Creatinine Height Index

Daily production of creatinine is related to the amount of lean body mass. Because of this, it may be useful for evaluating body composition. Creatinine is formed from the metabolism of creatine and phosphocreatine, which are

TABLE 16-4 Percentile Norms for Measurement of Upper Arm Triceps Skinfold Thickness

Sex, Age (Y) Group			Triceps Skinfold Thickness							
			Percentile						
	Sample	Mean	5th	10th	25th	50th	75th	90th	95th
			MM						
Women									
60–89	496	25.2	12.5	14.4	18.5	24.0	30.8	38.1	43.6
60–69	146	27.2 ± ~0.2*	13.0	14.7	20.7	26.2	33.0	40.3	47.2
70–79	239	25.1 ± .3	13.0	15.0	18.0	23.7	31.0	38.3	41.5
80–89	111	23.3 ± 9.7′	10.9	12.9	16.7	21.8	27.5	34.6	43.4
Men									
60–89	250	22.5	5.7	7.6	11.5	20.4	31.8	42.1	45.8
60–69	86	21.9 ± 13.6	4.9	6.9	10.8	18.0	31.9	45.1	49.3
70–79	115	23.5 ± 13.3	6.3	7.9	12.0	22.0	32.7	41.8	45.4
80–89	49	21.6 ± 11.0	5.8	8.0	11.5	21.0, 29.6		37.5	40.5

found primarily in muscle. Measurement of urinary creatinine excretion, therefore, can serve as a simple biochemical tool for assessing total body skeletal muscle mass or body composition.

Creatinine height index (CHI) is a measure of lean body mass that has been used to assess the nutritional status of older individuals. However, the method does have some limitations on its use with older adults. For example, CHI must be related to height, which is difficult to accurately obtain in some older adults due to their inability to stand straight. Collection of urine for 24 hours is also required, and this, too, can be difficult to achieve with older adults.

Explanations for the decline in creatinine excretion normally seen with age include the following:

1. Decrease in lean body mass
2. Decrease in proportion of muscle in lean body
3. Decrease in meat intake

Dual-Energy X-Ray Absorptiometry (DXA)

Dual-energy X-ray absorptiometry (DXA) is increasingly being used to assess body composition in older adults. DXA is a noninvasive method of determining body fat, fat distribution, and bone density. It involves passing two low-dose X-ray beams through the body that differentiate among fatfree tissue, fat tissue, and bone, providing a precise measurement of total body fat and its distribution.

DXA methods have been validated against other methods, and have good reported reproducibility. DXA is sensitive for capturing small changes in body composition. In addition, it requires very little effort by the subject. DXA has been used to determine long-term changes of body composition with age and short-term changes in body com-

position as a result of intervention. However, because DXA may underestimate age-related sarcopenia, these measurements should be interpreted with caution.

Biochemical Measures/Laboratory Data

Nutrition screening and assessment emphasize anthropometric and dietary data; however, biochemical measures are essential for assessing nutritional status, evaluating nutrition intervention programs, and predicting medical outcomes. Biochemical assessment of nutritional status may be employed to determine the level of recent intake of specific nutrients, to estimate nutrient stores in body fluids or tissues, to obtain functional measures of nutritional adequacy or deficiency, and to determine nutritional risk. In the development of nutritional deficiencies, biochemical changes precede clinical signs of deficiency. Biochemical assessment is used to confirm or refute a nutritional diagnosis based on clinical, dietary anthropometric, or hematological assessment. **Box 16-3** presents some limitations for the use of biochemical assessment as a means of establishing a nutritional diagnosis in older adults.

Factors that Influence Biochemical Markers

The appropriateness of each biochemical test must be evaluated for each individual patient. Many factors can influence biochemical markers of older adults (**Table 16-5**). Overall medical condition and metabolic stress, pharmacological interventions, and changes in hydration status must be considered when interpreting laboratory data. Differences in the procedures and equipment used at different facilities also must be considered. Lack of age-adjusted reference standards for the interpretation of laboratory results emphasizes the need for repeated measurements on an indi-

BOX 16-3 Limitations for Using Biochemical Assessment

1. Age-related changes in biochemical parameters

2. Lack of appropriate normative values for older age groups

3. Inadequate laboratory facilities in geriatric institutions

4. Problems collecting samples

5. Polypharmacy may interfere with biochemical assays

6. Difficulty in separating cause and effect

7. Multiple medical conditions may confound interpretation of results.

Source: Data from Roe DA. *Geriatric Nutrition.* 3rd ed. Englewood Cliffs, NJ: Prentice-Hall; 1992.

TABLE 16-5 Factors That Could Influence Lab Data and Lead to False Interpretation

- Overall medical condition, past and present diseases
- Use of prescription and over-the-counter medications
- Tobacco and alcohol use
- Hydration status
- Stress
- Medical interventions
- Reference standards
- Equipment calibration

vidual. Numerous factors could influence the lab data and lead to false interpretation of the results. Also note that no single laboratory test definitively evaluates an individual's nutritional status or short-term response to MNT. Physical findings, as well as dietary information and changes in reported symptoms, are necessary for the correct interpretation of laboratory data. Laboratory tests commonly used to evaluate nutritional status of the older adults as well as information on normal values, nutritional significance, and factors that may increase or decrease certain laboratory values are presented in the following discussion.

Protein Status. Biochemical measurements are available that reflect dietary protein intake as well as body protein stores. These measurements are useful for predicting protein-energy malnutrition in older adults. Serum albumin, prealbumin, retinol-binding protein, transferrin, hemoglobin, total lymphocyte count, cholesterol, and total iron-binding capacity (TIBC) are among the most widely available and useful measures for evaluating protein status. Many conditions and diseases common in older adults can alter plasma protein levels; therefore, an individual's entire medical status needs to be considered when interpreting these measures as indicators of nutritional status. While visceral proteins such as albumin, prealbumin, and Retinol binding protein seem to be useful indexes in detecting malnutrition in the elderly, low values still within the normal range should also

be carefully evaluated as part of a complete overall assessment because they could imply poor nutritional status.

Albumin. Albumin is the major visceral protein produced by the liver. Its synthesis is dependent on an adequate supply of protein and energy. Serum albumin is a reliable marker of protein energy malnutrition and is the most consistently used measure of visceral protein status. Albumin has a half-life of 12 to 21 days; therefore, it is a poor indicator of early malnutrition.

In healthy older adults, serum albumin levels do not decrease significantly. However, plasma protein concentrations can be affected by many diseases common in older adults. Hypoalbuminemia (low serum albumin levels, <3 g/dL) is a reliable predictor of malnutrition in older adults and an early indicator of increased risk of death. In addition to malnutrition, the following can also result in depressed albumin: liver disease, increased plasma volume due to coronary heart failure or renal disease, extended periods of confinement to bed, overhydration, acute inflammatory responses and infections, and gastrointestinal disease. Hydration status directly affects albumin and must be considered for correct interpretation of albumin measurement. Dehydration, which is common in older adults, will produce artificially high albumin.

Normal serum albumin levels are 3.5 to 5.0 g/dL. Serum albumin less than 3.5 g/dL is suggestive of protein-energy malnutrition and requires further investigation of nutritional status, which should include additional lab tests as well as anthropometry, clinical evaluation, and dietary assessment.

When evaluating a nutrition intervention, it is important to remember that it takes approximately two weeks for albumin levels to respond to nutrition therapy.

Serum Transferrin. Serum transferrin is another visceral protein used to assess nutritional status. Serum transferrin is an iron-transport protein that is considered a sensitive marker of protein status. Due to its half-life of eight to ten days and smaller body pool than albumin, serum transferrin responds more rapidly to changes in protein status.

However, as with serum albumin and many other biochemical measurements, use of serum transferrin is complicated in older adults. Serum transferrin levels can be affected by many conditions, including anemia, iron overload, gastrointestinal disorders, renal disease, liver disease, congestive heart failure, and inflammation. All of this should be considered when assessing protein nutrition.

Prealbumin. Prealbumin (PA) is a useful indicator of subclinical malnutrition and helpful for the long-term management and monitoring of older patients. PA is synthesized by the liver and functions as the protein carrier for thyroxine. PA has a rapid turnover rate with a half-life of just two to three days. In addition, PA has a small body pool which is sensitive to changes affecting its synthesis or catabolism.

The concentration of PA decreases in the presence of protein-energy malnutrition and responds quickly to nutrition interventions. Therefore, it is considered a useful biochemical indicator of nutritional status. Normal levels of PA are in the range of 15 to 40 mg/dL. When malnutrition is significant, PA will fall below 11 mg/dL. As with albumin, other medical conditions can influence PA levels and should be considered when using this biomarker to assess nutritional status. Dehydration will cause elevated PA levels. In addition to protein-energy malnutrition, PA levels will be decreased in acute inflammatory response and by infection.

Total Lymphocyte Count. A low total lymphocyte count (TLC) is an indicator of immunocompromise, which is commonly associated with malnutrition. TLC declines and lymphocyte response to antigens is impaired with malnutrition. TLC values lower than 1,500 cells/mm3 are indicative of protein depletion. TLC is affected by many other factors, so its usefulness as a measure of nutritional status in older adults is complicated.

Cholesterol. The National Cholesterol Education Program screening guidelines are considered appropriate for use with older adults. Elevated serum cholesterol has been associated with increased risk of cardiovascular disease. A total cholesterol level above 240 mg/dL and an LDL cholesterol level above 160 mg/dL indicate high risk. In older populations, lipoprotein levels may be more predictive of coronary events than total serum cholesterol and should be examined for more accurate assessment of cardiovascular risk. Cholesterol is also used as an indicator of malnutrition. When cholesterol levels decline along with other indicators of protein status, nutritional needs are not being met. A total cholesterol level below 160 mg/dL is a marker for protein-energy malnutrition and is used in level II screening of NSI and SCALES as an indication of the need for nutrition intervention. Low total cholesterol in older adults is associated with poor health sta-

tus and may be a predictor of mortality. Many factors affect total cholesterol and lipoprotein levels and these should be considered along with historic cholesterol values.

Iron Status/Anemias. In the older adult, hematological assessment can also be used to screen for malnutrition. The extent to which hematologic changes can be used in the diagnosis of nutritional deficiency depends on the duration of the deficiency, with consideration of potential confounding factors. Whether the anemia is related to the aging process or to nutritional factors is difficult to determine. To diagnose nutritional anemia, a complete blood count is necessary. Supportive evidence is usually required from additional biochemical measurements, dietary assessment, and from monitoring the older adult's response to nutritional therapy.

Iron deficiency is the most common nutrient deficiency in the world. Other common nutritional anemias include megaloblastic anemia (folate deficiency), pernicious anemia (vitamin B12 deficiency), and anemia of chronic disease. It should be noted that in some cases the causes of these anemias are different in the older adult than in younger people. In older adults, iron deficiency is often caused by blood loss resulting from chronic or excessive aspirin intake or anti-inflammatory medicine use. Many additional factors can result in low iron levels, including chronic disease, infection, protein-energy malnutrition, and vitamin B12 or folate deficiency. No single biochemical indicator has proven to be diagnostic of iron deficiency. In general, two or more abnormal values are considered indicative of impaired iron status.

Epidemiologic evidence indicates that anemia is fairly common in the older adult. In addition, cultural variations in dietary patterns may influence iron availability and body iron stores and contribute to an increased risk for iron deficiency anemia among older adults of different ethnic groups. For example, older adults of Caribbean origin, particularly women, may be significantly more likely than their non-Hispanic White neighbors to suffer from anemia and poor iron status.

Hemoglobin. Hematologic measures are routinely obtained and indices such as hemoglobin, hematocrit, and total lymphocyte count and should be followed regularly in the older adult. Most of the iron in the body is found in hemoglobin of red blood cells; therefore, hemoglobin can be used to detect iron deficiency anemia associated with malnutrition. Hemoglobin concentration is a measure of the total amount of hemoglobin in the peripheral blood and is a more direct measure of iron deficiency than hematocrit. A decline in hemoglobin may occur as a result of physiologic aging; however, nutrient deficiencies and chronic diseases may also be involved.

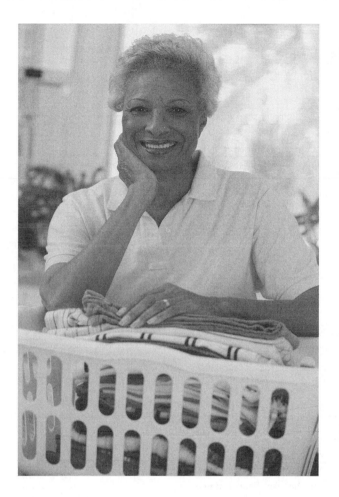

tion can also result in reduced folate levels. Folate levels are used to evaluate hemolytic disorders and to detect megaloblastic anemia. Serum and erythrocyte folate are the most frequently used biochemical indicators of folate status. Serum folate levels reflect recent dietary intake and acute folate status. Erythrocyte folate levels are used to reflect body stores and are reliable indices of folate status. Normal folate levels (5 to 25 g/mL) can be seen in iron deficiency anemia. Low folate levels (less than 5 g/dL) indicate folate deficiency anemia. Folate levels can increase (greater than 25 g/dL) in B12 deficiency anemia.

Of clinical significance is the ability of folate supplementation to mask a vitamin B12 deficiency. This can be of particular concern for older adults, for whom the symptoms of vitamin B12 deficiency can go undetected, resulting in irreversible neurological damage. For example, forgetfulness, changes in mental status, and moderate dementia may be overlooked as simple consequences of aging, yet in reality be symptoms of a vitamin B12 deficiency, which when detected early enough can be corrected. Older adults using folate supplements to reduce elevated homocystine levels should be encouraged to also supplement with vitamin B12.

Vitamin B12. Serum vitamin B12 is a measure used to identify pernicious anemia and megaloblastic anemia in older adults. Low levels may reflect poor intake; lack of stomach acid (HCL) to remove the vitamin from the bound state in the food source, making it available for absorption; or lack of intrinsic factor required for absorption, all of which are common possibilities in older adults.

Vitamin B12 deficiency is a common condition in older adults. When left untreated, it can lead to permanent degeneration of neurological status. Therefore, some studies suggest that a vitamin B12 level below 350 pg/mL should be considered a deficiency state and treated.

Clinical Assessment

The clinical assessment of older individuals is multifaceted and includes identification of physical, functional, cognitive, and social factors that may limit consumption of a nutritionally balanced diet. Early identification of barriers to a nutritious diet and appropriate intervention can prevent or delay the onset of malnutrition and related consequences.

Physical Assessment

Chronic inadequate intake of essential nutrients leads to malnutrition. When long-term inadequate intake of one or more essential nutrients exists, physical manifestations may result. **Table 16-6** contains a comprehensive list of clinical signs indicative of a nutritional disease. The goal of the clinical assessment is to reveal information about the individual's current state of health. The components of a clinical assessment include a medical history; a physical

Hematocrit. Hematocrit is the percentage of red blood cells in total blood volume and is used in conjunction with hemoglobin to evaluate iron status. It is common for individuals older than 50 years to have slightly lower hematocrit levels than younger adults. Individuals with anemia of chronic disease will not be able to maintain normal hematocrit levels because the body lacks the ability to use stored iron.

Mean Corpuscular Volume. Mean corpuscular volume (MCV) is a measure of the average volume of a single red blood cell. It is determined by dividing the hematocrit by the total red blood cell count. Increased MCV indicates that the red blood cells are macrocytic, as seen in megaloblastic anemia. This type of anemia can be caused by B12 and folate deficiencies. When MCV is low, the cells are microcytic, which is suggestive of iron deficiency anemia

Folate Status. Although folate deficiency can have many causes, low dietary intake is the most common cause in older adults. Malabsorption, medication, and alcohol inges-

TABLE 16-6 Clinical Signs of Nutritional Deficiencies

Nutrient	Clinical Deficiency Symptoms
Vitamin A	*Eyes*—Bitot's spots; conjunctival and corneal xerosis (dryness); keratomalacia *Skin*—follicular hyperkeratosis; xerosis *Hair*—coiled, keratinized
Vitamin D	*Bone*—bowlegs; beading of ribs; pain; epiphyseal deformities
Vitamin E	Possible Anemia
Vitamin K	*Skin*—subcutaneous hemorrhage; ecchymoses (bruises easily
Thiamine (vitamin B_1)	*Neurologic*—mental confusion; irritability; sensory losses; weakness, paresthesias; anorexia *Eyes*—ophthalmoplegia *Cardiac*—tachycardia; cardiomegaly; congestive heart failuree *Other*—constipation; sudden death
Niacin (vitamin B_2)	*Skin*—nasolabial seborrhea; fissuring eyelid corners; angular fissures around mouth; papillary atrophy; pellagrous dermatitis *Neurologic*—mental confusion *Other*—diarrhea
Riboflavin	*Skin*—nasolabial seborrhea; fissuring and redness around eyes and mouth; magenta tongue; genital deratosis *Eyes*—corneal vascularization
Pyridoxine	*Skin*—nasolabial seborrhea; glossitis
Vitamin B_6	*Neurologic*—paresthesias; peripheral neuropathy *Other*—anemia
Folic acid	*Skin*—glossitis; hyperpigmentation of tongue; pallor *Neurologic*—depression *Other*—diarrrhea; anemia
Pantothenic acid	*Other*—headache; fatigue, apathy; nausea; sleep disturbances
Ascorbic acid (vitamin C)	*Skin*—petechiae, purpura; swollen, bleeding gums *Other*—bone pain; dental caries; depression; anorexia; delayed wound healing
Vitamin B_{12}	*Skin*—glossitis; skin hyperpigmentation; pallor *Neurologic*—ataxia; optic neuritis; paresthesias; mental disorders *Other*—anemia; anorexia; diarrhea
Biotin	*Skin*—pluckable, sparse hair; pallor; seborrheic dermatitis *Neurologic*—depression *Other*—anemia; fatigue
Iron	*Skin*—pallor; angular fissures; glossitis; spoon nails; pale conjunctiva *Other*—enlarged spleen
Zinc	*Skin*—seborrheic dermatitis; poor wound healing *Eyes*—photophobia *Other*—dysgeusia
Iodine	*Other*—large swollen tongue; goiter
Protein	*Skin*—dull, dry easily pluckable hair; "flaky paint" dermatitis; edema
Protein/energy	*Skin*—loss of subcutaneous fat; dull, dry, easily pluckable hair; decubitis ulcers; muscle wasting

Source: Chernoff R. Geriatric Nutrition. 3rd ed. Sudbury, MA: Jones & Bartlett; 2006, p. 429. Reproduced with permission.

examination to determine which physical signs and symptoms of nutritional disease are present; an assessment of functional status, with particular attention to skills related to food acquisition, preparation, and consumption; and an oral health evaluation. Clinical assessment should also include a careful assessment of the hair, skin, nails musculature, eyes, mucosa, and other physical attributes. It is important to determine whether the clinical symptoms observed are part of normal physiologic aging or are related to nutritional inadequacies.

The following is a brief checklist of clinical symptoms that suggest nutritional problems for older adults:

- Wasted appearance
- Edema
- Pale color
- Bruises
- General weakness and fatigue
- Apathy, tremors
- Skin lesions
- Dry scaly skin
- Cracks or sores in the corner of the mouth and lips

Another clinical manifestation associated with nutritional deficiencies in older adults is fluid imbalances. Overrhydration that contributes to edema is probably less of an acute medical problem than dehydration. Dehydration, which is considered a form of malnutrition, is often caused by inadequate ingestion of fluids and is a common, potentially harmful, condition for older people. **Table 16-7** presents factors that contribute to risk of dehydration as well as presentation of symptoms in older adults.

Oral Status

Adequate oral health is essential for the ingestion of foods. Assessment of the oral status is therefore considered a critical feature of the nutritional status evaluation of older adults. Older adults often have a hard time eating because of poor oral health, including no teeth (affecting 14% to 48% of older adults); untreated conditions, such as cavities and crowns (30% of those with teeth); and periodontal disease (41%). One cause of unexplained weight loss in older adults is poor oral health.

Although often difficult to determine, poor oral status can be the cause or the result of poor nutrition. Many nutritional deficiencies are manifested in the mouth. Periodic examination of the oral cavity is an essential component of nutrition assessment. The condition of an individual's mouth should be evaluated as well as the older adult's ability to chew, swallow, and self-feed. This evaluation is most often performed by a dentist. Attention should also be given to the condition of the teeth, tongue, gums, and oral mucosa. Nutrition screening should attempt to determine the reasons for any oral problems, such as poor fitting dentures, absence of teeth, a sore mouth, swollen gums, glossitis (red tongue without papillae), ulcers in the mouth, paralytic disease involving the face, and dry mouth.

It is also important to consider that eating behavior is influenced by many factors, including taste, smell, and the ability to self-feed. Alterations in taste and smell contribute to decreased enjoyment of food. Appropriate interventions aimed at alterations in taste and smell have the potential to significantly improve food intake, nutritional status, and quality of life. Evaluation of swallowing should be per-

TABLE 16-7 Factors That Affect the Risk of Dehydration and Symptoms and Presentation of Dehydration in Older Adults

Risk Factors
· Reduced appetite/anorexia
· Laxative or diuretic abuse
· Confinement to bed or chair or disability
· Assistance required with feeding and drinking
· Difficulty eating, chewing, or swallowing
· Dementia, cognitive dysfunction, depression, mental confusion
· Central nervous system impairment
· Diarrhea, nausea, vomiting, incontinence, frequent urination, hemorrhage
· Tube feeding or parenteral feeding
· Chronic infection
· Presence of multiple chronic conditions
· Polypharmacy
· Social isolation
· Symptoms and Presentation of Dehydration
· Dry mouth and cracked lips
· Swollen tongue
· Sunken eyes
· Increased body temperature/fever
· Reduced urine output
· Constipation
· Nausea and vomiting
· Low blood pressure and postural hypotension
· Increased confusion
· Altered medicine response
· Electrolyte imbalances
· Weight loss
· Changes in balance or frequent falls
· Fatigue

Source: Adapted from Chernoff R. *Geriatric Nutrition.* 3rd ed. Sudbury, MA: Jones & Bartlett; 2006, p. 430.

formed by a speech and language pathologist, and an occupational pathologist should consider the need for thickened liquids, texture modification, and self-help feeding devices to improve food intake.

Medication Use

Chronic use of medication, either over-the-counter or prescription, have the potential to significantly affect nutritional status. Prescription medicines have a benefit in managing chronic diseases, but they also may contribute to decreased appetite or alterations in metabolism. Anorexia, nausea, altered bowel function, taste alterations, and medicine–nutrient interactions are just a few examples of the potential side effects of medication use. More detailed information on medications commonly used by older adults and how they may influence nutritional status can be found in Chapter 17.

Alcoholism

Alcoholism is more common in the older adult than it was once thought to be. With older adults, substance abuse is often harder to detect because it is masked and complicated by other health problems. Food intake, as well as vitamin and mineral status, may be compromised with chronic alcohol consumption. This is because alcohol intake often replaces consumption of nutrient-dense foods and beverages. Differences in body composition and metabolism that occur as part of the aging process increase risk at all levels of consumption for medical and psychological problems. Alcohol consumption should be assessed and intervention and treatment implemented, if necessary.

Physical Disabilities and Functional Status

Nutritional status can be affected by changes in physical ability to perform normal functions of life. Changes in functional status can dramatically affect nutritional intake and need to be monitored along with anthropometric, biochemical, and dietary measures. Functional status is an indicator of a person's ability to provide self-care. Impaired functional status is defined as an inadequate level of aerobic fitness, muscular strength or endurance, or flexibility, leading to an inability to perform those activities necessary for routine self-care and independent living.

Declines in food intake and sedentary lifestyle in older adults may increase the risk for malnutrition, decline in body functions, and the development of chronic diseases. The decreases in lean body mass that occur as a result of weight loss account for some of the decreased strength and activity levels in older adults. In addition, reduced strength in older adults is a major cause of disability and loss of independence.

Functional Declines

Declines in functional status were once considered to be a natural consequence of aging. However, maintaining or improving function can be achieved with regular physical activity, including aerobic and strength-training exercises. Most adults in the United States do not achieve the recommended amount of regular physical activity. Therefore, some of the "normal functional declines" that accompany aging may just be the result of years of physical inactivity, which leads to decreased strength, flexibility, and cardiorespiratory fitness. Regular physical activity in older adults is important for maintaining or improving function, preventing and/or delaying the onset of chronic diseases, and maintaining independence.

Functional Dependence

The term *dependence* is defined as requiring assistance with an activity most of the time. *Independence* implies that the activity can be performed without assistance. A general indication of functional status is often useful in determining increased nutritional risk.

Activities of Daily Living (ADLs) and Instrumental Activities of Daily Living (IADLs)

Two tools commonly used to measure independence/dependence and to assess functional status in older adults are the Activities of Daily Living (ADLs) and the Instrumental Activities of Daily Living (IADLs). These questionnaires measure the ability to perform the functional tasks necessary for daily living. ADLs include activities basic to self-functioning, such as the ability to toilet, feed, dress, groom, ambulate, and bathe. The IADLs assess skills needed to function independently in a community setting and include activities such as ability to use the telephone, shop, prepare food, perform housekeeping, do the laundry, travel, take medication, and pay bills.

The inability to perform the nutrition-related ADLs and IADLs suggest increased risk for poor nutritional status. Identification of limitations in these functional skills as part of nutritional screening and assessment can predict complications and serve as indication for nutrition intervention.

Reduced ability to perform the ADLs and IADLs often contributes to the institutionalization of older adults. Interventions designed to reduce functional disability provide an opportunity to target and improve nutritional intake. Difficulties related to eating, food preparation, or food procurement must be identified and documented early, so that appropriate community, social service, and therapeutic treatments can be implemented before these functional limitations lead to nutritional insufficiencies.

Cognitive and Psychological Function (Mental Status)

Changes in cognitive and psychological status can seriously affect quality of life, level of function, productivity, and perceived physical and emotional health. Dementia, depression, and insomnia can reduce the older adult's ability to access, prepare, and consume an adequate diet. Symptoms of mental illness as well as related changes in appetite and lack of interest in food, leading to inadequate food intake and subsequent weight loss, can result in nutrition deficiencies. Poor memory, loss of feeding skills, hyperactive behavior, anorexia, and depression may also contribute to poor dietary intake.

Declines in mental status can contribute to significant involuntary weight changes, and depression has been shown to be a leading cause of unexplained weight loss in older adults.

BOX 16-4 Common Adverse Side Effects of Medications Used to Treat Depression

- Oversedation
- Cognitive impairment
- Delirium
- Increased or decreased appetite
- Dry mouth
- Nausea
- Anorexia
- Constipation
- Dehydration
- Changes in bowel status
- Drowsiness

TABLE 16-8 Psychological and Social Risk Factors That Affect the Nutritional Status of Older Adults

Food security, income, resources for food preparation
Education level, literacy level, language barriers, lack of ability to communicate needs
Cultural factors, religious beliefs, food preferences
Caregiver, neighborhood, community resources or social support system
Transportation to obtain food

It is well recognized that weight loss occurs in patients with senile dementia, such as Alzheimer's disease. Depression occurs frequently in older adults in institutional settings and is recognized as a treatable cause of weight loss.

Many of the medications used to treat depression have side effects that may negatively affect nutritional status. **Box 16-4** lists common adverse side effects of these medications, and Chapter 17 discusses pharmacology in more detail.

Assessment of Mental Status

Depression in older adults is multifactorial. Depression can be caused by changes in health status, medication use, loss of a loved one, changes in lifestyle, and declining physical function. Causes of depression should be investigated so that appropriate interventions can be implemented.

The Folstein Mini Mental Examination (MME) is a screening tool commonly used to detect dementia, which is responsible for most of the loss of cognitive function in older adults. In addition, a DETERMINE checklist score of at least four has been found to be associated with more symptoms of depression and lower functional status. Therefore, the DETERMINE checklist may be useful for targeting older individuals likely to have problems affecting their food intake and therefore their nutritional status.

Social, Psychological, and Economic Factors

To gain a complete understanding of the many factors that influence an individual's food intake, it is important to assess the environment in which they live. Living situation, degree of independence, financial and social resources available, level of education, and social support are all factors that could influence food choice and nutritional intake. Additional psychological and social risk factors include culture, food resources, and support systems (**Table 16-8**). These factors help to determine an individual's risk level.

Income

A fixed income limits food purchasing power. Food consumption patterns show that low-income adults have consistently low intakes of many nutrients. Low-income older adults often have less access to food and have limited food choices. Their ability to purchase fresh fruits, vegetables, and meats may be limited and contribute to the consumption and reliance on higher-calorie, low-nutrient-dense foods. Single servings and small-portion-size packaged foods tend to be more costly. Ready-to-eat and convenience foods that make food preparation easier are often higher in calories and fat, are less nutrient dense, and are more expensive, thereby limiting their usefulness for low-income older adults. Food-assistance programs such as food stamps, home-delivered meals, congregate meals, or similar services are available to those older adults in need.

Social Isolation

Social isolation is broadly defined as the absence of social interactions. Social interactions have a positive impact on health, quality of life, and food intake. With advancing age, the loss of family and friends is inevitable. Many older adults experience declines in independence, functional ability, physical and mental health, self-esteem, and income, making maintenance of social contacts increasingly difficult. Attempts must be made to identify socially isolated people and increase their opportunity for social interactions. Use of senior centers, congregate feeding sites, meals-on-wheels, and similar community resources provide opportunities to promote social contacts as well as nutritious meals. Home-delivered meal programs not only provide nutritious meals, but also social interaction. In some cases, the meal delivery provides the only visitor some older adults receive on a daily basis.

Cultural Factors, Food Preferences, and Religious Beliefs

Cultural and religious beliefs as well as food preferences should be considered when evaluating social factors involved in nutritional status. Food programs that do not provide culturally acceptable foods may be poorly utilized. Food lists that do not include ethnically appropriate food choices may underestimate intake. Sensitivities to food preferences and ethnic food patterns are necessary for assessment and interventions to be successful.

Dietary Assessment

A **dietary assessment** is a comprehensive evaluation of the foods consumed and behaviors surrounding food consumption. The goal of dietary assessment is to identify foods consumed and eating patterns that contribute to nutritional status. A dietary assessment is often conducted to determine an estimate of the macronutrient and micronutrient content of the diet and to assist in providing dietary counseling and nutrition interventions as well as to examine the relationship between dietary behavior and health.

Purpose of Dietary Assessment

The purpose of dietary assessment in the older adult is to provide insight into past and current food-intake behaviors and their impact on health status. Assessing the dietary intake of older adults can be difficult for many reasons. Physical and mental impairments often present in older adults need to be considered when determining the best dietary assessment method for this group. Information obtained during a dietary assessment may be incomplete or not reflective of usual dietary intake; therefore, careful interpretation of the data collected is necessary. Many hospitalized and institutionalized older adults are not competent enough to provide accurate self-reported diet histories. In this case, dietary information should be obtained from a family member or caregiver who prepares meals or who is present at meal time.

Classifications

There are two main classifications of dietary assessment methods: retrospective and prospective. Methods of collecting dietary information in the older adult population include 24-hour recalls, diet histories, food-frequency questionnaires, and food records. Dietary assessment methods can be used to identify individuals at risk for nutrient deficiencies, those who are having trouble consuming an adequate diet, those who follow unusual dietary patterns, and those who exclude an important food or food group.

dietary assessment
A comprehensive evaluation of the foods consumed and behaviors surrounding food consumption to identify eating patterns that contribute to nutritional status.

Retrospective Methods

Retrospective methods rely on the ability of the person to recall food intake in the past.

24-Hour Recall

The 24-hour recall method asks the individual to recall all the foods and beverages consumed in the previous 24 hours. Short-term memory is therefore required for accurate reporting. Low respondent burden, short administration time, and the ability to assess larger number of people make 24-hour recall a widely accepted method for free-living as well as institutionalized or hospitalized older people. This method requires a trained interviewer to ask questions and to probe to determine portion sizes, preparation methods, and possibly forgotten foods.

In general, 24-hour recalls tend to underestimate mean intakes of older adults. It is widely accepted that a 24-hour recall does not represent an individual's usual intake because of day-day variability. Repeated or serial 24-hour recalls provide a better estimate of an individual's food intake. The 24-hour recall method is considered reliable and is often used in large population studies. However, the reliability of this method for use in older adults has been questioned due to changes in short-term memory with age.

Food Frequency Questionnaires

Food frequency questionnaires (FFQ) provide a qualitative description of how often foods are eaten in a specific time period. These questionnaires can be self-administered provided a person can read and write. FFQs are useful in large population studies. In addition, they are useful for describing food-intake patterns for diet and meal planning, for studying the association of foods and disease, and for developing nutrition education programs. Like the 24-hour recall, the subject's ability to remember foods eaten affects the accuracy of this method. Semiquantified food frequency questionnaires include an estimate of the amounts of foods consumed along with their frequency of use. A semiquantified food frequency questionnaire designed specifically for older populations has been developed to help minimize some of the limitations of this method in older adults.

Diet History

The diet history method provides a more complete and detailed description of both the qualitative and quantitative aspects of food intake. Dietary intake information collected with this method correlates well with nutritional status. Diet histories do have some limitations: Administration is time-consuming and requires a highly trained nutritionist and a highly motivated participant. In addition, similar to limitations of other methods, a diet history requires the patient to remember foods eaten in the past.

A diet history gathers information on the eating pattern on a typical day; occasional alternative foods; usual portion sizes; past changes in eating pattern; food likes, dislikes, and aversions; and ethnic as well as cultural preferences. Additional data regarding socioeconomic factors, transportation availability, cooking facilities, income status, health-related dietary restrictions, and medication and alcohol use can also be obtained. A diet history questionnaire for use with older adults should be representative of the usual diet, contain both qualitative and quantitative questions, and be objective, clear, valid, and reproducible. In general, although a simplified diet history is likely adequate due to the older adult's consumption of a less-varied diet, the questionnaire should include items representative of the subject's usual diet and should include clearly defined food sources and portion sizes to increase accuracy.

Prospective Methods

With a prospective dietary assessment method, a record of food intake is obtained at the time the food is consumed. Self-written food records are a diary of what, where, when, and how much food is eaten. To obtain a representative summary of usual intake and minimize burden on the respondent, dietary intake is usually recorded for three (include two weekdays and one weekend day) or seven days. This method requires a person to be able to read (education) and write (no physical limitations such as arthritis) to accurately record food intake and portion sizes. Errors associated with memory are minimized with this method, because intake is recorded immediately after eating. However, this method requires a great deal of cooperation on the part of the person to write down everything eaten. In addition, because recording of food has been shown to alter food intake, this method is also useful for monitoring the effectiveness of nutrition interventions.

Once dietary information has been obtained, food intakes of individuals or groups are then compared to various standards such as the 2005 Dietary Guidelines for Americans, the Modified MyPyramid for Older Adults, or the Dietary Reference Intakes (DRIs). The goal is to determine potential excesses and deficiencies of foods and nutrients and to identify those older adults who are at nutritional risk. Dietary assessment should then be repeated on a regular basis to continue to screen for nutritional deficiencies as well as to assess the impact of nutrition interventions.

Food Security

Food security means that a person has access to enough food for an active, healthy life at all times. Food insecurity is defined as the availability of safe foods or the ability to acquire acceptable foods in socially acceptable ways. Because homebound older adults are at greater risk for malnutrition, it is recommended that food security be examined when performing a dietary assessment.

Conclusion

In the United States, many older adults are at risk of nutritional deficits, excesses, or imbalances as a result of age-related changes, chronic diseases, or poor dietary patterns. Nutrition screening can be used as the basis for initiating a plan of care for the older adult. The assessment is a comprehensive integrative process that includes anthropometric measurements, biochemical laboratory values, clinical evaluation, and dietary assessment to determine the nutritional health of individuals and populations.

As disability tends to progress with age, this group becomes more heterogeneous with regards to nutritional needs and barriers to achieving optimal nutritional status. It is important to consider each older adult as unique with individual nutritional needs and concerns. Early identification of increased risk and timely, appropriate nutrition interventions can aid in the achievement and maintenance of optimal nutritional health and quality of life. The onset of disease and subsequent complications can be lessened by the early detection of risk factors or conditions and the initiation of nutritional interventions, thus or thereby enabling older adults to maximize their health and independence.

> **food security** Access to enough food for an active, healthy life at all times.

Activities Related to This Chapter

1. Contact a local senior center and ask the director if you can conduct nutrition screening at the center. Use the DETERMINE checklist to see if you can identify individuals at nutritional risk. Tell individuals identified as being "at risk" to follow up with their physician.

2. What are the different ways to complete a dietary assessment? Find an online dietary assessment program (for example, there is one at www.mypyramid.org). Enter the diet of an older friend or relative. Examine the results for excesses and deficiencies. What are some limitations in the analysis? What suggestions can you make for that person to improve his or her diet?

3. Visit a nursing home and ask the nurses if you can join them as they weigh and measure the height of their residents. What are some limitations you encounter? What factors may have influenced the measurements you obtained? Do you think your measurements are accurate? Explain.

REFERENCES

Abraham S, Lowenstein FW, Johnson CL. *Preliminary Findings of the First Health and Nutrition Examination Survey, United States, 1971–1972: Dietary Intake and Biochemical Findings*. National Center for Health Statistics: US Dept of Health, Education, and Welfare publication HRA 74-1219-1. Washington, DC: U.S. Government Printing Office; 1974.

Agarwal N, Acevedo F, Leighton LS, et al. Predictive ability of various nutritional variables for mortality in elderly people. *Am J Clin Nutr*. 1988;48:1173–1178.

Allad JP, Aghdassi E, McArthur M, et al. Nutritional risk factors for survival in the elderly living in Canadian long-term care facilities. *J Am Geriatr Soc*. 2004;52:59–65.

Allsion DB, et al. Body mass index and all-cause mortality among people age 70 and over: The Longitudinal Study of Aging. *Int J Obes Related Metabol Disord*. 1997;21:424–431.

American Academy of Family Physicians, American Dietetic Association, National Council on the Aging I. *Keeping Older Americans Healthy at Home: Guidelines for Nutrition Programs in Home Health Care*. Washington, DC: Nutrition Screening Initiative; 1996.

American Dietetic Association. ADA's definitions for nutrition screening and nutrition assessment. Identifying patients at risk. *JADA*. 1994;94(8):838–839.

American Dietetic Association. Position of the American Dietetic Association. The cost-effectiveness of medical nutrition therapy. *JADA*. 1995;95:88–91.

American Dietetic Association. Comments—HCFA Conditions of Participation for Home Health Agencies. Federal Register. 1997;65:46.

American Dietetic Association. Position of the American Dietetic Association. Nutrition, aging and the continuum of Care. *JADA*. 2000;100(5):580–595.

American Medical Directors Association. *Clinical Practice Guidelines: Altered Nutritional Status*. Columbia, MD: American Medical Directors Association; 2002.

Bailey RL, Mitchell DC, Miller CK, et al. A dietary screening questionnaire identifies dietary patterns in older adults. *J Nutr*. 2007;137:421–426.

BAPEN. Malnutrition Universal Screening Tool. Available at http://www.bapenorguk/must_toolhtml.

Bjornthorp P. Obesity and the risk of cardiovascular disease. *Ann Clin Res*. 1985;17:3.

Blackburn GL, Bistrian BR, Maini BS. Nutritional and metabolic assessment of the hospitalized patient. *J Parenter Enter Nutr*. 1977;1:11–22.

Boult C, Krinke UB, Urdangarin CF, Skarin V. The validity of nutritional status as a marker for future disability and depressive symptoms among high-risk older adults. *J Am Geriatr Soc*. 1999;47:995–999.

Bowman BB, Rosenberg IH. Assessment of the nutritional status of the elderly. *Am J Clin Nutr*. 1982;35:1142–1144.

Burt VL, Harris T. The third National Health and Nutrition Examination Survey: contributing data on aging and health. *Gerontologist*. 1994;34:486–490.

Butterworth CE, Blackburn GL. Hospital malnutrition and how to assess the nutritional status of a patient. *Nutr Today*. 1975;10:8–18.

Chernoff R. *Geriatric Nutrition Handbook*. Gaithersburg, MD: Aspen; 1991.

Chernoff R. *Geriatric Nutrition: The Health Professional's Handbook*. 3rd ed. Sudbury, MA: Jones and Bartlett; 2006.

Chumlea WC, et al. Bioelectrical and anthropometric assessments and reference data in the elderly. *J Nutr*. 1993;123:449.

Chumlea WC, Guo S, Wholihan K, Cockram D, Kuczmarski RJ, Johnson CL. Stature prediction equations for elderly non-Hispanic white, non-Hispanic black, and Mexican-American persons developed from NHANES III data. *JADA*. 1998;98(2):137–142.

Chumlea WC, Guo S. Equations for predicting stature in white and black elderly individuals. *J Gerontol*. 1992;47:197.

Chumlea WC, Guo SS, Vellas B, Guigoz Y. Assessing body composition and sarcopenia with anthropometry. Proceedings CERI Symposium. In: *Nutrition Et Personnes Agees Au-Dela Apports Recommandes*. Paris, France; 1997. pp. 161–169.

Chumlea WC, Guo SS, Vellas B. Anthropometry and body composition in the elderly. *Facts Res Gerontol*. 1994;2(suppl):61.

Chumlea WC, Roche AF, Makjerjee D. *Nutrition Assessment of the Elderly Through Anthropometry*. Columbus, OH: Ross Laboratories; 1990.

Chumlea WC, Roche AF, Steinbaugh ML. Estimating stature from knee height for persons 60–90 years of age. *J Am Geriatr Soc*. 1985;33:116–120.

Covinsky KE, Martin GE, Beyth RJ, et al. The relationship between clinical assessments of nutritional status and adverse outcomes in older hospitalized medical patients. *J Am Geriatr Soc*. 1999;47:532–538.

De Jong N, Paw MJ, de Groot LC, Hiddink GJ, van Staveren WA. Dietary supplements and physical exercise affecting bone and body composition in frail elderly persons. *Am J Public Health*. 2000;90:947–954.

de Onis M, Habicht JP. Anthropometric reference data for international use: recommendations from a World Health Organization Expert Committee. *Am J Clin Nutr*. 1996;64:650–658.

Dequeker JV, Baeyens JP, Classens J. Significance of stature as a clinical measurement of aging. *J Am Geriatr Soc*. 1969;17:169–179.

Detsky AS, Baker JP, O'Rourker K, et al. Predicting nutrition-associated complications for patients undergoing gastrointestinal surgery. *JPEN*. 1987;11:440–446.

Detsky AS, McLaughlin JR, Baker JP, et al. What is subjective global assessment of nutritional status? *JPEN*. 1987;11:8–13.

Deurenberg P, et al. Assessment of body composition by bioelectrical impedance in a population aged >60 years. *Am J Clin Nutr*. 1990;51:3.

Duerksen DR, Yeo TA, Siemens JL, O'Connor MP. The validity and reproducibility of clinical assessment of nutritional status in the elderly. *Nutrition*. 2000;16:740–744.

Durnin JV, Womersley S. Body fat assessed from total body density and its estimation from skinfold thickness: measurements of 481 men and women aged from 16–72 years. *Br J Nutr*. 1974;32:77–79.

Economos CD, Nelson ME, Fiatarone MA, et al. A multicenter comparison of dual-energy X-ray absorptiometers: in vivo and in vitro soft tissue measurement. *Eur J Clin Nutr*. 1997;51:312–317.

Elahi VK, Elahi P, Andres R. A longitudinal study of nutritional intake in men. *J Gerontol*. 1983;38:162–180.

Evans WJ, Cyr-Campbell D. Nutrition, exercise, and healthy aging. *JADA*. 1997;97:632–638.

Evans WJ. What is Sarcopenia? *J Gerontol*. 1995;50A:5–10.

Falciglia G, O'Connor J, Gredling E. Upper arm anthropometric norms in elderly white subjects. *J Am Dietetic Assoc*. 1988;88:569–574.

Fey-Yensan N, English C, Pacheco HE, Belyea M, Schuler D. Elderly food stamp participants are different from eligible nonparticipants by level of nutrient risk but not nutrient intake. *JADA*. 2003;103:103–107.

Fink A, Hays RD, Moore AA, JC B. Alcohol-related problems in older persons. Determinants, consequences, and screening. *Arch Intern Med*. 1996;156:1150–1156.

Fishcher J, Johnson MA. Low body weight and weight loss in the aged. *JADA*. 1990;90:1697–1706.

Folstein MF, Folstein SE, McHugh PR. "Mini-mental state." A practical method for grading the cognitive state of patients for the clinician. *J Psychiatr Res*. 1975;12(3):189–198.

Forbes GB. The adult decline in lean body mass. *Hum Biol*. 1976;48:161–166.

Fox EA, Boylan ML, Johnson L. Clinically applicable methods for body fat determination. *Top Clin Nutr*. 1987;2:1–9.

Fuller NJ, Hardingham CR, Graves M, Screaton N, Dixon AK, Ward LM. Assessment of limb muscle and adipose tissue by dual-energy X-ray absorptiometry using magnetic resonance imaging for comparison. *Int J Obes Relat Metab Disord*. 1999;23:1295–1302.

Galanos AN, Peiper CF, Cornono-Huntley JC, Bales CW, Fillenbaum GC. Nutrition and function: is there a relationship between body mass index and the functional capabilities of community-dwelling elderly? *J Am Geriatr Soc*. 1994;42:368–377.

Gallagher D, Kovera AJ, Clay-Williams G, et al. Weight loss in postmenopausal obesity: no adverse alterations in body composition and protein metabolism. *Am J Physiol Endocrinol Metab*. 2000;279:E124–E31.

Gallagher D, Ruts E, Visser M, et al. Weight stability masks sarcopenia in elderly men and women. *Am J Physiol Endocrinol Metab*. 2000;279:E366–E375.

Garth S, Young R. Concurrent fat loss and fat gain. *Am J Phys Anthropol*. 1956;14:497–504.

Goichot B, Schlienger JL, Gruenenberger F, et al. Low cholesterol concentrations in free-living elderly subjects: relations with dietary intake and nutritional intake. *Am J Clin Nutr*. 1995;62:547–553.

Gordon CC, Chumlea WC, Roche AF. Stature, recumbent length and weight. In: Lohman TG, Martorell R, eds. *Anthropometric Standardization Reference Manual*. Champaign, IL: Human Kinetics; 1988.

Guigoz Y, Lauque S, Vellas BJ. Identifying the elderly at risk for malnutrition. The Mini Nutritional Assessment. *Clin Geriatr Med*. 2002;18(4):737–757.

Guigoz Y, Vellas B, Garry PJ. Assessing the nutritional status of the elderly: the Mini-Nutritional Assessment as part of the geriatric evaluation. *Nutr Rev*. 1996;54(suppl):S59–S65.

Guigoz Y, Vellas B, Garry PJ. Mini Nutrition Assessment: a practical assessment tool for grading the nutritional state of elderly patients. *Facts Res Gerontol*. 1994;2(suppl):S15–S59.

Guigoz Y. The Mini Nutritional Assessment (MNA) review of the literature—what does it tell us? *J Nutr Health Aging*. 2006;10(6):466–485.

Hankin JH. Development of a diet history questionnaire for studies of older persons. *Am J Clin Nutr*. 1989;50:1121.

Hejda S. Skinfold in old and long-lived individuals. *Gerontology*. 1963;8:201–297.

Heymsfield SB, Arteaga C, McManus C, Smith J, Moffitt S. Measurement of muscle mass in humans: validity of the 24-hour urinary creatinine method. *Am J Clin Nutr*. 1983;37:478–494.

Heymsfield SB, McManus CB, Nixon DE, et al. Anthropometric assessment of adult protein-energy malnutrition. In: Wright RA HSe, ed. *Nutritional Assessment*. Boston: Blackwell Scientific; 1984.

Hickson M, Frost G. A comparison of three methods for estimating height in acutely ill elderly persons. *J Human Nutr Diet* 2003;16(1):13–20.

Houtkooper LB, Going SB, Sproul J, Blew RM, Lohman TG. Comparison of methods for assessing body composition over 1 y in postmenopausal women. *Am J Clin Nutr*. 2000;72:401–496.

Hudgens J, Langkamp-Henken B. The Mini Nutrition Assessment as an assessment tool in elders in long-term care. *Nutr Clin Prac.* 2004;19(5):463–470.

Institute of Medicine. *Dietary Reference Intakes for Energy, Carbohydrates, Fiber, Fat, Protein, and Amino Acids (Macronutrients) (2002/2005).* Washington, DC: National Academies Press; 2005.

Katz S, Ford AB, Moskowitz RW, et al. Studies of illness in the aged: the index of ADL; a standardized measure of biological and psychosocial function. *JAMA.* 1963;185:914–919.

Kuczmarski RJ. Need for body composition information in elderly subjects. *Am J Clin Nutr.* 1989;50:1150.

Kumanyika S, et al. Picture-sort method for administering a food frequency questionnaire to older adults. *JADA.* 1996;96:137.

Kwok T, Whitelaw MN. The use of arm span in nutritional assessment of the elderly. *J Am Geriatr Soc.* 1991;39:492.

Kyle UG, Kossovsky MP, Kasegard VL, Pichard C. Comparison of tools for nutritional assessment and screening at hospital admission: a population study. *Clin Nutr.* 2006;25(3):409–417.

Latin RW, Johnson SC, Ruhling RO. An anthropometric estimation of body composition of older men. *J Gerontol.* 1987;42:24–28.

Lauque S, Arnaud-Battandier F, Mansourian R, et al. Protein-energy oral supplementation in malnourished nursing-home residents: a controlled trial. *Age Ageing.* 2000;29:51–56.

Lawton MP, Brody EM. Assessment of elderly people: self-maintaining and instrumental activities of daily living. *Gerontologist.* 1969;9:179–186.

Lichtenstein AH RH, Yu WW, Epstein SR, Russell RM. Modified MyPyramid for Older Adults. *J Nur.* 2008;138(7):1400.

Lipschitz DA, Mitchell CO. Nutritional assessment of the elderly: special considerations. In: Wright RA HS, McMan CB, eds. *Nutritional Assessment.* Boston: Blackwell Scientific; 1984.

Lipschitz DA, Mitchell CO. The correctability of nutritional, immune, and hematopoietic manifestations of protein-calorie malnutrition in the elderly. *J Am Coll Nutr.* 1982;1:16–23.

Lipschitz DA. Nutrition and the aging hematopoietic system. In: Hutchinson ML; Munro HN, eds. *Nutrition and Aging.* New York: Academic Press; 1986.

Lipschitz DA. Nutrition, aging, and the immunohematopoietic system. *Clin Geriatr Med.* 1987;3(2):319–328.

Madden JP, Goodman SJ, Guthrie HA. Validity of the 24-hour recall: analysis of data obtained from elderly subjects. *JADA.* 1976;68:143.

McGee M, Jensen GL. Mini Nutrition Assessment (MNA): research and practice in the elderly. *Am J Clin Nutr.* 2000;71(1):158.

Meydani M. Nutrition interventions in aging and age-associated disease (Boyd Orr lecture). *Proc Nutr Soc.* 2002;61:165–171.

Miall WE, Ashcroft MT, Lovell HG, et al. A longitudinal study of the decline of adult height with age in two Welsh communities. *Hum Biol.* 1967;39:445–454.

Mitchell CO, Lipschitz DA. The effect of age and sex on the routinely employed measurements used to assess the nutritional status of hospitalized patients. *Am J Clin Nutr.* 1982;36:340–349.

Mitchell CO, Lipschitz DA. Arm length measurements as an alternative to height in nutritional assessment of the elderly. *J Parenter Enter Nutr.* 1982;6:226–229.

Mitchell CO, Lipschitz DA. Detection of protein-calorie malnutrition in the elderly. *Am J Clin Nutr.* 1982;35:398–406.

Morely JE, Miller DK, Perry HM III, Patrick P, Guigoz Y, Vellas B. Anorexia of aging, leptin and the Mini Nutritional Assessment. Nestle Nutrition Workshop Series Clinical Performance Programme. 1999;I:67–76.

Morely JE. Nutritional assessment is a key component of geriatric assessment. *Facts Res Gerontol.* 1994;2:5.

National Institutes of Health: Expert panel of detection, evaluation and treatment of high blood cholesterol in adults (Adult Treatment Panel II), NIH Publication NO. 93-3096. Bethesda, MD: U.S. National Heart, Lung, and Blood Institute; 1993.

Niedert KC, Dorner B. *Nutrition Care of the Older Adult.* 2nd ed. Chicago: American Dietetic Association; 2004.

Nutrition Screening Initiative. *Nutrition Interventions Manual for Professionals Caring for Older Adults.* Washington, DC: Nutrition Screening Initiative; 1992.

Nutrition Screening Initiative. DETERMINE Your Nutritional Health Checklist. 1991. Available at: http://www.aafp.org/x17367.xml.

Nutrition Screening Initiative. Level 1 Screen. 1991.

Nutrition Screening Initiative. Level 2 Screen. 1991.

Ostlund RE, et al. The ratio of waist-to-hip circumference, plasma insulin level and glucose intolerance as independent predictors of the HDL2 cholesterol level in older adults. *NEJM.* 1990;322:229.

Persson MD, Brismar KE, Katzarski KS, Nordenstrom J, Cederholm TE. The nutritional status using Mini Nutritional Assessment and Subjective Global Assessment predict mortality in geriatric patients. *J Am Geriatr Soc.* 2002;50:1996–2002.

Posner BM, et al. Nutrition and health risks in the elderly: the Nutrition Screening Initiative. *Am J Public Health.* 1993;83:972.

Ranhoff AH, Gjoen AU, Mowe M. Screening for malnutrition in elderly acute medical patients: the usefulness of MNA-SF. *J Nutr Health Aging.* 2005;9(4):221–225.

Remer T, Neubert A, Maser-Gluth C. Anthropometry-based reference values for 24-hour urinary creatinine excretion during growth and their use in endocrine and nutritional research. *Am J Clin Nutr.* 2002;75:561–569.

Roe DA. *Geriatric Nutrition.* 3rd ed. Englewood Cliffs, NJ: Prentice Hall; 1992.

Rosenberg IH. Summary comments. *Am J Clin Nutr.* 1989;50:1231–1233.

Rudman D, Feller AG. Protein-calorie undernutrition in the nursing home. *J Am Geriatr Soc.* 1989;31:173.

Rudman D, Mattson DE, Nagrai HS, et al. Prognostic significance of serum cholesterol in nursing home men. *J Parenter Enter Nutr.* 1988;12:155–158.

Sacks GS, Dearman K, Replogle WH, et al. Use of subjective global assessment to identify nutrition-associated complications and death in geriatric long-term care facility residents. *J AM Coll Nutr.* 2000;19:570–577.

Salamone LM, Fuerst T, Visser M, et al. Measurement of fat mass using DEXA: a validation study in elderly adults. *J Appl Physiol* 2000;89:345–352.

Salive ME, Cornoni-Huntley J, Phillips EL, et al. Serum albumin in older persons: relationship with age and health status. *J Clin Epidemiol.* 1992;45:213–221.

Schlenker ED. *Nutrition in Aging.* 3rd ed. Boston: McGraw-Hill; 1998.

Seaverson EL, Buell JS, Fleming DJ, et al. Poor iron status is more prevalent in Hispanic than non-Hispanic white older adults in Massachusetts. *J Nutr.* 2007;137:414–420.

Seiber CC. Nutritional screening tools—how does MNA compare? Proceedings of the session held in Chicago, May 2–3, 2006 (15 years of Mini Nutritional Assessment). *J Nutr Health Aging.* 2006;10(6):488–492.

Sergi G, Enzi G. Role of visceral proteins in detecting malnutrition in the elderly. *Eur J Clin Nutr.* 2006;60:203–209.

Steen B, Bfroce A, Isaksson B, et al. Body composition in 70-year-old males and females in Gothenburg, Sweden. *Acta Med Scand.* 1977;611(suppl):87–112.

Stoudt HW, Damon A, McFarland R, et al. Weight, height and selected body dimensions of adults, United States, 1960–1962. *Vital Health Stat.* 1963(11):35.

Stratton RJ, King CL, Stroud MA, Jackson AA, Elia M. 'Malnutrition Universal Screening Tool' predicts mortality and length of hospital stay in acutely ill elderly. *Br J Nutr.* 2006;95(2):325–330.

Sullivan DH, Sun S, Walls RC. Protein-energy undernutrition among elderly hospitalized patients: a prospective study. *JAMA.* 1999;281:2013–2019.

Svendsen OL, et al. Measurement of body fat in elderly subjects by dual-energy x-ray absorptiometry, bioelectrical impedance, and anthropometry. *Am J Clin Nutr.* 1991;53:1117.

U.S. Department of Agriculture and U.S. Department of Health and Human Services. *Dietary Guidelines for Americans 2005.* 6th ed. Home and Garden Bulletin no. 232; 2005.

Vellas B, Villars H, Abellan G, et al. Overview of the MNA—its history and challenges. *J Nutr Health Aging.* 2006;10(6):456–463.

Visser M, Fuerst T, Lang T, Salamone LM. Validation of fan-beam dual-energy X-ray absorptiometry for measuring fat-free mass and leg muscle mass. *J Appl Physiol.*1999;87:1513–20.

Visser M, Pahor M, Tylavsky F, et al. One and two-year change in body composition as measured by DXA in a population-based cohort of older men and women. *J Appl Physiol.* 2003;94:2368–2374.

Walser M. Creatinine excretion as a measure of protein nutrition in adults of varying age. *JPEN.* 1987;11(5 suppl):73S–78S.

Wang ZM, Gallagher D, Nelson ME, Matthews DE, Heymsfield SB. Total body skeletal muscle mass: evaluation of 24-h urinary creatinine excretion by computerized azial tomography. *Am J Clin Nutr.* 1996;63:863–869.

Wang ZM, Visser M, Ma R, et al. Skeletal muscle mass: evaluation of neutron activation and dual-energy X-ray absorptiometry methods. *J Appl Physiol.* 1996;80:824–831.

Welle S, Thornton C, Totterman S, Gilbert F. Utility of creatinine excretion in body-composition studies of healthy men and women older than 60 years. *Am J Clin Nutr.* 1996;63:151–156.

White JV, et al. Nutrition Screening Initiative: development and implementation of the public awareness checklist and screening tools. *JADA.* 1992;92:163.

Wilson MMG, Thomas DR, Rubenstein LZ, et al. Appetite assessment: simple appetite questionnaire predicts weight loss in community-dwelling adults and nursing home residents. *Am J Clin Nutr.* 2005;82:1074–1081.

Wolinsky FD, et al. Progress in the development of a nutrition risk index. *J Nutr.* 1990;120:1549.

Zhang C, Rexrode KM, van Dam RM, Li TY, Hu FB. Abdominal obesity and the risk of all-cause, cardiovascular, and cancer mortality. *Circulation.* 2008;117:1658–1667.

CHAPTER

17

Pharmacology, Nutrition, and the Older Adult: Interactions and Implications

Jill Arnold, PharmD, Julie L. Baron, PharmD, and
William Schwab, MD, PhD, AGSF

CHAPTER OBJECTIVES   Upon completion of this chapter, the reader will be able to:

1. Discuss the increasing role medications play in the health of older adults
2. Review the physiological changes that occur with aging that influence the pharmacokinetic effects of medications
3. List and describe the various classes of medications that facilitate adequate nutrition or interfere with the normal digestive and absorptive processes
4. Review the general effects medications have on the body systems, including the gastrointestinal system
5. Explain the basic features of Medical Part D and how it influences the availability of medications for older adults

KEY TERMS AND CONCEPTS

Appetite

Complementary and alternative medicine (CAM)

Consciousness

Dysgeusia

Peristalsis

Pharmacodynamics

Pharmacokinetics

Xerostomia

Medications play an ever-increasing role in the life and health of older adults, especially in the frailest of the elder cohort. Just as medications can affect basic functions such as balance and cognition, it can also affect obtaining and utilizing nutrition.

Although older adults comprise about 13% of the population, they consume over 30% of prescription medications, spending over $10 billion a year. Ninety percent of older adults take at least one medication, with 40% taking five or more, not including over-the-counter medications.

The average older person in America takes two to six medications, along with one to three over-the-counter medications. Obviously, the potential for medication interaction is immense. Medication interaction rate has found to be as high as 70% in patients on six medications.

Frailty increases with age, as does the number of co-morbidities. In the last British census, 72% of the older adult population had at least one chronic illness, with 21% having two and 11% having four or more. Heart disease, cancer, lung disease, and stroke have become the most prevalent serious health conditions affecting adults today. By age 65, individuals have at least one chronic disease and approximately 80% of older adults report at least one chronic condition resulting in pain and disability, loss of function, or limited activity. Older adults use the most drugs, have the highest number of physician visits, and

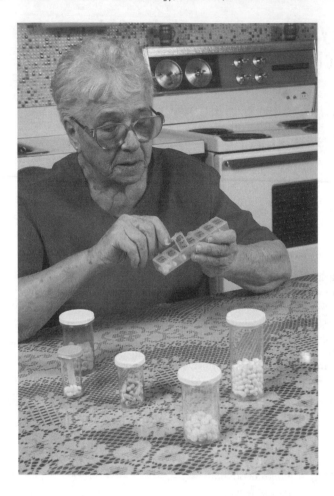

require care by a larger variety of specialists than any other age group.

Older adults are often found in venues of care where multiple medications are prescribed, such as outpatient medical offices, hospitals, and nursing homes. Oftentimes, the medications prescribed are inappropriate and have the potential to cause disorders in consciousness and physical injury. The high prevalence of drug-related problems occurring as a result of multiple drug use combined with age-related changes in pharmacokinetics and pharmacodynamics, is a well known occurrence in older adults.

Levinson and colleagues, 1990, found almost one out of ten medical visits resulted in the prescription of a psychotropic medication. Inappropriate medications are currently blamed for billions of dollars in excess medical costs and 100,000 excess deaths. Inappropriate medi-

appetite The desire to satisfy a bodily need.

dysgeusia Distorted or strange taste, which can be a side effect of some medications.

cation has been estimated to be the fifth leading cause of death in the United States. In the outpatient arena, an adverse medication event was found at as many as 25% of outpatient visits, with 13% of the events being serious. Obviously, awareness of the potential for harm in pharmacologic therapy is incumbent on all medical professionals and a serious consideration when working with older adults who are often on numerous medications.

Polypharmacy, when a patient is on multiple medications, is a significant problem in the geriatric population. Polypharmacy can be rational at times. For example, most cancer chemotherapeutic regimens involve deliberate polypharmacy to decrease doses of toxic medications by utilizing synergistic combinations of several medications at lower doses. Congestive heart failure is almost always treated with multiple medications in order to ameliorate multiple pathways that lead to illness and dysfunction. Although polypharmacy is, in general, harmful to the health of the patient, **Box 17-1** lists some examples of common, rational polypharmacy in selected disease states.

In most cases, however, older adults are at risk for polypharmacy that is accidental rather than rational. For instance, the average nursing home resident is on seven medications. The reasons for polypharmacy in older adults can include severity of illness, multiple coexisting comorbidities, multiple prescribing physicians, and a disorganized medical chart. The consequences of polypharmacy can include medication interactions, reduced compliance due to pill burden, and increased costs of medication.

Common Classes of Medications in the Older Adult

The four most common classes of medications used by older adults are cardiovascular and antihypertensive medications, hypoglycemics, analgesics, and psychiatric medications. Their common indications and diet-related concerns are as follows:

- **Cardiovascular/antihypertensives.** Common indications include hypertension and decreased heart contractility (cardiac systolic dysfunction). This class includes many different medications within this class. Of note, clonidine can depress **appetite** due to central nervous system effects as well as constipation and decreased salivation. Angiotensin-converting enzyme inhibitors (ACE inhibitors) can cause **dysgeusia** (strange taste). Diuretics can cause dehydration, which can manifest paradoxically in the demented older adult by causing decreased fluid intake.
- **Hypoglycemics.** These medications are used to treat diabetes. Hypoglycemics such as sulfonylureas and insulin itself increase serum insulin levels. They can cause increased fat formation and stability and can lead to worsening obesity.

> **BOX 17-1 Common, Rational Polypharmacy in Selected Disease States**
>
> 1. **Coronary artery disease (CAD):** Beta-blocker, ACE inhibitor, antiplatelet therapy, statin.
> 2. **Chronic obstructive pulmonary disease (COPD):** Inhaled beta agonist, inhaled anticholinergic, inhaled or oral steroid.
> 3. **Congestive heart failure (CHF):** Diuretic, beta-blocker, spironolactone, ACE Inhibitor.
> 4. **Diabetes mellitus:** Oral hypoglycemic or insulin, metformin, alpha-glucosidase inhibitor.
> 5. **Hypertension:** Monotherapy or combined therapy of thiazides, ACE inhibitors, calcium channel blockers, beta-blockers, vasodilators, and other classes.

- **Analgesics.** The class includes nonsteroidal anti-inflammatory medications (NSAIDs) and the opiates. NSAIDs can cause significant gastric and esophageal injury and bleeding and affect renal function. Opiates cause constipation and can depress consciousness. Inception of opiate therapy often results in nausea that subsides within a few days.
- **Psychiatric medications.** Common indications include depression and the behavioral symptoms of dementia. This class includes many medications. It is important to remember that any medication that is active in the central nervous system can affect consciousness and appetite.

Medicare Part D

January 1, 2006, saw the implementation of the Medicare Part D pharmacy plan as part of the sweeping Medicare Modernization Act that was signed into law in 2003 and implemented in 2004. Although it is part of the largest revision of the Medicare program since its inception, our discussion will be restricted to Part D and its impact on pharmacy utilization and the senior population.

All Medicare beneficiaries now have access to Part D prescription coverage. Beneficiaries may choose whether to enroll and are able to choose from a variety of different plans. The Part D benefit now assists those who were previously unable to get assistance with medication costs. Part D is a three-tiered approach to cost and cost-sharing. Older adults who join Part D are restricted to formulary medications, although it should be noted that the formulary

is quite extensive. Medications covered under Part B, such as nebulizers and chemotherapeutic agents, will continue to be covered under Part B.

There have been changes in the cost to patients for Medicare Part D since its inception in 2006. In 2008, after a $275 deductible, the patient paid 25% of medication costs until out-of-pocket expenses reached $2,510. Thus, the actual payout by the patient (TRue Out Of Pocket or TROOP) would be $558.75. After this amount is reached, the "doughnut hole" takes effect, whereby the patient pays the entire medication cost to a total of $5,726 (TROOP of $4,050). After the "doughnut hole," the patient pays a minimum co-pay of $2.25 for generics and $5.60 for all other medications. Neither the premium for Part D coverage nor excluded medications (medications not on the Part D formulary) count toward either the total medication cost or the TROOP.

The out-of-pocket threshold of $4,050 a year is a prohibitive sum for many older adults. The Center for Medicare and Medicaid Services (CMS), the administrative agency for Medicare, has set up programs to help those who cannot afford the medication costs under Part D. This has become especially important, because most of the pharmaceutical manufacturers do not provide medication assistance for people who have insurance with a medication benefit, such as Part D. Some of the drug companies are now offering assistance programs to those in the "doughnut hole." Anyone who cannot afford their medications should call Social Security at 800-772-1213.

CMS has estimated that it will need to provide assistance for all or part of the TROOP for about one-third of enrollees. Since Medicare Part D took effect in January 2006, it has been estimated that user costs have been reduced by 18.4%. In addition, there has been a 12.8% increase in prescription medications in the elderly, and increased total usage by 4.5%.

Attempts to assess the effects of shared prescription costs and the "doughnut hole" have been contradictory. In addition, it is important to assess whether patients have the funds to eat an appropriate diet. In many cases, it may be necessary to help older adults to obtain the resources to eat a nutritious diet and to receive necessary medications for good health.

Use of Complementary and Alternative Medicines

Interest in **complementary and alternative medicine (CAM)** has increased over the last several years. Although the use of CAM products varies by ethnicity, age, socioeconomic class, and education level, overall use of herbal remedies has

> **complementary and alternative medicine (CAM)** A broad range of healing philosophies, approaches, and therapies that include treatments and health care practices not widely taught in medical schools, not generally used in hospitals, and not usually reimbursed by medical insurance companies.

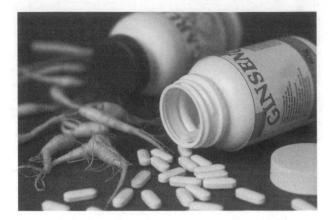

increased dramatically. Little is known about the potential for medication interactions and adverse reactions when CAM product are used with prescription medications. Although there is limited scientific literature available on CAM products, and even less information available on the interactions between CAM products and conventional medicines, their use is becoming increasingly popular in older adults; therefore, medical professionals must be aware of some of the more common CAM products.

It is important to keep in mind that older adults are at higher risk for potential problems with the concomitant use of CAM and conventional medicines because of polypharmacy and decreased metabolism and elimination of medications, which increases the older adult's sensitivity to the effects of medications. A study of a Medicare population by Elmer, Lafferty, Tyree, and Lind in 2007 revealed that after four years in the study, 15% of participants were using CAM products, 14% were concurrently taking conventional medications, and almost 6% were taking combinations considered to have a significant potential risk for an adverse reaction. Some CAM products, including garlic, gingko, ginseng, and St. John's wort, are known to interact with several medications, including digoxin, warfarin, and aspirin.

Many people mistakenly believe that CAM products are without risk. However, medication-related hospitalizations due to side effects of CAM products are becoming more common. Oftentimes, health care providers are unaware that the older adult is using CAM products. Health care providers need to ask questions that will elicit information on CAM product use so that comprehensive health care plans can be administered.

With the increasing costs of prescription medications, there is the potential for an increase in use of CAM products for common disease states. It is important for health care providers to be aware of CAM products their patients may be using and also to be knowledgeable on the efficacy of CAM products compared to conventional medications.

Food and Medication Interactions

A food–medication interaction is the effect of a food or a nutrient in a food on a medication. Dietary nutrients can affect medications by altering their absorption or metabolism. Food and nutrients can alter a medication's effectiveness in many ways. Foods can make medications work faster, slower, or even prevent them from working. Food can increase or decrease the absorption of a medication (absorbing less than the intended dose may decrease the medication's effect and absorbing more than the intended dose increases the chance for an overdose); interfere with a medication's metabolism or action in the body; or prohibit the removal of a medication from the body. For example, dietary calcium can bind to tetracycline. Thus, if a person consumes too much dietary calcium, the body does not absorb the amount of antibiotic intended.

Medications are absorbed more quickly into the body when the stomach is empty. Sometimes a medication should be taken with food. Others should be taken on an empty stomach or one hour before or two hours after eating.

The type of food or beverage consumed with a medication can affect the medication's absorption. For example, consumption of acidic soft drinks, juices, and foods may produce excess stomach acidity, which may destroy a medication or cause it to dissolve in the stomach instead the intestine. Acidic foods may also dissolve a timed-released medication all at once instead of over time.

Aged and fermented foods contain a chemical called tyramine that interacts with monoamine oxidase inhibitors. The interaction can result in dangerously high blood pressure. Vitamin K can decrease the effectiveness of certain anticoagulant medications. Liver enzymes prepare medications for removal from the body. These enzymes require nutrients to work properly. If the required nutrients are not present, medications may stay active in the body longer than they are supposed to and might cause an overdose effect. See **Table 17-1** for more specific examples of medication–nutrient interactions.

Risks of medication–nutrient interactions can be reduced by eating a healthy diet that follows MyPyramid, following the directions on how to take medications (prescription and over-the-counter); reading warning labels on both prescription and over-the-counter medications; and informing the physician and pharmacist about everything taken, including over-the-counter medications, alcohol, and herbal products.

Pharmacokinetic and Pharmacodynamic Changes in Aging

Age-related physiologic changes can affect the body's **pharmacokinetics** and **pharmacodynamics**. These changes can

TABLE 17-1 Medication–Nutrient Interactions‡

Nutrient/Food Item	Medication	Potential Interaction
Grapefruit juice	Statins, amiodarone, cyclosporine, carbamazepine, sirolimus, tacrolimus, calcium channel blockers (i.e., felodipine, amlodipine)	Increase effect of medications
Foods containing Vitamin K (brussels sprouts, cabbage, spinach, etc.)	Warfarin	Decrease INR
Salt	Lithium	Increased salt intake decreases lithium levels Decreased salt intake increases lithium levels
Tyramine-containing foods (aged, mature cheeses; aged, cured meats)	MAO-inhibitors (phenelzine, selegiline)	Hypertensive crisis
Folic acid	Cholestyramine,* phenytoin	Decreased folic acid concentrations
Sodium	Carbamazepine, thiazide diuretics, lactulose	Alter sodium balance
Potassium	Diuretics, corticosteroids, insulin, trimethoprim, heparin, amphotericin B, antipseudomonal penicillins, β_2 agonists	Alter potassium balance
Phosphorus	Antacids, sulcralfate	Hypophosphatemia
Magnesium	Diuretics, amphotericin B, cyclosporine, aminoglycosides	Hypomagnesemia
Calcium	Foscarnet, cholestyramine	Hypocalcemia
Glucose	Protease inhibitors, corticosteroids	Hyperglycemia
Vitamin D	Phenytoin, phenobarbital	Decreased vitamin D concentrations
Vitamin B12	Proton pump inhibitors	Decreased absorption of vitamin B12
Pyridoxine	Isoniazid	Induces pyridoxine deficiency
Calcium or calcium-containing foods	Tetracycline	Decreased absorption of tetracycline
Alcohol	Metronidazole	Nausea, vomiting, palpitations, flushing, headache
Any food	Bisphosphonates	Decreased absorption and effectiveness of the medication
High-fat meal	Theophylline	Increase theophylline levels
High-carbohydrate meals	Theophylline	Decrease theophylline levels
Vitamin E	Warfarin	High doses (>400 IU) can increase INR and increase risk of bleeding

*Cholestyramine decreases absorption of many vitamins and medications.

‡Not all-inclusive.

lead to a number adverse effects with many prescription and over-the-counter medications. Age-related changes that affect the body's pharmacokinetics include absorption, distribution, metabolism, and elimination (**Table 17-2**).

Absorption

The kinetics of solubilization of medications changes with age, leading to a decreased rate of absorption of certain prescription and over-the-counter medications.

Age-related changes in the gastrointestinal tract include slowed gastric emptying, increased intestinal transit time, and decreased production of saliva and gastric and intestinal fluids, and lowered splanchnic blood flow. The decrease in gastric fluids is directly related to an increase in gastric pH with age, which could potentially slow absorption of medicines normally soluble in acid. However, it is the increase in intestinal transit time that provides the potential for

pharmacokinetics The study of how drug levels are affected by absorption, distribution, metabolism, and elimination.

pharmacodynamics The study of the effect of drugs over time.

TABLE 17-2 Age-Related Changes in Pharmacokinetics and Pharmacodynamics

Pharmacokinetic	Physiologic Change	Clinical Significance
Absorption	Possible changes in gastric pH, absorptive surface and splanchnic blood flow; generally preserved gastric emptying	Little to none
Distribution	Increased body fat	Increased volume of distribution of lipid-soluble medications
	Decreased water compartment	Higher levels of water-soluble medications
	Decreased lean body mass	Serum creatinine becomes a less accurate indicator of medication elimination
	Decreased serum albumin	Increased level of free acidic medication
Hepatic metabolism	Decreased liver mass and hepatic blood flow	Phase I reactions altered (oxidation, reduction, hydrolysis)
Renal elimination	Creatinine clearance reduced (with aging or disease)	Dose adjustments required for medications excreted by the kidneys
Pharmacodynamics	Decreased beta-receptor response	Effect of beta-adrenergic agonists and beta-blockers decreased
	Increase receptor response	Effect of opiates and benzodiazepines increased

greater absorption of prescription and over-the-counter medicines. Clinicians continue to debate how age-related physiologic changes affect medicine absorption.

Skin changes that accompany aging may alter the absorption of topical medicines. The net effect on medicine absorption is variable. The older adult's skin may be fragile, and dermal patches should be used cautiously.

Medicines administered by intramuscular injection may be affected by a decrease in muscle mass, which reduces the number of possible injection sites.

Distribution

Age-associated changes in body composition, such as an increase in adipose tissue and decreases in lean body muscle and total body water, can alter the volume of distribution of prescription and over-the-counter medications. The volume of distribution (Vd) is the space in which a medication is stored in the body. Increased blood levels of medications distributed into muscle, as well as the medication-elimination indicator, serum creatinine, becoming less accurate, are the result of decreased lean body mass. The greater amount of body fat that often accompanies aging provides a larger area of distribution, which increases fat-soluble medication tissue levels and thus the duration of action. The decrease in total body water results in higher levels of water-soluble medications in the body. Serum levels of water-soluble medications, such as digoxin, lithium, and aminoglycosides, increase as the volume of distribution decreases.

Fat-soluble (nonpolar) medications (e.g., diazepam, haloperidol, amiodarone, and tricyclic antidepressants) readily cross membranes and are taken up by adipose tissue. Water-soluble (polar) medications (e.g., lithium, hydrochlorothiazide, digoxin, angiotensin-converting enzyme (ACE) inhibitors, and aminoglycosides) are typically confined to lean body tissue due to the decreased volume of distribution.

The distribution of medications is also affected by the decreases in cardiac output and plasma protein concentrations that occur with aging. The decrease in cardiac output leads to decreased perfusion of organs, which affects the body's ability to metabolize and excrete medications. Plasma protein concentrations decrease with age, causing highly protein bound medications (e.g., NSAIDs, furosemide, phenytoin, sulfonyureas, and coumadin) to have diminished binding. This leads to the increase of free medication circulating, which may put the older adult at an increased risk of developing toxic free (active) medication levels.

Metabolism

The liver is the primary site of medication metabolism in the body. With age, however, the liver's ability to metabolize medications becomes less efficient, leading to the possibility for increased concentrations of medications. Some medications are at an increased risk of accumulation due to decreases in liver mass and hepatic blood flow. The metabolism of other medications (e.g., acetylation, glucuronidation, sulfation, and glycine conjugation) are not affected by age-related changes to the liver.

Elimination

A high percentage of medications are excreted by the kidneys. Age-related decreases in kidney function can lead to increases in medication half-lives and serum levels. One example of this is digoxin, a medication used to treat atrial fibrillation. Medication adjustments for older adults should be considered for medications that are eliminated renally. Various factors, including lean body mass, obesity, congestive heart failure, and dehydration, among others, can lead to inaccuracies in estimating kidney function; therefore, kidney function needs to be considering carefully.

Effect of Medications on Target Cells
Homeostasis

The effect of medications on target cells is a pharmacodynamic change that occurs in older adults. These pharmacodynamic changes are related to homeostatic functions and receptor responses. Homeostatic mechanisms are altered with age. This means that older adults are more affected by medications due to their increased ability to penetrate into the central nervous system (CNS). Medications that could potentially penetrate into the CNS and put older patients at an increased risk of developing adverse effects include benzodiazepines, antidepressants, neuroleptics, and NSAIDs.

Receptors

The functionality of various tissue receptors also changes with advancing age. For example, the response of the beta-adrenergic system decreases with age, lowering the effect of some medications, such as beta-adrenergic agonists and beta-blockers. The total number of beta-receptors is not altered in the older patient; rather, there is an alteration of postreceptor events that lead to decreased effects. The alpha-adrenergic system does not seem to be affected by the increase in age.

Normal Physiology of Nutrition

To understand the role that medication can play in the maintenance of proper nutrition, one must understand the normal processes by which nutrition is obtained and utilized. The process can be thought of as a sequential chain where the interruption of any one site can result in inadequate intake of vital nutrients. Unless nutrition is being provided by enteral or parenteral means, the older adult must maintain a level of **consciousness** sufficient to obtain and ingest food. Beyond simple consciousness, there must be appetitiveness. The older adult must eat either from a sense of desire or from a sense that they have to eat. The older adult must also be able to locate and prepare the food and purposefully bring it to his or her mouth. Once in the mouth, the older adult must be able to chew and form the food and saliva into a bolus that is then swallowed. The bolus is carried by **peristalsis** to the stomach where it is further digested and emulsified. The food and digestive juices and enzymes are carried into duodenum and intestine where the nutrients are absorbed and the waste is

eliminated. At the same time, the nutrients absorbed into the bloodstream are carried to their sites of utilization. To summarize, nutrition can be thought of as flowing from appetitiveness, physical manipulation, chewing, bolus formation, swallowing, peristalsis, digestion, and absorption to the utilization of nutrients and the elimination of waste. Various medications used by older adults can affect these processes in both positive and negative ways, either by facilitating adequate nutrition or interfering with the normal digestive and absorptive processes.

Consciousness

The processes of consciousness are complex and are located within the CNS. Although many neurotransmitters are involved, GABA-nergic, noradrenergic, and acetylcholinergic receptors likely play a primary role.

Medications That Affect Consciousness

A common side effect of many medications that exert action on the CNS is sedation, which, in turn, can lead to a disinterest in eating. This may be particularly troublesome in older patients, who are more susceptible to adverse effects of medications due to a combination of factors such as pharmacokinetic changes, pharmacodynamic changes, and medication interactions related to polypharmacy. Many of the medications listed in **Table 17-3** that are known to cause sedation should be avoided in older patients due to increased frequency and severity of side effects.

Tricyclic antidepressants, atypical antipsychotics, gastrointestinal drugs, benzodiazepines, and antihistamines can interfere with food intake by causing sedation. Of the typical antipsychotics (i.e., haloperidol, fluphenazine, mellaril, etc.), those with lower potency are less likely to be associated with sedation. SSRIs may be associated with sedation, although most do not have the strong sedating effects of older classes of antidepressants.

Medications such as antidepressants, anxiolytics, and neuroleptics can cause an increase in food intake as a result of improved mood and psychological function in some patient populations; however, the opposite is often observed in the older adult population. Some antidepressants (e.g., nortriptyline, desipramine, imipramine) can stimulate appetite due to serotonergic activity in younger patients, but in older subjects behaviors such as agitation can interfere with eating.

The most important common medications that interfere with consciousness are those with anticholinergic activity. Unfortunately, anticholinergy is a very common

consciousness The awareness of one's existence.

peristalsis The rhythmic, coordinated contractions by which material is moved through the gastrointestinal tract.

TABLE 17-3 Medications Commonly Associated with Sedation

Medication Class	Examples
Tricyclic antidepressants	Amitriptyline, clomipramine, doxepin
Benzodiazepines	Chlordiazepoxide, diazepam, flurazepam, temazepam, triazolam
Muscle relaxants	Baclofen, carisoprodol, cyclobenzaprine, tizanidine
Atypical antipsychotics	Clozapine, olanzapine, quetiapine
Narcotics	Fentanyl, hydrocodone, methadone, morphine, oxycodone
Barbiturates	Phenobarbital, secobarbital
Antihistamines	Cyproheptadine, diphenhydramine, hydroxyzine, promethazinde
Gastrointestinal	Belladonna, dicyclomine, hyoscyamine, propantheline
Other	Meprobamate, mirtazapine, reserpine, trazodone

property in many medications, and as many as 14 of the 25 most commonly prescribed medications had significant anticholinergic effects.

Although a full discussion of the neurochemistry of consciousness is beyond the scope of this chapter, any medication that is active in the CNS has the capacity to disturb consciousness.

Appetite

Assuming an intact level of consciousness, food consumption requires both an appetite and a lack of nausea. Appetite is regulated by peripheral messengers, central messengers, and monoamines (serotonin and norepinephrine). In addition, intact sensation of taste and smell are important

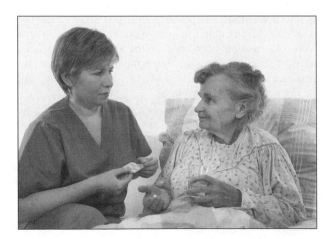

in stimulating appetite. Dysgeusia (taste disorder) can decrease the desire to eat by reducing the pleasure of eating. The dopaminergic and serotonergic receptors appear to play a primary role in satiety and nausea, although many classes of receptors have been implicated.

Older patients characteristically report concerns of gastrointestinal (GI) symptoms such as anorexia, diarrhea, constipation, decreased appetite, and weight loss. A review of prescription and over-the-counter medications can be conducted in order to rule out medications as the offending agent(s) along with a complete medical work-up, if necessary.

Several medications can influence appetite in a positive or negative manner. Currently, no medications have been approved by the Food and Medication Administration (FDA) specifically for the treatment of weight loss in older adults. Several agents that promote weight gain and that are utilized as a last-line in weight loss management include megestrol, cannabinoids (dronabinal), anabolic steroids (oxandrolone), corticosteroids, and human growth hormone (somatropin). Mirtazapine, a serotonin/norepinephrine reuptake inhibitor that is associated with increased appetite and weight gain, is commonly prescribed for older patients experiencing weight loss and depression.

SSRIs (e.g., fluoxetine, paroxetine, sertaline, citalopram, and escitalopram), tricyclic antidepressants (e.g., nortriptyline, desipramine, doxepin, and amitriptyline), and serotonin/norepinephrine reuptake inhibitors (e.g., venlafaxine), which are all commonly used for the treatment of depression, can produce side effects in the older patient that could potentially lead to decreased appetite. Venlafaxine is associated with dose-dependent weight loss and could potentially be the cause of an older patient's weight loss.

Careful attention to potential anticholinergic effects (such as decreased secretions, slowed gastrointestinal motility, blurred vision, increased heart rate, heat intolerance, sedation, and possibly mild confusion) of medications should be considered during a review of an entire medication regimen. Examples of medications with anticholinergic effects include TCAs, benztropine, dicyclomine, trihexphenidyl, and scopolamine. The anticholinergic potential of impaired GI motility and decreased secretions could lead to constipation or decreased food intake and, in turn, affect the patient's appetite; therefore, if possible, these drugs should be avoided in older patients.

GI adverse effects (nausea, vomiting, and diarrhea) are therapy-limiting for SSRIs and should be considered as a potential offending agent if GI concerns are expressed. The acetylcholinesterase inhibitors (AChE) used for the treatment of mild to moderate Alzheimer's disease have a procholinergic effect that can also manifest as nausea, diarrhea, and/or constipation. The monitoring of oral intake and weight should be part of the routine evaluation of AChE therapy.

Physical Manipulation

The patient must be able to move food to his or her mouth (unless an attendant is available for feeding). This activity requires the sensory ability to locate the food, the strength to transport it, and the physical coordination to reach the target (the mouth). Whereas the first two steps are generally not affected by medications, the extrapyramidal effects of dopamine-blocking medications can inhibit both the initiation and performance of the activities necessary to transport the food.

Chewing, Bolus Formation, and Swallowing

Once nonliquid food is in the mouth, it must be chewed, mixed with saliva, formed into a bolus, and swallowed. Both disordered consciousness and disordered coordination can affect the process. Decreased saliva production from anticholinergics can make swallowing more difficult, as well as diminish taste. In addition, a painful mouth (for example, thrush from antibiotic usage or inhaled steroids) can make the process less efficient.

Coordination and Motor Function

Older patients may be more predisposed to movement disorders caused by medications. This type of disorder is due to a decrease in levels of dopamine and acetylcholine in the central nervous system associated with advancing age.

Medications that block dopamine receptor include fluphenazine, haloperidol, trifluoperazine, and thiothixene. In addition, reserpine or tetrabenazine deplete dopamine levels. Atypical antipsychotics, such as olanzapine, risperidone, ziprasidone, and quetiapine, can also produce movement disorders, although the risk is lower than that with typical antipsychotics.

Antipsychotics (including antiemetics) can lead to a common side effect known as extrapyramidal symptoms (EPS). Symptoms of EPS include medication-induced parkinsonism, akathisia (motor restlessness), acute dystonia, and tardive dyskinesia. These movement disorders can cause significant barriers to maintaining adequate nutrition. Medications most often implicated in producing EPS are those that block the central dopaminergic receptors involved in motor function or that result in an imbalance of dopamine, acetylcholine, and other neurotransmitters. **Box 17-2** lists medications commonly associated with extrapyramidal symptoms. Extrapyramidal symptoms are often treated with anticholinergics, which pose additional risks (such as confusion) in older populations.

Tardive dyskinesia is characterized by unwanted movements of the lips, face, hands, arms, and feet. These side effects can cause patients to have difficulty with motor tasks such as talking or eating. First-generation antipsychotics have been associated with the incidence of tardive dyskinesia in approximately 25% to 30% of older patients. Atypical

BOX 17-2 Medications Commonly Associated with Extrapyramidal Symptoms

Amoxapine	Prochlorperazine
Chlorpromazine	Promazine
Fluphenazine	Reserpine
Haloperidol	Triflupromazine
Loxapine	Trifluoperazine
Molindone	Thiothixine
Metoclopramide	

Source: Data from Jenike MA. *Handbook of Geriatric Psychopharmacology.* Littleton, MA: PSG Publishing Company; 1985.

antipsychotics produce tardive dyskinesia in 2% to 13% of patients, depending on the specific agent.

Medication-induced parkinsonism is characterized by symmetrical stiffness, shuffling gait, masked face, or difficulty in arising from a sitting position. Symptoms of medication-induced parkinsonism, such as stiffness and shaking, can significantly impair a patient's ability to self-feed. As with tardive dyskinesia, medication-induced parkinsonism is much more common with older, high-potency antipsychotics, such as haloperidol or fluphenazine.

Acute dystonia as a result of antipsychotics is not often seen in the older adults and, therefore, is not likely to interfere with nutritional intake. Akathisia, presenting as agitation, anxiety, or restlessness, may cause the patient to become increasingly irritated, which can potentially lead to refusal of food.

Peristalsis

The coordinated movement of the bolus through the digestive tract involves both the peristalsis of the bolus as well as the appropriate relaxation of the muscular sphincters that separate regions of the digestive system. The propulsion of the bolus is dependent on the coordination of muscular contraction behind the bolus and relaxation ahead of it. This process is controlled by a complex system of neurotransmitters, which also mediate the relaxation of the gastrointestinal sphincters.

Medications That Have Gastrointestinal Effects

Medications can affect the digestion of food by causing dysphagia, affecting peristalsis, and altering the acidity in the stomach. Medications can induce dysphagia through three mechanisms: side effects of the medication, as a complication of the medication's therapeutic action, and by medication-induced esophageal injury. Medications such as neuromuscular blocking agents that have a direct effect on striated muscle can also cause dysphagia. These agents are typically used only during surgical procedures and with only short-term effects, and thus have very little effect on long-term nutritional intake.

Xerostomia (dry mouth) can also cause dysphagia and lead to changes in food intake. **Table 17-4** lists medications commonly known to cause xerostomia. This list includes medications anticholinergic effects, such as TCAs and antihistamines, but other classes can also cause xerostomia.

As a result of their dopamine-blocking activity, typical antipsychotics can cause swallowing dysfunction associated with medication-induced parkinsonism and tardive dyskinesia. Other medications that could cause difficulty swallowing include inhaled corticosteroids and antibiotics, which can lead to thrush. This can be avoided by advising patients to rinse the mouth after steroid use and to limit the use of antibiotics, if possible. Chemotherapeutic agents; antibiotics, such as metronidazole and clarithromycin; antidepressants, such as amitriptyline; and antidiabetic agents, such as metformin, are all known to cause bitter or metallic taste. Medication-induced changes in taste will often negatively impact food intake.

Medications That Cause Gastrointestinal Injury

Medications can cause esophageal, gastric, and duodenal injury. Medication-induced esophageal injury (**Table 17-5**) can result in weight loss, and, although not common, more serious complications such as malnutrition.

Older adults are more susceptible to medication-induced esophageal injury due to decreased saliva production and esophageal motility, which can cause pills to become lodged in the esophagus. Medications have different mechanisms for inducing esophageal injury. Antibiotics such as tetracycline, minocycline, and doxycycline have been implicated in medication-induced esophageal injury. Once dissolved in the saliva, tetracyclines are acidic and can cause erosive injury. Doxycycline capsules can be ulcerogenic, because they have the tendency to stick to the esophageal wall. Bisphosphonates also have been implicated in causing medication-induced esophageal injury as a result of prolonged contact with tissue leading to mucosal damage. This can be prevented by counseling patients to stay upright for at least 30 minutes after taking the medication and to avoid the use of bisphosphonates in patients with a history of esophageal disorders. Anti-inflammatories most likely to produce esophageal injury include aspirin, indomethacin, naproxen, and ibuprofen. The risk of esophageal injury appears to increase with advancing age.

Xerostomia Dry mouth due to inadequate saliva.

TABLE 17-4 Medications Associated with Xerostomia

Medication Class	Examples
Antihypertensive agents (ACE inhibitors, calcium channel blockers, diuretics)	Amlodipine, captopril, ethacrynic acid, lisinopril
Antiarrythmics	Meclizine, metoclopramide, odansetron, prochlorperazine, promethazine
Antihistamines/decongestants	Chlorpheniramine, cyproheptadine, diphenhydramine, hydroxyzine, pseudoephedrine
Selective-serotonin reuptake inhibitors (SSRIs)	Citalopram, fluoxetine, paroxetine, sertraline
Serotonin norephinephrine reuptake inhibitors	Venlafaxine
Tricyclic antidepressants (TCAs)	Amitriptyline, desipramine, imipramine, nortriptyline

Source: Data from Balzer KM. Drug-induced dysphagia. *Int J MS Care.* 2000 Mar;(3):29–34.

Medications That Affect Gastrointestinal Motility

Table 17-6 lists examples of medications that influence gastrointestinal motility. Of significant importance for older adults is the common use of medications that cause either diarrhea or constipation. Diarrhea can be a result of changes in intestinal motility due to decreased contact time in the small intestine, premature emptying of the colon, or bacterial overgrowth, all of which could be side effects of medications. Older patients often have diarrhea and/or constipation; the culprit in some cases being medication side effects rather

TABLE 17-5 Medications Associated with Esophageal Injury

Medication Class	Examples
Antibiotics	Clindamycin, doxycycline, erythromycin, minocycline, tetracycline
Antiarrythmics	Quinidine
Bisphosphonates	Alendronate, ibandronate, risedronate
Methylxanthines	Theophylline
Anti-inflammatory agents	Aspirin, ibuprofen, indomethacin, ketoprofen, naproxen
Other	Iron-containing products, potassium chloride, Vitamin C products

Source: Data from Balzer KM. Drug-induced dysphagia. *Int J MS Care.* 2000 Mar;(3):29–34.

TABLE 17-6 Medications That Affect Gastrointestinal Motility

- Dopamine receptor antagonists such as metoclopramidehave both direct GI prokinetic properties and CNS antiemetic effects.
- Metoclopramide works primarily in the proximal gut, stimulating esophageal contractions, gastric emptying, and small intestinal motor activity, with only limited effects in the colon.
- Tegaserod is indicated for the treatment of constipation predominant with irritable bowel syndrome.
- Antibiotics, such as erythromycin and clarithromycin, increase solid and liquid gastric emptying in a dose-dependent fashion.
- Nitrates are potent gastrointestinal smooth muscle relaxants.
- Nitroglycerin and long-acting nitrates decrease esophageal motor patterns and promote relaxation of gastric fundus.
- Calcium plays a role in esophageal muscle contraction. Calcium channel blockers, such as nifedipine, diltiazem, and verapamil, may cause constipation, because they have been shown to impair lower gut motility by inhibition of calcium uptake into smooth muscle cells and alteration of intraluminal electrolyte and water transportation.
- Octreotide affects motor function in different regions of the gastrointestinal tract by inhibiting small intestine transit and secretion and stimulating motor patterns in the small intestine.
- Anticholinergic medications inhibit bowel function. Medications such as TCAs and antispasmodics, such as dicyclomine and hyoscyamine, decrease peristaltic contraction and lower esophageal sphincter (LES) pressure.
- Cholinergic agents such as bethanecholincrease esophageal peristalsis and LES pressure, and neostigmine stimulates phasic contractile activity in the colon.

TABLE 17-7 Medications Causing Diarrhea

Medication Class	Examples
Laxatives	Bisacodyl, magnesium citrate, senna
Antacids	Magnesium-containing antacids
Antibiotics	Clindamycin, sulfonamides, tetracyclines, any broad-spectrum antibiotic
Antihypertensives	Guanethidine, methyldopa, reserpine
Cholinergics	Bethanechol, metoclopramide, neostigmine
Cardiac agents	Digoxin, quinidine

Source: Data from DiPiro JT, Talbert RL, Yee GC, Matzke GR, Wells BG, Posey LM. *Pharmacotherapy: A Pathophysiologic Approach.* New York: McGraw-Hill; 2002.

TABLE 17-8 Medications Causing Constipation

Medication Class	Examples
Narcotic analgesics	Codeine, morphine, oxycodone
Antihistamines	Chlorpheniramine, diphenhydramine
Antiparkinsonian agents	Benztropine, levodopa
Phenothiazines	Chlorpromazine, fluphenazine, prochlorperazine
Tricyclic antidepressants	Amitriptyline, desipramine, nortriptyline
Antacids	Calcium- or aluminum-containing antacids
Calcium channel blockers	Diltiazem, nifedipine, verapamil
Iron-containing products	Ferrous sulfate
Muscle blockers	Succinylcholine
NSAIDs	Diclofenac, ibuprofen, naproxen

Source: Data from DiPiro JT, Talbert RL, Yee GC, Matzke GR, Wells BG, Posey LM. *Pharmacotherapy: A Pathophysiologic Approach.* New York: McGraw-Hill; 2002.

than more serious underlying causes. Medications known to cause either constipation or diarrhea as a side effect have a dose-dependent effect; larger doses are associated with a higher incidence of constipation or diarrhea. **Tables 17-7** and **17-8** list classes of medications causing diarrhea and constipation, respectively. A thorough review of both prescription and over-the-counter medications can help identify medications associated with constipation or diarrhea.

Medications that affect the central nervous system, nerve conduction, and smooth muscle function may produce unwanted gastrointestinal side effects. For example, antacids can cause diarrhea or constipation. Diarrhea is a common side-effect of magnesium-containing antacids. Constipation is a common side-effect of antacids containing aluminum or calcium.

Opiates affect all parts of the intestine, although the major effects are largely on the colon. Opioids and opiates are commonly known to produce constipation. This occurs as a result of a delay in the transit of intraluminal content and an increase in gut capacity, prolonging contact and absorption. Loperamide and diphenoxylate, both peripherally acting opiate-based agents, are commonly used to treat

diarrhea. Docusate, a commonly used stool softener and emollient laxative, exerts its effect by promoting mixing of aqueous and fatty materials within the intestinal tract. In contrast, stimulant laxatives, such as senna or bisacodyl products, increase intestinal motility and secretion of water in the bowel. A side effect of stimulant laxatives is abdominal cramping due to increased peristalsis through the gastrointestinal tract.

Medications that Affect Gastric Acidity
Older adults are at an increased risk for peptic ulcer disease and gastroesphogeal reflux disease (GERD) symptoms for a variety of reasons, from age-related changes to medications. The following medications can contribute to GERD symptoms in older adults by decreasing lower esophageal sphincter pressure: anticholinergics, barbiturates, calcium-channel blockers, diazepam, estrogen, meperidine, nitrates, progesterone, somatostatin, and theophylline.

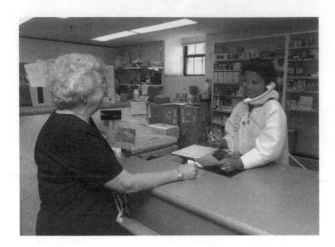

Medications that require an acidic environment for absorption, such as ketoconazole and ampicillin, may have decreased effect when administered with H2-antagonists (such as famotidine). However, caution should be exercised with higher-dose H2-antagonists in the older adult, because changes in mental status are a potential side effect due to renal and hepatic functional impairment.

Proton pump inhibitors (PPIs) differ from H2-antagonists in that their maximal effects occur at meal time. PPIs are activated by an acidic environment and work well for control of both daytime acid production and nocturnal acid production. PPIs cure approximately 95% of NSAID-induced ulcers. Chronic acid suppression can lead to increase growth of intragastric bacteria. The clinical significance of these alterations in gastric pH and increased bacteria growth on medication metabolism are not completely known, but they do have significant effects on nutrient digestion and absorption.

Absorption and Utilization of Nutrients

Absorption and utilization are generally not subject to pharmacological interaction. From a historical perspective, in the 1930s diet pills containing 2,4-dinitrophenol (DNP) were prescribed for weight control. DNP interferes with the normal metabolism of nutrients and causes the release of all the energy typically removed from glucose and fatty acids as heat. This agent was banned in 1938 due to concerns about carcinogenic mutations, increased health risk, and death from overdosing.

Conclusion

Awareness of medication–nutrient and medication–diet interactions by all members of the health care team caring for the older adult is fundamental to the delivery of sound medical treatment. Interaction of medications with dietary components has far-reaching implications on medication safety and efficacy and the overall health and well-being of individuals. Medication kinetics can vary widely within an individual with alterations in diet. Knowledge and application of the relationships among pharmacology, nutrition, and age-related physiological changes can reduce complications related to medication use and maximize overall health and well being. Clear communication must exist between older adults and/or their caregivers and medical professionals to avoid potential adverse consequences. This is of increasing importance with the increased use of over-the-counter medications and alternative/complementary supplements.

Activities Related to This Chapter

1. Try eating your meals with your nondominant hand for an entire day. How does this affect your food intake?
2. Visit your local nursing home and find a patient with an "allergy" to an antipsychotic (such as haldol) or an antiemetic (such as compazine or phenergan). Ask the patient to describe the side effects that occur with these drugs. Are they describing a true allergic reaction? If not, what explanation can you offer for their symptoms?
3. Call an older family member or friend and ask him or her to list all the medications he or she takes on a daily and weekly basis. Create a list of all the potential medication–food interactions, medication–nutrient interactions, and nutrition-related (dietary and physiologic) side effects of the medications.

REFERENCES

Anderson G. *Chronic care and the private sector: partnerships for solutions.* Paper presented at 2001 Health Sector Assembly; October 30, 2001; Baltimore, MD.

Anis AH, Guh DP, Lacaille D, Marra CA, Rashidi AA, Li X, Esdaile JM. When patients have to pay a share of medication costs: effects on frequency of physician visits, hospital admissions and filling of prescriptions. *CMAJ.* 2005;173(11):1335–1340.

Balzer KM. Medication-induced dysphagia. *Int J MS Care.* 2000;3:29–34.

Bates DW, Spell N, Cullen DJ, Burdick E, Laird N, Petersen LA, Small SD, Sweitzer BJ, Leape LL. The costs of adverse medication events in hospitalized patients. Adverse Medication Events Prevention Study Group. *JAMA.* 1997;277(4):307–311.

Castro-Alamancos MA, Calcagnotto ME. High-pass filtering of corticothalamic activity by neuromodulators released in the thalamus during arousal: in vitro and in vivo. *J Neurophysiol.* 2001;85(4):1489–1497.

Centers for Disease Control. *Healthy Aging: Preventing Disease and Improving Quality of Life Among Older Americans.* Atlanta, GA: Department of Health and Human Services, Centers for Disease Control; 2003.

Correll CU, Leucht S, Kane JM. Lower risk for tardive dyskinesia associated with second-generation antipsychotics: a systematic review of 1-year studies. *Am J Psychiatry.* 2004;161(3):414–425.

Delafuente JC. Understanding and preventing medication interactions in elderly patients. *Crit Rev Oncol Hematol.* 2003;48(2):133–143.

DiPiro JT, Talbert RL, Yee GC, Matzke GR, Wells BG, Posey LM. *Pharmacotherapy : A Pathophysiologic Approach.* New York: McGraw-Hill; 2002.

Eisenberg DM, Davis RB, Ettner SL, et al. Trends in alternative medicine use in the United States, 1990–1997: results of a follow-up national survey. *JAMA.* 1998;280:1569–1575.

Elmer, GW, Lafferty WE, Tyree PT, Lind BK. Potential interactions between complementary/alternative products and conventional medicines in a Medicare population. *Ann Pharmacother.* 2007;41(10):1617–1624.

Fernstrom JD, Fernstrom MH. Diet, Monoamine neurotransmitters and appetite control. In JD Fernstrom, R Uauy, P Arroyo (eds.), *Nutrition and Brain: Nestlé Nutrition Workshop Series Clinical & Performance Program*, Vol. 5. Basel: Nestec Ltd.; 2001; pp. 117–133.

Gandhi TK, Weingart SN, Borus J, Seger AC, Peterson J, Burdick E, Seger DL, Shu K, Federico F, Leape LL, Bates DW. Adverse medication events in ambulatory care. *N Engl J Med.* 2003;348(16):1556–1564.

Gurvich T, Cunningham JA. Appropriate use of psychotropic medications in nursing homes. *Am Fam Physician.* 2000;61(5):1437–1446.

Gurwitz JH, Field TS, Harrold LR, Rothschild J, Debellis K, Seger AC, Cadoret C, Fish LS, Garber L, Kelleher M, Bates DW. Incidence and preventability of adverse medication events among older persons in the ambulatory setting. *JAMA.* 2003;289:1107–1116.

Hasler WL. Pharmacotherapy for intestinal motor and sensory disorders. *Gastroenterol Clin North Am.* 2003;32(2):707–732.

Holloman LC, Marder SR. Management of acute extrapyramidal effects induced by antipsychotic medications. *Am J Health Syst Pharm.* 1997;54(21):2461–2477.

Hsieh C. Treatment of constipation in older adults. *Am Fam Physician.* 2005;72(11):2277–2284.

Jenike MA. *Handbook of Geriatric Psychopharmacology.* Littleton, MA: PSG Publishing; 1985.

Johnson JA, Bootman JL. Medication-related morbidity and mortality. A cost-of-illness model. *Arch Intern Med.* 1995;155(18):1949–1956.

Johnson RE, Goodman MJ, Hornbrook MC, Eldredge MB. The effect of increased prescription medication cost-sharing on medical care utilization and expenses of elderly health maintenance organization members. *Med Care.* 1997;35(11):1119–1131.

Jones EG. Thalamic circuitry and thalamocortical synchrony. *Philos Trans R Soc Lond B Biol Sci.* 2002;357(1428):1659–1673.

Levinson DF, Simpson GM, Singh H, Yadalam K, Jain A, Stephanos MJ, Silver P. Fluphenazine dose, clinical response, and extrapyramidal symptoms during acute treatment. *Arch Gen Psychiatry.* 1990;47(8):761–768.

Lichtenberg FR, Sun SX. The impact of Medicare Part D on prescription medication use by the elderly. *Health Aff.* 2007;26(6):1735–1744.

Lin SH, Lin MS. A survey on medication-related hospitalization in a community teaching hospital. *Int J Clin Pharmacol Ther Toxicol.* 1993;31(2):66–69.

Meunier P, Rochas A, Lambert R. Motor activity of the sigmoid colon in chronic constipation: comparative study with normal subjects. *Gut.* 1979;20(12):1095–1101.

Mort JR, Aparasu RR. Prescribing potentially inappropriate psychotropic medications to the ambulatory elderly. *Arch Intern Med.* 2000;160(18):2825–2831.

Motsinger CD, Perron GA, Lacy TJ. Use of atypical antipsychotic medications in patients with dementia. *Am Fam Physician.* 2003;67(11):2335–2340.

O'Neill JL, Remington TL. Medication-induced esophageal injuries and dysphagia. *Ann Pharmacother.* 2003;37(11):1675–1684.

Paykel PS, Mueller PS, and De La Vergne PM. Amitriptyline, weight gain, and carbohydrate craving: a side effect. *Br J Psychiatry.* 1973;123(576):501–507.

Perry E, Walker M, Grace J, Perry R. Acetylcholine in mind: a neurotransmitter correlate of consciousness? *Trends Neurosci.* 1999;22(6):273–280.

Storr M, Allescher HD. Esophageal pharmacology and treatment of primary motility disorders. *Dis Esophagus.* 1999;12(4):241–257.

Thumshirn M, Camilleri M, Choi MG, Zinsmeister AR. Modulation of gastric sensory and motor functions by nitrergic and alpha2-adrenergic agents in humans. *Gastroenterology.* 1999;116(3):573–585.

Traube M, McCallum RW. Calcium-channel blockers and the gastrointestinal tract. American College of Gastroenterology's Committee on FDA related matters. *Am J Gastroenterol.* 1984; 79(11):892–896.

Tune L, Carr S, Hoag E, Cooper T. Anticholinergic effects of medications commonly prescribed for the elderly: potential means for assessing risk of delirium. *Am J Psych.* 1992;149(10):1393–1394.

Vinks TH, Egberts TC, de Lange TM, de Koning FH. Pharmacist-based medication review reduces potential drug-related problems in the elderly: the SMOG controlled trial. *Drugs Aging.* 2009;26(2):123–133.

Woerner MG, Alvir JM, Saltz BL, Lieberman JA, Kane JM. Prospective study of tardive dyskinesia in the elderly: rates and risk factors. *Am J Psychiatry.* 1998;155(11):1521–1528.

Zagaria ME. Suppressing gastric acid in seniors with GERD: treatment risks and benefits. *US Pharmacist.* 2005;10:34–39.

Nutritional Support for the Older Adult

Colleen Tsarnas, MS, RD, CNSD, LDN

CHAPTER OBJECTIVES   Upon completion of this chapter, the reader will be able to:

1. Define nutrition support and explain its role in the older adult
2. Identify the pros and cons of the different types of nutrition support for the older adult
3. Determine specialized nutrition support needs for older adults

KEY TERMS AND CONCEPTS

Enteral nutrition

Oral nutrition support

Parenteral nutrition

Medical technologies continue to evolve, and the possibilities of improving quality of life for the aging population are promising. Stem cells, organ transplantation, therapeutic cloning, and gene-based therapies are all expected to benefit the health of the aging population. In addition, as pharmacological treatments for cancer and stroke (two leading causes of death) become streamlined, the use of nutrition support will likely expand.

Indications for Nutrition Support

The aging process, discussed in detail in Chapter 2, can ultimately progress to the need for nutrition support in older adults. *Nutrition support* can be defined as the provision of nutrients needed to optimize health and nutritional status that cannot be achieved through basic diet alone. According to the American Society for Parenteral and Enteral Nutrition, nutrition support is categorized as either parenteral or enteral. **Enteral nutrition** is provided by mouth (oral) or tube (enteral). **Parenteral nutrition** is the intravenous provision of nutrients via a central (large, usually the vena cava) or peripheral (hand or forearm) vein.

There are numerous indications for support in older adults. It is paramount to provide the least restrictive type of support and to attempt to upgrade the older adult to the highest functional level of nutrition support possible. For example, oral supplements should be considered prior to placing a feeding tube if the older adult is able to consume nutrients by mouth. **Figure 18-1** explains the methodology for determining the most appropriate form of nutrition support.

In general, older adults tend to consume fewer calories. Most 70-year-olds consume one-third fewer calories than the RDA, and 16% to 18% of community-dwelling older adults consume fewer than 1,000 calories per day. Decreased oral intake can ultimately progress to weight loss and malnutrition.

When evaluating nutritional intake, in addition to medical circumstances, it is

enteral nutrition The provision of nutrients using the gastrointestinal tract; includes oral diet and tube feedings.

parenteral nutrition Provision of nutrients by intravenous infusion.

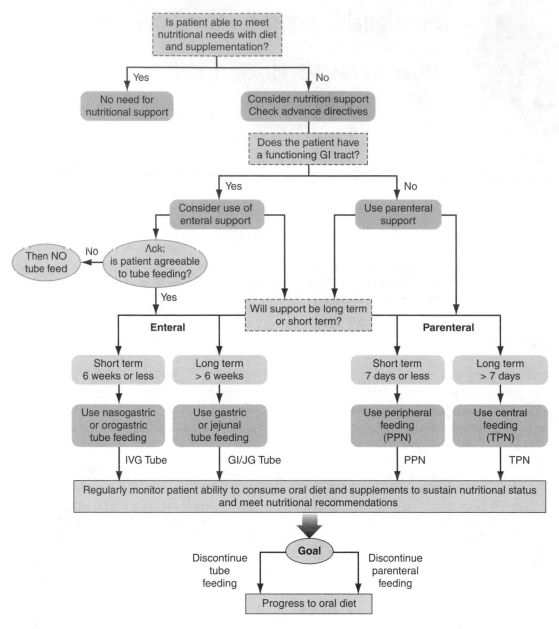

FIGURE 18-1 Nutrition Support Decision Algorithm

Source: Data from A.S.P.E.N. *Nutrition Support Core Curriculum.* 2nd ed. Silver Spring, MD: American Society for Parenteral and Enteral Nutrition; 1993.

also important to consider the many socioeconomic factors that also play a role in the development of malnutrition. Community-dwelling older adults identified to be at risk for malnutrition are often those with lower levels of social support, decreased life satisfaction, and depression. Dietitians employed in acute care and community settings can play a significant role in collaborating with social workers and nursing case managers to help prevent community-acquired

malnutrition. Several urban and rural programs exist to deliver hot or frozen meals to older adults, along with food banks for ambulatory older individuals. These services are discussed in Chapter 21, "Nutrition Services for Older Adults."

Weight loss and malnutrition are outcomes of preexisting conditions, including cardiopulmonary diseases, depression, anxiety, cancer, Parkinson's disease, and Alzheimer's

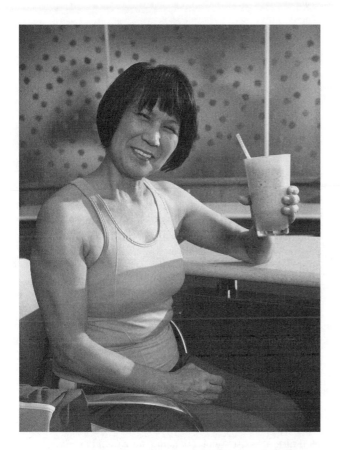

dementia, that are commonly seen in older adults who reside in long-term care facilities. These and other comorbidities have been found to contribute to severe undernutrition in 18% of residents of long-term care facilities and mild to moderate malnutrition in 27.5%. The high prevalence of malnutrition in the community and long-term care settings, coupled with the increasing elderly population, will increase the utilization of all types of nutrition support.

Oral Supplements

A wide variety of oral supplements are available today, in an assortment of flavors. **Table 18-1** lists selected oral supplements and their uses and contraindications. Oral supplements are commonly used in health care institutions to increase calorie and protein intake. Many are also easily accessible in drug stores and grocery stores and are available for home delivery to accommodate older adults who live at home or in assisted-living facilities. Disease-specific oral supplements, also listed in Table 18-1, are available for people with diabetes, chronic kidney disease, and disorders of the small bowel.

Oral supplements can play a significant role in the prevention of malnutrition in both free-living and institutionalized older adults. Nutrition supplementation in older adults can lead to significant improvement in nutritional status, increased energy intake and improvement in body weight, as well as a decreased utilization of health care services.

TABLE 18-1 Uses and Contraindications with Selected Oral Supplements Available on Today's Market

Type of Supplement	Examples and Manufacturers	Uses	Contraindications
Standard	Boost (Novartis); Ensure (Ross); Carnation Instant Breakfast (Nestle Nutrition)	Weight gain and anabolism of visceral protein stores; meal replacement	Disease-specific need; adequate oral intake with diet
High protein	Boost HP (high protein) (Novartis); Ensure Plus (Ross); NuBasics VHP (Nestle Nutrition)	Wound healing; anabolism of visceral protein stores	Protein restriction
High calorie	Boost Plus (Novartis); Nestle VCH 2.25 (Nestle Nutrition); Novasource 2.0 (Novartis); Ensure Plus (Ross); Two Cal HN (Ross)	Medication administration in health care facilities; weight gain; increase calorie intake with less intake than standard supplements	Disease-specific need; adequate oral intake with diet
Diabetic	Glucerna (Ross); Glytrol (Nestle Nutrition)	Blood glucose control; weight gain	Absence of diabetes mellitus
Kidney disease	Nepro (Ross); Nutri-Renal (Nestle Nutrition)	Weight gain; improve visceral protein stores; provide decreased fluid, vitamins, and minerals to meet needs with chronic kidney disease	Absence of chronic kidney disease
Modular	Promod (Ross)	Anabolism of visceral protein stores; wound healing; increase protein without promoting weight gain	Increased calorie needs (use standard or high-calorie supplement)

Source: Data from Novartis Nutrition Corporation. Your Source Chart—Product Reference Guide. 2004 Apr:1–55.

An important factor to consider when providing oral nutritional supplements is the acceptability factor. Before providing an oral supplement, patients should be screened for likes, dislikes, food allergies or intolerances, normal food intake, percent of ideal and usual body weight, and changes in dietary patterns. Once a supplement is provided, follow up is essential to ensure that a patient is consuming the supplement. Lack of acceptability has been associated with negative outcomes in older patients. A negative correlation between supplements consumed and weight loss in hip fracture patients has been attributed to lack of acceptability.

The nutritional status of individuals receiving oral nutritional supplements should be evaluated regularly. Individuals able to maintain visceral and somatic protein stores with diet alone are not candidates for oral supplements.

Obese individuals should be screened for appropriateness of supplements; these patients may fare better with a modular protein supplement versus a calorically dense supplement. Older obese adults, especially those with chronic disease, can lose interest in eating as easily as those of normal weight. It is important to evaluate food intake records and calorie needs relative to actual intake to assess the need for a high-calorie supplement in the obese older adult.

Enteral Nutrition Support

Enteral nutrition (EN) is often the next step after all **oral nutrition support** options have been exhausted. Additional factors to consider prior to considering enteral feeding are pain management, psychosocial factors, and appetite-stimulant use. The increase in the older adult population may be contributing to the increased use of feeding tubes in health care settings. For example, in North Carolina hospitals there has been a 60% increase in feeding tube placements, with the greatest increase in individuals aged 75 and older.

EN can be used in individuals deemed unable to consume nutrients by mouth for both the short and long term. Conditions warranting short-term EN are commonly seen in hospital settings in patients with increased calorie needs and/or inability to temporarily consume adequate oral intake. Diagnoses and conditions necessitating short-term EN include burns, trauma, mechanical ventilation, closed head injuries, and acute cerebrovascular accidents. Short-term EN for the critically ill can improve clinical outcomes, although despite all of the positive outcomes associated with EN in critical illness, mortality rates are high among older patients due to severity of illness associated with age.

oral nutrition support The provision of supplemental nutrition products to treat or prevent malnutrition in patients who can swallow safely and have a well-functioning gastrointestinal tract with the goal of ensuring that total nutrient intake meets individual needs.

Indications for long-term EN are usually due to the progression of chronic diseases such as Parkinson's disease, end-stage Alzheimer's disease, and certain types of cancers, including gastric, head and neck, and esophageal cancers, that cause functional swallowing impairments and/or decreased oral intake. Long-term EN can also be used for persons without a functional impairment for diagnoses such as depression with decreased oral intake and malnutrition and decreased oral intake with cancer cachexia. Individuals with nonhealing decubitus ulcers and decreased oral intake are also candidates for supplemental EN.

Long-term EN can improve the nutritional status of older adults. Nursing home residents fed via EN show a mean weight gain of 5 kg in the first year and sustained weight gain thereafter. However, as discussed later in the ethics portion of this chapter, controversy exists regarding the use of nutrition support to optimize nutritional status, improve quality of life, and decrease mortality among older adults.

Enteral Feedings Formulas

Many types of formulas are available for EN, accommodating virtually every disease state and nutritional need (**Table 18-2**). As with oral supplements, accurate nutrition assessment is the method of determining which formula is best suited for a particular patient. Factors to consider when deciding on a tube feeding include food allergies; body mass index; presence of decubitus ulcers, diabetes, or chronic kidney disease; and fluid, protein, and fiber requirements. Most standard enteral formulas can meet a patient's nutritional needs.

Not only are standard formulas likely to meet the patient's nutritional needs, they are also isotonic. An isotonic solution provided in the gastrointenstinal tract will decrease cell membrane permeability. Decreased permeability will decrease fluid and electrolyte shifts, which can ultimately decrease the risk of diarrhea. Standard isotonic formulas are also less costly than disease-specific formulas, primarily because they do not contain specialized nutrient compositions.

The nutrient composition of standard enteral formulas varies from product to product (**Table 18-3**). Generally, they are 14% to 18% protein in the form of soy protein isolates, calcium caseinates, and milk protein concentrates; 45% to 57% carbohydrate in the form of corn syrup, maltodextrin, and hydrolyzed corn starch; and 29% to 37% fat in the form of canola oil, safflower oil, and medium-chain triglycerides. The RDA for vitamins and minerals in enteral nutrition support is usually met with 1,500 calories/day. Additional vitamin and or mineral supplementation may be needed for patients with nonhealing wounds, B12 or folate deficiency, or anemia.

An integral component of enteral feeding for older adults is fiber. Fiber can assist with controlling blood glucose and lipid levels, as well as aid with constipation. Constipation is

TABLE 18-2 Examples and Uses of Enteral Feedings Used for Older Adults

Type of Tube Feeding	Key Elements	Product Examples and Manufacturer	Uses	Contraindications
Polymeric	Fiber free	Osmolite (Ross); Nutren (Nestle Nutrition)	Can be used for most standard enteral feedings.	Intolerance to feeding; food allergies
	Contains fiber	Jevity (Ross); Probalance (Nestle Nutrition)	Should be first choice in tube feeding for older adults.	Inability to digest intact proteins and long-chain triglycerides
	High protein	Promote (Ross); Replete (Nestle Nutrition)	Wound healing; need for increased protein without additional calories.	
	Fluid restricted	2 Cal HN (Ross); Novasource 2.0 (Novartis); Carnation Instant Breakfast VHC (Nestle Nutrition)	Conditions requiring fluid restrictions—SIADH, CHF.	Normal fluid requirements
Partially hydrolyzed	Elemental	Vivonex (Novartis)	Gastrointestinal impairments	Able to digest intact protein formulas
	Semi-elemental	Peptamen (Nestle Nutrition); Peptinex (Novartis)	Gastrointestinal impairments	
Disease specific	Diabetic	Glucerna (Ross); Glytrol (Nestle Nutrition)	Diabetes mellitus	Absence of diabetes mellitus
	Dialysis	Nepro (Ross); Nutri-Renal (Nestle Nutrition)	Chronic kidney disease	Absence of kidney disease
	Non-dialysis	Suplena (Ross)	Acute renal failure	Absence of acute renal failure
	Immune enhancing	Crucial (Nestle Nutrition); Pivot (Ross)	Increase immune response for immunocompromised persons.	Absence of critical illness
Modular	Protein	Promod (Ross)	Supplement protein intake with enteral feedings to aid with wound healing and/or anabolism of visceral protein stores.	Conditions that require protein restriction—acute renal failure, end-stage liver disease

Source: Data from Novartis Nutrition Corporation. Your Source Chart—Product Reference Guide. 2004 Apr:1–55; Kieft H, et al. Clinical outcome of immunonutrition in a heterogeneous intensive care population. *Intensive Care Med.* 2005;31(4):524–532.

often a painful condition in older adults, and the causes are multifactorial, including decreased mobility, medications, lack of fluid intake, and medical conditions affecting bowel motility, such as Parkinson's disease, amyotrophic lateral sclerosis (ALS), multiple sclerosis, and cerebrovascular accidents. Most fiber-containing formulas include a combination of soluble and insoluble fiber, ranging from 10 to 22 g/L.

Recent research has focused on the use of prebiotics, which are naturally occurring fibers, to support normal intestinal flora. Comparison of enterally fed individuals receiving a standard tube-feeding formula without fiber to one with fructo-oligosaccharides (FOS), a prebiotic, and fiber showed that the FOS/fiber group had significantly higher levels of *Bifidobacteria* (a probiotic bacteria shown to ben-

efit digestion) and decreased levels of *Clostridia* (a bacteria commonly found in intestinal flora, but that is more pathogenic) compared to the fiber-free group. Additional studies on the outcome of fiber-supplemented tube feedings in hospitalized older adults, such as that by Vandewoude and colleagues in 2005, suggest that individuals fed high-fiber formulas pass stool less often and have stool of a more solid consistency. Enteral formulas enriched with guar gum have been shown to decrease diarrhea among intensive care unit patients, and also have a trend for lowering glucose and cholesterol levels.

Fiber-supplemented formulas should be used when possible. However, at times, too much fiber can cause constipation or diarrhea in older adults. In such cases, fiber-free

TABLE 18-3 Nutrient Composition of Select Enteral Formulas

Formula	Calories/ mL	Protein g/L	Carbohydrate g/L	Fat g/L	% Calories from Protein	% Calories from Carbohydrate	% Calories from Fat	Osmolality mOsm/kg Water	g/Fiber/L
Standard									
Osmolite	1.06	37.1	151.1	34.7	14	57	29	300	0
Probalance	1.2	54	156	40.8	18	52	30	350-450	10
Jevity	1.06	44.3	154.7	34.7	16.7	54.3	29	300	14.4
Wound healing									
Replete	1.0	62.4	113	34	25	45	30	300-350	0
Semi-Elemental									
Peptamen	1.0	40	127	39	16	33	51	270	0
Vivonex Plus	1.0	45	190	6.7	18	76	6	650	0
Renal									
Nepro	1.8	81	166.8	96	18	34	48	585	15.6
Novasource Renal	2	74	200	100	15	40	45	700	0
Pulmonary									
Oxepa	1.5	62.5	105.5	93.7	16.7	28.1	55.2	493	0
Pulmocare	1.5	62.6	105.7	93.3	16.7	28.2	55.1	475	0
Diabetic									
Glucerna	1.0	41.8	95.6	54.4	20	34.3	49	470	14.1
Glytrol	1.0	45.2	100	47.6	18	40	42	280	15.2
Calorically Dense									
Nutren 1.5	1.5	60	169	67.6	16	45	39	430-510	0
Two Cal HN	2	83.5	218.5	90.5	16.7	43.2	40.1	725	5

Source: Data from Novartis Nutrition Corporation. Your Source Chart—Product Reference Guide. 2004 Apr:1–55.

formulas may be of benefit, and a gradual increase of supplemental soluble fiber may be better tolerated. Because fluid requirements are increased with increased fiber intake, fluid intake should be increased prior to discontinuing a fiber-containing formula in a patient with constipation, unless contraindicated.

Disease-specific formulas are used for diabetes, chronic obstructive pulmonary disease (COPD), acute and chronic kidney disease, wound healing, acute respiratory distress syndrome, GI impairments, and critical illness. For example, diabetic formulas have fewer carbohydrates and more protein than standard formulas. Diabetic formulas can improve long-term glucose control and thus may improve the long-term negative effects of diabetes. In a review of 25 studies associated with tube feeding and oral supplements, the majority of which compared diabetic formulas with standard formulas, diabetic formulas were found to significantly reduce postprandial blood glucose levels, decrease insulin

requirements, and result in fewer overall diabetic complications.

Formulas designed for acute and chronic kidney disease contain less fluid, phosphorus, and potassium. Their vitamin and mineral content is designed specifically for the chronic kidney disease patient. They are appropriate for elderly individuals receiving hemodialysis or for those with acute renal failure. Persons receiving peritoneal dialysis can usually tolerate a standard fluid-restricted formula due to daily filtration versus three times weekly during hemodialysis.

High-protein formulas are designed for individuals with normal or decreased calorie requirements and increased protein needs. High-protein formulas are used primarily to meet the heightened demands for wound healing and usually contain additional amounts of vitamin C, vitamin A, and zinc. High-protein enteral nutrition support can reduce the risk of developing pressure ulcers and aid with healing pressure ulcers.

Pulmonary formulas contain less carbohydrate than standard isotonic formulas. These formulas have been shown to decrease the respiratory quotient to improve ventilator weaning. However, many health care practitioners focus on meeting the nutritional needs of the ventilated patient and preventing overfeeding to optimize ventilator-weaning potential. Therefore, the consensus, among most practitioners, is that it is not necessary to use pulmonary formulas for nonventilated patients.

Partially hydrolyzed formulas are used for individuals with gastrointestinal impairments such as Crohn's disease, short bowel syndrome, pancreatitis, intractable diarrhea, and colitis. Partially hydrolyzed formulas contain "predigested" proteins and medium-chain triglycerides (MCTs) for optimal intestinal absorption. Protein components of hydrolyzed formulas are free amino acids, peptides, or a combination of both. Peptides have shown to be absorbed more rapidly than intact proteins across the gut mucosa. Partially hydrolyzed formulas play a role in the care of critically ill patients and have shown to increase rapid synthesis proteins (prealbumin) faster than intact proteins.

MCTs are an integral component of partially hydrolyzed formulas and are ideal for those with short bowel syndrome, pancreatitis, or hepatic disorders. MCTs are absorbed directly into the bloodstream from the small intestine into the portal circulation. MCTs do not require pancreatic enzymes or bile salts for digestion, thus making digestion easier. Decreased pain in persons receiving a peptide-based formula with MCTs has been attributed to decreased release of cholecystokinin. Formulas are not prepared exclusively with MCTs, because long-chain triglycerides are needed to provide essential fatty acids.

As life span increases, so does the likelihood of becoming critically ill due to respiratory failure or sepsis. Current trends in specialized nutrition support formulations are focusing on immune-enhancing formulas. Immune-enhancing enteral formulas have been created to inhibit the negative consequences associated with the stress response, thus improving patient outcome. Specialized formulas commonly include additional antioxidants, omega-3 fatty acids, arginine, and glutamine. Studies of these specific nutrients have shown promise in reducing the complications of critical illness. Omega-3 fatty acids provided preoperatively have been shown to have an impact on the postoperative inflammatory response. Recent research has found mixed results in critically ill patients, which suggests that the use of immune-enhanced formulas requires additional investigation.

Enteral Feeding Delivery and Access Devices

Choosing the proper feeding-delivery mechanism and access device is as important as deciding on an enteral formula. Along with the planned duration of feeding as well as the patient's diagnosis and personal preferences, possible complications should be anticipated. Short-term enteral access devices are used for patients with a projected tube-feeding duration of six weeks or less. These devices are usually placed through the nostril into the stomach, duodenum, or jejunum (nasogastric, nasoduodenal, or nasojejunal, respectively). **Table 18-4** lists common enteral feeding administration routes used for geriatric patients.

The most common delivery mechanism is nasogastric feeding. A small-bore feeding tube is inserted into the nostril and then passed through the esophagus and into the stomach, duodenum, or jejunum. The placement of the tube must be checked before feeding can begin. Correct placement is usually confirmed with an X-ray. Tube placement can also be checked via air auscultation. With this method, a large syringe of air is pumped into the tube, and if no air is heard in the lungs, the tube is properly placed. Recently, the development of external magnetic guidance has ensured more accurate tube placement without the need for an X-ray. With this method, a small magnet is placed on the feeding tube and an external magnet is placed on the upper right quadrant of the patient's abdomen. A small screen displays the migration of the tube.

Nasoduodenal and nasojejunal feedings are used primarily to prevent aspiration and to provide nutrition to patients with poor gastrointestinal motility. In these instances, tube placement can be complicated and may possibly require the assistance of motility agents and video fluoroscopy.

Long-term enteral access devices are used for patients with an expected feeding duration of longer than six weeks. These devices are similar to short-term access devices with regards to the distal feeding site, but the tubes are permanently placed. However, feeding tubes occasionally need to be replaced because of corrosion, leakage, or skin irritations.

Long-term gastric feedings are most commonly provided via a percutaneous endoscopic gastrostomy (PEG) tube. PEG tubes are less costly than gastrostomy tubes and do not require surgical placement.

Long-term jejunal feedings are used for persons with gastric obstructions, enterocutaneous fistulas, or high pulmonary aspiration risk. Jejunostomy tubes are usually placed in adjunct with abdominal surgeries; percutaneous endoscopic jejunostomy (PEJ) tubes do not require surgical placement.

Most enteral feeding tubes are made of silicone and polyurethane and are designed for optimal flexibility and comfort while maintaining resistance to gastric secretions and tube occlusions. The unit of measurement used with these tubes—"French"—refers to the outer lumen tube diameter. Small-bore feeding tubes are used for nasogastric, nasoduodenal, and nasojejunal feedings and are usually 8 to 12 French units. Gastrostomy and PEG tube sizes usually

TABLE 18-4 Common Enteral Feeding Administration Routes in the Geriatric Population

Type of Feeding				
Gastric	**Indications**	**Contraindications**	**Advantages**	**Disadvantages**
Nasogastric	Short-term feeding; normal gastric emptying	Able to consume adequate calories by mouth; high pulmonary aspiration risk	Easily inserted and removed	Can be uncomfortable for patient; increased risk of sinusitis; smaller bore size, should use pump for administration; tube can become displaced
Gastric (PEG)	Long-term feeding; normal gastric emptying	Able to consume adequate calories by mouth; high pulmonary aspiration risk	No surgery required with percutaneous endoscopic gastrostomy (PEG)	Potential pulmonary aspiration risk
Small Bowel				
Nasoduodenal	Short-term feeding; gastroparesis or impaired gastric emptying	No pulmonary aspiration risk	Decreases pulmonary aspiration risk	Tube can become displaced
Nasojejunal	Short-term feeding; pulmonary aspiration risk; impaired gastric emptying; gastroparesis	No pulmonary aspiration risk; no difficulties with gastric emptying	Able to use gastrointestinal tract	Small bore size usually requires pump; hyperosmolar formula can cause diarrhea; tube can become displaced
Jejunal (PEJ)	Long-term feeding; gastric obstruction; gastroparesis; impaired gastric emptying; pulmonary aspiration risk	No pulmonary aspiration risk; no difficulties with gastric emptying	Allows feeding into the small bowel if unable to feed into the stomach	Small bore size usually requires pump; hyperosmolar formula can cause diarrhea

Source: Data from A.S.P.E.N. *Nutrition Support Core Curriculum: A Case-Based Approach—The Adult Patient.* Silver Spring, MD: American Society for Parenteral and Enteral Nutrition; 2007.

are 18, 22, 24, or 28 French. Jejunostomy tubes are typically 5 to 7 French.

The nutritional supplement formula can be delivered via pump, bolus, or gravity drip. Determining the method of delivery depends on the feeding type, the size of the feeding tube, and the patient's state of health and feeding preferences. Gravity-drip feedings are used to minimize the infusion flow without the use of a pump. Feedings are poured directly into a feeding set and hung to gravity drip. A similar mechanism is used with feeding pumps, but the feeding is infused at a set continuous or intermittent rate ranging from 10 to 295 mL/hour.

Bolus feedings are delivered via syringe several times daily. Typically one or two cans of formula are delivered during each feeding. Bolus delivery methods may be more advantageous in older adults. Bolus delivery simulates actual meal consumption because the boluses are delivered in larger amounts several times daily. They are also convenient for individuals in a home health setting who do not want to wait an hour or two to administer their feedings.

Pumps should be used in older adults with a high pul-

monary aspiration risk. Bedridden, long-term PEG patients fed via pump have been found to have better glucose control and less diarrhea, vomiting, reflux, and aspiration. Although feeding pumps have been shown to decrease aspiration, they have not been shown to positively affect diarrhea.

Tube size is an important consideration when choosing a feeding modality. Large-bore tubes can accommodate viscous formulas and medications that are directly bolused, whereas small-bore tubes often clog with a large infusion of a similar formula. Thus, feeding pumps should be used with nasogastric and jejunal feeding tubes due to their smaller size and increased risk of clogging. PEG and gastrostomy tubes, which are large-bore feeding tubes, present less clogging risk with bolus feedings.

Complications with Enteral Nutrition Support

Many complications are associated with enteral nutrition support. However, it is important to rule out other causes of complications prior to arbitrarily changing enteral nutrition support formulations.

Nausea	Residuals	Diarrhea	Constipation
Checklist ✓ Is the head of the bed elevated 45 degrees during and one hour after tube feeding	*Checklist* ✓ Is the head of the bed elevated 45 degrees during and one hour after tube feeding	*Checklist* ✓ Was patient checked for Clostridium Difficile ✓ Are medications causing diarrhea ✓ Does the patient have any gastrointestinal disorders ✓ Are proper handling techniques being used	*Checklist* ✓ Is patient on fiber containing formula ✓ Is patient receiving adequate fluid
Still with Nausea	**Still with residuals**	**Still with Diarrhea**	**Still with Constipation**
• If nausea or vomiting, hold tube feeding for 30–60 minutes	• Stop tube feeding for 30–60 minutes and restart at 20–25 mL/hours	• Add fiber containing formula • Consider closed system formula • If patient on high fiber formula, consider fiber free formula • Consider peptide formula for optimal absorption	• Patient may be receiving too much fiber, consider fiber free formula • Fiber source may need to be changed, or provided as a medication flush
Medication Interventions	**Medication Interventions**	**Medication Interventions**	**Medication Interventions**
• Consider anti-emetics	• Consider anti-motility agents	• Consider anti-diarrheals	• Consider stool softeners, enemas

FIGURE 18-2 Management of Enteral Gastrointestinal Complications

Source: Data from A.S.P.E.N. *Nutrition Support Core Curriculum: A Case-Based Approach—The Adult Patient.* Silver Spring, MD: American Society for Parenteral and Enteral Nutrition; 2007; Heimburger DC, et al. Effects of small peptide and wholeprotein enteral feedings on serum proteins and diarrhea in critically ill patients: a randomized trial. *JPEN.* 1997;21(3):162–167, Ross Laboratories. *Tube Feeding Complications: A Guide to Problem Solving;* 1990; Novartis Medical Nutrition, *At Home, Living with Tube Feeding;* 2005.

Complications of enteral feeding can be manual, gastrointestinal, infectious, or metabolic. Whereas enteral feedings may or may not be the catalyst for the aforementioned reactions, formulas may need to be changed to accommodate a patient's needs. It is important to discuss the patient's nutritional care with all members of the health care team to develop the most appropriate plan of care.

Gastrointestinal complications are common in the older adult population and include nausea, vomiting, diarrhea, constipation, and increased residuals. **Figure 18-2** provides suggestions regarding management of gastrointestinal complications in the enterally fed patient.

Causes of diarrhea not related to enteral feeding include medications (especially antibiotic therapies); *Clostridium difficile* bacteria; and gastrointestinal disorders, such as colitis, short bowel syndrome, and Crohn's disease. Diarrhea may be caused by microbial contamination of the formula, food allergies, lactose intolerance (most enteral formulas are lactose free), hyperosmolar formula, or inadequate or too much fiber intake.

As with diarrhea, causes of nausea, vomiting, and increased residuals can be multifactorial. Conditions that can delay gastric emptying, especially in a critically ill patient, include sepsis, hypotension, anesthesia, and medications such as opiates (codeine, fentanyl) and anticholinergics (clidinium bromide). For vomiting, feedings should be withheld for at least 1 hour, restarted at a low rate of 20 to 25 mL/hour, and gradually increased 10 to 25 mL/hour every 8 to 24 hours. Motility agents such as erythromycin and metoclopramide may be beneficial in decreasing residuals.

Infectious causes of enteral feeding intolerance are usually improper handling techniques and microbial contamination of enteral formula. The innovative closed-system enteral feeding has decreased the risk of cross-contamination. Closed enteral feeding systems contain 1,000 to 1,500 mL of formula ready for infusion with a spike set, as opposed to pouring cans into a feeding container. In a comparison of closed versus open systems, the open system took almost twice as much nursing time, and 16 of 17 nurses preferred the closed system. Closed systems are advantageous for patients on long-term enteral feedings with a standard prescription and minimal interruptions in infusion rates. Patients requiring frequent interruptions and changes in enteral feeding may fare better with open-system enteral feedings, which produce less waste.

Metabolic complications associated with enteral feeding are most likely not caused by the enteral feeding itself. However, changes may need to be made to correct metabolic abnormalities. Patients who are fluid overloaded may benefit from a calorically dense, low-fluid formula. In contrast, dehydrated patients should be provided with a formula with a higher fluid content, along with water flushes. Low-potassium formulas should be used in persons with or at high risk for hyperkalemia, as in the chronic kidney disease patient.

Manual complications of enteral feeding are primarily due to dislodging or clogging of the tube and skin irritations. Enteral feeding tubes should be cleaned and checked regularly by nurses and physicians to prevent manual complications. Tube positioning should be monitored by marking the external bolster with a nontoxic marker close to the abdomen and then checking the spot daily for tube migration. To prevent clogging, feeding tubes should be flushed with 30 mL of water before and after medication administration. Medications should not be added directly to the tube feeding, because it can cause clogging. If an enteral feeding tube becomes completely blocked, a physician should be contacted immediately to dislodge the contents. If the tube is partially clogged, it should be flushed with 60 mL of warm water. Pancreatic enzymes may be used if water does not unclog the tube.

Parenteral Nutrition

Total parenteral nutrition (TPN) should be used when enteral feeding is not an option. Common uses for parenteral nutrition in health care settings are short bowel syndrome, ileus, severe malnutrition, inability to feed enterally within five days, large-output enterocutaneous fistula, bowel obstruction, massive gastrointestinal bleeding, intractable diarrhea, and vomiting.

Parenteral nutrition should be managed by a health care team consisting of a pharmacist, a nutrition support nurse, a physician, a social worker, and a nutrition-support dietitian. Parenteral nutrition management is complex, and it should not be administered arbitrarily, because significant metabolic and infectious complications can arise.

Vascular access route needs to be determined prior to initiating parenteral nutrition. Ideally, central access is preferred to peripheral access to optimize the ability to provide adequate nutrients with a higher osmotic load, to decrease the risk of infectious complications, and to enable longer feeding durations, if needed. The most common proximal sites for central access include the subclavian, jugular, femoral, cephalic, and basilica veins. To decrease the risk of inflammation and infection, it is recommended that the peripheral solution contain no more than 900 m/Osm (milliosmoles). Thus, peripheral solutions are limited in the amount of amino acids and dextrose they can contain and therefore rarely will meet the nutritional needs of patients.

Central access devices can be used for the short or long term feeding. The PICC (peripherally inserted central catheter) is probably the most common short-term central catheter due to ease of placement. A PICC is also often used for medication administration, such as intravenous antibiotic therapy. Surgically implanted ports can also be used for TPN, but a port is often placed for another type of long-term intravenous therapy, such as chemotherapy.

Once access is obtained, the composition of the TPN formula must then be determined. Every TPN order should be individualized, reflecting the patient's macro- and micronutrient needs. Calories and protein are considered macronutrients, whereas electrolytes, vitamins, and minerals are considered micronutrients. Fluid needs must also be assessed, because, quite often, TPN is the sole source of fluid intake.

Calorie and protein needs should be assessed using standardized equations for determining enteral and oral intake. However, it is important to ensure that calories are equally distributed between protein, fat, and carbohydrate. Overfeeding of TPN patients can cause fatty liver, hypertriglyceridemia, and hyperglycemia.

Patients receiving TPN have complex medical problems and will likely not fit the standard when determining fluid requirements. It is essential for all of the health care providers involved in the patient's care to work as a team to review any factors that may contribute to fluid requirements, such as diuretic therapy, surgical drain and fistula output, cardiac status, and renal function.

Once nutrient requirements have been determined, the macronutrient components of parenteral nutrition can be calculated. Nutrients are provided in the form of free amino acids, providing 4 calories per gram, and dextrose monohydrate, providing 3.4 calories per gram. Lipids are administered in a separate solution, known as 2 in 1 TPN, or compounded by a pharmacy in the same solution along with the dextrose and amino acids, known as 3 in 1 TPN. Lipid solutions for 2 in 1 TPN are 10% lipids, providing 1.1 calories/mL, or 20% lipids, providing 2 calories/mL. It should be noted that 3 in 1 solutions use 20% lipids. Lipids may be withheld from patients with serum triglycerides greater than 400 mg/dl. **Figure 18-3** provides examples for calculating TPN calories.

Protein needs should always be met first to ensure adequate protein intake. For example, if a patient needs 2,000 calories daily, and 120 grams of protein, a patient should

Calculate total calories for the following TPN solutions

	Answers
Case 1	
250 grams of dextrose	850 calories
500 milliliters of 20% lipid	1000 calories
75 grams of protein	300 calories
Case 2	
300 grams of dextrose	1020 calories
500 milliliters of 10% lipid	550 calories
90 grams of protein	360 calories
Case 3	
350 grams of dextrose	1190 calories
250 milliliters of 20% lipid	500 calories
80 grams of protein	320 calories
Case 4—3 in 1 solution	
300 grams of dextrose	1020 calories
60 grams of lipid	600 calories
120 grams of protein	480 calories
Case 5	
1600 calories	
50 % calories from carbohydrate	200 grams of dextrose
25 % calories from protein	100 grams of protein
25% calories from fat (use 20% lipids)	40 grams of lipid

FIGURE 18-3 Parenteral Nutrition Calculations

receive 480 calories from protein, and 1,520 calories from dextrose and lipid.

Medications should be reviewed when determining TPN nutrient composition. Diuretics can deplete the body of vital electrolytes such as potassium. ACE inhibitors used to treat hypertension can cause hyperkalemia. Steroids can cause hyperglycemia and could increase the patient's insulin requirements.

Diprivan (propofol) is a sedative/hypnotic agent used in intensive-care settings that is based in a 10% lipid emulsion. Thus, patients receiving this medication usually have lipids excluded from their TPN. Diprivan is also dosed based on patient weight; thus it can be a challenge to feed obese patients receiving large amounts of the sedative. Serum triglycerides are frequently monitored in patients receiving Diprivan, because hypertriglyceridemia can occur.

TPN additives may include potassium, sodium, phosphate, calcium, magnesium chloride, or acetate, depending on the patient's renal function and respiratory status.

Frequent laboratory monitoring is essential to ensure adequate provision of additives to prevent serious metabolic complications. Prior to providing electrolyte additives, medications that could affect serum levels of potassium, such as ACE inhibitors and diuretics, should be noted, and TPN solutions should be adjusted accordingly. Phosphorus and calcium can form a precipitate in TPN, which could be harmful to patients, so patients with depleted levels may need additional supplementation beyond TPN. Standard multivitamin and mineral solutions are available for TPN and should be added daily to the formulas. Unlike enteral nutrition formulas, medications such as Pepcid can be added to parenteral nutrition, but most medications are not compatible with TPN solutions. Insulin is another common medication used in parenteral nutrition solutions that is often essential to aid with glucose control.

Home Nutrition Support

The primary benefit of home nutrition support is to give the caregiver, usually a family member, ultimate responsibility for the patient's care. Home care companies are often used to provide care in conjunction with a family caregiver. Home health care organizations are a key component to success of the provision of home health care. They provide support staff such as nurses, dietitians, and pharmacists to conduct home visits, educate patients and families, and obtain and provide durable medical equipment and supplies.

Home enteral nutrition is mostly prescribed for older adults. Several factors should be considered when deciding on a home enteral nutrition regimen. Lifestyle, education level, patient and caregiver motivation, resource accessibility, and cost all impact home enteral nutrition. Enteral feedings in the home setting differ primarily from the hospital and acute care setting due to the type and administration of formula. Bolus feedings are often preferred in the home setting to save time and to allow individuals to maintain an active lifestyle. Patients also often prefer to use a calorically dense formula to decrease the number of feedings throughout the day.

It is imperative to ensure adequate monitoring of patients receiving home enteral nutrition. Caregivers should be trained to note any changes in enteral feeding tube function, weight, bowel habits, and hydration status, because some studies have shown some negative outcomes associated with home enteral nutrition. Complications seen in older adults receiving home enteral nutrition include gastrointestinal complications that interrupt daily enteral feeding infusions, tube clogging or displacement, inadequate water intake, decreased urination, weight loss, and limited dietitian follow up.

Home parenteral nutrition is limited to individuals with a functional impairment of the small bowel that significantly decreases the ability of the body to absorb and metabolize nutrients. Persons with short bowel syndrome, Crohn's disease, and certain malignancies are often candidates for home TPN. Parenteral nutrition in the home setting differs from that provided in acute care in that laboratory values are monitored less frequently, because patients are less prone to metabolic complications. In the home setting, patients are more likely to receive 3 in 1 TPN, due to ease of administration, and feedings are often cycled during the night to enable freedom and flexibility throughout the day.

Ethics and Nutrition Support

As modern medicine has advanced, the possibilities for extending life have increased. These advances do not surface without controversy and ethical dilemmas. Controversies exist with regards to the use of both parenteral and enteral nutrition for end-of-life care. Several factors facilitate ongoing ethical debates, including cost-effectiveness, medical necessity, and cultural and religious beliefs.

Many patients requiring long-term TPN are younger adults with short bowel syndrome or other gastrointestinal impairments who can lead normal lives. Ethical issues arise when TPN is used by terminally ill oncology patients who have a year or less to live, for example. TPN is most likely used at end of life for persons who are unable to tolerate or who refuse enteral nutrition support. TPN may be used in patients with suboptimal oral intake due to inoperable bowel obstructions, nausea, vomiting, and generalized weakness. Most studies regarding TPN and end-of-life care show marginal, if any, differences in survival rates.

One of the most difficult things one must face in life is the death of a loved one. Patients, especially those with cancer, often refuse to eat or drink significant amounts toward the end of life and can lose a significant amount of weight. This can be quite disconcerting for a loved one to watch. Consequently, patients and family members often request TPN and intravenous fluids to prevent further weight loss and dehydration to make the patient more comfortable. Paradoxically, the provision of TPN and intravenous fluids may actually worsen the dying experience. As a possible explanation for this, some evidence suggests that the effects of ketosis and opioids released during starvation prior to death block pain and discomfort.

Cost is another factor to consider when using TPN during end-of-life care. An entire health care team is responsible for the provision and maintenance of TPN. Physicians place catheters, nursing staff administers TPN and provides catheter care, dietitians assist with order writing and determining nutrient needs, phlebotomists draw blood levels to monitor the need to adjust TPN, and pharmacists prepare and distribute parenteral nutrition solutions. Many insurance companies will not provide coverage for TPN in end-

of-life situations, simply because it is not been proven to have a significant impact on patient longevity. Too often, financially volatile health care institutions absorb the financial burdens of these patients.

Finally, the use of TPN can increase risk of infectious and metabolic complications. Catheters can become infected, resulting in catheter-related sepsis, which can be deleterious to an already immunocompromised patient. Individuals who are not monitored for laboratory changes or who experience excessive fluid and electrolyte losses can have serious complications while receiving supplemental TPN.

Unlike TPN, enteral nutrition is provided to those with a functional gastrointestinal system as either a sole source of nutrition due to a patient's inability to consume food or as supplemental nutrition support in those unable or unwilling to consume adequate oral intake. Persons receiving long-term EN may be suffering from illnesses with a gradual decline in activities of daily living, such as Parkinson's disease, Alzheimer's disease, chronic obstructive pulmonary disease requiring ventilator support, multiple sclerosis, or ALS. Acute scenarios that may require long-term EN include stroke, spinal cord injuries, and closed head injuries.

Without EN, persons unable to eat would eventually die. The advent of EN showed great promise in prolonging the lives of individuals with chronic conditions, perhaps even long enough to develop a cure. Many people with chronic illnesses resulting in functional impairments still have intact minds and are able to enjoy a longer life with the assistance of EN. Probably one of the most famous of these individuals is Christopher Reeve. A debilitating spinal cord injury inhibited his ability to consume food, thus requiring a feeding tube. His story has been an inspiration to millions that one can live a fulfilling life and help others with disabilities.

The story of Christopher Reeve does not involve an ethical dilemma, because his mental faculties were intact. Nutrition support is an ethical issue when it is provided to individuals who lack the functional capacity to care for themselves and make informed decisions, thus requiring a health care proxy (or spokesperson) to make decisions for them. As the population of older adults increases, more and more individuals may be forced to make the difficult decision regarding continuation of nutrition support.

Deciding on long-term enteral feeding at the end of life can be difficult. Five concerns of older adults regarding receipt of enteral nutrition support include the nature of illness, preservation of quality of life, dependency concerns, personal experiences, and religion.

Religion is an integral component of life values for millions of persons, so it is no wonder the people struggle with deciding whether to place a feeding tube. Being forced to decide whether to implement enteral feeding can be quite daunting for the patient and his or her loved ones.

If there are no clear advanced directives regarding end-of-life care, it can be difficult for caregivers to make decisions that they believe are in their loved ones' best interests. Advanced directives are legally binding documents that explain an individual's desires regarding life-saving treatments in the event that he or she would be deemed unable to make a decision.

In the event that an advanced directive is not in place, decisions are often left to the patient's health care proxies and the legal system. Further complicating the decision-making process, legal outcomes regarding cessation of EN vary from case to case. Examples of this occcasionally reach public attention. For example, the parents of Nancy Cruzan wanted to halt their daughter's enteral feedings because she was in a vegetative state. The Missouri supreme court ruled that no one may order discontinuation of life sustaining treatment without a living will or clear and convincing evidence of patient wishes. More recently, with the case of Terry Schiavo, the Florida courts allowed Schiavo's husband to make the ultimate decision with regard to withdrawing enteral feeding, despite her parents insistence on continuing feeding. In a third example, a New York State supreme court denied a hospital the right to place a PEG feeding tube in a 79-year-old woman with Alzheimer's disease based simply on a statement that the son claims his mother had made.

The probabilities of being alive at one month, one year, and five years have been found to be 80%, 41.7%, and 25%, respectively, for patients receiving home enteral nutrition. Other reports also suggest no increased chances in survival and no differences in wound healing. Perhaps the real solution regarding withdrawing of EN is not to place a feeding tube at all. Many studies show many negative outcomes associated with EN, such as reduced quality of life. However, persons receiving long-term home enteral nutrition are likely to already have functional impairments limiting their quality of life.

Most studies showing positive outcomes with enteral nutrition have looked at critically ill patients, not the geriatric patient with dementia, who is the typical recipient of enteral nutrition. Therefore, it is important to consider some drawbacks of long-term enteral nutrition in older patients with dementia. Patients may require wrist restraints to prevent pulling on the tube. They may also require nursing home placement, which can be devastating to those previously living independently, as well as their family members. Long-term care facilities, unless equipped with hospice units, will not admit a resident who is unable to consume adequate oral intake without a permanent long-term feeding mechanism intact. Thus, many family members see no solution but to place a feeding tube if they are unable to care for their loved one.

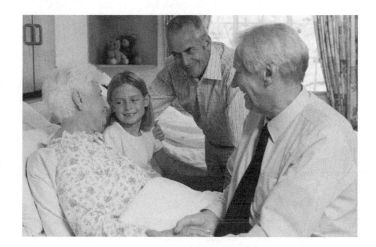

The best way one can limit inappropriate use of EN is to have the support staff, including physicians, nurses, dietitians, clergymen, and case managers, work as a team to educate patients and families on the risks and benefits of EN to help them make an informed decision. Palliative care consulting and education programs have been shown to reduce the number of feeding tubes placed.

In general, chronically ill older adults with intact minds and an inability to consume food benefit from EN. Those adults with debilitating chronic illness who often become bedbound and unaware of their surroundings will likely not experience improved quality of life. As the population of older adults increases, it will become imperative to better address death and dying and to develop alternate means to caring for individuals approaching the end of life. Death is as much a fact of life as birth. Health care employees, patients, and families should be educated regarding end-of-life care options, hospice programs should be utilized, and cultural and religious factors should be considered in end-of-life care. In a culturally diverse society, the probability of establishing a common ground on end-of-life care is unlikely, but increased education can possibly allow a more peaceful transition to the inevitable afterlife.

Conclusion

The future of nutrition support in the geriatric population will continue to grow more complex. More research is needed to determine when nutrition support, both enteral and parenteral, is best used, and when nutrition support should be avoided. Biological needs, as well as emotional and social needs, must be considered to provide optimal patient care. It is an exciting time for patients and health care providers alike to promote disease prevention and maintenance with the rapidly growing geriatric population.

Activities Related to This Chapter

1. Develop advanced directives for yourself and/or loved ones.
2. Browse through the dietary supplements aisle at your local drug store or grocery store. Compare supplements and decide which you would recommend to your patients and why.
3. Travel to a local hospital or long-term care facility. Review their enteral nutrition formulary and observe a tube feeding being administered.

REFERENCES

ASPEN. *Adult Patient.* Silver Springs, MD: ASPEN; 2007.

ASPEN. *Nutrition Support Dietetics Core Curriculum: A Case-Based Approach–The Adult Patient.* Silver Springs, MD: ASPEN;2007.

ASPEN. Definition of terms used in ASPEN guidelines and standards. *Nutr Clin Pract.* 1995;10:1–3.

Arnaud-Battandier F, Malvy D, Jeandel C, Schmitt C, Aussage P, Beaufrere B, Cynober L. Use of oral supplements in malnourished elderly patients living in the community: a pharmaco-economic study. *Clin Nutr.* 2004;23(5):1096–1103.

Bengmark S, Martindale R. Prebiotics and synbiotics in clinical medicine. *Nutr Clin Pract.* 2005;20:244–261.

Brard L, et al. The effect of total parenteral nutrition on the survival of terminally ill ovarian cancer patients. *Gynecol Oncol.* 2006;103(1):176–180.

Bruce D, et al. 2003. Nutritional supplements after hip fracture: poor compliance limits effectiveness. *Clin Nutr.* 2003;22:497–500.

Ciocon JO. Indications for tube feedings in elderly patients. *Dysphagia.* 1990;5(1):1–5.

De Rooij SE, et al. Factors that predict outcome of intensive care treatment in very elderly patients: a review. *Crit Care.* 2005;9(4):R307–R314.

Elia M, et al. Enteral nutritional support and use of a diabetes-specific formulas for patients with diabetes: A systematic review and meta-analysis. *Diabetes Care.* 2005;28(9):2267–2279.

Fairrow AM, et al. Preferences of older African-Americans for long-term tube feeding at the end of life. *Aging Ment Health.* 2004;8(6):530–534.

Gabriel SA, Ackermann RJ. Placement of nasoenteral feeding tubes using external magnetic guidance. *JPEN.* 2004;28(2):119–122.

Grossman T. Latest advances in anti-aging medicine. *Keio J Med.* 2005;54(2):85–94.

Heimburger DC, et al. Effects of small peptide and whole-protein enteral feedings on serum proteins and diarrhea in critically ill patients: a randomized trial. *JPEN.* 1997;21(3):162–167.

Hoda D, et al. Should patients with advanced incurable cancers be sent home with total parenteral nutrition? A single institution's 20-year experience. *Cancer.* 2005;103(4):863–868.

Hurley AC, Volicer L. Alzheimer disease: "It's okay, mama, if you want to go, it's okay." *JAMA.* 2002;288(18):2324–2331.

Johnson CS. Psychosocial correlates of nutritional risk in older adults. *Can J Diet Pract Res.* 2005;66(2):95–97.

Joyner J. Terry Schiavo Case Revisited. *Outside the Beltway.* February 14, 2005. Available from: http://www. outsidethebeltway.com/archives/background_terry_schiavou2019s_right_to_live_or_die_revised_terrys_right_to_die_and_her_parents_fight_against_euthanasia/. Accessed on Feb 24, 2009.

Keller HH. Malnutrition in institutionalized elderly: how and why? *J Am Geriatr Soc.* 1993;41(11):1212–1218.

Kieft H, et al. Clinical outcome of immunonutrition in a heterogeneous intensive care population. *Intensive Care Med.* 2005;31(4):524–532.

Koretz RL. Do data support nutrition support? Part II. Enteral artificial nutrition. *JADA.* 2007;107(8):1374–1380.

Lauque S, et al. Protein-energy oral supplementation in malnourished nursing-home residents. A controlled trial. *Age Ageing.* 2000;29(1):51–56.

Lauque S, et al. Improvement of weight and fat-free mass with oral nutritional supplementation in patients with Alzheimer's disease at risk of malnutrition: a prospective randomized study. *J Am Geriatr Soc.* 2004;52(10):1702–1707.

Lee JS, Auyeung TW. A comparison of two tube feeding methods in the alleviation of diarrhea in older tube fed patients: a randomized controlled trial. *Age Ageing.* 2003;32(4):388–393.

Levison Y, et al. Is it possible to increase weight and maintain protein status of debilitated elderly residents of nursing homes? *J Gerontol A Biol Med Sci.* 2005;60(7):878–881.

Lewis CL, et al. Trends in the use of feeding tubes in North Carolina hospitals. *J Gen Intern Med.* 2004;19(10):1066–1067.

Loeser C, et al. Quality of life and nutritional state in patients on home enteral tube feeding. *Nutrition.* 2003;19(7–8):5–11.

Luther H, et al. Comparative study of two systems of delivering supplemental protein with standardized tube feedings. *J Burn Care Rehabil.* 2003;24(3):167–172.

McMahon KT. Catholic moral teaching, medically assisted nutrition and hydration, and the vegetative state. *Neuro Rehabilitation.* 2004;19(4):373–379.

Mitchell SL, et al. The risk factors and impact on survival of feeding tube placement in nursing home residents with severe cognitive impairment. *Arch Intern Med.* 1997;157(3):327–332.

Monteleoni C, Clark E. Using rapid-cycle quality improvement methodology to reduce feeding tubes in patients with advanced dementia: before and after study. *BMJ.* 2004;321:491–494.

Morita T, et al. Association between hydration volume and symptoms in terminally ill cancer patients with abdominal malignancies. *Ann of Oncology.* 2005;16(4):640–647.

New York Supreme Court, Queens County. West's NY Supplement. In Re: Christopher. 1998;675:807–810.

Novartis Nutrition. Your source chart: product reference guide. Available at: http://www.abbottnutrition.com/products/roducts.aspx?pld = 264.

Rushdi TA, et al. Control of diarrhea by fiber-enriched diet in ICU patients on enteral nutrition: a prospective randomized controlled trial. *Clin Nutr.* 2004;23(6):1344–1352.

Saalwachter AR, et al. A nutrition support team led by general surgeons decreases inappropriate use of total parenteral nutrition on a surgical service. *Am Surg.* 2004;70(12):1107–1111.

Schneider SM, et al. Outcome of patients treated with home enteral nutrition. *JPEN.* 2001;25(4):203–209.

Senkal M, et al. Preoperative oral supplementation with long-chain omega-3 fatty acids beneficially alters phospholipids fatty acid patterns in liver, gut mucosa, and tumor tissue. *JPEN.* 2005;29(4):236–240.

Shang E, et al. Pump-assisted enteral nutrition can prevent aspiration in bedridden percutaneous endoscopic gastrostomy patients. *JPEN.* 2004;28(3):180–183.

Shea J, et al. An enteral therapy containing medium chain triglyceride and hydrolyzed peptides reduces postprandial pain associated with chronic pancreatitis. *Pancreatology.* 2003;3:36–40.

Silver AJ, et al. Older adults receiving home enteral nutrition: enteral regimen, provider involvement, and health care outcomes. *JPEN.* 2004;28(2):92–98.

Slomka J. Withholding nutrition at the end of life: clinical and ethical issues. *Cleveland Clin J Med.* 2003;70(6):548–552.

Soo I, Gramlich L. Use of parenteral nutrition in patients with advanced cancer. *App Physiol Nutr Metab.* 2008;33(1):102–106.

Stratton RJ, et al. Enteral nutritional support in prevention and treatment of pressure ulcers: a systematic review and meta-analysis. *Ageing Res Rev.* 2005;4(3):422–450.

Thomas, DR. Are older people starving to death in a world of plenty? Nestle Nutrition Workshop Series: Clinical and Performance Program. 2005;10:15–29.

U.S. Census Bureau. http://www.census.gov/Press-Release/www/releases/archives/facts_for features_special_editions/004210.html.

U.S. Supreme Court, West's Supreme Court Report. *Cruzan v. Director, Missouri Dept. of Health.* 1990;110:2041–2092.

Vandewoude MF, et al. Fibre-suppplemented tube feeding in the hospitalized elderly. *Age Ageing.* 2005;34(2):120–124.

Whelan K, et al. Fructooligosaccharides and fiber partially prevent the alterations in fecal microbiota and short chain fatty acid concentrations caused by standard enteral formula in healthy humans. *J Nutr.* 2005;135(8):1896–1902.

Exercise for the Older Adult: Nutritional Implications

Maria A. Fiatarone Singh, MD, FRACP and
Melissa Bernstein, PhD, RD, LD

CHAPTER OBJECTIVES   Upon completion of this chapter, the reader will be able to:

1. Describe the physiologic changes of aging that affect exercise capacity
2. List examples of nutritional disorders in the older adult and describe their impact on exercise capacity
3. Outline the benefits of an exercise prescription for a geriatric patient
4. Discuss the various forms of exercise appropriate for older adults and describe how they benefit body composition
5. Identify the key features in the assessment of an older individual for exercise
6. List the necessary components of an exercise prescription
7. Discuss the medical screening process for exercise prescription
8. List nutritional considerations of an exercising older adult
9. Discuss the practical implications of exercise programs

KEY TERMS AND CONCEPTS

Aerobic exercise

Anaerobic exercise

Disability

Exercise prescription

Behavior modification

Frailty

Functional dependency

Lean body mass

Functional status

Progressive resistance training

Sarcopenia

Sedentariness

"We don't stop playing because we grow old; we grow old because we stop playing."

—George Bernard Shaw

Exercise and nutrition are an integral part of the medical management of many chronic and complex conditions, and they are becoming increasingly important in the care of geriatric patients. Age-related changes in body composition and exercise capacity have significant implications for health and functioning. Many of these changes are associated with chronic diseases and geriatric syndromes such as metabolic syndrome, mobility impairment, falls,

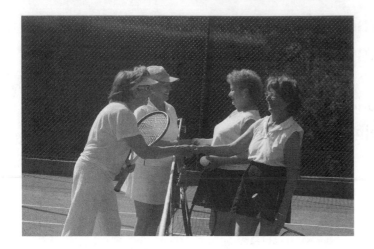

frailty, and functional decline. It is well accepted that physical activity and exercise are central in the promotion of health and prevention of disease for individuals of all ages. In aging individuals, genetic susceptibility, lifestyle choices, accumulated burden of disease, accidents, and iatrogenic misfortunes all intersect to determine both current health status as well as the prognosis for the coming years. Therefore, understanding the preventative and therapeutic options for optimizing body composition and exercise capacity in aging adults is central to geriatric care. Sufficient evidence exists to support the idea that a substantial portion of what historically has been thought of as "normal

frailty The condition of being weak or vulnerable in health or body. Factors such as unintentional weight loss (10 pounds or more in a year); general feelings of weakness and exhaustion; physical weakness (as measured by grip strength, decreased walking speed, and low levels of physical activity) are indicators of frailty.

exercise prescription
A program of exercises designed to meet desirable individual objectives for fitness. Includes specific recommendations for types of activities as well as the intensity, duration, and frequency of each exercise.

progressive resistance training A method of strength training based on the principle of overload, which states that a greater-than-normal load on the body requires the body to adapt. Once the adaptation takes place, the stress is gradually increased. In strength training, this involves the continuous attempt to increase weight or resistance designed to maximize gains in muscle growth and strength.

aging," especially with regard to changes in muscle, fat, and bone, are in fact related to an energy imbalance resulting from either excess or insufficient energy consumption, decreased energy expenditure from physical activity, or both factors in combination.

This chapter discusses the ability of physical activity and exercise patterns to influence health and quality of life. Physical fitness and habitual activity levels in old age have been shown to be directly related to functional limitations, as well as indirectly related through diseases associated with inactivity. Health care practitioners in all disciplines will be better able to serve their older clientele if they understand the theoretical basis for and the practical implementation of an **exercise prescription** for this population.

Importance of Exercise for Older Adults

The benefits of physical activity are numerous and far-reaching. Individuals who engage in regular physical activity report better health, improved self-esteem, and an overall sense of higher quality of life and social well-being. Evidence suggests that compared to their less active counterparts, physically active older men and women have lower rates of all-cause mortality, coronary heart disease, high blood pressure, stroke, type 2 diabetes, metabolic syndrome, colon cancer, breast cancer, and depression. They exhibit higher levels of cardiorespiratory and muscular fitness, have healthier body mass and composition, and have better quality sleep. The biomarker profile of physically active older adults is more favorable for preventing cardiovascular disease and type 2 diabetes and for enhancing bone health. They also have higher levels of functional health, a lower risk of falling, and better cognitive function.

As listed in **Table 19-1**, physical activity exerts benefits at multiple levels, including amelioration of the biological changes of aging; prevention or delay in the development of risk factors for chronic diseases; primary prevention of some of the most common chronic diseases in the older adult; treatment for disabling geriatric syndromes not well addressed by standard medical practice; and adjunctive treatment for established disease.

In addition, the pharmacotherapy offered for chronic disease management may carry with it a burden of side effects, including often unrecognized nutritional consequences in the older patient. In these situations, a novel combination of exercise and standard care may shift the risk/benefit ratio of treatment significantly (**Table 19-2**). For example, **progressive resistance training** (PRT) has been shown in both animals and humans to reverse losses of both muscle (sarcopenia) and bone mass (osteopenia), which are common side effects of long-term corticosteroid treatment for chronic obstructive pulmonary disease (COPD) or inflammatory

TABLE 19-1 Benefits of Exercise in the Older Adult

1. Exercise aids in minimizing physiological changes of aging:
   - Atrophy of tendons and ligaments
   - Decreased aerobic and glycolytic enzyme capacity
   - Decreased bone mass and fracture threshold
   - Decreased capillary density
   - Decreased glycogen storage, insulin sensitivity, glucose tolerance
   - Decreased maximal aerobic capacity and cardiovascular efficiency
   - Decreased muscle mass and strength
   - Decreased tissue elasticity, joint flexibility
   - Endothelial cell dysfunction
   - Immunosenescence
   - Increased fat mass
   - Impaired gait and balance
   - Increased visceral adiposity

2. Exercise aids in decreasing risk factors for chronic disease:
   - Glucose intolerance
   - Hyperinsulinemia and insulin resistance
   - Hyperlipidemia
   - Hypertension
   - Inflammatory cytokinemia (CRP, IL-6, etc.)
   - Obesity, visceral obesity
   - Osteopenia
   - Sarcopenia

3. Exercise aids in preventing or delaying onset of chronic diseases:
   - Breast cancer
   - Colon cancer
   - Coronary artery disease
   - Endometrial cancer, prostate cancer
   - Hypertension
   - Osteoporosis, fracture
   - Stroke
   - Type 2 diabetes mellitus
   - Dementia

4. Exercise provides adjunctive treatment for established diseases:
   - Chronic obstructive pulmonary disease
   - Congestive heart failure
   - Coronary artery disease
   - Depression
   - Diabetes mellitus
   - Hypertension
   - Inflammatory arthritis
   - Obesity
   - Osteoarthritis
   - Parkinson's disease
   - Peripheral vascular disease
   - Stroke
   - Varicose veins
   - Chronic renal failure
   - Congestive heart failure
   - Organ transplant
   - Chronic HIV infection

5. Exercise aids in preventing and/or treating common geriatric syndromes:
   - Anorexia/nutrient deficiencies
   - Constipation
   - Functional decline
   - Gait and balance disorders/falls
   - Incontinence
   - Insomnia
   - Low self-efficacy
   - Low self-esteem
   - Social isolation, loneliness, low morale
   - Weakness, fatigue, low exercise tolerance
   - Musculoskeletal pain

arthritis. Loss of muscle and bone secondary to hypocaloric dieting, low-protein diets in chronic renal failure, or the disuse that accompanies bed rest or decreased mobility with any acute or chronic illness may all be similarly minimized by an appropriate prescription of resistive exercise.

A common side effect of some chronic diseases and many medications is anorexia and subsequent weight loss. It is often difficult to treat such patients with nutritional interventions alone, because their energy requirements are markedly blunted by both decreased muscle mass (and therefore decreased basal metabolic rate) and reduced energy expenditure from low levels of physical activity. Attempts at nutritional supplementation with additional energy are often not successful in these situations; however, individuals who begin an exercise regimen along with supplementation have been shown to be able to significantly augment their total energy intake. The combination of multinutrient supplementation and anabolic exercise has also been shown to improve adaptations to resistance training, including greater strength gain. In addition to stimulating appetite, initiation of resistance training has been shown to enhance nitrogen retention in older adults.

TABLE 19-2 Counteracting Adverse Consequences of Chronic Disease Treatment with Exercise

Common Disease Treatments for Chronic Conditions	Adverse Consequence	Effective Exercise Modalities to Reduce Adverse Consequences
Anorexogenic drug therapy (digoxin; serotonin reuptake inhibitors; theophylline; anticholinergic medications; or polypharmacy causing nausea, dry mouth, or anorexia)	Weight loss Sarcopenia	Progressive resistance exercise*
Corticosteroid treatment for chronic pulmonary disease or inflammatory arthritis	Myopathy Osteopenia, Osteoporotic fracture	Progressive resistance exercise, high-impact exercise, or weight-bearing aerobic exercise
Hypocaloric dieting for obesity	Loss of lean body mass (muscle and bone)	Progressive resistance exercise
Low-protein diet for chronic renal failure or liver failure	Weight loss Sarcopenia	Progressive resistance exercise*
Postural hypotension secondary to drug therapy (diuretics, antihypertensives, Parkinsonian drugs, antidepressants)	Postural symptoms, falls, fractures	Endurance exercise
Slowed gastrointestinal motility secondary to anticholinergics, narcotics, calcium channel blockers, iron therapy	Constipation, fecal impaction, reduced food intake	Progressive resistance exercise or endurance training*
Thyroid replacement for hypothyroidism	Osteopenia	Progressive resistance exercise, high-impact exercise, or weight bearing aerobic exercise
Treatment with beta blockers or alpha-methyldopa for hypertension or heart disease	Depression	Progressive resistance training or endurance training*

*For these conditions, the benefit of exercise remains to be tested in controlled trials in patients receiving the indicated treatment. For example, exercise has been shown to speed gastrointestinal transit time and thus theoretically would counteract the constipating effect of listed medications.

Nitrogen retention may be especially important for older adults in catabolic situations, such as those recovering from surgery or trauma or having catabolic illnesses, hepatic diseases, or low protein intake.

The interdependence of nutritional requirements, energy expenditure in physical activity, body composition, and the health and medication profile in geriatric practice emphasizes the importance of implementing a multidisciplinary approach to the management of medical and nutritional disorders in the older patient.

Physiologic Changes of Aging That Affect Exercise Capacity

Table 19-3 lists the important physiologic alterations in the older patient that affect exercise capacity. Note that although these changes affect peak athletic performance, they do not prevent physiologic adaptation to an appropriate exercise stimulus, even in individuals of very advanced age. In other words, an individual is never too old to gain benefits from an appropriately designed exercise prescription.

The ability of exercise training to slow the progression or even reverse some of these commonly accepted "signs of aging" suggests that a proportion of what we know of as "aging" is not inevitable biologic progression but is attributable to disuse of organ systems over time.

For example, a comparison of two MRI scans of middle-aged women clearly shows a very different body composition profile in the thigh muscle of a sedentary verses an active woman (**Figure 19-1**). Unquestionably, certain age-related phenomena would persist despite athletic training, such as the decline in maximal heart rate and motor neuron death. However, the impact of such "unavoidable" physiologic aging is primarily limited to performance in athletic competitions and will cause little **disability** in daily functional activities for the otherwise healthy older adult.

Nutritional Disorders in the Older Adult and Their Impact on Exercise

Functional Capacity

Physiologic aging and chronic diseases are not the only factors that limit functional capacity in the older adult. Exer-

disability General term used to refer to deficits in an individual's overall health (physical or psychological) that affects that person's ability to perform the tasks of everyday living.

TABLE 19-3 Physiologic Changes of Aging That Impair Exercise Capacity

Physiologic Change	Habitual Exercise Minimizes Change
Decreased glucose transport and glycogen storage capacity in skeletal muscle	Yes
Decreased capillary density in skeletal muscle	Yes
Decreased ligament and tendon strength	Yes
Decreased maximal aerobic capacity	Yes
Decreased maximal heart rate	No
Decreased maximal muscle strength	Yes
Decreased muscle endurance	Yes
Decreased muscle mass	Yes
Decreased muscle power	Yes
Decreased nerve conduction velocity	Yes
Decreased skeletal oxidative muscle and glycolytic enzyme capacity in skeletal muscle	Yes
Decreased pulmonary flow rates	No
Decreased stroke volume	Yes
Decreased tissue elasticity and joint range of motion	Yes
Degeneration of cartilage	Yes*
Increased general and visceral fat mass and percent body fat	Yes
Increased heart rate and blood pressure response to submaximal exercise	Yes
Loss of motor neurons and motor units	Unknown
Prolonged neural reaction time	Yes

*Although exercise-related injuries may result in chronic damage and degeneration of cartilage, habitual weight-bearing exercise without injury is protective to cartilage viability.

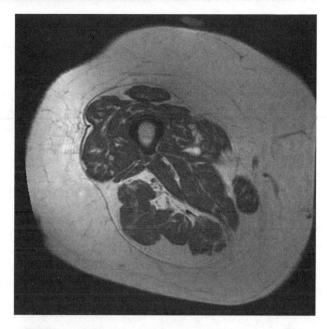

FIGURE 19-1A MRI Scan of a Sedentary Woman

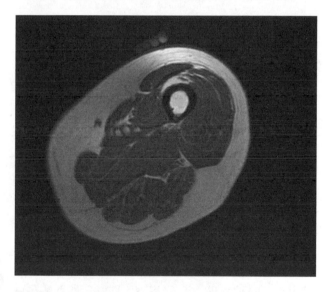

FIGURE 19-1B MRI Scan of an Active Woman

Source: Courtesy of Professor Maria A. Fiatarone Singh.

lean body mass The portion of the body exclusive of stored fat, including muscle, bone, connective tissue, organs, and water.

sarcopenia Age-associated loss of muscle mass, associated with muscle weakness, functional limitations, and disability, as well as impairments in cardiovascular capacity and metabolic health.

cise and nutrition are interrelated and share many common pathways that may affect disease processes as well as their management. When nutritional deficiencies exist, such as those listed in **Table 19-4**, in addition to physical degeneration, the potential for clinically overt consequences for functional capacity is even greater.

Protein-calorie malnutrition, alone or in combination with catabolic diseases, will lead to loss of **lean body mass**, and is thus one of the most important sequelae of malnutrition in the older adult. Loss of muscle mass, known as **sarcopenia** or "loss of flesh" from undernutrition, physical inactivity, or other causes, may result in weakness, gait and balance disorders, falls and fractures, functional decline,

TABLE 19-4 Nutritional Deficiencies That Impair Exercise Tolerance

Deficiency	Physiologic Consequence	Primary Exercise Capacity Affected
B12	Central and peripheral nervous system dysfunction	Muscle strength and power
Calcium	Muscle contractile dysfunction, cardiac conduction disturbance	Aerobic capacity; muscle strength, power, and endurance
Carbohydrate	Reduced glycogen storage	Aerobic capacity, musculoskeletal endurance
Energy	Sarcopenia, osteopenia	Aerobic capacity; muscle strength, power, and endurance
Iron	Decreased oxygen carrying capacity	Aerobic capacity
Magnesium	Muscle contractile dysfunction, cardiac conduction disturbance	Aerobic capacity; muscle strength, power, and endurance
Potassium	Muscle contractile dysfunction, cardiac conduction disturbance	Aerobic capacity; muscle strength, power, and endurance
Protein	Sarcopenia, osteopenia	Aerobic capacity; muscle strength, power
Thiamin	Nerve conduction impairment, myopathy, cardiac dysfunction	Aerobic capacity; muscle strength, power, and endurance
Vitamin D	Muscle contractile dysfunction and atrophy, impaired balance	Aerobic capacity; muscle strength, power, and endurance, gait and balance

disability, reduced quality of life, and insulin insensitivity. Such sarcopenia is often "masked" in older adults, because concomitant adipose mass accretion results in weight stability or increase, a common body composition presentation in the older adult known as *sarcopenic obesity*. The causes of sarcopenia are multifactorial, but fortunately the most common etiological factors (undernutrition and inactivity) are treatable with lifestyle modification and supportive nutritional and social services.

Micronutrient status is also important for physical function. Even with adequate protein intake, decreased protein synthesis rates in older adults may lead to gradual loss of lean mass over time. Evidence suggests that protein supplementation, particularly if taken in the hour following weight-lifting exercise, may lead to increased uptake of amino acids into skeletal muscle, providing the substrate for the enhanced protein synthesis rate associated with acute bouts of anabolic exercise. However, greater accretion of skeletal muscle in response to training (hypertrophy) or functional and health benefits have not yet been unequivocally linked to augmentation of protein intake from dietary sources or supplements. Thus, current evidence suggests that dietary protein should be maintained at or slightly above the RDA of 0.8 g/kg/day during resistance training in older adults.

Skeletal muscle has receptors for 1,25 dihydroxyvitamin D, which appears to be necessary for muscle to fully relax and therefore be able to subsequently produce maximal force during the contractile phase. Vitamin D deficiency results in clinical muscle weakness, particularly of the proximal muscles of the lower extremities, and even subclinical deficiency (determined by blood tests) has been associated with falls and fractures. Homebound or institutionalized elders without exposure to ultraviolet light, as well as individuals abstaining from dairy products because of lactose intolerance or other reasons, are at high risk for vitamin D deficiency. Because older skin does not optimally synthesize vitamin D from cholesterol precursors, even "adequate" exposure to sunlight (15 minutes of exposure of the upper extremities, face, and neck in the mid-morning to early afternoon period) may be unable to prevent vitamin D deficiency. Vitamin D is typically not part of the food supply in large quantities; therefore, the older adult may require vitamin D supplementation.

Nutritional deficiencies of calcium, magnesium, and potassium impair muscle contractile activity and result in clinical weakness. Patients on long-term or high-dose diuretic therapy are at highest risk for deficiencies of these nutrients. However, because serum levels of these minerals remain normal even when tissue stores are quite low, they are an insensitive index of deficiency states and should not be relied upon to determine the need for supplementation. Patients with no other definable cause for muscle weakness and fatigue who have risk factors for these mineral losses should be considered candidates for replacement or alternative drug therapy. Sometimes in the older adult fatigue may be a more prominent complaint than actual muscle weakness in these conditions, so a thorough history and a high index of suspicion are essential to early diagnosis and treatment.

Optimizing Body Composition with Exercise in Older Adults

One of the most direct pathways from physical activity to health status involves the ability of regular exercise to alter body composition and partially offset adverse body composition changes associated with aging. In "usual aging" typical changes observed in body compartments are decreased muscle and bone mass and increased total and central fat mass. The extent to which these changes occur in an individual depend on a combination of interrelated genetic, lifestyle, and disease-related factors. Nutritional and body composition changes may negatively impact metabolic, cardiovascular and musculoskeletal function, even in the absence of overt disease, and therefore it is important to anticipate them and optimize lifestyle choices and medical treatments that can counteract the negative effects of aging and/or disease on body composition.

Beginning the fourth decade of life, body composition changes often include a decrease in muscle and bone mass and an increase and redistribution of adipose tissue. Exercise is able to partially offset all of the adverse body composition changes associated with aging. For example, a stabilization or increase in bone mass may be important for both prevention and treatment of osteoporosis and related fractures and disability, and should complement the provision of adequate calcium, vitamin D, protein, and energy, which are also required for adequate bone health. Age-related declines in muscle power may be an early indicator of "subclinical" gait and balance defects and may predict an increased risk of falls in older adults. Low-intensity, high-velocity (explosive) power training improves balance performance as well as power in older adults. The combination of exercise effects on bone strength, muscle mass, muscle strength, power, and balance should theoretically lower the risk of injurious falls substantially in physically active individuals.

Obesity is one of the most important nutritional problems in older adults, with prevalence estimates for combined overweight and obesity exceeding 60% in many Western countries. Obesity is defined as a body mass index (BMI) of greater than 30.0 kg/m² in White populations, the level at which associated morbidity and mortality rise substantially. Overweight status is generally defined as the range between 25 and 30 kg/m², although obesity-associated risks tend to rise at a higher threshold of 27.5 kg/m² in

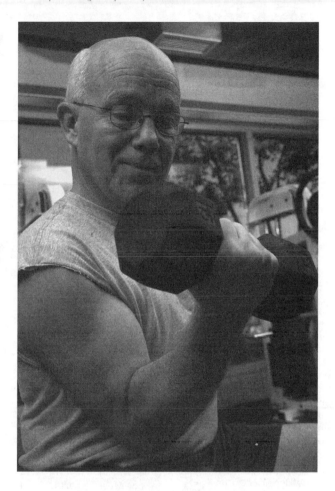

older adults. Obesity is linked to increased rates of insulin resistance, hypertension, type 2 diabetes, atherosclerosis, depression, osteoarthritis, sleep apnea, mobility disorders, and functional impairment with aging. Prevention of excess adiposity is both protective and therapeutic for many common chronic diseases, for example, offering significant risk reduction in the cases of osteoarthritis; cardiovascular disease; gallbladder disease; type 2 diabetes; breast, colon, and endometrial cancer; hypertension; stroke; and vascular impotence.

Visceral obesity (excess accumulation of intra-abdominal adipose tissue) is even more metabolically risky than generalized obesity. It may be defined by image analysis studies such as computerized technology or magnetic resonance imaging or in clinical practice by a waist circumference (WC) greater than 102 cm in White males or 88 cm in White females.

Although generalized obesity is associated with excess mortality, cardiovascular disease, osteoarthritis, mobility impairment, and disability, it is predominantly excess visceral fat that is associated with the derangements of dyslipidemia, elevated fibrinogen, hyperinsulinemia, glucose intolerance or diabetes, vascular insulin resistance, hypertension, and cardiovascular disease. An increase in central distribution of fat with advancing age is associated with chronic metabolic and cardiovascular abnormalities. The relationship between excess abdominal adipose tissue and cardiovascular health risk has recently stimulated interest in the efficacy of physical activity in the treatment of this condition.

Evidence suggests a beneficial influence of physical activity on the reduction of abdominal and visceral fat in overweight and obese individuals. The amount of exercise necessary to maintain a constant body weight increases with age and depends on a variety of physiological and lifestyle factors. Decreases in both total adipose tissue accumulation and its abdominal (visceral) deposition are achievable through both aerobic and resistance training. Significant changes in total body fat are usually only seen with exercise in conjunction with an energy-restricted diet, further emphasizing the importance of both exercise and nutritional interventions in health management. Lifestyle modification programs have recently been shown to decrease weight, blood pressure, and insulin resistance. Most important, five separate randomized, controlled trials, such as those by Ramachandran and colleagues in 2007 and Mayor in 2007, have found that lifestyle modification can prevent the progression to type 2 diabetes in high-risk individuals with impaired glucose tolerance. In these studies, the introduction of aerobic and resistance training or **aerobic exercise** alone, combined with modest dietary energy and fat restriction and increase in fiber, fruits and vegetables, were effective in preventing incident diabetes. The relative risk reductions in middle-aged and older adults ranged from 28% in India to 63% in Japan. In the U.S. Diabetes Prevention Program, lifestyle modification was approximately twice as effective as metformin administration, and older adults achieved the greatest risk reduction in incident diabetes, compared to younger individuals.

An increase in strength and muscle mass achieved through progressive resistance training (PRT) has a potential role in prevention of **functional dependency**, and falls and fractures, as well as being important in the prevention and treatment of chronic diseases and disabilities that are accompanied by disuse, catabolism, and sarcopenia. For some diseases, such as type 2 diabetes mellitus, there are potential advantages to both minimizing fat tissue and maximizing muscle tissue, because these compartments have opposite, and likely independent, effects on insulin resistance and metabolic syndrome in older individuals. In another example, a small number of clinical trials involving patients with chronic renal disease, progressive resistance training programs have been shown to be safe, feasible, and efficacious in the improvement of clinical, physical, and functional outcomes.

The use of **anaerobic exercise**, including weight lifting and PRT, to combat sarcopenia in older adults is one of the most important applications of exercise science to clinical medicine and gerontology in recent years. The remarkable responsiveness of this syndrome of muscle atrophy and weakness with a targeted exercise prescription, even among those over the age of 90 with advanced disability, underscores the importance of the assessment and treatment of remediable conditions and maintenance of preventive health strategies at all ages.

Assessing the Exercise Capacity and Needs of the Older Patient

Older adults are the least active age group of Americans. National survey data from 2005 show that an average of only 21% of those aged 65 years and older report meeting recommended levels of physical activity, and some evidence suggests that actual levels may be substantially lower than what is reported. Therefore, as with many adults, the majority of older patients in any geriatric clinical setting will not be physically active or have optimized their physical fitness level and physical activity habits when they present to their health care professional.

As a first step, it is critical to assess current level of fitness as well as deficits in order to set appropriate goals and develop a rational and feasible exercise prescription individualized for the older patient. **Box 19-1** outlines the stages necessary for the adequate assessment and recommendation of exercise modalities for the older patient. Question the patient about previous involvement in sport,

aerobic exercise The term *aerobic* refers to the presence of or a need for oxygen. The complete breakdown of glucose, fatty acids, and amino acids to carbon dioxide and water occurs only via aerobic metabolism. The citric acid cycle and electron transport chain are aerobic pathways. Therefore, aerobic exercise is any activity, such as running, walking, dancing, or biking, that requires the presence of sufficient oxygen. Also referred to as *cardiorespiratory exercise*.

functional dependency Requiring assistance for activities related to the functions of the body usually involving activities of daily living.

anaerobic exercise The term *anaerobic* refers to the absence of oxygen or the ability of a process to occur in the absence of oxygen. Therefore, anaerobic exercise is any activity that does not require the presence of oxygen. This includes is short-term, high-intensity activities such as sprinting, weightlifting, and jumping.

1. Assess exercise needs/goals on the basis of history and physical and individual preferences.

2. Identify behavioral readiness to change; provide appropriate counseling for current stage.

3. Identify potential risk factors for exercise-related adverse events.

4. Prioritize physical activity needs in relation to risks.

5. Prescribe the specific exercise modality and dose desired.

6. Provide or refer for specific training, equipment advice, facility options, and safety precautions.

7. Set up behavioral program for adoption, adherence, and relapse prevention.

8. Monitor compliance, benefits, and adverse events over time.

9. Modify exercise prescription as health status/goals/behavioral stage changes.

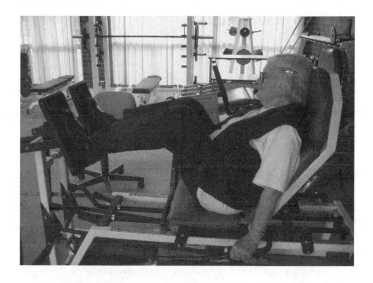

sity exercise will be required if new or unstable cardiac symptoms are present.

For completely sedentary adults and novices to regular exercise, suggesting only one new physical activity at a time is likely to enhance compliance. Simply identifying the appropriate exercises and establishing goals is not sufficient. As with dietary counseling and intervention, **behavior modification** is a central component to successful exercise program adherence.

Some of the most often cited barriers to appropriate physical activity in the older adult are listed in **Box 19-2**. It is of critical importance to identify the barriers for each individual and to design a plan to change or maintain desired behavior and prevent relapse. As with adults of all ages, perceived lack of time is frequently cited, even by nursing home residents, when asked why they do not exercise. It is helpful to go through a daily schedule, pointing out times when watching television or other sedentary activities can be combined with flexibility, resistive, or even stationary aerobic exercise or when stairs can be substituted for elevators and escalators.

Extensive sedentary time, particularly if uninterrupted by physical activity episodes, is an independent risk factor for insulin resistance and type 2 diabetes. Thus, both behaviorally and metabolically, inserting physical activity "breaks" into sedentary activities such as computer work or TV watching may be an extremely efficient and effective approach to combating obesity and associated metabolic disease. Breaking down the exercise prescription into small components that can

recreational, and competitive activities, and ask about any remote or chronic exercise-related injuries. As part of a complete exercise history, gather information on current household, work-related, and recreational activities. This information can be quantified in terms of days per week, weeks per year, average length of each session or activity, and how long this pattern has been followed. In addition, specific questions about distances walked per week (in miles or blocks) and number of flights of stairs climbed per week will provide useful information upon which to build the prescription and an index of current capacity. Standardized scales such as the Harvard Alumni Questionnaire or the Physical Activity Scale for the Elderly (PASE), as well as questions about the need for human or mechanical assistance with daily activities and household tasks, will also point out the greatest physiologic deficits. Take into account the person's activity preferences as well as potential limitations. Before beginning any exercise program, an older patient should undergo a complete physical exam to identify physiologic deficits. In some cases, exercise stress testing prior to the initiation of a physical activity prescription of moderate-to-high inten-

behavior modification A systematic method for changing a behavior to a more desirable one by learning new lifestyle techniques and skills.

BOX 19-2 Barriers to Appropriate Physical Activity in the Older Adult

- Acute and chronic medical problems and disabilities
- Caregiving role for sick spouse or family member
- Lack of interest
- Exaggerated perception of risk/fear of injury
- Financial limitations
- Geographical constraints and environmental design features
- Institutional/residential policies
- Lack of advocacy by family and health care community
- Lack of appropriately designed exercise equipment
- Lack of health care professional/caregiver/family education about exercise
- Perceived lack of time
- Psychological issues (depression, dementia, bereavement, self-efficacy, fear of falling, low self-esteem, social isolation)
- Reduced appreciation of benefit
- Societal norms/expectations of sedentariness (ageism)
- Transportation difficulties

The initial challenges must be overcome with a creatively designed, medically sound exercise prescription. This includes monitoring the patient, if needed; providing adequate lighting; strengthening muscles around arthritic joints before prescribing weight-bearing exercise; and keeping intensity levels below those that produce cardiopulmonary or musculoskeletal symptoms. For example, if the risk of ischemia is very high with aerobic exercise, then prescribing resistance exercises may offer similar benefits in terms of health and functioning with far less potential to provoke cardiac symptoms. If an older runner who likes competition is getting into difficulty with knee and ankle injuries, substituting a lower impact yet intense activity such as race walking can provide all of the physical and psychological benefits desired with a reduced risk of musculoskeletal trauma. In all cases, it is important to balance the pleasurable components of exercise for the individual with the health-maintaining aspects important to the practitioner, maximizing enjoyment, and therefore compliance, so that both short- and long-term health benefits can be achieved.

Exercise prescriptions sometimes fail because they are too vague to be useful. The exercise prescription needs to be clearly written and treated like a medication prescription. The patient needs to know the indication, type, dose, frequency, potential side effects, alternatives, and interactions with other nutritional or pharmaceutical preparations that he or she is already taking.

Guidelines to Physical Activity and Exercise

All adults can benefit from integrating more exercise into their lives.

Older adults, in particular, are a heterogeneous group with varied levels of physical activity or inactivity, and they face diverse social, economic, and environmental challenges, and often at least one or more chronic conditions. The American College of Sports Medicine (ACSM), the Centers for Disease Control (CDC), and the American Heart Association (AHA) recently joined together to update recommendations regarding physical activity for adults ages 65 and older and adults aged 50–64 with clinically significant chronic disease or functional limitations that affect movement ability, fitness, or physical activity. Their recommendation states: "Regular physical activity, including aerobic activity and muscle-strengthening activity, is essential for healthy aging." **Table 19-5** outlines the ACSM/CDC and the AHA's most recent recommendations for healthy adults over age 65. These guidelines have been shown to have benefit in terms of disease prevention and treatment as well as maintenance of cardiovascular and musculoskeletal fitness. A total of about three hours per week (approximately 30 minutes per day) is sufficient to meet the requirements for

be incorporated into the daily routine is the most effective way to encourage long-term adherence to a healthy lifestyle. For example, simple balance exercises, such as standing on one leg, can be practiced whenever one is standing in line at a bank or supermarket or at the sink or counter at home doing daily chores.

To add to the challenge that practitioners face when designing exercise programs for older adults, older patients often will have medical problems that place them at higher risk for exercise-related adverse events. Some conditions that may impair exercise that may not be obvious include visual impairment, balance disorders, osteoarthritis of the shoulder or weight-bearing joints, low thresholds for ischemia or bronchospasm, peripheral vascular disease, and peripheral neuropathy. If carefully monitored, these conditions need not be a contraindication to exercise. In fact, some of these problems and conditions, such as poor balance, are actually primary indications for beginning the correct exercise program.

TABLE 19-5 Exercise Recommendations for Older Adults

The ACSM/CDC and AHA basic recommendation is that older adults

1. "Do *moderately intense aerobic* exercise for 30 minutes a day, five days a week"

or

2. "Do vigorously intense aerobic exercise for 20 minutes a day, 3 days a week"

Notes: *Aerobic activity.* Aerobic exercise increases oxygen use to improve heart and lung function. These activities are important for their cardiovascular benefits such as strengthening of the heart and lungs as well as lowering blood pressure and cholesterol. Aerobic activities have also been shown to improve mood and sleep. Walking, swimming, dancing, aerobic exercise classes, climbing stairs, pushing a lawn mower, biking to the store, playing with children, gardening, and even heavy housework are also types of activity that count, as long as activity is moderate or vigorous for at least 10 minutes at a time.

Intensity. Intensity is how hard the body is working during an activity. Older adults should aim to include 150 minutes of moderate intensity physical activity each week. *Moderate-intensity* aerobic exercise means working at a 5 or 6 on a 10 point scale, with 0=sitting, and 10= as hard as possible. As a rule of thumb the exerciser should still be able to carry on a brief conversation but not sing a song. For those with a higher level of fitness and limited time to be active, older adults could include 75 minutes of vigorous activity weekly or an equivalent amount of time by combining moderate and intense activities. *Vigorous-intensity* activity produces larger increases in breathing and heart rate. The activity should rate a 7-8 on the 10 point scale. Breathing will be hard enough so that the exerciser cannot say more than a few words without catching their breath.

and

3. "Do 8-10 strength-training exercises, 10-15 repetitions of each exercise twice-three times per week"

Notes: *Muscle strengthening activities* are strength training exercises designed to increase muscle strength and endurance. These activities prevent loss of muscle and bone and thereby help to maintain health and physical independence. To gain the health benefits of muscle strengthening exercises, the activities need to be done to the point where it becomes difficult to finish the repetitions without help. There are many ways older adults can strengthen their muscles such as lifting weights, working with resistance bands, doing exercises that use body weight for resistance such as sit ups and push ups, and yoga. The activities should work all the major muscle groups in the body including the chest, shoulders, arms, legs, hips, abdomen, and the muscles of the back.

An additional bonus for older adults is the beneficial effects of physical activity for their *functional health.* Improvements in functional health contribute to the ease of performing everyday activities such as walking, grocery shopping, food preparation, and housekeeping.

and

4. "If you are at risk of falling perform balance exercises"

Notes: *Balance exercises* are recommended for community-dwelling adults with a history of falling or trouble walking. The activity plan for these adults should include exercise specifically designed to maintain or improve balance.

Flexibility activities such as stretching large muscle groups are also recommended. Stretching helps to maintain the necessary range of motion for the performance of everyday activities.

and

5. "Have a physical activity plan"

Notes: Experts also recommend that older adults have an *activity plan* developed with a health professional. This plan should be designed to maximize physical activity while managing risks, take therapeutic needs into account, and ensure safety.

Source: Data from American College of Sports Medicine. Physical activity and health guidelines. Available at: http://www.acsm.org. Accessed January 19, 2009; Nelson ME, Rejeeski WJ, Blair SN, Duncan PW, Judge JO, et al. Physical activity and public health in older adults: recommendations from the American College of Sports Medicine and the American Heart Association. *Med Sci Sports Exerc.* 2007 Aug;39(8):1435–1445; Centers for Disease Control. Physical activity for everyone; how much physical activity do older adults need? Available at: http://www.cdc.gov/physical activity/everyone/guidelines/olderadults.html. Accessed January 19, 2009.

all four modes of exercise (aerobic, strengthening, balance, flexibility), which is feasible for most individuals of retirement age. Higher intensities or greater amounts of exercise may be undertaken for competitive purposes or in highly athletic individuals, but they are not required for general health in the older adult and are associated with greater risk of injury and higher dropout rates. These recommendations are similar to those made recently in the *2008 Physical Activity Guidelines for Americans*. These comprehensive guidelines by the U.S. Department of Health and Human Services include a chapter specific to older adults.

While more activity is better, all adults should strive to avoid inactivity. Not doing any physical activity is bad for health regardless of the age or physical condition of the person. When an older adult cannot meet these recommendations or needs to take a break due to vacation or illness, it is critical to remember that some activity is better than nothing. Everyone should be encouraged to be as physically active as their situation allows. Taking a gradual stepwise approach is especially important for those beginning a physical activity program. Breaking activities up throughout the day, choosing safe and social environments, with well fitting, comfortable shoes and clothes will also help to ensure successful adoption of a more physically active lifestyle. Simply reducing sedentary behavior is an appropriate starting point for many older adults. This can be accomplished by choosing a variety of enjoyable activities to make fitness a part of everyday life.

Most older patients unfamiliar with exercise programs will require more training than can be provided by the average health care professional without special exercise knowledge. Therefore, it of critical importance that a referral is made to a qualified fitness instructor, exercise physiologist, or physical therapist. In addition, many older adults, especially those with mental impairments, will benefit from supervised, personalized instruction along with unambiguous illustrated instructions or videotapes, particularly in the first six months of the initiation of an exercise program. Such materials provide both knowledge and motivation for the novice exerciser and having them on hand in the waiting room or office setting reinforces the power of the prescription and emphasizes the commitment of the practitioner to healthy lifestyle principles.

Health professionals should set up the personalized behavioral program at the same time that the exercise prescription is given. Clients can be given a written copy of their short- and long-term goals broken down into measurable components, in addition to an exercise calendar or diary to fill out each week, motivational tokens, and a plan for feedback on his or her progress at frequent intervals. Anticipate potential circumstances such as illness, caregiving responsibilities, and travel, and create a plan to man-

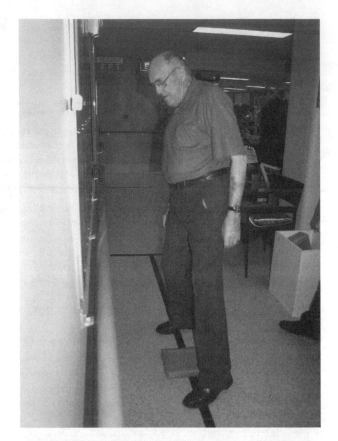

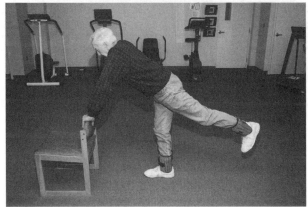

age them early before setbacks occur. Compliance with the exercise program should be assessed at every visit so that problems and barriers can be identified early and resolved before they hinder adherence. A review of perceived benefits and recent adverse events should also be part of the routine compliance assessment.

Repeating the physical function testing that was used to generate the initial prescription can be very motivating. In this way, the patient can be given direct feedback on the specific physical benefits attributable to his or her new physical activity pattern. It is of utmost importance that as **functional status** improves, the exercises and goals be modified to emphasize new areas of fitness once the routine of regular physical activity has been firmly established. Shaping behavior in small increments is more likely to be successful than overwhelming an adult who has been sedentary for 50 years with an overly ambitious plan of physical activity.

Medical Screening for the Exercise Prescription

Exercise carries with it the possibility of complications and adverse events; the most important of which are outlined in **Table 19-6**. The most feared events are those of a cardiovascular nature, although they are relatively rare even in cardiac rehabilitation settings. The most common complications are minor musculoskeletal injuries. Many injuries can be prevented by paying attention to proper technique; slowly progressing in intensity, as tolerated; avoiding ambulatory activities until strength and balance are adequate to safely support the body weight; and abstaining from exercise during acute illness, extremes of temperature or humidity, or the appearance of new, unidentified medical symptoms.

Many sets of recommendations have been created in an attempt to make exercise as safe as possible for adults. As with any person, complete medical screening of older adults should occur prior to the onset of a new exercise program. Physicians should be aware of any new exercise prescription that may affect medication requirements or cause exacerbation of underlying conditions.

A broader use and definition of medical screening for exercise for the geriatric patient is suggested. It is important to keep in mind that **sedentariness** itself is a risk factor for disease and disability. Habitual exercise protects against many major chronic diseases and is indicated in medical treatment. Therefore, health professionals working with older adults should reframe past thinking. Rather than asking, "Is this patient safe to exercise?" pose the question "Is this patient safe to be sedentary?" In general, hypertension, cardiovascular disease, diabetes, pulmonary disease, obesity, neurologic disease, chronic renal failure, chronic arthritis, and even cancer are indications for exercise in medically stable older adults, rather than contraindications, to more activity.

Some specific areas of concern in the older adult include cardiopulmonary status, musculoskeletal integrity, mental status, podiatric problems, and vision. For most cardiopulmonary symptoms, activity should be stopped at their on-

TABLE 19-6 The Risks of Exercise in the Older Adult

Musculoskeletal	Cardiovascular/ Cardiopulmonary	Metabolic
Falls	Arrhythmia	Dehydration
Fatigue	Bronchospasm	Electrolyte
Foot ulceration	Claudication	imbalance
Fracture,	Cerebrovascular	Energy imbalance
osteoporotic or	accident	Heat stroke
traumatic	Cardiac failure	Hyperglycemia
Hemorrhoids	Hypertension	Hypoglycemia
Hernia	Hypotension	Hypothermia
Joint or bursa	Ischemia	Seizures
inflammation,	Pulmonary	Weight loss
exacerbation of	embolism	
arthritis	Retinal hemorrhage	
Laceration/soft-	or detachment,	
tissue injury	lens detachment	
Ligament or	Ruptured aneurysm	
tendon strain or	Syncope or	
rupture	postural	
Muscle soreness	symptoms	
or tear		

set. Some patients, such as those with advanced chronic pulmonary disease, may not tolerate aerobic activity at all; however, they often are able to perform resistance, balance, and flexibility exercises without difficulty. The catabolic effects of chronic pulmonary disease, often accompanied by anorexia, malnutrition, and corticosteroid treatment, produce severe losses of lean tissue (muscle and bone). It is important to remember that the adaptive response to resistive exercise is required to reverse this wasting process. Therefore, patients with the most severe lung disease, who are least likely to be able to tolerate aerobic activities, in fact are more likely to benefit in terms of body composition and function from weight lifting exercise. Instruct the patient to avoid exercise during febrile episodes or acute flares of disease, because the risk of complications is higher during this period.

Identification of depression, anxiety, or insomnia on screening is important, because these conditions all benefit from both resistive and aerobic exercise. There

functional status The ability of an individual independently to perform a task, activity, or behavior related to daily living.

sedentariness A state of low level of energy expenditure in voluntary physical activity; an overall lifestyle characterized by a habitual low level of movement in daily activities and occupational or recreational pursuits.

are numerous conditions that many health professionals consider contraindications to exercise, for example, severe withdrawal or lethargy and cognitive impairment. However, the patient may simply require additional treatments and safety precautions and closer supervision for the exercise prescription to be successful. In these circumstances, group activity or the assistance of a nonimpaired spouse, exercise trainer, or home care worker may be helpful. Screen for aggressive or disruptive behavior, poor safety awareness and judgment, or uncontrolled alcohol intake, because these will dictate the feasibility of group or isolated activity.

Contrary to common belief, in an institutional setting with an adequate staff-to-patient ratio all but the most severely cognitively impaired patients can successfully participate in exercise. Exercise is currently being explored as a preventive and therapeutic treatment for both mild cognitive impairment and established dementia. This comes in response to a host of epidemiological studies that have identified a protective effect of higher physical activity levels on brain structure and function, reducing the risk and rate of incident cognitive decline. The mechanisms underlying this benefit are currently unknown, but some researchers suggest that exercise decreases visceral fat and associated inflammatory cytokines and cortisol that are destructive to neurons. They also suggest that exercise may decrease cardiovascular disease and insulin resistance and improve cerebral blood flow and nerve growth factors and neural networks.

Patients with peripheral vascular disease (PVD) or neuropathy need to be particularly careful about sudden increases in weight-bearing activities. If ulcers develop on the foot or ankle and ambulation is temporarily restricted, patients may substitute seated weight-lifting exercises to prevent disuse atrophy from occurring during a period of reduced activity. Additionally, PRT has been shown to improve claudication, although probably less than those accruing from aerobic exercise.

Visual problems are common in the geriatric patient. Optimal lighting, exercise during the day, and use of corrective lenses at all times will minimize safety problems associated with visual problems. Blind individuals should not be automatically denied an exercise prescription. Substitution of stationary bikes, rowers, and steppers for other aerobic activities allows even these patients to exercise vigorously without supervision. As with any exercising individual, older patients who experience changes in chronic patterns warrant referral to a medical practitioner.

The Use of Exercise in the Prevention and Treatment of Common Geriatric Symptoms

It is not necessary to develop a specific exercise prescription for every medical condition that a person may have. Most individuals with one or more chronic diseases and their associated disabilities will benefit from both resistance training and aerobic training at the dosages indicated in **Table 19-7**. The four major components of fitness—strength, endurance, flexibility, and balance—should be incorporated into the exercise prescription for general health.

The goal should be to gradually get individuals to incorporate most or all of these modalities into their weekly routine, regardless of their specific medical history. This is particularly important for individuals who cannot participate in one mode of exercise at all. For example, older adults living in a retirement village demonstrated a decrease in depressive symptoms with a multimodal exercise program that included progressive resistance training, aerobic training, and progressive balance training proportional to their improvements in muscle strength. Older adults who are unable or unwilling to regularly attend exercise classes can still gain improvements in functional performance by combining weight training with functional training, thus minimizing a potential barrier to program adherence.

In addition to isolated diseases, older patients commonly present with multifactorial syndromes for which standard medical treatment often has little to offer. For these syndromes, exercise may be very therapeutic and have far fewer side effects than attempts at pharmacological management, which may contribute to polypharmacy and iatrogenic disease. For example, an obese older woman with severe degenerative disease of the knees who cannot ambulate without severe pain will benefit in terms of mood, arthritis pain, mobility, and weight loss from resistive exercises, which can be performed without standing. Some of the most commonly encountered scenarios and suggested approaches to exercise management are listed in Table 19-7.

Nutritional Considerations

Older adults who engage in regular exercise have some differences with regards to nutritional requirements compared to their sedentary counterparts. Energy requirements may increase with exercise if sufficient volumes and intensities are achieved and can work to an individual's advantage in numerous ways depending on the patient's BMI and medical condition. For those individuals who start an exercise regimen when they are advised to lose weight, the incorporation of nutritional recommendations with activity suggestions is critical to the success of attempts to achieve a negative energy balance. The caloric deficit created by the increased activity can aid weight loss without necessitating unrealistically large or unsustainable dietary energy restrictions. Alternatively, older individuals who need to improve their dietary quality or maintain body weight can use the appetite stimulation created by exercise as an opportunity to add a variety of nutritious foods to their diet without

TABLE 19-7 Choice of Exercise for Common Geriatric Syndromes

Syndrome	Therapeutic Exercise Recommendation
Anorexia	Endurance or resistance training before meals
Constipation	Endurance or resistance exercise
Depression, anxiety, low self-efficacy	Individual or group exercises, including endurance, resistive, and callisthenic activities, as preferred
Fatigue	Endurance training in the morning hours; increase duration and intensity, as tolerated
Functional dependency	Walking, stair climbing for endurance; resistance training of upper and lower extremities
Incontinence (stress)	Pelvic muscle strengthening (Kegel exercises); mobility improvement with endurance, balance, and resistance training, as needed
Insomnia	Endurance or resistance exercise in mid-afternoon (4 to 6 hours before bedtime)
Low back pain, spinal stenosis	Resistance training to strengthen the back extensor muscles, rectus abdominus, and hip and knee extensor muscle groups
Recurrent falls, gait and balance disorders	Lower extremity resistance training for hip, knee and ankle; balance training, Tai Chi, yoga, ballet; walking in safe or supported environment; training in use of ambulatory device as needed
Weakness	Moderate- to high-intensity resistance training for all major muscle groups

overconsumption of energy, which could contribute to undesirable adipose tissue gain. Increased protein intake may be required for anabolic adaptation (muscle hypertrophy) to resistance training, given the marginal protein intake in some older cohorts and the reduced protein synthesis rate observed in even healthy older individuals. In most older adults, however, this should be achieved with standard dietary plans, without requiring specialized dietary protein supplements. **Box 19-3** outlines guidelines for commonly encountered exercise–nutrition interactions.

Older adults are often victims of nutrition quackery. They can easily fall prey to the false promises of good health, longevity, and symptom relief of nutritional supplements, which seem too good for many individuals to resist. Education is often required for older adults regarding overstated advertising claims for many expensive "nutrition" products. Often, these individuals will have questions about what to eat when exercising or the need for special drinks, supplements, or protein sources. In general, individuals should be advised that food sources are preferable to packaged supplements, because this encourages greater dietary diversity. Concerns regarding the efficacy and safety of these products as well as the potential for drug interactions must also be discussed with the individual.

Practical Implementation of Exercise Programs

Because the exercise prescription will affect functional capacity, health status, nutritional requirements, psychological status, and other lifestyle changes, it will be most effective if it is integrated with the other components of the individual's care plan. All members of the health care team should be educated on the goals of the exercise program, the patient's physical activity patterns, and exercise prescription. Easily completed forms for patient assessment in terms of exercise history, physical performance, exercise prescription, and activity logs should be made available to the health care team.

Most environments can be modified to encourage rather than restrict activity; this is as true of the doctor's or nutritionist's office as it is of the nursing home. Creativity in implementing the program will go a long way. Community-dwelling older adults who are unable to get out frequently to exercise or who are self-conscious about exercising in public or group settings can exercise in their own home with relatively little equipment or training. Minimally supervised exercise is safe and has been shown to improve functional performance and balance in older individuals. However, compliance, adherence, and progression are difficult to achieve in totally unsupervised home-based programs, and adaptations and health benefits may therefore be compromised. Intermittent supervision and a strong behavioral change program with ongoing support, feedback, and self-monitoring of behavior may optimize this mode of delivery.

Institutional settings can provide a health library with reference works on major exercise techniques. Waiting rooms or lobbies should have tables with educational materials to read and videos showing various exercises. The videos could also be available to view on demand in the waiting room or even borrowed from the library for home use. Stairways should be accessible (rather than prohibited

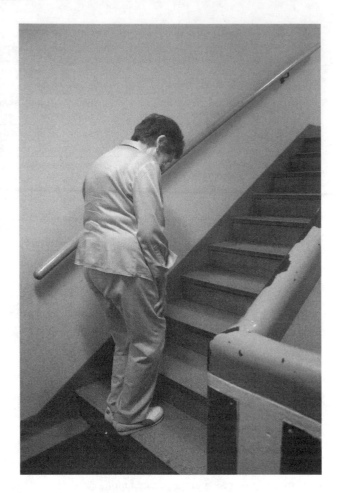

> ◗ **BOX 19-3 Nutritional Recommendations for the Physically Active Older Adult**
>
> 1. Encourage extra water intake (500–1,000 mL) on exercise days, especially by those on diuretics or very low-sodium diets, during high ambient temperatures or humid conditions, and after recovery from dehydrating illnesses or fevers. Sports drink formulations are unnecessary for fluid replacement under normal conditions and in noncompetitive athletes.
>
> 2. If a goal is fat/weight loss, combine exercise with a balanced hypocaloric diet and supplement with a multivitamin at RDA levels.
>
> 3. If a goal is weight maintenance, counsel on increased energy intake (with normal ratios of fat/carbohydrate/protein) through food rather than supplements. Encourage dietary diversity to fulfill energy requirements and supply micronutrient needs.
>
> 4. If a goal is weight gain, add nutrient- and energy-dense food snacks between meals and after exercise sessions.
>
> 5. There is generally no need to supplement protein beyond 1.0 to 1.2 g/kg/per day, which can be achieved with diverse dietary sources rather than amino acid or protein supplements. However, for sarcopenia, intake of high-protein foods or supplements within the one-hour period following resistance-training exercise may increase lean mass accretion and associated functional benefits.
>
> 6. In diabetics, time exercise sessions for the postprandial peaks in blood glucose (1.5 to 2 hours after a meal); keep high carbohydrate and concentrated sugar snacks available during exercise sessions for brittle or insulin-dependent diabetics; advise against exercise after prolonged fasting or skipping meals. Increased intake of foods with a low glycemic index and complex carbohydrates may assist in minimizing blood glucose excursions.
>
> 7. Increase dietary or pharmacological sources of potassium and magnesium if levels are marginal or low, particularly in high-risk coronary artery disease or arrhythmia-prone patients on diuretics or digoxin.

from use by patients) and marked clearly to encourage use, be well lighted, and have sturdy handrails. Provide incentives for exercise adherence in the form of reduced fees, free exercise equipment, lottery tickets, or whatever is meaningful to the clientele and staff in a particular setting. Even video games designed to increase physical activity have been marketed with increasing popularity to older adults and nursing home residents. The video games provide not only mechanisms for increasing movement but also active socialization and neurocognitive rehabilitation after stroke, brain injury, or disuse. Interactive video games such as the Nintendo Wii and the Sony PlayStation have become common features of physical therapy and activities departments in a growing number of facilities. Although the scientific literature has not established their benefit in older adults, the use of such game systems in a supervised and safe environment may benefit energy expenditure, flexibility, balance, mental status, and program compliance, as seen in younger adults and rehabilitation patients.

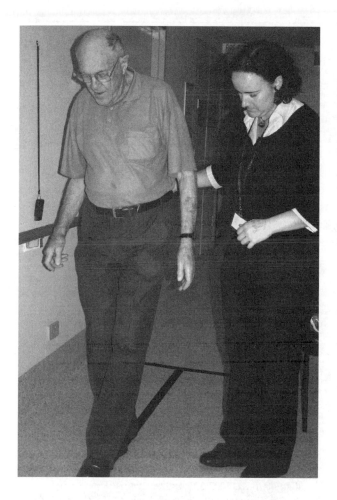

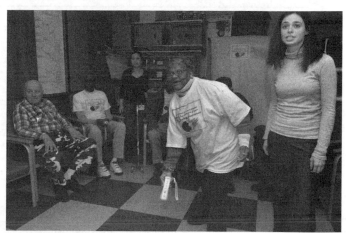

Physical activity and age-appropriate exercise interventions have the potential to increase and preserve skeletal muscle mass, to improve physical functioning, and to prevent disability across the lifespan.

Caregivers, family members, and volunteers are responsible for providing education, opportunity, and access to even the eldest members of our communities. Health care practices and policies for older adults must be enlarged to promote fitness, activity, and independence to the fullest extent possible for each individual as an important component of overall quality of life. Additional research needs to be carried out to identify ways to disseminate the robust findings of randomized controlled trials of exercise and aging to real-world, community-based settings.

Encouraging practitioners to become more physically active will be the most successful way to ensure that they encourage their older patients to exercise. The exercise prescription will carry a lot more credibility if a patient sees his or her practitioner following an exercise prescription too.

Conclusion

Physical fitness is not merely a medical prescription or treatment; it is a right of individuals, both fit and frail, to minimize and delay what was once considered "normal aging."

Activities Related to This Chapter

1. Briefly describe the importance of exercise to older adults. Be sure to discuss the benefits of the various forms of exercise and the related benefits for older adults.
2. Explain how exercise can be used in the prevention and treatment of common geriatric syndromes.
3. If you are not already physically active or in a formal exercise program, try following one for one month. Chart your weekly progress in strength, flexibility, and endurance.

REFERENCES

American College of Sports Medicine. *ASCM's Resource Manual for Guidelines for Exercise Testing and Prescription*. 5th ed. Baltimore, MD: Lippincott Williams and Wilkins; 2005.

American College of Sports Medicine. Physical activity and public health guidelines. Available at: http://www.acsm.org/AM/Template.cfm?Section = Home_Page&TEMPLATE = /CM/HTMLDisplay.cfm&CONTENTID = 7764. Accessed July 7, 2009.

Baker MK, Kennedy DJ, Bohle PL, et al. Efficacy and feasibility of a novel tri-modal robust exercise prescription in a retirement community: a randomized, controlled trial. *J Am Geriatr Soc.* 2007;55(1):1–10.

Ballor DL, Harvey-Berino JR, Ades PA, Cryan J, Calles-Escandon J. Contrasting effects of resistance and aerobic training on body composition and metabolism after diet-induced weight loss. *Metab Clin Exp.* 1996;45(2):179–183.

Betker AL, Szturm T, Moussavi ZK, et al. Video–game-based exercises for balance and rehabilitation: a single-subject design. *Arch Phys Med Rehabil.* 2006;87(8):1141–1149.

Bortz WM. Redefining human aging. *J Am Geriatr Soc.* 1989;37(11):1092–1096.

Braith R, Mills R, Welsch M, Keller J, Pollock M. Resistance exercise training restores bone mineral density in heart transplant recipients. *J Am Coll Cardiol.* 1996;28(6):1471–1477.

Braith R, Welsch M, Mills R, Keller J, Pollock M. Resistance exercise prevents glucocorticoid-induced myopathy in heart transplant recipients. *Med Sci Sports Exerc.* 1998;30:483–489.

Campbell W, Crim M, Dallal G, Young V, Evans W. Increased protein requirements in the elderly: new data and retrospective reassessments. *Am J Clin Nutr.* 1994;60:501–509.

Campbell WW, Crim MC, Young VR, Evans WJ. Increased energy requirements and body composition changes with resistance training in older adults. *Am J Clin Nutr.* 1994;60:167–175.

Castaneda C, Gordon P, Uhlin K, et al. Resistance training to counteract the catabolism of a low protein diet in chronic renal insufficiency: A randomized controlled trial. *Ann Intern Med.* 2001; 135:965–976.

Centers for Disease Control. Physical activity for everyone: how much physical activity do older adults need? Available at: http://www.cdc.gov/physicalactivity/everyone/guidelines/olderadults.html. Accessed July 7, 2009.

Chan M, Cheema BS, Fiatarone Singh MA. Progressive resistance training and nutrition in renal failure. *J Ren Nutr.* 2007;17(1):84–87.

Chandler JM, Hadley EC. Exercise to improve physiologic and functional performance in old age. *Clin Geriatric Med.* 1996;12(4):761–784.

Chumlea W, Guo S, Glaser R, Vellas B. Sarcopenia, function, and health. *Nutr Health Aging* 1997;1(1):7–12.

Despres JP, Lemieux I, Prud'homme D. Treatment of obesity: Need to focus on high risk abdominally obese patients. *Br Med J.* 2001;322(7288):716–720.

Evans WJ, Campbell WW. Sarcopenia and age-related changes in body composition and functional capacity. *J Nutr.* 1993;123:465–468.

Fiatarone MA, O'Neill EF, Ryan ND, et al. Exercise training and nutritional supplementation for physical frailty in very elderly people. *New Engl J Med.* 1994;330:1769–1775.

Fiatarone Singh M, Ding W, Manfredi T, et al. Insulin-like growth factor I in skeletal muscle after weight-lifting exercise in frail elders. *Am J Physiol (Endo and Metab).* 1999;277:E136–E43.

Fiatarone Singh M. Combined exercise and dietary intervention to optimize body composition in aging. *Ann of the New York Acad Sci.* 1998;854:378–393.

Fiatarone Singh MA. Benefits of exercise and dietary measures to optimize shifts in body composition with age. *Asia Pac J Clin Nutr.* 2002;11(suppl 3):S642–S52.

Flynn S, Palma P, et al. Feasibility of using the Sony Playstation 2 gaming platform for an individual poststroke: a case report. *J Neurol Phys Ther.* 2007;31(4):180–189.

Folsom A, Kay S, Sellers T. Body fat distribution and 5-year risk of death in older women. *JAMA.* 1993;269:483–487.

Graves L, Stratton G, Ridgers ND, Cable NT. Comparison of energy expenditure in adolescents when playing new generation and sedentary computer games: cross-sectional study. *BMJ.* 2007;335:1282–1284.

Healy GN, Dunstan DW, Salmon J, Shaw JE, Zimmet PZ, Owen N. Television time and continuous metabolic risk in physically active adults. *Med Sci Sports Exer.* 2008;40(4):639–645.

Healy GN, Dunstan DW, Salmon J, et al. Breaks in sedentary time. *Diabetes Care.* 2008;31:661–666.

Henwood TR. Short-term resistance training and the older adult: the effect of varied programmes for the enhancement of muscle strength and functional performance. *Clin Physiol Funct Imaging.* 2006;26(5):305–313.

Huang Y, Macera C, Blair S, Brill P, Kohl H, Kronenfeld J. Physical fitness, physical activity, and functional limitations in adults aged 40 and older. *Med Sci Sports Exer.* 1998;30(9):1430–1435.

Hughes VA, Roubenoff R, Wood M, Frontera WR, Evans WJ, Fiatarone Singh MA. Anthropometric assessment of 10-y changes in body composition in the elderly. *Am J Clin Nutr.* 2004;80(2):475–482.

Journal of the American Medical Association. Fitness for older adults. Available at: http://jama.ama-assn.org/cgi/content/full/296/2/242. Accessed July 7, 2009.

Jurca R, Lamonte MJ, Barlow CE, Kampert JB, Church TS, Blair SN. Association of muscular strength with incidence of metabolic syndrome in med. *Med Sci Sports Exer.* 2005;37(11):1849–1855.

Kay SJ, Fiatarone Singh MA. The influence of physical activity on abdominal fat: a systematic review of the literature. *Obes Rev.* 2006;7(2):183–200.

Kempen GI, van Heuvelen MJ, van Sonderen E, van den Brink RH, Kooijman AC, Ormel J. The relationship of functional limitations to disability and the moderating effects of psychological attributes in community-dwelling older persons. *Soc Sci Med.* 1999;48(9):1161–1172.

Kohrt WM, Obert KA, Holloszy JO. Exercise training improves fat distribution patterns in 60- to 70-year-old men and women. *J Gerontol.* 1992;47(4):M99–M105.

Koop C. *The Surgeon General's Report on Nutrition and Health: U.S. Department of Health and Human Services.* Report No.: DHHS Publ. No. 88-50210; 1988.

Mayor S. International Diabetes Federation consensus on prevention of type 2 diabetes. *Int J Clin Pract.* 2007;61(10):1773–1775.

Miller M, Rejeski W, Reboussin B, TenHave T, Ettinger W. Physical activity, functional limitations and disabilities in older adults. *JAGS.* 2000;48:1264–1272.

Morley JE. Anorexia, sarcopenia and aging. *Nutrition.* 2001;17(7–8):660–663.

Nelson ME, Layne JE, Bernstein MJ, et al. The effects of multidimensional home-based exercise on functional performance in elderly people. *J Gerontol A Biol Sci Med Sci.* 2004;59(2):154–160.

Nelson ME, Rejeeski WJ, Blair SN, Duncan PW, Judge JO, et al. Physical activity and public health in older adults: recommendations from the American College of Sports Medicine and the American Heart Association. *Med Sci Sports Exerc.* 2007 Aug;39(8):1435–1445.

Orr R, de Vos NJ, Singh NA, Ross DA, Stavrinos TM, Fiatarone-Singh MA. Power training improves balance in healthy older adults. *J Gerontol A Biol Sci Med Sci.* 2006;61(1):78–85.

Paddon-James D, Short KR, Campbell WW, Volpi E, Wolfe RR. The role of dietary protein in the sarcopenia of aging. *Am J Clin Nutr.* 2008;87(suppl):1562S–1566S.

Paffenbarger R, Hyde R, Wing A, Hsieh C-C. Physical activity and longevity of college alumni. *N Engl J Med.* 1986;315:399–401.

Physical Activity Guidelines Advisory Committee. *Physical Activity Guidelines Advisory Committee Report, 2008.* Washington, DC: U.S. Department of Health and Human Services; 2008.

Prevalence of regular physical activity among adults—United States, 2001 and 2005. *MMWR Morb Mortal Wkly Rep.* 2007;56(46):1209–1212.

Ramachandran A, Snehalatha C, Yamauna A, Mary S, Ping Z. Cost-effectiveness of the interventions in the primary prevention of diabetes among Asian Indians: within-trial results of the Indian Diabetes Prevention Programme (IDPP). *Diabetes Care.* 2007;30(10):2548–2552.

Rogers MA, Hagberg JM, III WHM, Ehsani AA, Holloszy JO. Decline in VO2 max with aging master athletes and sedentary men. *J Appl Physiol.* 1990;68(5):2195–2199.

Schwartz RS, Shuman WP, Larson V, et al. The effect of intensive endurance exercise training on body fat distribution in young and older men. *Metab Clin Exp.* 1991;40(5):545–551.

Seynnes O, Fiatarone Singh MA, Hue O, Pras P, Legros P, Bernard PL. Physiological and functional responses to low-moderate versus high-intensity progressive resistance training in frail elders. *J Gerontol A Biol Sci Med Sci.* 2004;59(5):503–509.

Shephard RJ. Physical activity and reduction of health risks: how far are the benefits independent of fat loss? *J Sports Med Physical Fitness.* 1994;34(1):91–98.

Singh NA, Stavrinos TM, Scarbek Y, Galambos G, Liber C, Fiatarone Singh MA. A randomized controlled trial of high versus low intensity weight training versus general practitioner care for clinical depression in older adults. *J Gerontol A Biol Sci Med Sci.* 2005;60(6):768–776.

Stuck A, Walthert J, Nikolaus T, Bula C, Hohmann C, Beck J. Risk factors for functional status decline in community-living elderly people: a systematic literature review. *Soc Sci Med.* 1999;48:445–469.

Treuth M, Ryan A, Pratley R, et al. Effects of strength training on total and regional body composition in older men. *J Appl Physiol.* 1994;77:614–620.

Troiano RP, Berringan D, Dodd KW, Masse LC, Tilert T, McDowell M. Physical activity in the United States measured by accelerometer. *Med Sci Sports Exercise.* 2008;40(1):181–188.

U.S. Department of Health and Human Services and U.S. Department of Agriculture. *Dietary Guidelines for Americans, 2005.* Washington, D.C.: U.S. Department of Health and Human Services and U.S. Department of Agriculture.

U.S. Department of Health and Human Services. Physical activity and health: A report of the Surgeon General. Atlanta: U.S. Dept of Health and Human Services, Centers for Disease Control and Prevention, National Center for Chronic Disease Prevention and Health Promotion; 1996.

U.S. Department of Health and Human Services. 2008 Physical Activity Guidelines for Americans, At-A-Glace: A Fact Sheet for Professionals. Available at: http://www.health.gov/PAGuidelines/factsheetprof.aspx. Accessed July 7, 2009.

U.S. Department of Health and Human Services. 2008 Physical Activity Guidelines for Americans, Chapter 5: Active Older Adults. Available at: http://www.health.gov/

PAGuidelines/guidelines/Chapter5.aspx. Accessed July 7, 2009.

Visser M, Langlois J, Guralnik J, et al. High body fatness, but not low fat-free mass, predicts disability in older men and women: the Cardiovascular Health Study. *Am J Clin Nutr.* 1998;68:584–590.

Wang X, Perry AC. Metabolic and physiologic responses to video game play in 7- to 10-year-old boys. *Arch Pediatr Adolesc Med.* 2006;160(4):411–415.

Warburton DE, Bredin SS, Horita LT, et al. The health benefits of interactive video game exercise. *Appl Physiol Nutr Metab.* 2007;32(4):655–663.

Washburn R, Smith K, Jetter A, Janney C. The physical activity scale for the elderly (PASE): development and evaluation. *J Clin Epidemiol.* 1993;46(2):153–162.

CHAPTER 20

Diet and Cultural Diversity in Older Adults

Odilia I. Bermudez, PhD, MPH, LDN

....

CHAPTER OBJECTIVES   Upon completion of this chapter, the reader will be able to:

1. Illustrate how cultural values influence food choices made by elderly people
2. Demonstrate how cultural variances that exist among older adults from different cultures and generations influence how they fulfill their nutritional needs
3. Show basic knowledge and skills necessary to work with older adults from different cultural backgrounds
4. Understand the implications in risk of chronic disease with inadequate food choices that may be acquired by older adults when adjusting to a different, new culture

KEY TERMS AND CONCEPTS

Acculturation

Core Foods

Eating patterns

Foodways

....

The United States is a multicultural country; different ethnic groups have been entering the United States since pre-colonial periods. The United States was initially colonized by Europeans, particularly those from England, France, and Spain. Since that time, a multitude of ethnic groups have migrated here from all continents. Each of these groups has brought cultural characteristics that together have shaped what is today known as the American culture, transforming the United States into a diverse and multicultural nation. In the United States, older adults are the fastest growing population group, and one that is becoming more ethnically diverse. In 2006, about 19% of older adults belonged to a minority group (**Figure 20-1**).

Cultural differences impact food patterns and eating behaviors. At the most basic level, people need food to sustain basic physiological functions. However, what, when, and how to eat is based on acquired eating behaviors. The cultural and social influences that contribute to the food choices we make are complex and multifaceted. Acceptance or rejection of edible products is a learned behavior. Different cultures classify edible products as food based on learned experiences and transmitted myths and beliefs. Thus, the desire to eat a specific food, such as a piece of bread, a potato, or a tortilla, can thereby be considered to be a cultural behavior.

Older adults have developed lifelong **eating patterns** based on socio-demographic and psychosocial determinants as well as by the environmental circumstances associated with food access and availability. However, how cultural factors specifically influence food choices is still incompletely understood.

In this chapter, we attempt to critically assess some documented experiences related to food choices made by older adults from different cultures in order to highlight when such deci-

eating patterns The foods and beverages a person consumes on a regular basis; also includes behaviors surrounding eating events.

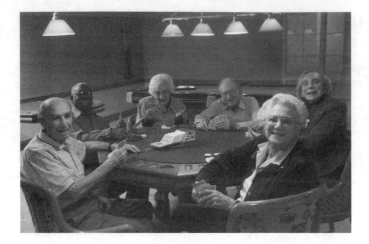

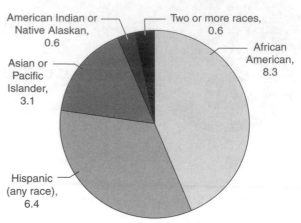

American Indian or Native Alaskan, 0.6

Asian or Pacific Islander, 3.1

Hispanic (any race), 6.4

Two or more races, 0.6

African American, 8.3

Total proportion of ethnic minority elderly adds up to 19% of elderly people (65 years of age and over). Non-Hispanic Whites represented 81% of the elderly population in 2006.

FIGURE 20-1 Ethnic Minority Population in the United States, 2006

Source: Administration on Aging and U.S. Department of Health and Human Services. A Profile of Older Americans: 2006. Washington, DC; 2007.

sions result in favorable (or unfavorable) outcomes and to elaborate on strategies and approaches to take into account when working with older adults in multicultural settings.

Food Choices and Older Adults

For many individuals, food is selected, prepared, served, and eaten based on culture. Limited information is available about culture and food choices among older adults. However, from that limited information it is clear that the interactions between food choices and the **acculturation** process that affects diverse ethnic groups in the United States are complex and dynamic.

In the United States, individuals from different ethnic groups start replacing traditional foods from the first to the second generation. For some Hispanic groups, such as Puerto Ricans and Dominicans, nutrient intake and dietary diversity improve with acculturation, whereas for others (e.g., Mexican American adult women) nutrient intake is negatively affected by acculturation.

Older individuals are more likely to maintain traditional food choices compared to younger individuals, because older adults' food preferences are well established. People arrive at their aging stage with strong, and sometimes lifelong, eating behaviors and patterns for food choices. Within their culture and their individual characteristics, they have already defined what their core foods are and what the various meanings of those foods

are. Individual **foodways** (traditions, beliefs, and myths around food) may include categorizations of core and secondary foods; religious and profane foods; healthy and unhealthy foods; foods of opposing categories, such as the hot–cold system developed by some Hispanic groups or the yin–yang (cold–hot) Chinese principles; and many other categorizations that orient their food choices.

Older adults' strong attachment to their food-related behaviors is multidimensional. It includes their cultural beliefs about appropriate food use in the presence of health and disease, beliefs about healing properties of foods, and attitudes as gatekeepers of cultural traditions, particularly those associated with their foodways.

The motivations for individuals to move into new cultures are often associated with economic, political, or educational factors. Rarely is the motivation associated with nutrition. However, a host culture will invariably affect the food choices made by those individuals. Some factors that may contribute to changes in food choices include, among others, access and availability of their cultural foods. Puerto Rican older adults, for example, grew up with a special appreciation for root crops (e.g., cassava, yautia, malanga and others). However, those who migrated to the Northeast United States use those products infrequently due to their high costs and low availability.

Changes in Food Selection with Age

Although most people reach older age with well-established food patterns, changes in food choices that occur later in

acculturation Process whereby a group or individual's culture is modified while adapting to another culture. With regards to diet, acculturation can be seen with immigrants who after years (and generations) of living in a new country begin to adopt food patterns similar to those of the host country.

foodways Food traditions or customs of a group of people; involves how foods are obtained, prepared, served, and consumed. Encompasses beliefs about food, food preferences, and customs; has cultural, social, and economic components as well.

life are most often a result of physiological, medical, or social factors. For example, medical conditions that may modify food choices include sensory losses with age (e.g., the taste and smell could become less intense); frailty, making shopping and food preparation more challenging; and other physical and mental health and medical changes that may force them to reluctantly alter their food preferences to accommodate those changes.

Although some older adults adapt to lower sensory stimulus, others compensate by eating more flavorful foods or adding enhancers (e.g., adding more table salt or more sweeteners) to their meals. Older adults with functional declines tend to eat less and more slowly. Dietary variety may decrease, because older adults may become attached to a limited number of foods that are easier to prepare, cook, and eat. There is little information about how they manage to maintain their attachment to their cultural foods under such circumstances.

Dietary Patterns of Different Ethnic/Racial Older Adults

The traditional food system is one of individual characterizations that are more resilient to the effects of the acculturation process in diverse ethnic groups. **Table 20-1** shows traditionally common foods (**core foods**) for various ethnic groups. Maintenance of traditional eating patterns usually persists beyond the first generation of immigrants or after extended periods of residence in the host society. For example, older Puerto Ricans living in Massachusetts, including those less and more acculturated to the mainstream American culture, tend to maintain their traditional foods, including rice, beans, cooking oil, and coffee with milk, as their main sources of dietary energy and macronutrients, even though the diets of more acculturated older adults tend to resemble the standard American diet. One explanation for this is that older adults maintain their attachment to their food systems as a source of cohesion and comfort.

Dietary Patterns: Implications for Nutrition Education and Intervention

The aging process, especially if it is not free of damaging events, may force the older adult to restructure his or her foodways. If drastic changes in older adults' eating practices go undetected for extended periods of time, their health and well-being could be affected, because nutritional imbalances could occur. Therefore, culturally appropriate nutrition education and intervention for older adults needs to take into account their individual characteristics while maintaining a focus on the prevention and alleviation of nutrition-related chronic conditions that affect important proportions of the older population in the United States. Some of those chronic conditions, including obesity and obesity-related chronic conditions, are listed in **Table 20-2**.

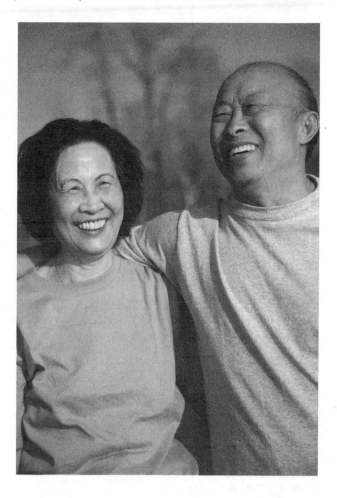

Food-related behaviors that are important to address in nutrition education and promotion efforts include the practice of healthy eating patterns with the inclusion of cultural foods, the use the Nutrition Fact Labels, the incorporation of more physical activity, and the avoidance of alcohol and tobacco. Successful communication with ethnic populations can be enhanced by not only developing awareness of their individual cultural and circumstances, but also "speaking their language." More and more organizations working with older adults are engaged in the incorporation of cultural aspects and the use of different languages to improve their educational efforts and better meet the needs of their target groups.

The Administration on Aging recognizes that, compared to the older adult in general, those from minority groups are at greater risk for social, economic, nutrition, and health-related problems. To alleviate those problems, the agency has included on its website a section addressing diversity among older adults in the

core foods The most commonly consumed foods for a population or group or people.

TABLE 20-1 Common Foods for Various Ethnic Groups and Vegetarians

Asian
Pineapples, bananas, mangos, tangerines, watermelon, grapes, pears, carrots, broccoli, mushrooms, bok choy, cabbage, bamboo shoots, chilies, bean sprouts, scallions, onion, leafy greens, nori, peppers, millet, rice, noodles, breads, soybeans, peanuts, dried beans, ginger root, garlic, salted pickles, soybeans, miso, tofu, vegetable oils, fish/shellfish, egg, poultry, pork, red meat, ice cream, sorbets, tea
Latin American
Maize, potatoes, rice, bread, taro, tortillas, arepa, black beans, seeds, quinoa, malanga, peanuts, amaranth, legumes, cassava, pecans, potatoes, sweet potatoes, pumpkin, plantains, yucca, garbanzo beans, pinto beans, limes, bananas, avocados, cacao, breadfruit, plums, apples, berries, papayas, mangos, cherimoya, guanabana, pineapple, melon, tamarind, quince, grapes, guava, oranges, kiwi, kale, cactus, eggplant, turnip, chard, squash, hot peppers, cilantro, zucchini, onions, broccoli, okra, spinach, lettuce, tomatoes, tomatillos, sweet peppers, chilies, plant oils (soy, corn, olive), milk, cheese, shrimp, salmon, snapper, mussels, fowl, turkey, chicken, eggs
African American
Root vegetables, taro roots, manioc, beets, eggplant, yam, peas, sweet potatoes, white potatoes, collards, black-eyed peas, okra, tomatoes, corn, watermelon, lemons, oranges, peaches, pears, dates, figs, grapes, pomegranates, melons, peanuts, salt pork, bacon fat, lard, shortening, cornmeal, biscuits, fried chicken, fatty pork chops, bacon, sausages, spareribs, nuts, pecan pie, butter-filled pastry, syrup, catfish, bread pudding, cornbread, biscuits, rice pilafs, cooked cereal, puddings, fruit pies, sweet potato pie, deep-fried breaded meat, barbecued ribs, wheat, barley, rice, millet, dried beans, fava beans, lentils, goat, chicken, fish, beef, wild game, coffee, olives, fruit cobbler, rice corn, bread, eggs, cookies, chocolate, hard candy, soda, sweetened drinks
Native American*
Acorns, pumpkin, hominy corn, beans, carrots, onion, celery, corn, peas, green beans, squash, onion, sunflower seeds, legumes, cactus leaves, cactus fruit, apricots, melons, peaches, figs, fish, deer, seeds, mesquite pods, wild rice, sunflower oil, pigweed flour, wheat, mint, lamb, currents, blueberries, raspberries, blackberries, chokecherries, pin cherries, strawberries, cranberries, and rosehips wild meats, poultry, fish, deer meat, walleye pike, northern pike, sucker fish, whitefish, and rabbit, maple syrup, tea.
(*Traditional foods will vary by tribal custom and food availability.)
Vegetarian
Corn, grapes, raisins, pears, avocados, oranges, melon, apples, bananas, plums, cherries, dried fruits, mushrooms, tomatoes, kale, broccoli, collards, sweet potatoes, peppers, asparagus, cucumber, potatoes, onions, carrots, cabbage, squash, leeks, eggplant, celery, lettuce, various beans, legumes, oats, wheat, rice, buckwheat, soy flour, flax, bulgur, quinoa, seitan, tempeh, tofu, textured vegetable protein, barley, bread, pita, tortilla, couscous, noodles, kasha, pasta, eggs, soy milk, cheese, yogurt, nuts, peanut butter, plant oils pie, custard, ice cream, cake, cookies
(*Products are often organic and actual foods included depend on vegetarian classification.)

Sources: Data from U.S. Departamento de Agricultura. MiPirámide: pasos hacia una mejor salud (Spanish). 2008. Available at: http://www.mypyramid.gov/sp-index.html. Accessed April 29, 2008; U.S. Department of Agriculture. MyPyramid: steps to a healthier you. 2006. Available at http://www.mypyramid.gov/. Accessed February 15, 2008; Oldways Preservation Trust. Available at: http://www.oldwayspt.org/. Accessed May 22, 2008.

United States. The section includes a cultural competency module, program modules, and various helpful resources. The Office of Minority Health of the U.S. Department of Health and Human Services offers important resources on minority populations, cultural competency, and a Spanish-language website. Another organization, the American Diabetes Association, has developed educational materials in Spanish to address the growing number of Hispanics, including older adults, affected by type 2 diabetes. The American Dietetic Association offers a diversity resource list and its Nutrition Care Manual offers detailed information on the food practices of many ethnic groups. The WIC Works Resource System offers consumer-friendly factsheets, a valuable resource for any health care provider working with culturally diverse populations.

Factors that may increase older adults' cultural acceptability of nutrition education are listed in **Table 20-3**. Specific tools are available to support nutrition education efforts for older adults, including the Dietary Guidelines for Americans and similar guidelines issued in many other countries, which could be useful when dealing with ethnic groups in need of specific culturally sensitive approaches. Pictorial representations of food guidelines specific for older adults also are available, such as the Tufts Food Guide Pyramid for people over 70 years of age. Many other pictorial representations that could also facilitate nutrition education efforts for ethnically diverse older adults are available from other countries. As an example, **Figure 20-2** shows the Spanish version of MyPyramid, which is available at *www.mypyramid.gov.*

TABLE 20-2 Nutrition-Related Chronic Conditions That May Require Culturally Sensitive Nutrient Adaptations

Obesity, particularly abdominal obesity

Diabetes, particularly type 2 diabetes

Cardiovascular disease

Certain cancers (lung, breast, colorectal, prostate, pancreas, and brain)

Osteoporosis

Physical impairment, including age-associated frailty

Cognitive impairment and dementia, particularly Alzheimer's disease

Behavioral and psychological disorders

Source: Bermudez OI, Tucker KL. Total and central obesity among elderly Hispanics and the association with type 2 diabetes. *Obes Res.* 2001;9(8):443–451; Harris MI, et al. Prevalence of diabetes, impaired fasting glucose tolerance in U.S. adults: the Third National Health and Nutrition Examination Survey, 1988–1994. *Diabetes Care.* 1998;21(4):518–524; Must A, et al. The disease burden associated with overweight and obesity. *JAMA.* 1999;282(16):1523–1529; Ogden CL, et al. Prevalence of overweight and obesity in the United States, 1999–2004. *JAMA.* 2006;295(13):1549–1555.

TABLE 20-3 Factors Associated with Increasing Cultural Acceptability of Nutrition Education

Acknowledge the older adult's role as an active participant in his or her own diet-related care.

Promote foods that are culturally appropriate.

Be sensitive to food traditions and beliefs.

Be sensitive to the inclusion of religion in food selection and preparation.

Avoid making requests for radical changes in dietary practices.

Identify positive dietary patterns and promote them.

Encourage the use of healthy traditional foods.

Use appropriate language in delivering the messages.

Interpret verbal and nonverbal diet-related behaviors in a culturally relevant manner.

Be aware of the culture shock experienced by the recent older adult immigrant.

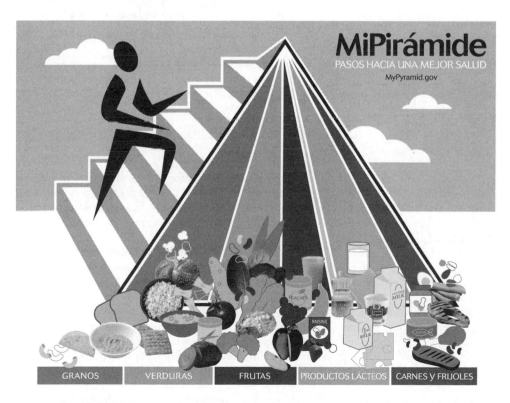

FIGURE 20-2 MyPyramid for Spanish-speakers

Source: U.S. Departamento de Agricultura. MiPirámide: pasos hacia una mejor salud (Spanish). 2008. Available at: http://www.mypyramid.gov/sp-index.html. Accessed April 29, 2008.

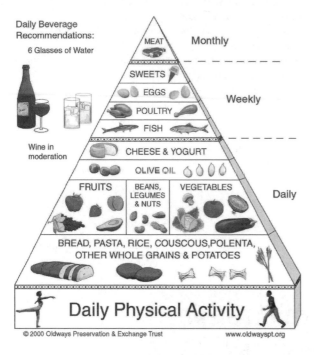

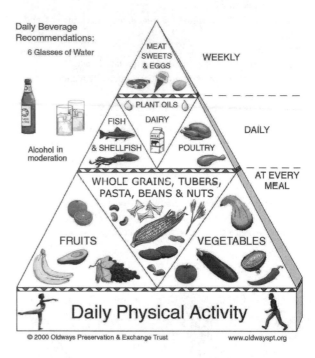

FIGURE 20-3 The Mediterranean Diet Pyramid, Latin American Diet Pyramid, Asian American Diet Pyramid, and Vegetarian Diet Pyramid

Source: Oldways Preservation and Exchange Trust.

Oldways Preservation and Exchange Trust has developed food pyramids to reflect the foodways of various cultural groups. The Mediterranean Diet Pyramid, the Latin American Diet Pyramid, and the Asian Diet Pyramid, found in **Figure 20-3**, are based on the dietary traditions of these regions. Although variations of a healthy vegetarian diet exist throughout the world, the Vegetarian Diet Pyramid, also shown in Figure 20-3, represents a traditional healthy vegetarian diet. Because these diet pyramids describe diets for healthy adults, adjustments must be made to meet the nutritional requirements, health status, and functional limitations of older adults.

Culturally Appropriate Programs for the Older Adult

Ethnic minority older adults are a special population group, because, in addition to being in a minority group, they have the double jeopardy of also being old. Healthy People 2010 states that special population groups often require targeted preventive efforts and that such efforts involve understanding the needs and the particular disparities experienced by those groups. The two overarching Healthy People 2010 goals specific to ethnic older adults: (1) to increase quality and years of healthy life and (2) to eliminate health disparities. These two goals should be addressed when considering food and nutrition and health programs for ethnically diverse older adults.

As the United States becomes increasingly culturally and linguistically diverse, disparities in health care access and status and nutrition-related services are becoming major issues. To work in solving these disparities, health and nutrition professionals working with older adult groups must become culturally sensitive and competent, because there is a direct relationship between the level of competence of health and nutrition professionals and their ability to provide culturally responsive health care services. A

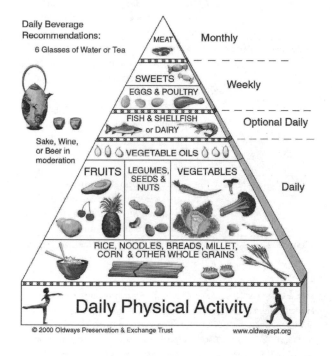

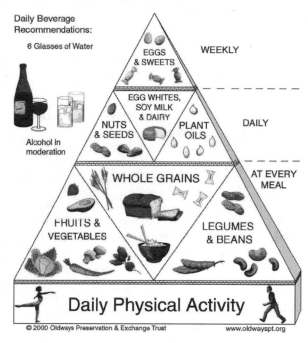

FIGURE 20-3 The Mediterranean Diet Pyramid, Latin American Diet Pyramid, Asian American Diet Pyramid, and Vegetarian Diet Pyramid (Continued)

Source: Oldways Preservation and Exchange Trust.

culturally competent professional is aware of, supportive of, and respectful of the cultural differences among diverse racial, ethnic, and other minority groups and is proactive in bringing that knowledge to the professional practice. Those working with ethnically diverse elders need to pursue a satisfactory level of cultural competence, as their respect and understanding of cultural diversity in food choices and eating patterns is critical for successful delivery of the planned activities.

When designing nutrition guidance for older adults, health care providers must understand the underlying motivations and decision-making processes that influence food choices. Food choices are influenced by individual and situational factors as well as by cultural influences. A professional's respect and understanding of cultural diversity in food choices and eating patterns is critical for successful delivery of planned activities. **Table 20-4** lists intercultural

concepts, knowledge, skills, and attitudes that illustrate the need for culturally competent care for the older adults. As shown in **Table 20-5**, culturally competence includes five constructs: cultural awareness, cultural knowledge, cultural skill, cultural encounters, and cultural desire.

Institutions dealing with ethnic minority older adults should create a sensitive and inclusive environment where diverse older adults can engage and participate in positive ways. Institutions and organizations need to incorporate various components such as those found in **Table 20-6** to demonstrate a culturally competent environment. A partial list of organizations and programs that provide insights, materials, and resources about cultural competence for the nutrition and health professional can be found in **Table 20-7**.

Several approaches could be tested when working on designing professional and work-related settings where older adults from diverse ethnic and cultural backgrounds could

TABLE 20-4 Becoming Culturally Competent: Intercultural Areas and Learning Objectives

Intercultural Areas	Learning Objectives
Basic concepts	Culture is important in every subject's identity, particularly in older adults from minority groups or recent immigrants.
	Culture-related stresses and tensions can affect eating practices and induce illness.
	Culture-related behaviors can affect the older adult's acceptance of and compliance with prescribed therapy or dietary regimen.
	Nonverbal and verbal communication may differ from culture to culture.
Knowledge to be acquired	Culture-specific dietary habits, foods, and their nutritional components
	Predominant cultural values, health practices, and traditional health beliefs
	Impact of religion on health beliefs and practices.
	Significance of common verbal and nonverbal communication
Skills to be developed	Interpret verbal and nonverbal behaviors in a culturally relevant manner.
	Recognize culture-related eating patterns.
	Respect differences in eating behaviors.
	Have basic or essential language proficiency.
	Negotiate a culturally relevant care plan with the older adult as a partner.
Intercultural attitudes	Recognize the importance of the older adult's cultural background and environment when constructing a dietary plan.
	Acknowledge possible changes in eating practices due to the aging process, along with culture-specific attributes.

Source: Data from Office of Minority Health. Teaching cultural competence in health care: a review of current concepts, policies and practices. Available at: http://www.omhrc.gov/assets/pdf/checked/em01garcia1.pdf. Accessed July 15, 2009.

TABLE 20-5 Interdependent Constructs of Cultural Competence

Constructs	Conceptualization
Cultural awareness	The health/nutrition care provider becomes appreciative and sensitive to the values, beliefs, lifestyles, practices, and problem-solving strategies of the older adult's culture.
Cultural knowledge	Seeks and obtains a solid educational foundation about the commonalities and differences of diverse cultures and ethnic groups.
Cultural skill	Is able to collect and interpret data regarding the older adult's dietary patterns, health behaviors, situation within a culturally appropriate framework.
Cultural encounters	The health/nutrition care provider engages directly in cross-cultural interactions with older adults from culturally diverse backgrounds.
Cultural desire	The health care provider "wants to" engage in the process of cultural competence.

Source: Data from Office of Minority Health. Teaching cultural competence in health care: a review of current concepts, policies and practices. Available at: http://www.omhrc.gov/assets/pdf/checked/em01garcia1.pdf. Accessed July 15, 2009; Campinha-Bacote J. The process of cultural competence in the delivery of healthcare services: a model of care. *J Transcultural Nursing.* 2002;13(3):181–184.

TABLE 20-6 Components of a Culturally Competent Organization

A Culturally Competent Organization:
Values diversity.
Implements cultural self-assessment.
Is conscious of the dynamics inherent when cultures interact (how and where the service is provided must also be taken into consideration).
Has institutionalized cultural knowledge.
Develops adaptations of service delivery based on understanding of cultural diversity.

Source: Data from Administration on Aging. Available at: http://www.aoa.gov/prof/adddiv/adddiv.asp.

find services and support tailored to their health, nutritional, socioeconomic, and cultural needs. A solid knowledge of the cultural characteristics of the target populations is invaluable, as demonstrated with the successful delivery of some interventions targeting minority groups that could serve as models when working with minority older adults. For example, changes in fat consumption in culturally diverse populations were achieved with a culturally sensitive nutrition intervention. In another example, the Traditional Hawaiian Diet (THD) program for adults, developed as a

TABLE 20-7 Online Resources Addressing Cultural Competence

Organization
Center for Linguistic and Cultural Competency in Health Care, Office of Minority Health (OMH), Dept. of Health and Human Services (DHHS)
Office of Minority Health National Culturally and Linguistically Appropriate Services (CLAS) Standards
Agency for Healthcare Research and Quality, DHHS
National Center for Cultural Competence, Georgetown University Center for Child and Human Development
National Standards for Culturally & Linguistically Appropriate Services in Health Care, OMH, DHHS
Think Cultural Health, OMH, DHHS
Multicultural Health Clearinghouse, McKinley Health Center, University of Illinois at Urbana-Champaign
Diversity Rx
EthnoMed
Cross Cultural Health Care Program
The American Dietetic Association Diversity Resource List
Oldways
American Dietetic Association Nutrition Care Manual
WIC Works

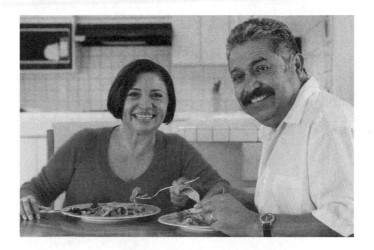

culturally appropriate community intervention, demonstrated high success, as indicated by the reported increases in intakes of all major nutrients, including key vitamins and minerals. Finally, the Strong Heart Diet Study continues to add to the knowledge of dietary patterns of Adult American Indians and the relationship to cardiovascular disease, metabolic syndrome, and insulin resistance.

If cultural and language-related barriers are not taken into consideration in the design of nutrition interventions for minority older adults, the implementation of those programs could risk failure and create disillusion among the targeted individuals. Examination of fat-related dietary behaviors of Hispanic and non-Hispanic White and African American adults, suggests important differences in the behaviors among those ethnic groups. Understanding the ethnic aging process can provide insight on health and longevity and information for better programs and services.

Conclusion

Food choices of older adults from different cultural backgrounds are dictated not only by their social, economic, and physiological needs, but also by their culture of origin and the degree to which they have been acculturated into mainstream America. The identification of cultural foods by ethnic groups changes over time, as acculturation takes place. The present challenge is how to overcome the many limitations in the current understanding of culture, acculturation, and aging as dynamic processes that modulate the demands of the older adult target groups.

Aging populations are increasing rapidly, requiring more and better care and services. Older adults may have high levels of illness and lifestyle change that significantly affect their eating patterns. They may also be immersed in their cultural environments and demand that their foodways be addressed and respected. However, the scarcity of tested materials and strategies that could guide culturally appropriate programs for older adults could limit health care providers' responses to meeting those demands. Such limitations need to be overcome with more resources and efforts from health and nutrition service providers. In addition, research is needed on dietary behaviors and the appropriate channels, theories, and messages for delivery of culturally sensitive nutrition education.

The ultimate goal in attending to the food and nutritional needs of minority older adult groups is to bring programs and services that respond to the cultural diversity and the health and social characteristics of such groups in a sensitive and timely manner.

Activities Related to This Chapter

1. Interview three ethnically different older adults and ask them for a "family" recipe or a "typical" recipe from their background. Prepare one or more of the recipes for the class to try.
2. Research a particular way of eating. What are the motivations behind the diet? How does following this diet affect participation in social events? What adaptations, compromises, and so on, must be made in order to follow the diet? What special food purchase and preparation patterns are required?

3. Adopt the diet you studied in question 2 for a week. Keep track of everything you eat. Write a summary of the week. How easy or hard was it to follow this diet? If it was hard, did you cheat? Why? What did your friends and family say? How did you manage to follow the diet while away from home?

4. Try one new food each day for a week. This may require some advance planning and menu research. Keep a journal of your experience, barriers you encounter, and any assistance you receive.

5. What are your core foods? Create a list that records everything you eat for a month. After a food appears once, make a tic mark next to it each time you choose it again in that month. Your core foods will be the ones with the most tic marks.

REFERENCES

Administration on Aging and U.S. Department of Health and Human Services. *A Profile of Older Americans: 2006.* Washington, DC: Administration on Aging; 2007.

American Dietetic Association. Nutrition care manual. Available at: http://www.nutritioncaremanual.org/index.cfm?Page = Intro&NextPage = Home&CFID = 770714&CFTOKEN = 84743841. Accessed May 22, 2008.

American Institutes for Research. Teaching cultural competence in health care: A review of current concepts, policies and practices. Available at: http://www.omhrc.gov/assets/pdf/checked/em01garcia1.pdf.

Bermudez OI, Tucker KL. Total and central obesity among elderly Hispanics and the association with type 2 diabetes. *Obes Res.* 2001;9(8):443–451.

Bermudez OI, Falcon LM, Tucker KL. Intake and food sources of macronutrients among older Hispanic adults: association with ethnicity, acculturation, and length of residence in the United States. *J Am Diet Assoc.* 2000;100(6):665–673.

Bermudez OI, Tucker KL. Cultural aspects of food choices in various communities of elders. *Generations: J Am Society Aging.* 2004;28(3):22–27.

Broussard-Marin L, Hynak-Hankinson MT. Ethnic food: the use of Cajun cuisine as a model. *J Am Diet Assoc.* 1989;89(8):1117–1121.

Campinha-Bacote J. The process of cultural competence in the delivery of healthcare services: a model of care. *J Transcultural Nursing.* 2002;13(3):181–184.

Coates RJ, et al. The Women's Health Trial Feasibility Study in Minority Populations: changes in dietary intakes. *Am J Epidemiol.* 1999;149(12):1104–1112.

Conti K. Nutrition status of American Indian Adults and impending need in view of the Strong Heart Dietary Study. *J Am Diet Assoc.* 2008;108(5):781–784.

Dwyer J, Bermudez O. Ethnic foods. In B Caballero (ed.), *Encyclopedia of Food Sciences and Nutrition,* 2nd ed. Philadelphia: Elsevier; 2003.

Eilat-Adar S, et al. Sex may modify the effects of macronutrient intake on metabolic syndrome and insulin resistance in American Indians: The Strong Heart Study. *J Am Diet Assoc.* 2008;108(5):794–802.

Fanelli MT, Stevenhagen KJ. Characterizing consumption patterns by food frequency methods: core foods and variety of foods in diets of older Americans. *J Am Diet Assoc.* 1985;85(12):1570–1576.

Fernandez-Mendez E. *Historia cultural de Puerto Rico.* San Juan, Puerto Rico: E.E. Cemi; 1971.

Gans KM, et al. Baseline fat-related dietary behaviors of white, Hispanic, and black participants in a cholesterol screening and education project in New England. *J Am Diet Assoc.* 2003;103(6):699–706.

Guendelman S, Abrams B. Dietary intake among Mexican-American women: Generational differences and a comparison with White Non-Hispanic women. *Am J Pub Health.* 1995;85(1): 20–25.

Harris MI, et al. Prevalence of diabetes, impaired fasting glucose tolerance in U.S. adults: the Third National Health and Nutrition Examination Survey, 1988–1994. *Diabetes Care.* 1998;21(4):518–524.

Jones DV, Darling ME. *Ethnic Foodways in Minnesota: Handbook of Food and Wellness Across Cultures.* St. Paul: University of Minnesota; 1996.

Kaufman-Kurzrock DL. Cultural aspects of nutrition. *Top Clin Nutr.* 1989;4(2):1–6.

Khan LK, Martorell R. Diet diversity in Mexican Americans, Cuban Americans and Puerto Ricans. *Ecol Food Nutr.* 1997;36:401–415.

Koehler KM. Core, secondary, and peripheral foods in the diets of Hispanic, Navajo, and Jemez Indian children. *J Am Diet Assoc.* 1989,89(4):538–540.

Lee SK, Sobal J, Frongillo EA Jr. Acculturation and dietary practices among Korean Americans. *J Am Diet Assoc.* 1999;99(9):1084–1089.

Lee SK, Sobal J, Frongillo EA Jr. Acculturation and health in Korean Americans. *Soc Sci Med.* 2000;51(2):159–173.

Leslie JH. Uli'eo Koa Program: incorporating a traditional Hawaiian dietary component. *Pac Health Dialog.* 2001;8(2):401–406.

Must A, et al. The disease burden associated with overweight and obesity. *JAMA.* 1999;282(16):1523–1529.

Nalbandian A, Bergan JG, Brown PT. Three generations of Armenians: food habits and dietary status. *J Am Diet Assoc.* 1981;79(6):694–699.

Newman JM. Cultural, religious and regional practices of the elderly. *J Nutr for the Elderly.* 1985;5(1):15–19.

Ogden CL, et al. Prevalence of overweight and obesity in the United States, 1999–2004. *JAMA.* 2006;295(13):1549–1555.

Oldways Preservation and Exchange Trust. Available at: http://www.oldwayspt.org. Accessed May 22, 2008.

Painter J, Rah JH, Lee YK. Comparison of international food guide pictorial representations. *J Am Diet Assoc.* 2002;102(4):483–489.

Russell RM, Rasmussen H, Lichtenstein AH. Modified food guide pyramid for people over 70 years of age. *J Nutr.* 1999;129:751–753.

Sanjur D. *Hispanic Foodways, Nutrition, and Health.* Boston: Allyn and Bacon; 1995.

Sigman-Grant MJ. Food choice: balancing benefits and risks. *J Am Diet Assoc.* 2008;108(5):778–780.

U.S. Department of Agriculture. MiPirámide: Pasos Hacia una Mejor Salud. Available at: http://www.mypyramid.gov/sp-index.html. Accessed on April 29, 2008.

U.S. Department of Agriculture. MyPyramid: Steps to a healthier you. Available at: http://www.mypyramid.gov/. Accessed February 15, 2008.

U.S. Department of Health and Human Services. Healthy People 2010. Available at: http://www.healthypeople.gov. Accessed October 15, 2005.

U.S. Department of Health and Human Services and U.S. Department of Agriculture. *Dietary Guidelines for Americans, 2005*. Washington, DC: U.S. Government Printing Office; 2005.

U.S. Department of Health and Human Services and U.S. Department of Agriculture. *Finding Your Way to a Healthier You: Based on the Dietary Guidelines for Americans*. Washington, DC: U.S. Government Printing Office; 2005.

Whitney ER, Rolfes SR. *Understanding Nutrition*. 8th ed. Belmont, CA: West/Wadsworth; 1999.

Yohai F. Dietary patterns of Spanish-speaking people living in the Boston area. *J Am Diet Assoc.* 1977;71:273–275.

CHAPTER 21

Nutrition Services for Older Americans

Joseph R. Sharkey, PhD, MPH, RD, and
Barbara Kamp, MS, RD

CHAPTER OBJECTIVES   Upon completion of this chapter, the reader will be able to:

1. Explain why nutrition is important to older adults' health and quality of life
2. List and describe the major food-assistance programs for older adults
3. Describe how optimal nutrition promotes healthy aging
4. Describe how nutritional deficiencies and inadequacies influence older adults' health and quality of life
5. List areas of nutritional concern for older adults and describe methods to promote their nutritional well-being
6. Review the key features in providing nutrition services for older adults

KEY TERMS AND CONCEPTS

Food insecurity

Nutrient deficiency

DETERMINE Checklist

Older Americans Act Nutrition Programs
    (OAANP)

Quality of life

Senescence

Title III of the Older Americans Act

The older population (those aged 65 years and older) is growing rapidly both in absolute numbers and as a proportion of the total population. Life expectancy has increased by 30 years since the early twentieth century. Not only are older adults in the United States living longer, they are living healthier and more functionally fit lives than ever before. Fewer than 5% of adults aged 65 and older are institutionalized, and most nursing home residents are aged 85 and older.

Of the 95% of older adults residing in the community setting, over half (54%) live with a spouse. Although many older persons have at least one or more chronic health conditions, approximately four in every five older adults are healthy enough to engage in their normal activities.

The Role of Nutrition in Healthy Aging

Although aging is a normal biological process, poor health is not an inevitable consequence of aging. Nevertheless, there are alterations in physiological function and organ systems that are linked to aging. The rate of change differs among individuals as well as within organ systems. These changes are called **senescence**; the organic process of growing older and displaying the effects of increased age. It is important to distinguish between normal changes of aging versus changes due to disease, such as atherosclerosis, with an onset seen as early as 5 years of age. In addition, although approximately 87% of older

> **senescence** The process of growing older and displaying the effects of increased age.

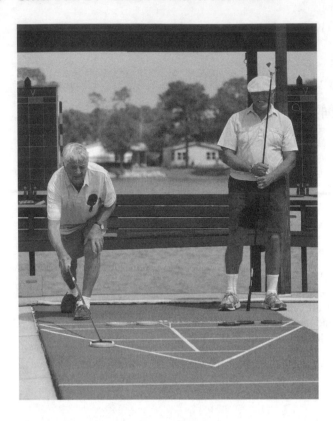

adults have one or more chronic diseases, older adults suffer fewer acute illnesses and accidents than younger adults.

Nutrition Challenges of Aging

Caloric needs decrease with age, while some micronutrient needs increase. Therefore, it is essential that older adults be educated on the importance of choosing nutrient-dense foods. Poor nutrition can be a concern for many older adults, especially minorities. Malnutrition occurs at both ends of the body weight spectrum—underweight and obesity.

Malnutrition, underweight, overweight, obesity, **food insecurity**, and hunger are all linked to decreased **quality of life**, increased morbidity, and premature mortality. Although most older adults do not show signs of overt **nutrient deficiencies**, surveys show that older adults eat inadequate diets and are at risk of malnutrition. The subsequent nutrient deficiencies may affect function and quality of life.

Food insecurity The state of, or risk of, being unable to obtain, prepare, chew, or swallow food.

Quality of life An individual's perception of well-being regarding his or her physical and mental health as well as his or her satisfaction with life as a whole.

nutrient deficiency A shortfall of any nutrient that may result in suboptimal health.

Nutrient Deficiency: Underweight

Although there is no uniform definition of undernutrition, it is often thought of occurring when the intake of dietary nutrients is less than that required to sustain health. The identification of undernutrition is complex and may differ across settings, such as independent living, home care, hospitalization, adult daycare, institutionalized long-term care, and hospice. Common indicators of undernutrition are body mass index (BMI), nutrient intakes, and weight loss. A BMI less than or equal to 18.5 kg/m² is considered to represent undernutrition.

Undernutrition is more prevalent in the nursing home population than among community-dwelling older adults. Various nursing home resident characteristics (problems chewing or swallowing or leaving at least 25% of food uneaten) as well as facility characteristics (for-profit facility or urban location) are associated with undernutrition.

One type of nutrient deficiency is protein-energy undernutrition (PEU). PEU is diagnosed based on the presence of clinical signs that include wasting or involuntary weight loss; low BMI; biochemical evidence, such as low serum albumin; and insufficient nutrient intake. PEU increases the likelihood of complications, mortality, and hospital care costs. Hospital stays are longer and home care needs are greater for older patients who are malnourished. Research suggests that 20% to 60% of homebound older adults have PEU and that PEU is predictive of mortality.

Other consequences of undernutrition are sarcopenia and cachexia. Sarcopenia is not just seen in those with low BMI. Those with morbid obesity can also suffer, and, in fact, muscle loss may be more severe due to immobility in addition to advancing age. Cachexia, which is often referred to as "wasting" or "the anorexia of aging," is a cytokine-mediated response to injury due to insufficient calories. Cachexia is not a normal characteristic of aging.

Undernutrition places additional demands, such as infections, pressure ulcers, electrolyte imbalances, altered skin integrity, and overall weakness and fatigue, on individuals. This results in increased use of health services and programs.

Nutrient Excess: Obesity

Obesity is the most common nutritional disorder in older adults. It is associated with an increased risk of myocardial infarction, stroke, hypertension, type 2 diabetes, osteoarthritis of the lower extremities, and several types of cancer. Another effect of obesity on older adults is on function (e.g., mobility, balance, leg strength). In studies of homebound older adults, it was found that severe obesity (i.e., BMI ≥ 35 kg/m²) was associated with decline in lower-extremity physical performance (balance, mobility, and strength) and increased disability in basic activities of daily living (ADLs) over one year.

Distribution of fat in the abdomen is an important risk factor for diabetes, hypertension, heart attack, and stroke. With increased abdominal fat, there is increased prevalence of glucose intolerance, insulin resistance, elevated blood pressure, and elevated blood lipids.

Epidemiological studies, such as that by Luchsinger and colleagues, suggest that the connection between BMI and mortality decreases as age increases, especially among persons aged 75 and older. BMI is not a predictor of mortality or hospitalization for most individuals aged 75 and older.

Nutritional Concerns of Older Adults

Several areas of nutritional concern are relevant to older adults. The older adult's ability to consume the appropriate quality and quantity of foods is influenced by food accessibility (i.e., they are obtainable), availability (i.e., they are suitable or ready for use), acceptability (i.e., they are agreeable), preparation, and consumption. Whether healthful foods are accessible and available depends to some degree on marital status and household roles, health behaviors, socioeconomic status, housing, neighborhood and community factors, geographic location, transportation, and social support.

The acceptability of foods may be the result of such psychosocial factors as culture, ethnic background, food faddism, food temperature, food texture or appearance, perceived intolerance, motivation, cognitive function, depression, and life stresses. Physiologic factors that influence acceptability of food include health, individual and multiple diseases, and altered sense of taste, smell, or oral status.

Acceptability may also be affected by the aging process, food intolerance, or medications. Medications may decrease appetite, diminish taste, alter salivation, or impair swallowing. Preparation and consumption are influenced by physiologic factors such as mobility, balance, nutritional status, sight and hearing, cognitive deficits, or physical limitations, such as difficulty opening containers or packages.

Overall food intake is also influenced by the number of meal occasions, meal size, and food choice. Studies, including a 2004 study by Sharkey and colleagues, have shown that almost 20% of older adults do not usually eat breakfast, which is usually a nutrient-dense meal. Older adults who do not regularly eat breakfast have lower nutrient intake than those older adults who do eat breakfast. Many older adults face the risk of not having enough food; they may adopt such strategies such as limiting the size of meals or portions to stretch the money available for food. The literature suggests that this may be the result of having to choose between competing demands for limited resources; that is, choosing between spending money on medications, bills, or food. In this case, older adults may choose cheaper or smaller meals, which limits the quality and quantity of food and increases the risk for low nutrient intake.

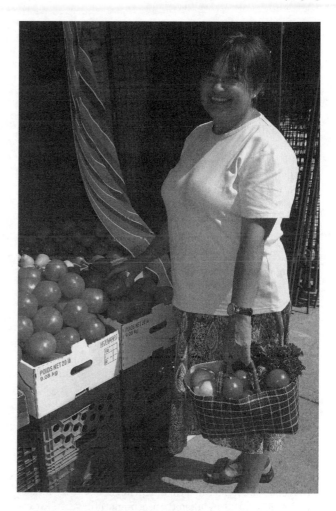

Healthful eating relies on making the right food selections. Food selection is influenced by personal factors, individual and community resources, social context, and the food environment and involves decisions made on the basis of convenience and quality. Individual and community resources may be inadequate for older adults to be able to choose the foods that are optimal for nutritional health. Food assistance programs may be inadequate in light of expected and unexpected out-of-pocket expenses. Other community programs, such as meal-delivery programs, may not be available due to lack of money or volunteer resources. Many of these programs have long waiting lists.

Other community factors, such as neighborhood safety, lack of business community involvement, geographic isolation, and minimal or no transportation make it difficult for some older adults to shop. This is exacerbated by a lack of supermarkets or grocery stores in certain areas, especially in rural or impoverished urban areas, and by challenges of the home environment, such as inadequate refrigeration. Inadequate refrigeration or storage means that some older adults must shop more frequently for fresh groceries or make other choices.

Convenience stores stock limited quality food options, offering few or no fresh fruits or vegetables, processed meats, canned vegetables high in sodium, and limited low-fat or fat-free dairy products. Furthermore, convenience store foods are often more expensive than grocery stores, so older adults who rely on convenience store foods have higher average food costs, reducing their overall food-purchasing power. In addition, fees needed for public transportation in order to reach a grocery store further reduces the amount of money available for food purchases.

Older Adult Nutrition: A Public Health Issue

What makes nutrition in older adults a difficult public health issue is the complex interaction of overall health and nutritional requirements merged with ethnic, racial, economic, and educational diversity of this cohort. First, there are many different indicators of deficiency, excess, or both, in nutritional health. Overall nutritional deficiency or excess can be shown through a variety of different measures: anthropometric (BMI or body circumference); clinical (unintended weight change, bone density, or muscle strength); biochemical (serum levels of specific markers); or dietary (usual dietary intake). In combination, these measures may describe both deficiency and excess. For example, some studies suggest that some older adults may be obese *and* nutritionally deficient, because of the consumption of less nutrient-dense (empty calorie) foods.

Second, nutritional health, independent of dietary intake, may be influenced by altered absorption, utilization, or excretion as a result of underlying health conditions, physiological changes, or medication use—all of which are more prevalent in older adults. For example, the use of diuretics increases the excretion of fluids and water-soluble vitamins, such as numerous B vitamins and vitamin C. In another example, as a result of physiologic changes, the body's synthesis of vitamin D may be decreased, resulting in reduced ability of the body to absorb calcium.

Nutrition as Part of the Health Care Continuum

Nutrition plays a critical role in the primary, secondary, and tertiary prevention of disease. This occurs in a variety of settings: from independent and living in the community to frail and in the community, hospitalized, adult day care, and institutionalization. In primary prevention, overall good nutrition helps to promote health, function, and the prevention of nutrition-related disease. In secondary and tertiary prevention, nutrition is a major component of the management of disease conditions and prevention of disability.

Nutrition Services for Older Persons

The achievement and maintenance of good nutritional health and a longer and healthier life requires efforts at the individual, family, organization, community, and policy levels. Public nutrition policy with regards to older adults takes many forms, including national goals, the development and dissemination of nutritional recommendations, and nutrition assistance programs.

Care for the nation's older adults falls under several systems. One is the health care system, which is composed of individual private health insurance, health maintenance organizations, and Medicare. The focus of this system is the promotion of health through the treatment of disease. In spite of the link between nutrition and health in older persons, major financing mechanisms, such as Medicare, limit coverage for nutrition services. The lack of funding for nutrition services, especially for primary prevention, creates a barrier for many older adults and contributes to high levels of nutritional risk.

The other system is home and community-based long-term care (HCBS). The focus of HCBS is to promote health through an array of services, including nutrition, that help maintain the quality of life and independence of older adults and prevent or delay institutionalization. Within HCBS there are two main government-supported systems that provide service to older adults: public health departments and aging services providers. Each delivers services to ensure optimal health and independence for the nation's older adults; however, they accomplish this goal through different networks.

In 1961, the first White House Conference on Aging was held. This citizen's forum was established to highlight the problems facing older Americans and to make policy recommendations on how best to improve the lives of this growing cohort. The forum resulted in the passage of Social Security Amendments, the Senior Citizen Housing Act, the Community Health Services and Facilities Act, Medicare, Medicaid, and the Older Americans Act.

The Older Americans Act (OAA) established the Administration on Aging (AoA). The AoA, a branch of the U.S. Department of Health and Human Services (USDHHS), is responsible for administering nutrition services to America's older adults. The mission of the act is:

> ...to promote the dignity and independence of older people, and to help society prepare for an aging population...by serving as an advocate for older people, and by overseeing the development of a comprehensive and coordinated system of care that is responsive to the needs and preferences of older people and their family caregivers.

To achieve this mission, the OAA funds six core service areas (**Table 21-1**). The passage of the OAA established a

TABLE 21-1 Core Service Areas Funded by OAA

Title		Services Provided
IIIB.	Support Services	Transportation to medical appointments and grocery and drug stores. Supportive services provide handyman, chore, and personal care services.
IIIC.	Nutrition Services	Congregate and home-delivered meals; nutrition screening, assessment, education, and counseling.
IIID.	Preventive Health Services	Education to enable older adults to make healthy lifestyle choices.
IIIE.	National Family Caregiver Support Program	Respite care or time off for the caregiver in several forms, including companions, homemakers, home health aides, adult day care, in-facility care, and chore services.
VI.	Service to Native Alaskans, Native Hawaiians and Native Americans	Nutrition and supportive services designed to meet the unique cultural and social traditions of tribal organizations and organizations serving Native Hawaiians.
VII.	Elder Rights Services	Long-Term Care Ombudsman program; programs for the prevention of abuse, neglect, and exploitation; state elder rights and legal assistance development programs; insurance/benefits outreach, counseling, and assistance programs.

Source: Data from Administration on Aging. Outline of 2006 amendments to the Older Americans Act. Available at: http://www.aoa.gov/AoARoot/AoA_Programs/OAA/oaa.aspx. Accessed July 15, 2009.

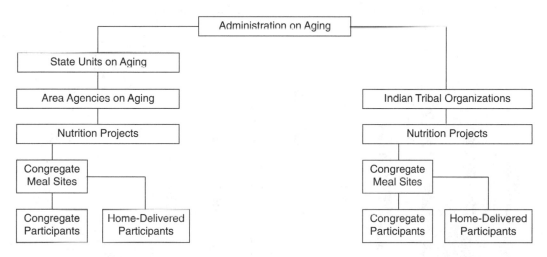

FIGURE 21-1 Title III and VI Nutrition Program Structure

national goal to promote better health through improved nutrition and to help older adults to remain independent in their own homes.

The OAA programs are implemented by the Aging Network (**Figure 21-1**). This national network consists of 56 State Units on Aging, providing services through 655 Area Agencies on Aging; 241 Tribal and Native American organizations, representing 300 American Indian and Alaska Native Tribal organizations; and two organizations serving Native Hawaiians. The network also includes thousands of service providers; adult care centers, caregivers, and volunteers. An estimated 12,000 senior centers serve approximately 10 million older adults annually.

Title IIIC consists of congregate (C1) and home-delivered (C2) meals. *Congregate meals* are served at community centers such as "senior" dining centers, faith-based settings, schools, and adult day centers. Initially designed to provide nutritious meals in a social setting, congregate sites also provide an opportunity for socialization, mental stimulation, and community involvement. The Nutrition Program serves approximately 3 million participants annually.

Congregate meals provide an estimated 40% to 50% of daily nutrients and calories. Many eat more food at congregate sites than they would eat at home. **Figure 21-2** shows a comparison of nutrient intakes as a percentage of RDA for

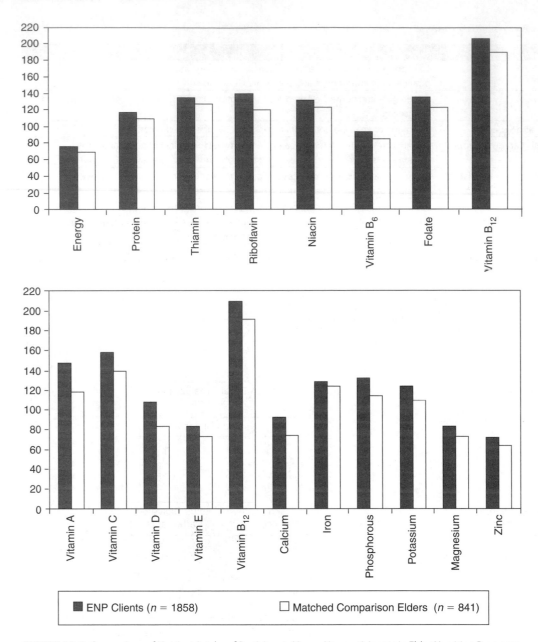

FIGURE 21-2 Comparison of Nutrient Intake of Participants Versus Nonparticipants in Elder Nutrition Programs

participants in older adult nutrition programs as compared to age-matched nonparticipants.

In 1978, the nutrition program was expanded to integrate nutrition and social ser-

Title III of the Older Americans Act Includes congregate and home delivered meals.

vices, transportation services, and a home-delivered meals component (Title III C-2) for the growing number of frail and homebound older adults unable to travel to a congregate site. This service is frequently referred to as *Meals on Wheels*. These meals provide more than just food: volunteers who deliver meals provide social interaction, especially for the 59%

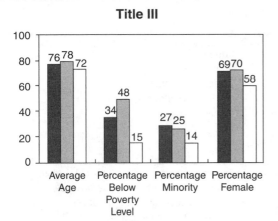

Title III

Title VI

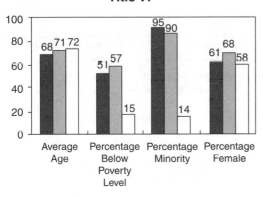

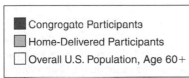

Congregate Participants
Home-Delivered Participants
Overall U.S. Population, Age 60+

FIGURE 21-3 Socioeconomic Characteristics of Title III and Title VI Nutrition Program Participants

of older adults who live alone. Volunteers can help monitor the health of the homebound and make sure they are getting the services and help they need.

At the current funding level, **Older Americans Act Nutrition Programs (OAANPs)** reach about 7% of the older individuals who need them. The socioeconomic characteristic of participants in Title III and Title VI Elder Nutrition Programs are shown in **Figure 21-3**.

Both congregate and home-delivered nutrition programs provide services to adults who are at least 60 years of age; neither program restricts eligibility to individuals with financial need. However, 84 percent of homebound and 65 percent of congregate program participants are poor or near

poor. All OAANP meals must provide at least one-third of the RDA and use the Dietary Guidelines for Americans as a framework. In addition, OAANP regularly screens their participants for nutritional risk based on the **Nutrition Screening Initiative's DETERMINE Checklist**, a 10-item instrument that focuses on food-group intake, adequacy of resources, eating in isolation, medication use, weight change, and physical limitations. Despite participation in food assistance programs, many older adults still consume less than adequate diets, and many experience food insufficiency and worsening of food sufficiency status over time.

OAANP is being challenged by a convergence of many factors, including (1) an overall demand that outstrips allocated resources, (2) the increasing numbers of older adults who will be living longer with chronic conditions, (3) a decreasing numbers of volunteers, (4) the location of congregate meal sites in older parts of the community, (5) earlier hospital discharges of older individuals to the community with a need for immediate home-based services, and (6) waiting lists for nutrition services. Over the years, the OAANP has found that many participants remain on the home-delivered meals program for longer than ten years.

Another source of funding is the Nutrition Services Incentive Program (NSIP). NSIP rewards effective performance by states and tribal organizations for the efficient delivery of nutritious meals to older Americans. Awards can be cash or food commodities. The goal of NSIP is to expand Older Americans Act services to include more older adults. **Table 21-2** provides a summary of U.S Department of Health and Human Service Administration on Aging programs.

Medicaid Waiver Program

Medicaid is a state–federal partnership that pays for health and long-term care services for low-income individuals who are aged, blind, disabled, or members of families with disabled dependent children, or who meet certain other criteria for need. In 1981, federal legislation established the Home- and Community-Based Care Service (HCBS) Waiver program under Section 1915(c) of the Social Security Act. States can allow community-based services to be care providers by waiving certain Medicaid statutes and regulations. This allows individuals at risk of being placed in long-term care facilities to receive care at home, preserving their independence and ties to family and friends. Approved nutrition services include home-delivered meals, nutrition risk-reduction coun-

Older Americans Act Nutrition Program (OAANP) The law that established the Administration on Aging; insures that all Americans age 60 and over receive necessary services to maintain health, independence, and dignity.

Nutrition Screening Initiative's DETERMINE Checklist
A 10-question tool to evaluate the nutrition risk of older adults.

TABLE 21-2 U.S. Department of Health & Human Services Administration on Aging Programs

Program	Purpose	Appropriations	Target Population	Services	Participation
Older Americans Act: Titles I–VII	Grants to state, tribal, and community programs on aging; research, demonstration projects, etc.	$1.42B (FY 2008)	Age 60+ in greatest economic need &/ or social need, with particular attention to low-income minorities, those in rural areas, and those with limited English proficiency.	Nutrition services, supportive and health services, protection of vulnerable older Americans.	9.5M older adults (FY 2006)
Older Americans Act: Title III	Nutrition services to older adults	$604M (FY 2008)	Age 60+, <60yrs and disabled who live in elderly housing, disabled living at home, and those who eat at congregate sites or who receive home-delivered meals.	Congregate and home-delivered meals; nutrition screening, assessment, education, counseling.	2.6M older adults, 238.3M meals (FY 2006)
Office of the Assistant Secretary for Planning and Evaluation: Title VI	Tribal and Native organizations for aging programs and services	$27M (FY 2008)	Age requirement determined by Tribal organizations or Native Hawaiian program.	Congregate and home-delivered meals; nutrition screening, education, counseling; array of other supportive and health services.	70,000 older adults, 4M meals (FY 2006)
Nutrition Services Incentive Program (NSIP)	Provides proportional shares to states and tribes based on number of meals served in prior year.	$153M (FY 2008)	Same as Title III.	Cash and/or commodities to supplement meals.	

seling, and nutritional supplements, as appropriate. Each state determines and implements its own benefits package. Currently, 38 states include meals and/or nutrition services among the specified benefits available.

The U.S. Department of Agriculture (USDA) has several programs designed to fight hunger that serve older adults, including the Federal Supplemental Nutrition Assistance Program (formerly the Food Stamp Program), Food Stamp Nutrition Education, Commodity and Supplemental Foods, The Emergency Food Assistance Program, the Child and Adult Care Food Program, and the Seniors' Farmers Market Nutrition Program. All of these USDA programs are means tested.

The Supplemental Nutrition Assistance Program (SNAP), the largest of the USDA food-assistance programs, provides electronic benefit transfer (EBT) cards or coupons to eligible low-income individuals and families. This is an entitlement program; participants who meet the requirements set by law are guaranteed benefits. Congress has no discretion as to how much money to appropriate; entitlement programs

are funded to meet the needed amount and are a legal right. Eligibility requires that the individual or household's gross monthly income not exceed 130% of the federal poverty guidelines and that participants' assets do not exceed set limits. There are few restrictions on food purchases, but alcohol, tobacco, and other nonfood items are excluded.

Although many older adults are eligible for food stamps, less than 30 percent of eligible older adults choose to participate in the program. A variety of reasons have been cited for lack of participation in the SNAP, including the stigma attached to receiving benefits, the difficult and demeaning application process, and minimal benefits. The average benefit for an older adult living alone is $65 per month, and $152 per month if they live with others.

The goal of Food Stamp Nutrition Education is to improve the likelihood that SNAP participants and applicants will make healthy choices within a limited budget and choose active lifestyles consistent with the current Dietary Guidelines for Americans and MyPyramid. Although optional, the USDA's Food and Nutrition Service actively encourages

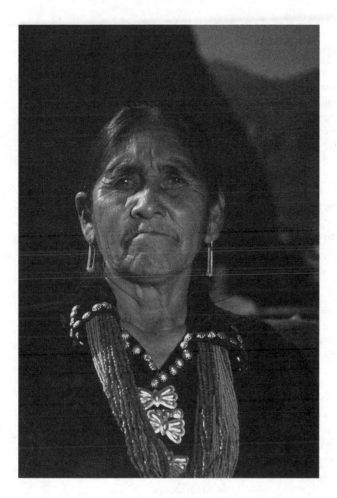

states to provide nutrition education for food-stamp participants and others who are eligible, but emphasis on reaching older adults is limited.

The Commodity Supplemental Food Program (CSFP) works to improve the health of low-income Americans by supplementing their diets with nutritious USDA commodity foods. Currently, 33 states and 2 tribal organizations participate. Targeted populations include adults older than age 60 with incomes less than 130% of the federal poverty guidelines. Others (some mothers, infants, and children) qualify at higher incomes. Local agencies determine eligibility, distribute the foods, and provide nutrition education. CSFP food packages do not provide a complete diet, but they may be good sources of nutrients typically lacking in diets. In 2007, 466,180 eligible participants were served; approximately 92% of CSFP clients were older adults.

The Emergency Food Assistance Program (TEFAP) is a commodity-food distribution program. The USDA buys food, including processed and packaged items, and ships it to states. Each state's allotment is based on its low-income

and unemployed population. States provide the food to local agencies, usually food banks, which, in turn, distribute the food to soup kitchens and food pantries that serve the public. These direct-service organizations distribute the commodities for household consumption or use them to prepare and serve meals in congregate settings.

The Child and Adult Care Food Program (CACFP) serves nutritious meals and snacks to eligible adults in participating adult day centers. Meals must meet minimum nutrition requirements. Each day, 86,000 adults receive meals and snacks at nonresidential adult day centers. This number represents only 3% of CACFP meals served, but the number of meals served in adult day centers is growing faster than the number served in childcare centers.

The Senior Farmers' Market Nutrition Program awards grants to states, U.S. territories, and federally recognized Indian tribal governments to provide low-income older adults with coupons that can be exchanged for eligible foods at farmers' markets, roadside stands, and community-supported agriculture programs. The program is designed to improve health by providing access to fresh fruits, vegetables, and herbs. It is also designed to increase domestic consumption of agricultural commodities and to help support and create more of these venues and community-supported agriculture programs. Currently, the program is available in 40 states, the District of Columbia, and Puerto Rico and through five Indian tribal organizations. Annual benefits are modest and are available only during the local growing season. Coupons range in size from $15 to $315; the average benefit level is between $40 and $50. The coupon amounts are determined by individual state agencies, not by recipient income levels.

Table 21-3 provides a summary of the USDA nutrition programs, including their purpose, target populations, and services.

Conclusion

A new paradigm of nutrition and aging recognizes a number of key nutritional issues. Good nutrition is a critical component of healthy aging, and good nutritional health plays a role in maintaining physical and cognitive function. The maintenance of good nutritional health for a growing older population requires approaches that recognize multiple levels of influence on the individual—from social networks to organizations, communities, and policy. OAANP congregate and home-delivered meals programs provide a critical source of nutrition support for many older adults. More attention, more resources, and more nutrition expertise are needed to meet the food and nutrition requirements of vulnerable older adults to enable them to live independently with a good quality of life. The challenges to healthy eating of various subgroups of older adults—namely, those with individual and multiple chronic conditions, racial and

TABLE 21-3 USDA Programs

Program	Purpose	Appropriations	Target Population	Services	Participation
Supplemental Nutrition Assistance Program (SNAP)	Helps low-income families buy nutritionally adequate food.	$41B (FY 2006)	U.S. citizens and legal residents who are most in need, gross income ≤130% federal poverty level; up to $2,000 countable resources, $3,000 if age 60+ or disabled.	Coupons or electronic benefits to purchase breads, cereals, fruits, vegetables, meats, fish, poultry, and dairy products or seeds and plants that produce food for households.	28M monthly 51% children, 41% adults, 8% age 60+ (FY 2006).
Commodity Supplemental Food Program	Food and administrative funds to states and tribes to supplement diets. Available in 33 states and through 2 tribes.	$140M (FY 2008)	Pregnant and breastfeeding women, mothers up to 1 year postpartum, infants, children up to age 6.	Participants receive a monthly food package.	466,180 (FY 2007); 92% of those served are 60+.
Senior Farmers' Market Nutrition Program	Grants to states and tribes to provide fresh foods and nutrition services while providing the opportunity for farmers to enhance their business.	$15M (FY 2002–2007)	Low-income older adults 60 years and older who have household incomes of not more than 185% federal poverty.	Coupons or vouchers to be exchanged for fresh fruits and vegetables at local farmers markets.	46 agencies (FY 2006); 825,691 older adults (FY 2006)
The Emergency Food Assistance Program	Provides food to local agencies that serve the public directly.	$189.5M (FY 2008), plus $67M worth of surplus commodity foods. $250 million annually in Farm Bill.	Adults aged 60+ who meet state criteria based on income, including homeless, low-income older adults.	Emergency food for low-income needy persons, including older adults. States provide food to local agencies, usually food banks, which, in turn, distribute food to soup kitchens and food pantries that serve the public directly.	3.8M households
Child and Adult Care Food Program	Healthy, nutritious meals for children and adults in day centers.	$2.2B (FY 2007)	Children younger than 12 years, homeless children, migrant children younger than 15yrs. Disabled citizens regardless of age. Age 60+; functionally impaired; reside with family members.	Nutritional meals and snacks.	1.85B meals served (FY 2007) 2.9M children, 86,000 older adults (FY 2007)

ethnic minorities, and those who reside in different settings (rural, community, or institutions)—need to be better understood. Greater efforts need to be made by those administering nutrition programs to identify and measure program outcomes; that is, the difference their programs make in the lives of older adults.

Activities Related to This Chapter

1. Contact a local senior center that participates in the Title III or VI congregate meal program or home-delivered meal program and volunteer for one month.
2. Visit a nursing home in your area and observe the dining

room during mealtime. Are the residents enjoying their meals and companionship? Is an aide present to help residents in need? How much of the meal are the residents consuming? Then visit residents who eat in their rooms and compare their experience.

3. Contact your local senior center and find out what activities it provides to older adults in your community. What activities could potentially affect nutritional status? What suggestions could you make to improve the delivery of nutritious foods to the older adults who use this center?

REFERENCES

Administration on Aging, U.S. Department of Health and Human Services. A Profile of Older Americans 2007. Available at: http://www.aoa.gov/prof/statistics/profile/2007/profiles2007.aspx.

American Dietetic Association. Position paper of the American Dietetic Association: nutrition across the spectrum of aging. *J Am Diet Assoc.* 2005;105:616–633.

Anderson SA. Core indicators of nutritional state for difficult-to-sample populations. *J Nutr.* 1990;120:1559–1600.

Blaum CS, Xue QL, Michelon E, Semba RD, Fried LP. The association between obesity and the frailty syndrome in older women: the Women's Health and Aging Studies. *J Am Geriatr Soc.* 2005;53:927–934.

Browne JP, O'Doherty VA, McGee HM, McLaughlin B, O'Boyle CA, Fuller R. General practitioner and public health nurse views of nutritional risk factors in the elderly. *Ir J Med Sci.* 1997;166:23–25.

Centers for Medicare & Medicaid Services. Home and community-based 1915(c) waivers. Available at: http://www.cms.hhs.gov/medicaid/1915c/default.asp

Challa S, Sharkey JR, Chen M, Phillips C. Association of resident facility, and geographic characteristics with chronic undernutrition in a nationally represented sample of older residents in U.S. nursing homes. *J Nutr Health Aging.* 2007;11(2):179–184.

Elia M. Obesity in the elderly. *Obes Res.* 2001;9:244S–248S.

Ferraro K, Su Y, Gretebeck R, Black D, Badylak S. Body mass index and disability in adulthood: a 20-year panel study. *Am J Public Health.* 2002;92:834–840.

Friedmann J, Jensen G, Smiciklas-Wright H, McCamish M. Predicting early nonelective hospital readmission in nutritionally compromised older adults. *Am J Clin Nutr.* 1997;65:1714–1720.

Institute of Medicine, Committee on Nutrition Services for Medicare Beneficiaries. *The role of nutrition in maintaining health in the nation's elderly: evaluating coverage of nutrition services for the Medicare population.* Washington, DC: National Academies Press; 1999.

Jensen GL. Obesity and functional decline: epidemiology and geriatric consequences. *Clin Geriatr Med.* 2005;21:677–687.

Jensen GL, Friedmann JM. Obesity is associated with functional decline in community-dwelling rural older persons. *J Am Geriatr Soc.* 2002;50:918–923.

Lee JS, Frongillo EA. Nutritional and health consequences are associated with food insecurity among U.S. elderly persons. *J Nutr.* 2001;131:1503–1509.

Lee JS, Weyant RJ, Corby P, et al. Edentulism and nutritional status in a biracial sample of well-functioning, community-dwelling elderly: the Health, Aging, and Body Composition Study. *Am J Clin Nutr.* 2004;79:295–302.

Luchsinger JA, Lee W, Carrasquillo O, Rabinowitz D, Shea S. Body mass index and hospitalization in the elderly. *J Am Geriatr Soc.* 2003;51:1615–1620.

National Heart Lung and Blood Institute (NHLBI). Association of body mass index with mortality in older adults. Available at: http://www.nhlbi.nih.gov/guidelines/obesity/e_txtbk/ratnl/2222.htm.

Ostir GV, Markides KS, Freeman DH, Goodwin JS. Obesity and health conditions in elderly Mexican Americans: The Hispanic EPESE. *Ethn Dis.* 2000;10:31–38.

Perkowski LC, Stroup-Benham CA, Markides KS, et al. Lower-extremity functioning in older Mexican Americans and its association with medical problems. *J Am Geriatr Soc.* 1998;46:411–418.

Poikolainen A. Characteristics of food stamp households: fiscal Year 2004. Alexandria, VA: U.S. Department of Agriculture, Food and Nutrition Service, Office of Analysis, Nutrition and Evaluation; September, 2005. FSP-05-CHAR.

Ponza, M, Ohls JC, Millen BE. Serving elders at risk: the Older Americans Act Nutrition Programs, National Evaluation of the Elderly Nutrition Program, 1993–1995 Princeton, NJ: Mathematica Policy Research, Inc.; 1996.

Rose D, Richards R. Food store access and household fruit and vegetable use among participants in the U.S. Food Stamp Program. *Pub Health Nutr.* 2004;7:1081–1088.

Schlenker ED. Nutrition and the continuum of care for older adults. In Schlenker ED (ed), *Nutrition in Aging.* Boston: WCB McGraw-Hill; 1998:355–383.

Sharkey JR. Longitudinal examination of homebound older adults who experience heightened food insufficiency: effect of diabetes status and implications for service provision. *Gerontologist.* 2005;45:773–782.

Sharkey JR. Risk and presence of food insufficiency are associated with low nutrient intakes and multimorbidity among homebound older women who receive home-delivered meals. *J Nutr.* 2003;133:3485–3491.

Sharkey J, Ory M, Branch L. Severe elder obesity and 1-year diminished lower extremity physical performance in homebound older adults. *J Am Geriatr Soc.* 2006; in press.

Sharkey JR, Branch LG, Giuliani C, Haines PS, Zohoori N. Nutrient intake and BMI as predictors of severity of ADL disability over 1 year in homebound elders. *J Nutr Health Aging.* 2004;8:131–139.

Sharkey JR, Branch LG, Zohoori N, Giuliani C, Busby-Whitehead J, Haines PS. Inadequate nutrient intake among homebound older persons in the community and its correlation with individual characteristics and health-related factors. *Am J Clin Nutr.* 2002;76:1435–1445.

Sturm R, Ringel JS, Andreyeva T. Increasing obesity rates and disability trends. *Health Affairs*. 2004;23:199–205.

Sullivan D. Risk factors for early hospital readmission in a select population of rehabilitation patients. *J Am Geriatr Soc*. 1992;40:792–798.

U.S. Department of Health and Human Services, Office of the Assistant Secretary for Planning and Evaluation. Understanding Medicaid home and community services: a primer. October 2000. Available at: http://www.aspe.hhs.gov/daltcp/projects.htm#GWo4.

USDA Food and Nutrition Service. Child and Adult Care Food Program. Available at: http://www.fns.usda.gov/cnd/Care/

USDA Food and Nutrition Service. Commodity and Supplemental Foods. Available at: http://www.fns.usda.gov/fdd/programs/csfp/pfs-csfp.pdf.

USDA Food and Nutrition Service. Food Stamp Nutrition Education. Available at: http://www.csrees.usda.gov/nea/food/fsne/fsne.html.

USDA Food and Nutrition Service. Food Stamp Program. Available at: http://www.fns.usda.gov/fsp/.

USDA Food and Nutrition Service. Senior Farmers' Market Nutrition Program. Available at: http://www.fns.usda.gov/wic/SeniorFMNP/SFMNPmenu.htm.

USDA Food and Nutrition Service. The Emergency Food Assistance Program. Available at http://www.fns.usda.gov/fdd/programs/tefap.

Watts ML. Improving nutrition for American seniors: a new way to look at the Older Americans Act. *J Am Diet Assoc*. 2005;105:527–529.

Weddle DO, Wellman NS, Bates GM. Incorporating nutrition screening into three Older Americans Act Elderly Nutrition Programs. *J Nutr Elder*. 1997;17:19–37.

Wellman N, Rosenzweig L, Lloyd J. Thirty years of the Older Americans Nutrition Program. *J Am Diet Assoc*. 2002;102:348–350.

Wellman NS, Kamp B. Federal Food and Nutrition Assistance Programs for older people. *Generations*. 2004;Fall:78–85.

Wilde P, Dagata E. Food Stamp participation by eligible older Americans remains low. *Food Rev*. 2002;25:25–29.

22

Health Promotion and Disease Prevention in the Older Adult

Timothy J. Legg, PhD, GNP-BC, CHES and Melissa Bernstein, PhD, RD, LD

. . . .

CHAPTER OBJECTIVES   Upon completion of this chapter, the student will be able to:

1. Explore the role of nutrition in the prevention of disease
2. Identify key terms related to health and health promotion in older adulthood
3. Elucidate common myths of aging associated with health promotion and disease prevention
4. Provide an overview of strategies for older adults for the prevention of disease and chronic conditions

KEY TERMS AND CONCEPTS

Complementary and alternative nutrition

Disease prevention

Frailty

Health promotion

Healthy aging

Pathological aging

Wellness

. . . .

This chapter explores the relationship between **health promotion** and positive aging. A necessary underpinning to the topics encompassing this chapter is that it is never too late to implement even small changes directed toward improving health and quality of life. Although not all diseases can be prevented, a considerable body of evidence supports the efficacy of health promotion activities. The role of nutrition in geriatric health promotion and disease prevention is an evolving practice with guidelines that need to be tailored to meet the needs of the aging individual. Stereotypes or preconceived notions about appropriate care of the older adult (not based in fact) can result in failure to offer the older adult the full range of options and services that he or she may benefit from.

Healthy Aging

What is **healthy aging**? When defining *healthy aging*, it is important to consider the terms *health* and *aging* inde-

pendently and then explore how these two terms come together to describe the older adult. Although these terms would seem straightforward, actually defining them can become complicated and cumbersome.

The World Health Organization (WHO) defines *health* as "a state of complete physical, mental, and social well-being and not merely the absence of disease or infirmity." Just as *health* incorporates many concepts within its definition, so, too, the definition of aging is

health promotion Deliberate actions that are taken with the intent of moving an individual to a higher level of wellness.

healthy aging Development and maintenance of optimal mental, social, and physical well-being and function in older adults. Most likely achieved when communities are safe and promote health and well-being and the older adult uses health services and community programs to prevent or minimize disease.

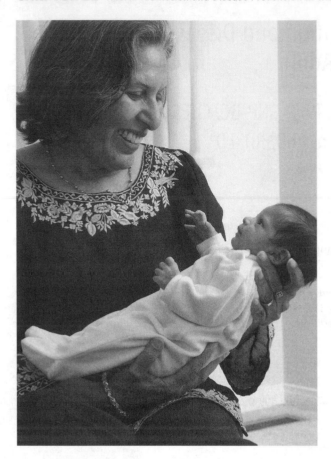

multifaceted. When discussing aging, it is important to distinguish among *chronological aging*, *biological aging*, *social aging*, and *psychological aging*.

Chronological aging refers to the actual number of years that a person has lived. This measure serves as an important criterion in contemporary society. Certain benefits and privileges are based on a person's chronological age (i.e., minimum age for operation of a motor vehicle, ability to purchase and consume alcoholic beverages, or obtain Social Security benefits).

The aging population is extremely heterogeneous, and therefore it is important to keep in mind that the term *old*, itself, can be quite subjective. Even though the term *young-old* refers to those individuals aged 65 to 74 years, *middle-old* refers to those aged 75 to 84 years, and *old-old* is sometimes

wellness A state of well-being achieved by a combination of emotional, environmental, mental, physical, social, and spiritual health, especially when maintained by proper diet, exercise, and habits.

pathological aging The etiologies, mechanisms, and manifestations of disease as they influence the aging process.

used to refer to individuals aged 85 and above, chronological age is often a poor indicator of health and well-being.

Biological aging encompasses changes in the individual's anatomy and physiology that affects all body systems and occurs over time. *Social aging* refers to the social habits and roles of an individual with respect to his or her culture. *Psychological aging* deals with the interchanges between the person and the psychological or social environments. It is also concerned with an individual's adaptation to both the internal and external experiences of the world.

When considering the multiple constructs involved in appropriately defining healthy aging, it becomes clear that there is some variability in the definition. A concise definition proposed by the West Virginia Rural Healthy Aging Network, defines *healthy aging* as "the development and maintenance of optimal mental, social, and physical well-being and function in older adults."

It is important to consider that although an individual may demonstrate attributes of healthy aging, alterations in **wellness** can result in disease or disability. Alternatively, it has been suggested that aging should be considered as the individual existing along a continuum. One side of the continuum is healthy aging; on the opposing end of the scale is pathological aging, which we will examine next.

Pathological Aging

The opposite of health aging is **pathological aging**. *Pathological* refers to an unhealthy or "disease" state. Pathological aging encompass disease processes that can occur in older adults that are not related to normal aging. The importance of being able to distinguish between normal and pathological aging is essential. Misconceptions about what is "normal" aging can result in failures to treat and the subsequent physical deterioration in the older client.

As we provide services to older adults, it is essential to consider all individuals along the continuum of aging—from healthy aging to pathological aging. Evaluation of where along the continuum each individual is currently situated and suggestions of ways to help move them along the continuum closer to healthy aging must be considered prior to implementing nutrition services. It is also critical to reevaluate older adults frequently to assess fluctuating health status.

Health Promotion Versus Disease Prevention

It is also important to consider health promotion and disease prevention—two key concepts that are important in moving aging individuals closer toward the healthy end of the continuum. The focus of health promotion is the achievement of optimal levels of wellness. Wellness is a multidimensional approach that incorporates spiritual, social, emotional, intellectual, and physical dimensions to obtaining quality of life.

At first glance, the terms *health promotion* and *disease prevention* seem like two different ways of saying essentially the same thing; however, they are quite different in their primary focus. **Health promotion** is a broad term used to describe those actions that are deliberately taken with the intent of moving an individual to a higher level of wellness. In our conceptual example of the continuum of healthy aging–pathological aging, the goal is to move the older adult closer to healthy aging. Eating a healthy diet, exercising, quitting smoking, obtaining appropriate levels of sleep/rest, reducing stress, and participating in leisure time help to move the older adult toward healthy aging.

When working with younger individuals, it is easier to recognize the importance of health promotion behaviors. The younger client (from a life-expectancy perspective) has many years of life ahead of him or her, and health-promoting behaviors are essential to achieve a long, productive, and healthy life. However, health-promotion activities in the older adult and the benefits of health promotion are often the subject of debate. One of the myths of aging is that health-promotion activities will have little benefit or that older adults have no interest in health-promotion activities. These myths, however, are not supported by the literature.

Alternatively, **disease prevention** can be considered those activities that an individual deliberately takes to prevent illness or disease. It is best conceptualized by stages or levels of prevention, as shown in **Table 22-1**. Prevention can be primary, secondary, or tertiary. *Primary prevention* refers to those actions taken to prevent disease or injury. This is accomplished by reduction of risk factors or exposure to illness or injury. An example of primary prevention would be immunization against disease (such as influenza). In *secondary prevention*, attempts are made to identify disease in the earliest stages and to control or reduce the impact on the individual. An excellent example of secondary prevention is mammography. Finally, *tertiary prevention* seeks to prevent disability and attempts to restore the individual to optimal levels of functioning after the disease has been treated. An example of tertiary prevention would be rehabilitation following a fractured hip.

Both health promotion and disease prevention seek to prevent disease; however, health promotion considers parameters not included in most disease-prevention models, specifically the spiritual, social, emotional, and intellectual realms.

Frailty and Disability in Pathological Aging

In order to assess pathological aging, it is important to consider frailty and disability. Another popular myth associated with aging is that older adults are (or will become) frail and sickly. Defining the term *frailty* is challenging, and therefore is often loosely used to imply declines in both health and functional status in geriatric literature. **Frailty** was recently defined by Rockwood as the "multidimensional syndrome of loss of reserves (energy, physical ability, cognition, health) that gives rise to vulnerability." Other definitions include such characteristics as the older adult being withdrawn, unsteady, and weak and tending to have more complications as they age, coupled with a higher rate of hospitalization. Despite much interest in the concept of frailty, consensus is lacking as to the term's actual definition. Although many experts have posed various constructs to explain the concept of frailty, one theme remains consistent—it is a state of vulnerability.

In its most fundamental terms, disability can be thought of as a decline in physical ability or mental capacity to the extent that the individual cannot perform the usual activities of daily living without great difficulty. Similar to frailty, disability is not a normal part of aging.

Gerontologists have explored the relationship between frailty and disability and the resultant consequences for older adults. Disability has been linked with negative consequences to society, such as increased service utilization in the form of nursing home placement, burdens on families, and as a barrier to the preservation of autonomy. It is important not to wait until the older adult is hospitalized and in need of health care services,

health promotion Deliberate actions that are taken with the intent of moving an individual to a higher level of wellness.

disease prevention The deferral or elimination of medical illnesses and conditions through appropriate interventions for an individual or group with the goal of improving the health of the individual or population and thereby improving quality of life. Often categorized as primary, secondary, and tertiary.

frailty The condition of being weak or vulnerable in health or body. Factors such as unintentional weight loss (10 pounds or more in a year); general feelings of weakness and exhaustion; physical weakness (as measured by grip strength, decreased walking speed, and low levels of physical activity) are indicators of frailty.

TABLE 22-1 Levels of Prevention

Level of Prevention	Definition	Examples
Primary	Actions taken to prevent a disease or injury.	Vaccination
Secondary	Actions taken to identify a disease at the earliest stage possible.	Mammogram
Tertiary	Prevent or limit disability; restore individual to optimal level of functioning.	Rehabilitation following a fractured hip

because by this point the spiral of decline may have already begun. This unfortunate "spiral of decline" moves the older adult closer to the pathological aging end of the aging spectrum.

Quality of Life

Wellness, health promotion, disease prevention, frailty, and disability are key concepts that ultimately impact the quality of life of the older adult. Similar to those concepts discussed previously, quality of life is not easily defined (**Figure 22-1**). It encompasses many dimensions—physical, emotional, psychological, and spiritual.

Another myth associated with aging is that quality of life will inevitably decline. Quality of life conveys an overall sense of well-being, including aspects of happiness and satisfaction with life as a whole. It is imperative for those working with older adults to recognize that although this population is at risk for experiencing a decrease in the quality of life, one should not assume that this is simply a consequence of aging.

Many experts have proposed definitions of quality of life; developed instruments, such as questionnaires, to "measure" quality of life; and focused on quality of life in specific settings (such as nursing homes) as well as with regards to specific diseases and disorders, such as dementia or terminal illnesses.

In public health nutrition practice and research, the concept of health-related quality of life refers to a person or group's perceived physical and mental health over time. The health-related quality of life (HRQOL) is often used to measure the effects of chronic illness and to better understand how an illness interferes with a person's day-to-day life as well as to measure the effects of numerous disorders, short- and long-term disabilities, and diseases in different populations. Tracking health-related quality of life in older adults can identify subgroups with poor physical or mental health and can help guide policies or interventions to improve their health. Three questionnaires have been developed and are used together by the CDC to comprise the full HRQOL-14 measure. These include the standard four-item set of Healthy Days core questions (CDC HRQOL-4), which has been in the State-based Behavioral Risk Factor Surveillance System (BRFSS); the CDC HRQOL-4 in the National Health and Nutrition Examination Survey (NHANES), and the CDC HRQOL-4 in the Medicare Health Outcome Survey (HOS) (**Table 22-2**). More information on the topic of health-related quality of life (HRQOL) surveillance can be found on the CDC's website.

One instrument designed specifically to measure quality of life for older adults was developed by researchers at University of Toronto to be used for a variety of purposes, including assessment, program evaluation, planning, and stimulation of discussion for community action. An impor-

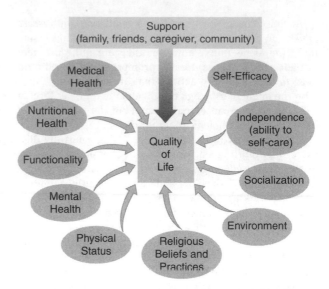

FIGURE 22-1 Factors that Influence Quality of Life

Source: Adapted from the Position Paper of the American Dietetic Association: nutrition across the spectrum of aging. *J Am Diet Assoc.* 2005; 105(4):616–633.

tant application of a quality-of-life assessment is its use in determining health and service needs of individuals at the community level and program evaluation. Quality of life is, however, highly subjective in that it can only truly be determined by the individual.

Successful Aging as the Product of Health Promotion and Disease Prevention

It is beyond the scope of this chapter to attempt to contribute to the already extensive body of literature that exists on the subject of which constructs should be included in a definition of successful aging. The concepts of health, health promotion, disease prevention, frailty, disability, and quality of life are multifaceted concepts. For the purposes of our exploration of health promotion in older adults, it is important to consider successful aging to be the product of effective health promotion activities coupled with evidence-based disease prevention strategies that are tempered with individual's needs. Activities should be aimed at the promotion of optimal levels of health and well-being, while at the same time avoiding making a negative impact on quality of life.

The Role of Nutrition in Geriatric Health Promotion and Disease Prevention

Whereas not all diseases can be prevented, there is a considerable body of literature that supports the efficacy of

TABLE 22-2 Centers for Disease Control and Prevention: Health-Related Quality-of-Life 14-Item Measure

Healthy Days Core Module (CDC HRQOL-4)

1. Would you say that in general your health is:

   Please Read

a. Excellent	1
b. Very good	2
c. Good	3
d. Fair	4

   or

e. Poor	5

   Do not read these responses

Don't know/Not sure	7
Refused	9

2. Now thinking about your physical health, which includes physical illness and injury, for how many days during the past 30 days was your physical health not good?

a. Number of Days	_ _
b. None	8 8
Don't know/Not sure	7 7
Refused	9 9

3. Now thinking about your mental health, which includes stress, depression, and problems with emotions, for how many days during the past 30 days was your mental health not good?

a. Number of Days	_ _	**If both Q2 AND**
b. None	8 8	**Q3 ="None," skip**
Don't know/Not sure	7 7	**next question**
Refused	9 9	

4. During the past 30 days, for about how many days did poor physical or mental health keep you from doing your usual activities, such as self-care, work, or recreation?

a. Number of Days	_ _
b. None	8 8
Don't know/Not sure	7 7
Refused	9 9

Activity Limitations Module

These next questions are about physical, mental, or emotional problems or limitations you may have in your daily life.

1. Are you LIMITED in any way in any activities because of any impairment or health problem?

a. Yes	1	
b. No	2	**Go to Q1 of Healthy Days Symptoms Module**
Don't know/Not sure	7	**Go to Q1 of Healthy Days Symptoms Module**
Refused	9	**Go to Q1 of Healthy Days Symptoms Module**

2. What is the MAJOR impairment or health problem that limits your activities?

   Do Not Read. Code Only One Category.

a. Arthritis/rheumatism	0 1
b. Back or neck problem	0 2
c. Fractures, bone/joint injury	0 3
d. Walking problem	0 4
e. Lung/breathing problem	0 5
f. Hearing problem	0 6
g. Eye/vision problem	0 7
h. Heart problem	0 8
i. Stroke problem	0 9
j. Hypertension/high blood pressure	1 0
k. Diabetes	1 1
l. Cancer	1 2
m. Depression/anxiety/emotional problem	1 3
n. Other impairment/problem	1 4
Don't know/Not sure	7 7
Refused	9 9

3. For HOW LONG have your activities been limited because of your major impairment or health problem?

   Do Not Read. Code using respondent's unit of time.

a. Days	1 _ _
b. Weeks	2 _ _
c. Months	3 _ _
d. Years	4 _ _
Don't know/Not sure	7 7 7
Refused	9 9 9

4. Because of any impairment or health problem, do you need the help of other persons with your PERSONAL CARE needs, such as eating, bathing, dressing, or getting around the house?

a. Yes	1
b. No	2
Don't know/Not sure	7
Refused	9

5. Because of any impairment or health problem, do you need the help of other persons in handling your ROUTINE needs, such as everyday household chores, doing necessary business, shopping, or getting around for other purposes?

a. Yes	1
b. No	2
Don't know/Not sure	7
Refused	9

(continues)

TABLE 22-2 Centers for Disease Control and Prevention: Health-Related Quality-of-Life 14-Item Measure *Continued*

Healthy Days Symptoms Module		
1. During the past 30 days, for about how many days did PAIN make it hard for you to do your usual activities, such as self-care, work, or recreation?		
a. Number of Days	_ _	
b. None	8 8	
Don't know/Not sure	7 7	
Refused	9 9	
2. During the past 30 days, for about how many days have you felt SAD, BLUE, or DEPRESSED?		
a. Number of Days	_ _	
b. None	8 8	
Don't know/Not sure	7 7	
Refused	9 9	
3. During the past 30 days, for about how many days have you felt WORRIED, TENSE, or ANXIOUS?		
a. Number of Days	_ _	
b. None	8 8	
Don't know/Not sure	7 7	
Refused	9 9	

4. During the past 30 days, for about how many days have you felt you did NOT get ENOUGH REST or SLEEP?
  a. Number of Days   _ _
  b None   8 8
     Don't know/Not sure 7 7
     Refused   9 9

5. During the past 30 days, for about how many days have you felt VERY HEALTHY AND FULL OF ENERGY?
  a. Number of Days   _ _
  b. None   8 8
     Don't know/Not sure 7 7
     Refused   9 9

Source: Data from National Center for Chronic Disease Prevention and Health Promotion. Centers for Disease Control and Prevention: health-related quality-of-life 14-item measure. Available at: http://www.cdc.gov/hrqol/hrqol14_measure.htm. Accessed July 15, 2009.

health promotion activities. The role of nutrition in health promotion and disease prevention of older adults is an evolving practice with guidelines and recommendations that necessitate being individualized to meet the individual needs of the older adult.

Heart Disease

Heart disease (sometimes referred to as cardiovascular disease) is an umbrella term that encompasses many different disorders. Some diseases included under this term include hypertension (HTN), coronary artery disease (CAD), myocardial infarction (MI), and heart failure (HF). **Box 22-1** briefly defines each disorder and more detailed information about heart disease can be found in Chapter 8.

When discussing many disease states, such as those affecting the heart, it is important to consider that there are factors that place individuals at risk for developing these disorders. These risk factors, which include lifestyle behaviors, current health status, age, and family history, can be separated into two groups: modifiable and nonmodifiable risk factors (**Table 22-3**).

Modifiable risk factors are those over which the individual has some control, whereas nonmodifiable risk factors are those that cannot be altered but must be considered in assessment and intervention.

Health Promotion and Disease Prevention in Heart Disease

Several risk factors associated with heart disease can be modified through health promotion/disease prevention activities. Primary prevention activities include discouraging older adults from engaging in activities that could increase the risk of heart disease and encouraging them to not smoke, to maintain a healthy weight, and to engage in physical activity for at least 30 minutes per day, most days of the week. Secondary prevention includes such activities as screening for high blood pressure through blood pressure monitoring, screening for elevated cholesterol through blood studies, quitting smoking, and reducing stress through stress management techniques. Tertiary prevention is aimed at controlling and monitoring the disease to limit damage to the heart muscle as well as other organs (such as the kidneys) as a result of the heart disease.

Cholesterol and Dietary Fat

Hypercholesterolemia is the condition of having elevated levels of serum cholesterol. Nutritional counseling should focus on teaching the older adult sources of dietary fat and cholesterol as well as strategies for decreasing their consumption. Increasing consumption of whole grains should also be encouraged (at least three servings per day). The consumption

BOX 22-1   Conditions Affecting the Heart

- **Hypertension (HTN).** Refers to an increase in systolic or diastolic blood pressure. Hypertension can be primary (essential hypertension) or secondary (secondary to another cause, such as renal disease, hyperaldosteronism, or pheochromocytoma).

- **Coronary artery disease (CAD).** Narrowing of the coronary arteries, the arteries that supply blood to the heart muscle, due to plaque formation. Incidence of CAD increases with age, but it is not *caused* by old age.

- **Myocardial infarction (MI).** What is commonly referred to as a "heart attack." This occurs when areas of the heart muscle are deprived of blood, resulting in ischemia and cell death.

- **Heart failure.** Sometimes referred to as *congestive heart failure*, this occurs when the heart cannot adequately pump blood, resulting in pulmonary or systemic circulatory congestion. This can be a direct result of CAD, MI, or HTN or secondary to lung diseases. The incidence of heart failure increases with aging.

TABLE 22-3 Risk Factors for Heart Disease

Modifiable Risk Factors	Nonmodifiable Risk Factors
Obesity	Gender (men are at greater risk than women)
Cholesterol (this includes lowering LDL and increasing HDL)	Age (incidence increases with advancing age, but is NOT caused by old age)
Sedentary lifestyle	
Smoking	Race (African Americans have twice the risk of Whites for developing hypertension)
High blood pressure	
Stress	
	Menopause (after menopause, a woman's risk for heart disease increases, but still does not reach the same level as a man's)
	Family history (increased risk for heart disease if parents, brothers, or sisters have heart disease)

Source: Data from Cleveland Clinic. Preventing and reversing cardiovascular disease. 2005. Available at: http://www.clevelandclinic.org/heartcenter/pub/guide/prevention/riskfactors.htm. Accessed July 8, 2006.

of whole grains has been associated with decreased plasma cholesterol levels and lowered risk of heart disease. Not all hypercholesterolemia is related to diet. Familial hypercholesterolemia, a hereditary type of hypercholesterolemia, requires pharmacologic intervention in addition to dietary modifications in order for treatment to be effective.

One area of growing interest and research is the relationship between heart disease and folic acid status. Standard nutritional counseling for the patient with heart disease now includes information about the necessity of adequate folate intake. Folate consumption for older adults is beneficial for the prevention and management of heart disease, vascular disease, cancer and overall health promotion and, therefore, nutrition counseling for heart disease should emphasize adequate consumption. Fruits, vegetables, fortified breads and grains, as well as breakfast cereals fortified with folate can help meet daily requirements.

Exercise

The recommendation that every American accumulate at least 30 minutes of exercise on most, but preferably all, days of the week applies to older adults as well. This recommendation is based on evidence that moderate physical activity is associated with a decrease in overall mortality, regardless of cause. Despite the several myths of aging and exercise

that exist, older adults can and do benefit from carefully designed exercise programs. Current research consistently supports the recommendation. More can be found on the topic of exercise for older adults in Chapter 19.

Smoking Cessation

The risk factors associated with smoking have been well documented over many years in multiple studies. It is the responsibility of each and every member of the interdisciplinary health care team to inquire about smoking and encourage the older adult to quit. The dietitian should consider the medication–nutrient interactions associated with cigarette smoking and make necessary adjustments in dietary recommendations. For example, cigarette smoke is associated with a release of free radicals that results in the oxidation of low-density lipoproteins (LDLs), which leads to atherosclerotic changes. Therefore, the dietitian should recommend increased consumption of those foods that contain vitamin C in clients who smoke.

Diabetes

Diabetes mellitus is a disorder resulting from deficiency of or resistance to the hormone insulin. Once thought to be a disorder of carbohydrate metabolism, diabetes is a generalized disorder of carbohydrate, fat, and protein metabolism.

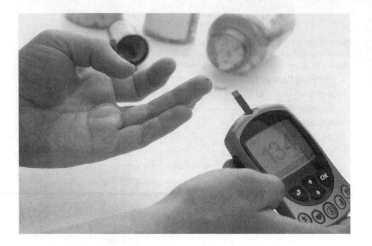

Diabetes results in microvascular as well as macrovascular complications if blood glucose levels are not maintained within acceptable parameters. These complications can manifest themselves in many ways, such as cardiovascular disease; retinopathy, which can lead to blindness; and nephropathy, which can lead to kidney failure; as well as generalized nerve damage. Diabetes and its clinical implications are discussed in more detail in Chapter 11.

According to the American Diabetes Association, more than 18% of those aged 60 and older have diabetes. Diabetes accounts for at least 3.6% of all deaths and 5.2% of cardiovascular disease deaths among U.S. adults. In considering these statistics, it is imperative that nutritionists understand the importance of nutritional health promotion as it relates to the diabetic older adult.

Primary prevention against the development of type 2 diabetes begins at an early age and should include counseling all adults to maintain a healthy weight and to engage in regular physical activity. Secondary prevention activities include screening for diabetes either through wellness clinics or through the older adult's primary care provider. Nutrition counseling is a key feature of primary and secondary prevention. Working with the older adult diabetic also often involves tertiary prevention in an effort to limit damage associated with diabetes.

Diet planning should include adequate calories to maintain or reduce weight in circumstances when the individual is noted to be overweight. Modest reductions in weight have been associated with improved control of blood glucose levels in those individuals with diabetes. The approach to dietary counseling should be individualized to the patient with diabetes—simply handing out an ADA diet sheet is rarely effective. The dietitian should help the older adult to identify eating patterns and assist him or her through nutritional counseling to make smart food choices.

Diabetes and Exercise

Exercise has been shown to improve insulin sensitivity in diabetics, in addition to medication and dietary interventions. Although many studies have demonstrated a clear benefit of aerobic activity in patients with diabetes, such activity may not be possible due to other comorbid conditions. Weight lifting or progressive resistance training (PRT) is a safe and effective alternative. PRT has been shown to improve glucose disposal rates, increase glycogen storage capacity, and improve insulin sensitivity. Exercise is discussed in detail in Chapter 19.

Pulmonary Disease

The term *pulmonary disease*, like heart disease, is a broad term that encompasses many disorders with the commonality that they affect the lungs. Most commonly, older adults are affected by a pulmonary disorder known as chronic obstructive pulmonary disease (COPD). COPD is characterized by chronic airflow limitation. Diseases such as chronic bronchitis, emphysema, and asthma are all types of COPD.

Cigarette smoking is the single most important risk factor for development of COPD. Approximately 80% of patients with COPD are current or former smokers. However, not all patients with COPD were cigarette smokers. Multiple theories have been developed to explain how COPD develops in nonsmokers; one such theory identifies viral infections in childhood (group C adenovirus in particular) as an independent risk factor for the development of COPD.

Nutritional Interventions

The Nutrition Screening Initiative provided interventions applicable to the client with COPD. Some key interventions to help ensure adequate nutritional status are listed in **Box 22-2**. Pharamacologic interventions are an important part of the medical care of the client with COPD. It is important to conduct a comprehensive review of an individual's medications and be aware of potential nutritional side effects of medications commonly used to treat COPD.

Smoking Cessation

As a priority, assessment of COPD patients should include eliciting whether the client smokes. Smoking cessation is considered to be one of the most essential parts of therapy in the treatment of COPD. In addition to smoking cessation, appropriate nutritional counseling should be included in the client's overall plan of care. Counseling should include replacement of vitamins that may have been depleted by cigarette smoking. The dietitian may also consider counseling specific to dietary antioxidants. Smoking has been found to result in oxidative stress, and antioxidant therapy is currently being considered in terms of its benefits in treating COPD.

Weight Control

Approximately one-third of all patients with COPD demonstrate some degree of malnutrition. Malnutrition is more common among patients with emphysema than those with chronic bronchitis. The malnutrition in this group is the result of impaired pulmonary status, reduced diaphragmatic mass, and decreased exercise capacity. Whether the individual is overweight or underweight, a nutrition care plan and medical nutrition therapy should include realistic goals that are mutually agreed upon with the older adult.

Osteoporosis

Bone mass is constantly being broken down and rebuilt as calcium is exchanged in the bloodstream in relation to hormones secreted by the parathyroid glands (parathormone increases calcium resorption, whereas calcitonin inhibits calcium resorption). In osteoporosis, there is a reduction of total bone mass, which predisposes the individual to bone fractures. Bones that are affected lose calcium and phosphate salts, resulting in porous and brittle bones. A more in-depth discussion of bone health can be found in Chapter 11.

Nutritional Intervention in Patients with Osteoporosis

Primary prevention of osteoporosis beginning in childhood and adolescence ensures that individuals achieve peak bone mass. Adequate diet and regular physical activity are important in the attainment as well as maintenance of healthy bone status throughout the later years.

Older adults should be encouraged to increase intake of foods high in calcium to a target of 1,000 to 1,200 mg of calcium per day. Ideally, 75% of calcium intake should come from milk products.

Foods rich in vitamin D to achieve a daily intake of 200 to 400 IUs should also be encouraged. Caution should be taken when encouraging patients to increase sunlight exposure. Reduced skin thickness secondary to normal aging decreases the epidermal concentrations of vitamin D precursors in older adults. Due to the frequency of inadequate dietary intake in older adults as well as limited sunlight exposure, supplemental calcium and vitamin D may be indicated.

Weight-Bearing Exercise

The association between mechanical stress and bone mass was first realized by Galileo in 1683. Since that time, the body of knowledge related to exercise and bone mass has expanded considerably. The role of exercise in the prevention and treatment of osteoporosis has been well documented, with particular emphasis on weight-bearing and resistance exercise. In addition to nutritional counseling, the dietitian should include recommendations for exercise, including weight-bearing activities (walking, mild-to-moderate-impact aerobics, and resistance exercise). Regular exercise increases muscle mass and strength, improves balance and coordination, and has been shown to reduce the risk of falls in frail elderly persons by approximately 25%, which in turn helps to prevent fractures.

Drugs That May Worsen Osteoporosis

Similar to chronic pulmonary disease, it is important to keep in mind that the medications used to treat one chronic condition may worsen another. Steroids, anticonvulsants, as well as some antineoplastic agents (used in the treatment of cancer) have the potential to worsen osteoporosis. The benefits of conducting a complete assessment that includes a medication history cannot be overemphasized. Discussion of medications commonly used by older adults can be found in Chapter 17.

Obesity

In the United States, obesity is becoming a public health epidemic. Twenty-three percent of adults aged 20 and older have been identified as being obese (defined as a BMI of 30 or greater). Adults aged 60 and older have a rate of obesity of 24%. Obesity is responsible for many billions of dollars in direct costs to the U.S. health care system on an annual basis. It has been noted that due to high costs and ineffectiveness of programs to treat obesity, the solution to the obesity epidemic may very well be found in targeting young people.

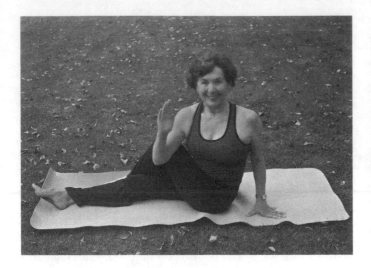

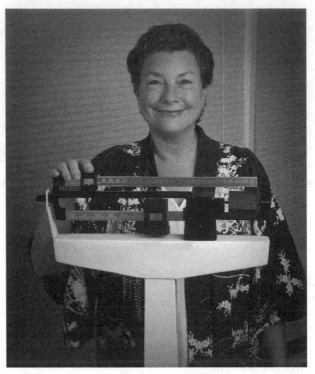

It has also been noted that a high proportion of people who were overweight or obese at young ages who survive past age 65 experience adverse consequences related to obesity. Studies have shown that obesity-related disability is of greater concern than obesity-related death in older adults. For example, new research suggests that overweight and obesity beginning early in life contribute to an increased risk of mobility limitation in old age. Notwithstanding, there are special considerations when working with the older adult to help reduce weight through mutual goal setting in order to avoid or limit the effects of disability secondary to obesity. Care should be used when working with obese older adults. Overweight and obesity can mask underlying malnutrition due to consumption of a poor quality diet. This compounds the conditions that accompany obesity with additional problem nutrient deficiencies for the older adult.

Obesity and Diet

As individuals age, the overall number of calories that are required to maintain body weight decreases. This is related to both decreased metabolic demand as well as increased sedentary activities that are associated with aging. It is of high importance when working with older adults to consider individualized strategies to achieve weight management through dietary and physical activity interventions. Special attention should be paid to comorbidities when providing dietary counseling. A comprehensive nutritional assessment should be conducted to assess current calorie needs as well as energy expenditure through daily lifestyle and physical activity.

Obesity and Exercise

Exercise is essential to weight loss and long-term maintenance of weight loss. Even small changes in daily activ-

ity levels have been shown to be extremely important to the achievement of sustained weight loss. The benefits of regular physical activity and exercise are far-reaching in older adults and include not only disease risk reduction and weight management, but also maintenance of functional independence and improved quality of life.

Nutritional Products and Dietary Supplements

It is difficult to pick up a newspaper or to watch a television program without being exposed to information about the "latest and greatest" discoveries in health care. Television "infomercials" have been developed to tell consumers about the latest diet or supplement that will enhance their well-being, extend their longevity, or improve their quality of life. Multiple local and national chain stores committed to the promotion and sale of nutritional supplements have proliferated over the past several years as our society seeks to enhance health, longevity, and well-being.

Health care providers should not discount the appropriate use of alternative nutrition therapies and nutritional supplementation. When working with adults, health care providers must educate themselves on the benefits and risks of supplement use specific to this population from a scientific perspective. Reliable guidance is challenging, however, be-

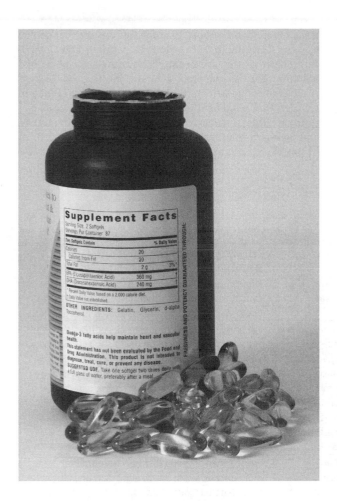

cause scientific evidence is in many cases still in its infancy with regards to supplement use in this population.

The use of nutritional supplements to achieve the health-related goals is part of a larger conglomeration of practices often referred to as **complementary and alternative medicine (CAM)**. The White House Commission on Complementary and Alternative Medicine Policy defined CAM as "a group of medical, health care and healing systems other than those included in mainstream health care in the United States. CAM includes the worldviews, theories, modalities, products, and practices associated with these systems and their use to treat illness and promote health and well-being."

A recent survey found that 88% of respondents older than age 65 reported using at least one form of CAM. Of this group, 65% reported using dietary supplements. Interestingly, individuals with advanced education used even more dietary and herbal supplements. In practical terms, this means that it is likely that many older adults are taking some type of

nontraditional supplementation. Therefore, when providing nutrition services, assessment of supplement use should be considered and evaluated for safety and efficacy.

Individuals working with older adults should be aware of the use of CAM, specifically the use of dietary supplements. Older adults may not always be forthcoming about taking supplements, because they feel that they are not medications. It is also important to determine if the use of CAM preparations can result in interactions with other medications that the older adult is taking. For example, St. John's Wort, an herb that has been demonstrated to be "superior" to placebo and "equivalent" to standard antidepressant therapies in the treatment of mild to moderate depression, can interfere with the action of many prescription medications.

Older adults faced with multiple chronic medical conditions, as well as declines in independence and functional capabilities and social changes, are often susceptible to believe advertisements for the "pill" that will fix any problem. Supplements are difficult to regulate, and many manufacturers of these products deliberately mislead consumers. As a result of the increased vulnerabilities, the potential exists for the older adult to fall prey to misleading claims about the "extraordinary" healing abilities of certain dietary supplements and this must be handled with sensitivity by informed nutrition counselors.

Food Safety

Regardless of age, foodborne illnesses can and do occur. The potential for foodborne illnesses are seldom considered and only capture the attention of the public when an outbreak occurs and generates a media sensation. Older adults are at particular risk for suffering extreme consequences of foodborne illnesses for several reasons, including comorbidities (such as diabetes or heart disease) and immunosenescence (the aging immune system).

The potential hazards to food safety are commonly divided into three categories: (1) biological hazards from bacteria and other microorganisms; (2) chemical hazards, such as pesticides used where foods are grown to prevent crop damage; and (3) physical hazards, such as hair, dirt, or other nonfood items. This chapter will examine only biological hazards.

Biological Hazards

Biological contamination can occur from a variety of sources, including bacteria, toxins, and viruses. Not all bacteria are harmful to humans. Some bacteria actually enhance digestion, for

> **complementary and alternative medicine** A broad range of healing philosophies, approaches, and therapies that include treatments and health care practices not taught widely in medical schools, not generally used in hospitals, and not usually reimbursed by medical insurance companies.

example, *Lactobacillus*, which are added to yogurt to enhance digestion. However, some types of bacteria are harmful to humans, such as those listed in **Table 22-4**, which provides an overview of common infectious agents, the disorders that they cause, and their symptoms.

Viruses pose another biological threat to food safety. Viruses are unable to replicate independently and, therefore, require a host. Although they cannot reproduce in or on food, they may survive in or on food long enough to be transmitted to a new host. Examples of viruses that can be transmitted through food include Hepatitis A and Novovirus. These viruses are usually transmitted via poor food handling, such as inappropriate hand washing.

Biological threats can result in contamination of food in a variety of ways. The three main "abuses" to food that can result in illness—time–temperature, cross-contamination, and poor personal hygiene by food handlers—are outlined in **Box 22-3**. Careful attention to safe food handling is es-

TABLE 22-4 Common Pathogenic Bacteria and Their Consequences

Infectious Agent	Comments	Symptoms
Campylobacter, which causes camplyobacteriosis	Common in poultry. Some experts suggest that approximately one-half of all raw chicken is contaminated by this bacteria. Can also be acquired from unpasteurized milk and contaminated water.	Fever, diarrhea, and bloody stool two to five days after eating a contaminated food. Usually mild, the infection can trigger Guillain-Barre syndrome, a condition whereby the immune system attacks the body's nerves and may cause paralysis or even death.
Clostridium botulinum, which causes botulism	Foodborne botulism is rare because the organism needs specific conditions in order to produce toxins; namely a temperature above 38°F and a lack of oxygen. Poorly canned vegetables and fruits are a potential source for this type of food poisoning, but modern canning methods have almost done away with the problem. Sometimes, older adults purchase dented cans, which are often reduced in price for quick clearance. Older adults should be counseled to avoid this practice.	Eye problems such as double vision, drooping eyelids and an inability to focus on nearby objects; difficulty swallowing or breathing; nausea, vomiting, cramps, and diarrhea, usually within 18–36 hours of eating a contaminated food. The infection is very serious and can be fatal.
Escherichia coli, which causes gastroenteritis	Most common cause of traveler's diarrhea. Can be acquired from drinking water, including ice cubes; peeled fruit; undercooked ground beef; and unpasteurized milk.	Nausea, vomiting, and diarrhea; headaches and muscle aches within one to eight days of eating a contaminated food.
Listeria monocytogenes, which causes *Listeriosis*	Acquired from soft cheeses and undercooked meats.	Fever, muscle aches, fatigue, and nausea. Some victims develop meningitis.
Salmonella, which causes *Salmonellosis*	Commonly found in raw or undercooked meat, poultry, and raw eggs.	Nausea, vomiting, cramps, and diarrhea within 48 hours of eating the offending food. The illness can be fatal in infants, older adults, and people with weakened immune systems.
Shigella, which causes *Shigellosis*	These bacteria thrive in food that is left out for long periods.	Abdominal cramps and pain, nausea and vomiting, watery diarrhea, bloody stool, and fever within one to seven days. The infection can be serious in infants, older adults, and people with weakened immune systems.
Staphylococcus	Usually picked up from mayonnaise-based salads (tuna salad, potato salad, egg salad) and cream-filled desserts.	Diarrhea and nausea/vomiting within two to eight hours after consumption.
Vibrios	Usually acquired by eating raw mollusks.	Diarrheal illness or sepsis syndrome in compromised hosts.

Source: Adapted from Physician's Desktop Reference. Food poisoning. Available at: http://www.pdrhealth.com/disease/disease-mono.aspx?contentFileName= BHG01GA29.xml&contentName=Food+Poisoning&contentId=56&TypeId=1. Accessed July 15, 2009.

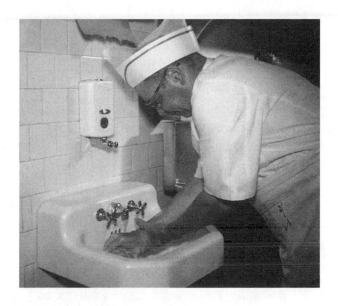

sential to the primary prevention of food-related illness. Food safety education and regular staff in-service programs should be a mandatory component of training for all individuals working in food service.

Preventing Foodborne Illnesses

Increased awareness of the dangers associated with food-borne illnesses and anticipatory guidance to older adults helps to protect them. Providing practical advice on food safety can help prevent sickness, or even death. Food safety experts recommend that consumers follow four rules (**Figure 22-2**)—clean, separate, cook, and chill—to ensure food safety.

Food Handling and Preparation

Hand washing is the single most important means of preventing the spread of infection. Meal preparation should begin with a thorough hand washing using soap and running water. Various types of antibacterial soaps are available; however, plain soap is also quite effective. The use of mechanical friction and running water will help minimize the likelihood of transmitting infectious agents.

Food Storage

Hot foods should be kept hot and cold food should be kept cold. The following guidelines should be used when working with food. Bacteria grow most rapidly in the "danger zone," temperatures between 40° and 140°F. It is essential to keep foods out of this temperature range for extended periods of time. The only way to evaluate temperature prop-

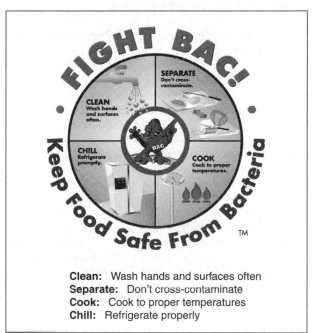

Clean: Wash hands and surfaces often
Separate: Don't cross-contaminate
Cook: Cook to proper temperatures
Chill: Refrigerate properly

FIGURE 22-2 Food Safety

Source: Courtesy of the Partnership for Food Safety Education. www.fightbac. org.

erly is with a food thermometer. Color is not a reliable indicator of doneness or food safety.

Refrigerate or freeze perishables, prepared foods, and leftovers within two hours of purchase or preparation, or within one hour if the temperature is above 90°F. Foods should be marinated in the refrigerator. Meats, such as roasts or steaks, should be cooked until their internal temperature (measured by a cooking thermometer) reaches a minimum of 145°F. Poultry should be cooked to a minimum internal temperature of 165°F. Special precautions need to be taken with ground meats, because bacteria could be spread to the center of the meat while it is being ground. Therefore, ground meats should be cooked to at least 160°F. Eggs should be cooked until the yolk and white are firm, not runny. Fish should be cooked to 145°F or until the flesh is opaque and separates easily with a fork. Older adults or individuals with a compromised immune system should be discouraged from using recipes in which eggs, any animal product, or fish remains raw or only partially cooked.

Microwave ovens are a source of convenience for many older adults. For best results when using a microwave oven, cover food, stir, and rotate for even cooking. If there is no turntable, the dish should be rotated by hand once or twice to ensure complete and even cooking.

Specific Strategies for Disease Prevention and Health Promotion

Nutritional requirements change with age and life circumstance. Older adults have special nutritional needs, and it is important for health professionals working in the field of geriatrics to have a working knowledge of these unique needs. Changes in specific nutrient requirements were discussed in preceding chapters. When providing nutrition counseling aimed at promoting health in older adults, the specialized considerations discussed briefly here should be integrated into the overall health care plan.

American Diabetes Association

People with diabetes have the same nutritional requirements as everyone else; however, careful attention should be given to their diet to reduce the likelihood of medical consequences of diabetes. The American Diabetes Association is a valuable source of nutrition information for those with diabetes and prediabetes and even those at risk for developing the disease.

The American Diabetes Association's recommendations for choosing healthy foods and recipes and exercise guidelines are clearly explained for children and adults of all ages. Suggestions for weight loss, dining out, reading food labels, grocery shopping, use of sweeteners and desserts are easily accessible from its website.

National Cancer Institute and the American Institutes for Cancer Research

Based on the 1982 National Academy of Sciences Committee report on Diet, Nutrition, and Cancer, the National Cancer Institute (NCI) released dietary guidelines for the public.

> **BOX 22-4   National Cancer Institute's Nutrition Guidelines for Cancer Prevention**

- Choose a diet rich in a variety of plant-based foods.
- Eat plenty of vegetables and fruits.
- Maintain a healthy weight and be physically active.
- Drink alcohol only in moderation, if at all.
- Select foods low in fat and salt.
- Prepare and store foods safely.
- Do not use tobacco in any form.

Source: Data from The American Institute for Cancer Research. Diet and health guidelines for cancer prevention. 2006. Available at: http://www.aicr.org/site/PageServer?pagename=dc_home_guides/. Accessed July 15, 2009.

These guidelines are geared toward cancer prevention, but they are also consistent with the USDA's Dietary Guidelines for Americans.

The American Institute for Cancer Research has published practical guidelines for cancer prevention, some of which are outlined in **Box 22-4**.

American Heart Association

The American Heart Association (AHA) advocates a healthy diet and lifestyle as the "best weapons to fight cardiovascular disease." The AHA's 2006 Diet and Lifestyle Recommendations suggest the following for preventing heart disease:

- **Use at least as many calories as you take in.** Individuals should start by knowing how many calories they should be eating and drinking to maintain their weight. The amount and intensity of physical activity should gradually be increased, with a goal of 30 minutes each day.
- **Eat a variety of nutritious foods from all the food groups.** Choose foods such as vegetables, fruits, whole-grain products, and fat-free or low-fat dairy products most often. Eating fish high in omega-3 fatty acids (e.g., salmon, trout, and herring) at least twice a week may help lower the risk of death from coronary artery disease.
- **Eat fewer nutrient-poor foods.** Older adults may be eating plenty of food, but their body may not be getting the nutrients it needs to be healthy. Limit foods and beverages high in calories but low in nutrients, and limit saturated fat, *trans*-fat, cholesterol, and sodium. Read food labels; the Nutrition Facts panel tells how much of those nutrients each food or beverage contains.

- **Do not smoke tobacco, and stay away from tobacco smoke.** Older adults who smoke should be encouraged to quit.

Specific recommendations for daily food choices are listed in **Table 22-5**. These recommendations can be applied to adults of all ages with cardiovascular disease or those at risk for cardiovascular disease.

National Cholesterol Education Program by NHLBI

The National Heart, Lung, and Blood Institute (NHLBI) initiated the National Cholesterol Education Program (NCEP) in November 1985. The goals of this program are to reduce the risk of illness and death from coronary heart disease by reducing the percentage of Americans with high blood cholesterol. The NCEP guidelines are available at the National Heart, Lung, and Blood Institute website.

Exercise

Older adults are never "too old" to enjoy the numerous beneficial effects of regular exercise. Participation in a regular exercise program is an effective method for minimizing the functional declines commonly associated with aging. Exercise recommendations as well as exercise prescriptions for older adults were discussed in detail in Chapter 19. Activities should be incorporated into an individual's habitual lifestyle. Aerobic exercises can help maintain and improve various aspects of cardiovascular function; reduce risk factors associated with disease states, such as heart disease and diabetes; improve overall health status; and contribute to an increase in life expectancy. Muscle weakness and sarcopenia are commonly seen with advancing age, and, therefore, strategies such as strength training for preserving or increasing muscle mass in the older adult should be implemented.

Together, aerobic activities and strength training greatly improve the functional capacity of older men and women and therefore successfully improve well-being and quality of life in this population.

Medical Nutrition Therapy

Nutrition plays an important role in the treatment of several diseases. The Centers for Medicare and Medicaid Services (CMS) reimburses medical nutrition therapy for patients with diabetes or renal diseases. The goal of the Medical Nutrition Therapy (MNT) program is to prevent or reduce complications from these conditions that can be modifiable. Medicare coverage for MNT includes:

TABLE 22-5 American Heart Association Recommendations: Base Your Eating Pattern on These Recommendations for Daily Food Choices

Limit how much saturated fat, trans fat and cholesterol you eat.
Choose lean meats and poultry without skin and prepare them without added saturated and trans fat.
Select fat-free, 1 percent fat, and low-fat dairy products.
Cut back on foods containing partially hydrogenated vegetable oils to reduce *trans* fat in your diet.
Cut back on foods high in dietary cholesterol. Aim to eat less than 300 milligrams of cholesterol each day.
Cut back on beverages and foods with added sugars.
Choose and prepare foods with little or no salt. Aim to eat less than 2,300 milligrams of sodium per day.
If you drink alcohol, drink in moderation. That means one drink per day if you're a woman and two drinks per day if you're a man.
Follow the American Heart Association recommendations for when you eat out, and keep an eye on your portion sizes.

Source: Data from American Heart Association. Diet and lifestyle recommendations. Available at: http://www.americanheart.org/presenter.jhtml?identifier=851. Accessed May 21, 2008.

- Initial assessment of nutrition and lifestyle
- Nutritional counseling
- Information regarding managing lifestyle factors that affect diet
- Follow-up visits to monitor progress of diet

Specifically, Medicare covers three hours of one-on-one counseling the first year and two hours each year thereafter. Changes in the beneficiary's condition/treatment/diagnosis can result in additional hours of treatment with physician referral. Physician referral is needed for initiation of MNT and must be renewed each calendar year for services to continue.

Other Nutrition Interventions

Those working with older adults should be familiar with the programs in the geographic area in which they practice. State and local governments as well as private sources provide a large number of programs and resources, many of which were introduced in Chapter 21. Practitioners are encouraged to seek out these resources.

Conclusion

This chapter has explored several important topics relating to promotion of health in the older adult. Some of the myths of aging were identified and replaced with fact-based knowledge. A major goal of this chapter was to demonstrate that the nutritionist is part of the health care team responsible for assessing and implementing those activities aimed at health promotion and disease prevention.

Activities Related to This Chapter

1. Contact your local office of aging and inquire about food assistance programs designed to meet the needs of older adults.
2. Contact a registered dietitian or licensed nutritionist in your area and ask him or her how they incorporate health-promotion and disease-prevention activities into their clinical practice.
3. Volunteer to give a presentation on "Healthy Aging" for local nursing home residents or older adults group at a local community center.

REFERENCES

American College of Sports Medicine (ACSM). ACSM position stand on exercise and physical activity for older adults. *Med Sci Sports Exerc.* 1998;30(6):992–1008.

Aldwin CM, Gilmer DF. *Health, Illness, and Optimal Aging.* Thousand Oaks, CA: Sage; 2004.

American Diabetes Association. Diagnosis and classification of diabetes mellitus. *Diabetes Care.* 2004;27:S5–S12.

American Dietetic Association. How did the RDAs become the DRIs? Available at: http://www.eatright.org/cps/rde/xchg/ada/hs.xsl/nutrition_5347_ENU_HTML.htm. Accessed August 5, 2006.

American Dietetic Association. Position paper of the American Dietetics Association: nutrition across the spectrum of aging. *J Am Diet Assoc.* 2005;105:616–633.

American Heart Association. What are healthy levels of cholesterol? Available at: http://www.americanheart.org/presenter.jhtml?identifier = 183. Accessed August 7, 2006.

American Heart Association. Our 2006 diet and lifestyle recommendations. Available at: http://www.americanheart.org/presenter.jhtml?identifier = 851. Accessed May 21, 2008.

American Institute for Cancer Research. Diet and health guidelines for cancer prevention. Available at: http://www.aicr.org/site/PageServer?pagename = home_guides. Accessed August 10, 2006.

Anspaugh DJ, Dignan MB, Anspaugh SL. *Developing Health Promotion Programs.* Boston: McGraw-Hill; 2000.

Avlund K, Vass M, Hendriksen C. Onset of mobility disability among community-dwelling old men and women: the role of tiredness in daily activities. *Age and Ageing.* 2003;32(6):579–584.

Bales CW, Fischer JG, Orenduff MC. Nutritional interventions for age related chronic disease. *Generations.* 2004;28(3):54–60.

Bloomgarden ZT. Diabetes and nutrition. *Diabetes Care.* 2002;25(10):1869–1875.

Butrum RR, Clifford CK, Lanza E. NCI dietary guidelines: rationale. *Am J Clin Nutr.* 1988;48(3):888–895.

Carlson JE, Ostir GV, Black SA, Markides KS, Rudkin L, Goodwin JS. Disability in older adults 2: physical activity as prevention. *Behav Med.* 1999;24(4):157–168.

Centers for Disease Control and Prevention. Measuring healthy days. Available at: http://www.cdc.gov/hrqol/hrqol14_measure.htm#1.

Centers for Medicare and Medicaid Services. Draft guidance to surveyors on F-31: sanitary conditions. Available at: http://www.ascp.com/resources/nhsurvey/upload/F371SanitaryConditionsJuly06.pdf. Accessed August 10, 2006.

Centers for Medicare and Medicaid Services. Medical nutrition therapy services—overview. Available at: http://www.cms.hhs.gov/MedicalNutritionTherapy/. Accessed August 6, 2006.

Cleveland Clinic. Preventing and reversing cardiovascular disease. Available at: http://www.clevelandclinic.org/heartcenter/pub/guide/prevention/riskfactors.htm. Accessed July 8, 2006.

Cote CG, Celli BR. New treatment strategies for COPD. *Postgrad Med.* 2005;117(3):27–35.

Daviglus ML. Health care costs in old age are related to overweight and obesity earlier in life. *Health Affairs* 2005;24:97–101.

Donahue JF. Still looking for answers in COPD. *Lancet.* 2005;365:1518–1520.

Drewnowski A, Evans WJ. Nutrition, physical activity and quality of life in older adults: summary. *J Gerontology, Series A.* 2001;56:89–94.

Ferreira IM, Brooks D, Lacass Y, Goldstein RS. Nutritional support for individuals with COPD. *Chest.* 2000;117(3):672–678.

Ferrins CE, Zerwic JJ, Wilbur JE, Larson JL. Conceptual model of health related quality of life. *J Nurs Scholarship.* 2005;37(4):336–342.

Fox S. Preliminary psychometric testing of the Fox Simple Quality-of-Life Scale. *J Neurosci Nurs.* 2004;36(3):157–166.

Ham RJ. Illness and aging. In Ham RJ, Sloane PD, Warshaw GA (Eds.). *Primary care geriatrics* (4th ed.). Philadelphia: Mosby; 2002; 29–50.

Healthy People 2010. Nutrition and overweight. Available at: http://www.healthypeople.gov/document/HTML/Volume2/19Nutrition.htm. Accessed August 1, 2006.

Hoe J, Katona C, Roch B, Livingston G. Use of the QOL-AD for measuring quality of life in people with severe dementia—the LASER-AD study. *Age and Ageing.* 2005;34(2):130–135.

Holick MF. Environmental factors that influence the cutaneous production of vitamin D. *Am J Clin Nutr.* 1995;61(3):638–646.

Houston DK, Ding J, Nicklas BJ, Harris TB, Lee JS, Nevitt MC, Rubin SM, Tylavsky FA, Kritchevsky SB, Health ABC Study. Overweight and obesity over the adult life course and incident mobility limitation in older adults. The Health, Aging and Body Composition Study. *Am J Epidemiol.* 2009;169(8)927–936.

International Food Safety Council. Chill facts. Available at: http://www.foodsafety.gov/ ~ fsg/f01chill.html. Accessed July 30, 2006.

Lawyere S, Mahoney MC. St. John's wort. *Am Fam Physic.* 2005;72(11):2249–2255.

Lichtenstein AH, Mayer J. Whole-grain plaque fighters. *Agri Res.* 2006;54(2):23.

Malinow MR, Duell PB, Hess DL, Anderson PH, Kruger WD, Phillipson BE, et al. Reduction of plasma homocystine levels by breakfast cereal fortified with folic acid in patients with coronary heart disease. *New England J Med.* 1998;338(15):1009–1015.

Maramaldi P, Berkman B, Barusch A. Assessment and the ubiquity of culture: threats to validity in measures of health related quality of life. *Health Soc Work.* 2005;30(1):27–38.

McIntosh CN. Report on the construct validity of the temporal satisfaction with life scale. *Soc Indicators Res.* 2001;54(1):37–56.

Mauck KF, Clarke BL. Diagnosis, screening, prevention and treatment of osteoporosis. *Mayo Clin Proceed.* 2006;81(5):662–672.

Mayer BH (Ed). *Better elder care.* Springhouse, PA: Springhouse; 2002.

National Heart, Lung, and Blood Institute. Third report of the expert panel on detection, evaluation, and treatment of high blood cholesterol in adults (Adult treatment panel III). Available at: http://www.nhlbi.nih.gov/guidelines/cholesterol/index.htm. Accessed August 6, 2006.

National Restaurant Association Education Foundation. *ServSafe essentials* (4th ed.). Chicago: Author; 2006.

Ness J, Cirillo DJ, Weir DR, Nisly NL, Wallace RB. Use of complementary medicine in older Americans: results from the health and retirement study. *The Gerontologist.* 2005;45(4):516–524.

Nutrition Screening Initiative. A physician's guide to chronic disease management in older adults. [Brochure]. Washington, DC: Author; 2002.

Partnership for Food Safety Education. Safe food handling: Cook to proper temperatures. Available at: http://www.fightbac.org/content/view/172/96/. Accessed July 30, 2006.

Reagan PA, Brookins-Fisher J. *Community health in the 21st century* (2nd ed.). San Francisco: Benjamin Cummings; 2002.

Rennard SI. Treatment of stable chronic obstructive pulmonary disease. *Lancet.* 2004;364(9436):791–802.

Reynolds SL, Saito Y, Crimmins EM. The impact of obesity on active life expectancy in older American men and women. *The Gerontologist.* 2005;45(4):438–444.

Rockwood K. What would make a definition of frailty successful? *Age and Ageing.* 2005;34:432–434.

Rockwood K, Song X, MacKnight C, Bergman H, Hogan D, et al. A global clinical measure of fitness and frailty in elderly people. *Can Med Assoc J.* 2005;173(5):489–496.

Rozzini R, Sabatini T, Cassinadri A, Boffelli S, Ferri M, Barbisoni P, et al. Relationship between functional loss before hospital admission and mortality in elderly persons with medical illness. *J Gerontology.* 2005;60A(9):1180–1183.

Ruser CB, Federman DG, Kashaf SS. Whittling away at obesity and overweight. *Postgrad Med.* 2005;117(1):31–40.

Saydah SH, Eberhardt MS, Loria CM, Brancatl FL. Age and the burden of death attributable to diabetes in the United States. *Am J Epidemiol.* 2002;156(8):714–719.

Stein K. Interaction of vitamin C and cigarette smoke. *J Am Dietetic Assoc.* 2000;100(8):880.

Thompson Healthcare. PDR health: food poisoning. Available at: http://www.pdrhealth.com/disease/diseasemono.aspx?contentFileName = BHG01GA29.xml&contentName = Food + Poisoning&contentId = 56&TypeId = 1. Accessed April 12, 2003.

Todd JA, Robinson RJ. Osteoporosis and exercise. *Postgrad Med.* 2003;79(932):320–426.

Turnock BJ. *Public health: what it is and how it works* (2nd ed.). Gaithersburg, MD: Aspen; 2001.

U.S. Department of Health and Human Services and the U.S. Department of Agriculture. Dietary Guidelines for Americans. Available at: http://www.health.gov/Dietary Guidelines/. Accessed August 5, 2006.

Vladeck DC. Truth and consequences: the perils of half-truths and unsubstantiated health claims for dietary supplements. *J Pub Policy Marketing.* 2000;19(1):132–139.

West Virginia Rural Healthy Aging Network. What is healthy aging? Available at: http://www.hsc.wvu.edu/coa/rhan/. Accessed June 16, 2006.

White House Commission on Complimentary and Alternative Medicine Policy. Final report, March 2002. Available at: http://www.whccamp.hhs.gov/finalreport.html. Accessed August 1, 2006.

Wiley KA, Fiatarone Singh MA. Battling insulin resistance in elderly obese people with type 2 diabetes. *Diabetes Care.* 2003;26(5):1530–1588.

Wilson JF. Frailty and its dangerous effects might be preventable. *Ann Int Med.* 2005;141(6):489–492.

World Health Organization. Definition of health. Available at http://www.who.int/about/definition/en/. Accessed June 16, 2006.

Glossary

Acculturation Process whereby a group or individual's culture is modified while adapting to another culture. With regards to diet, acculturation can be seen with immigrants who after years (and generations) of living in a new country begin to adopt food patterns similar to those of the host country.

Actinic keratoses Premalignant lesions that appear in areas of skin exposed to sunlight. Most common in adults after long exposure to ultraviolet light; especially common in those with fair complexion, blue eyes, and light hair. Rare in people with dark skin.

Acute renal failure Acute renal failure is an abrupt decrease in renal function usually associated with lessened urine output (oliguria). It may be caused by vascular obstruction, hypotension, or after administration of radiocontrast media when doing X-rays. It is reversible if diagnosed early.

Administration on Aging The Administration on Aging (AoA) is one of the nation's largest providers of home- and community-based care for older adults and their caregivers. It awards annual grants to state governments to support programs mandated by Congress in the Older Americans Act. The six core services funded by the AoA are: supportive services, nutrition services, preventive health services, the National Family Caregiver Support Program (NFCSP), services that protect the rights of vulnerable older adults, and services for Native Americans.

Adrenal glands Two organs located close to the upper pole of each kidney. Each gland has two separate parts: a cortex and a medulla. The cortex produces the mineralocorticoid aldosterone, estrogen, androgens, and glucocorticoids. The medulla secretes epinephrine and norepinephrine.

Aerobic exercise The term *aerobic* refers to the presence of or a need for oxygen. The complete breakdown of glucose, fatty acids, and amino acids to carbon dioxide and water occurs only via aerobic metabolism. The citric acid cycle and electron transport chain are aerobic pathways. Therefore, aerobic exercise is any activity, such as running, walking, dancing, or biking, that requires the presence of sufficient oxygen. Also referred to as *cardiorespiratory exercise*.

Ageusia Loss of taste.

Alpha-tocopheral A potent form of vitamin E found in germ oils or via synthesis.

Alzheimer's disease Progressive and fatal neurological disorder occurring primarily in older adults. Characterized by problems with memory, physical function, and behavior. It is the most common form of dementia.

Amyloid Insoluble proteins that aggregate abnormally. They are associated with a number of diseases, including Alzheimer's disease.

Anaerobic exercise The term *anaerobic* refers to the absence of oxygen or the ability of a process to occur in the absence of oxygen. Therefore, anaerobic exercise is any activity that does not require the presence of oxygen. This includes short-term, high-intensity activities such as sprinting, weightlifting, and jumping.

Anemia Abnormally low concentration of hemoglobin in the bloodstream; can be caused by impaired synthesis of red blood cells, increased destruction of red cells, or significant loss of blood.

Anorexia Loss of interest in eating.

Anorexins Anything causing anorexia (loss of appetite).

Anosmia Loss of smell.

Anthropometry The measurement of body size, weight, and proportions to assess the physiologic effects of undernutrition or overnutrition.

Antioxidant A substance that combines with or otherwise neutralizes a free radical, thus preventing oxidative damage to cells and tissues.

Apoptosis Programmed cell death. In humans, about 50 to 70 billion cells die each day. When apoptosis is excessive, cancers may occur.

Appetite The desire to satisfy a bodily need.

Apraxia Speech disorder whereby the person is unable to say what he or she wishes to say. There are two types: one occurs after a stroke in the area of the brain where speech originates, rending the patient unable to speak or unable to say what he wishes to say. The second type is caused by muscle weakness affecting the muscles used in speech.

Arteriosclerosis Blood vessel walls become hardened and thickened with lipid deposits and lose their natural elasticity. This causes an increase in blood pressure and narrowing of the arteries of the heart and legs.

Aspiration (1) Abnormal entry of food or fluid into the airway. (2) Withdrawal of fluid or substance by suction from the airway to promote breathing when the airway is obstructed.

Atherosclerosis Deposition of fatty plaques within artery walls. Medium and large arteries acquire yellowish deposits (atheromatous plaques) composed of cholesterol, fat, cellular debris, and calcium. These plaques cause vessel walls to become thick and hardened.

Behavior modification   A systematic method for changing a behavior to a more desirable one by learning new lifestyle techniques and skills.

Benign prostatic hyperplasia (BPH)   Enlarged prostate gland of the male. Very common in older men. May be problematic when it causes compression of the urethra. This can result in urinary retention, incomplete emptying of the bladder, urinary overflow incontinence, nocturia (waking up at night to urinate), and hesitancy.

Beta-carotene   Yellow carotenoid in vegetables and fruits that contain vitamin A.

Biological value (BV)   Extent to which the protein in a food can be incorporated by the body. Expressed as the percentage of the absorbed dietary nitrogen retained by the body.

Body mass index (BMI)   Ratio of weight in kilograms to height (in meters) squared.

Bone mineral density (BMD)   Measured by a DEXA scan. Measures minerals in bone. The higher the bone mineral content, the less likely one is to fracture a bone. Used in diagnosis of osteoporosis, a common problem of older adults.

Cachexia   Loss of weight and muscle mass, often due to loss of appetite. One may be cachectic without stopping eating; frequently indicates a medical problem, often cancer.

Calcitonin   A hormone secreted by the thyroid gland in response to elevated blood calcium. It stimulates calcium deposition in bone and calcium excretion by the kidneys, thus reducing blood calcium.

Calculi   Urinary stones composed of crystals, protein, and other substances that may form and obstruct the urinary tract. The most common minerals in the stones are calcium phosphate and calcium oxylate. They occur more frequently in men than women and in warmer climates over colder ones.

Caries   Tooth disease that causes cavities and tooth decay.

Carotenoids   A group of yellow, orange, and red pigments found in plants. Many of these compounds are precursors of vitamin A.

Cholesterol   A waxy lipid (sterol) whose chemical structure contains multiple hydrocarbon rings.

Chronic renal failure   Chronic renal failure is an irreversible loss of renal function. It is progressive to end-stage renal disease. It is usually caused by long term hypertension and diabetes mellitus.

Cirrhosis   Severe, life-threatening problem related to alcohol abuse (usually). Leads to end-stage liver disease, jaundice, esophageal varices with bleeding, ascites (abdominal fluid), coma, and death.

Coenzymes   Organic compounds, often B-vitamin derivatives that combine with an inactive enzyme to form an active one. Coenzymes associate closely with these enzymes, allowing them to catalyze certain metabolic reactions in a cell.

Collagen   Main content of connective tissue and much of the whole body protein content.

Complementary and alternative medicine (CAM)   A broad range of healing philosophies, approaches, and therapies that include treatments and health care practices not widely taught in medical schools, not generally used in hospitals, and not usually reimbursed by medical insurance companies.

Consciousness   The awareness of one's existence.

Copper   Along with iron, it helps form RBCs. Good sources include dried fruits such as prunes, dark green leafy vegetables, cocoa, and black pepper.

Core foods   The most commonly consumed foods for a population or group or people.

Cytokines   Low-molecularweight proteins or glycoproteins. Function as chemical signals between cells. They play an important role in inflammation and in the acquired immune response.

Dementia   Progressive decline of cognitive function that occurs most often in very old adults. There is loss of memory, attention, and problem solving abilities. There are many types of dementia, the most common being Alzheimer's disease.

Diabetes mellitus, types 1 (T1DM) and 2 (T2DM)   A chronic disease in which uptake of blood glucose by body cells is impaired, resulting in high glucose levels in the blood and urine. Type 1 is caused by decreased pancreatic release of insulin. In type 2, target cells (e.g., fat and muscle cells) lose the ability to respond to insulin.

Dietary assessment   A comprehensive evaluation of the foods consumed and behaviors surrounding food consumption to identify eating patterns that contribute to nutritional status.

Dietary fiber   Plant carbohydrates that are not digestible by the gastrointestinal tract.

Dietary Guidelines for Americans 2005   Foundation of federal nutrition policy; they are developed by the U.S. Department of Agriculture (USDA) and the Department of Health and Human Services (DHHS). These science-based guidelines are intended to reduce the number of Americans who develop chronic diseases such as hypertension, diabetes, cardiovascular disease, obesity, and alcoholism.

Dietary Reference Intakes (DRIs)   A framework of dietary standards that includes Estimated Average

Requirement (EAR), Recommended Dietary Allowance (RDA), Adequate Intake (AI), and Tolerable Upper Intake Level (UL).

Disability   General term used to refer to deficits in an individual's overall health (physical or psychological) that affects that person's ability to perform the tasks of everyday living.

Discretionary calories   Extra calories above the minimum required to meet essential nutrient needs.

Disease prevention   The deferral or elimination of medical illnesses and conditions through appropriate interventions for an individual or group with the goal of improving the health of the individual or population and thereby improving quality of life. Often categorized as primary, secondary, and tertiary.

Diverticulitis   Infection and inflammation of the diverticula. The patient will have fever, leftsided pain, constipation, and diarrhea. The worst possibility is that it perforates the wall of the colon. The best preventative measure is eating fiber, which keeps the colon active.

Diverticulosis   Small outpouchings in the colon and large intestine. They increase with age, so that most 80-year-olds have diverticula. They may be asymptomatic or there may be cramping and bloating.

Dopamine   A hormone and neurotransmitter in the brain. It is also in a medication used to treat Parkinson's disease.

Dysgeusia   Distorted or strange taste, which can be a side effect of some medications.

Dysphagia   Difficulty swallowing. It may result from a neurological disorder that impairs esophageal motility or a mechanical obstruction of the esophagus.

Eating patterns   The foods and beverages a person consumes on a regular basis; also includes behaviors surrounding eating events.

Electrolytes   Substances that dissolve into charged particles (ions) when dissolved in water or other solvents and thus are capable of conducting an electrical current. The terms electrolyte and ion are often used interchangeably.

Endocrine glands   Glands of the endocrine system that synthesize and release special chemical messengers known as *hormones*. The endocrine glands include the thyroid, parathyroid, pancreas, adrenal, pituitary, hypothalamus, pineal, thymus, ovaries, and testes.

Enteral nutrition   The provision of nutrients using the gastrointestinal tract; includes oral diet and tube feedings.

Erythrocytes or red blood cells (RBCs)   Derived from erythroblasts in the bone marrow. Production is stimulated by the glycoprotein erythropoietin. An erythrocyte enters the blood as a reticulocyte after losing its nucleus. It then matures in the bloodstream. The number of reticulocytes is used as a clinical index of erythropoietic activity to determine whether new red blood cells are being produced.

Erythropoietin   Produced by the kidney and essential for normal erythropoiesis. It regulates red blood cell production in the bone marrow.

Essential fatty acids   Fatty acids that the body needs but cannot synthesize and must obtain from diet.

Exercise prescription   A program of exercises designed to meet desirable individual objectives for fitness. Includes specific recommendations for types of activities as well as the intensity, duration, and frequency of each exercise.

Fecal incontinence   The inability to hold a bowel movement until one is able to get to the toilet. It may occur when passing gas. Occurs in those with dementia and those with neurological damage. It occurs more frequently in older adults and in women.

Ferritin   A complex of iron and apoferritin that is a major storage form of iron.

Folate   *See* Folic acid

Folic acid (folate)   A form of vitamin B9. Required for production and maintenance of new cells and DNA synthesis. Deficiency causes slowed red blood cell production. Appears in laboratory tests as a macrocytic anemia.

Folic acid deficiency   Lack of folic acid. Folic acid is found naturally in dark green leafy vegetables, citrus fruits, beans, and whole grains.

Food insecurity   The state of, or risk of, being unable to obtain, prepare, chew, or swallow food.

Food security   Access to enough food for an active, healthy life at all times.

Foodways   Food traditions or customs of a group of people; involves how foods are obtained, prepared, served, and consumed. Encompasses beliefs about food, food preferences, and customs; has cultural, social, and economic components as well.

Fortification   The addition of vitamins or minerals to a food that were not originally present in the food.

Frailty   The condition of being weak or vulnerable in health or body. Factors such as unintentional weight loss (10 pounds or more in a year); general feelings of weakness and exhaustion; physical weakness (as measured by grip strength, decreased walking speed, and low levels of physical activity) are indicators of frailty.

Functional dependency   Requiring assistance for activities related to the functions of the body, usually involving activities of daily living.

Functional status   The ability of an individual independently to perform a task, activity, or behavior related to daily living.

Gamma aminobutyric acid (GABA)   Main inhibitory neurotransmitter in central nervous system. Regulates excitation of neurons. Implicated in such disorders as anxiety, epilepsy, and addiction.

Gastroesophageal reflux disease (GERD)   A condition in which the gastric contents move backward (reflux) into the esophagus, causing pain and tissue damage.

Gastrointestinal (GI) tract   The connected series of organs and structures used for digestion of food and absorption of nutrients; also called the *alimentary canal* or the *digestive tract*. The GI tract includes the mouth, esophagus, stomach, small intestine, large intestine (colon), rectum, and anus.

Gingivitis   Oral condition that causes red, bleeding gums. It is less serious than periodontal disorders, but it will lead to serious disease if neglected.

Gluconeogenesis   Formation of glucose by the liver from noncarbohydrate sources.

Glucose intolerance   Impaired glucose tolerance; pre-diabetes state; associated with insulin resistance and increased risk of cardiovascular pathology.

Glutamate (glutamic acid)   Excitatory neurotransmitter. Excitotoxicity is associated with stroke, amyotrophic lateral sclerosis, and other disorders.

Glycoslated hemoglobin   *See* Hemoglobin A1C

Health promotion   Deliberate actions that are taken with the intent of moving an individual to a higher level of wellness.

Healthy aging   Development and maintenance of optimal mental, social, and physical well-being and function in older adults. Most likely achieved when communities are safe and promote health and well-being and the older adult uses health services and community programs to prevent or minimize disease.

Healthy People 2010   A nationwide health-promotion and disease-prevention program that includes a set of health objectives for the United States to achieve over the first decade of the new century.

Heart failure (HF)   A progressive disorder of the heart in which the heart is unable to pump sufficient blood for the body's metabolic demands. Results from such disorders as hypertension, rheumatic heart disease, coronary artery disease, and valve insufficiency.

Hematopoiesis   Production of blood cells in the bone marrow. It is a two-stage process of mitosis (division) and maturation (differentiation). The cells undergo these stages prior to entering the blood system. Each blood cell has a parent cell called a stem cell that determines what kind of blood cell it will be.

Hemoglobin   The oxygen carrying protein in red blood cells. Consists of four heme groups and four globin polypeptide chains. The presence of hemoglobin gives blood its red color.

Hemoglobin A1C (glycoslated hemoglobin)   Glucose–hemoglobin complex that lasts the life of the red blood cell (90 to 120 days). It is a laboratory test used to assess average glucose levels over three months and does not fluctuate as does blood tests in daily testing.

Hepatitis   Inflammation of the liver. It has many causes, however, in Chapter 15 it is associated with alcohol abuse.

Heterocyclic amines   Carcinogens found in cooked muscle meats such as those from beef, pork, fowl, and fish.

Hiatal hernia   A physical abnormality that allows the stomach to protrude through the diaphragm and up into the chest. Often caused by weakened musculature.

High density lipoprotein (HDL)   Blood lipoproteins that contain high levels of proteins and low levels of triglycerides. Synthesized primarily in the liver and small intestine, HDL picks up cholesterol released from dying cells and other sources and transfers it to other lipoproteins.

Homocysteine   An amino acid precursor of cysteine and a risk factor for heart disease.

Hypercalcemia   Abnormally high concentrations of calcium in the blood.

Hyperkalemia   Abnormally high potassium concentrations in the blood.

Hypernatremia   Abnormally high sodium concentrations in the blood due to increased kidney retention of sodium or rapid ingestion of large amounts of salt.

Hypertension   When resting blood pressure persistently exceeds 140 mm Hg systolic or 90 mm Hg diastolic.

Hyperthyroidism   Overproduction and release of thyroid hormones. May result in heart palpitations and atrial fibrillation. Symptoms include tremors, nervousness, anxiety, weight loss, and diarrhea. There may be intolerance to heat and hair loss. It is very serious and may result in death if not diagnosed and treated.

Hypocalcemia   A deficiency of calcium in the blood.

Hypogeusia   Reduced ability to taste; ageusia is total loss of taste.

Hypoglycemia   Abnormally low concentration of glucose in the blood; any blood glucose value lower than 40 to 50 mg/dL.

Hypokalemia   Inadequate levels of potassium in the blood.

Hyponatremia   Abnormally low sodium concentrations in the blood due to excessive excretion of sodium (by the kidney), prolonged vomiting, or diarrhea.

Hypothalamus   Link between the central nervous system and the endocrine system. Synthesizes and secretes neurohormones. Responsible for regulation of body temperature, hunger, thirst, and anger.

Hypothyroidism   Insufficient production of thyroid hormone. Fairly common disorder; incidence is higher in older adults. Iodine deficiency can increase the risk.

Early symptoms include poor muscle tone, fatigue, cold intolerance, depression, constipation, muscle cramps, arthritis, goiter, brittle fingernails and hair, dry itchy skin, and weight gain. Late symptoms include dry puffy skin, loss of hair in outer one-third of eyebrows, slow speech with hoarse voice, and low body temperature.

Incontinence Loss of the ability to control the elimination of urine. May be occasional or consistent loss of control. Very common in older adults. *Stress* incontinence, which is common in older women, occurs when intra-abdominal pressure exceeds urethral resistance. Urethral muscles become weakened and small amounts of urine are passed. *Urge* incontinence, which is more common in younger women, is an overactive bladder. It is caused by urinary tract infections or central nervous system lesions. The woman feels that she must urinate but cannot control the urine until the time it takes to reach the toilet. *Functional* incontinence occurs when the urinary tract is intact but incontinence occurs due to dementia, musculoskeletal disability, or environmental factors. *Overflow* incontinence is caused by spinal cord abnormalities that affect the detrusor muscles of the bladder.

Insulin sensitivity A measure of one's risk for heart disease. The more sensitive one is, the lower the risk for heart disease. Can be used to regulate insulin dosages.

Formula for measurement:

(1) weight (lbs)/4 = _____ units of insulin
(2) total daily dose of insulin (all types of insulin) = _____ units

Line 1 is the estimated need for insulin; if the actual insulin dose on line 2 is close to this number, and patient has good control, insulin sensitivity is normal. If line 2 is *less* than line 1 and control is good, insulin sensitivity is excellent. If line 2 is much *greater* than line 1, the patient is probably getting too much insulin and may have insulin reactions.

Iron A trace element incorporated into the theme complex that carries oxygen to parts of the body. It is heavily regulated because it is toxic.

Irritable bowel syndrome (IBS) A disruptive state of intestinal motility of unknown cause. Symptoms include constipation, abdominal pain, and episodic diarrhea.

Isoflavones Plant chemicals that include genistein and daidzein and may have positive effects against cancer and heart disease. Also called *phytoestrogens*.

Lean body mass The portion of the body exclusive of stored fat, including muscle, bone, connective tissue, organs, and water.

Lentigines Harmless flat sunspots seen on the sun-exposed skin of older adults. Freckles.

Limbic system Area of the brain that controls emotion, behavior, and long-term memory. It is also associated with the olfactory system.

Low density lipoprotein (LDL) Cholesterol-rich lipoproteins generated from the breakdown and removal of triglycerides from intermediate-density lipoprotein in the blood.

Lymphocytes White blood cells. Include T cells, B cells, and killer cells, all of which are important in immunity. Killer cells defend the body from tumors and viruses. T and B cells work against antigens, which are foreign substances in the body. They produce antibodies that fight the antigen.

Lymphoid stem cells These give rise to progenitor cells: T, B, and null cells.

Macrocytosis Enlarged red blood cells. Seen in certain anemias, vitamin B12 deficiency, and alcohol abuse.

Major minerals A major mineral is required in the diet and is present in the body in large amounts compared with trace minerals.

Malnutrition Failure to achieve nutrient requirements, which can impair physical and/or mental health. May result from consuming too little food or a shortage or imbalance of key nutrients.

Mastication Chewing.

Melanocytes Cells in the skin that produce and contain the pigment melanin.

Methylmalonic acid (MMA) A laboratory test, rarely performed today, that is elevated in persons with vitamin B12 deficiency.

Modified MyPyramid for Older Adults A modification of the MyPyramid educational tool that translates the principles of the 2005 Dietary Guidelines for Americans and other nutritional standards to help consumers age 70 and older in making healthier food and physical activity choices.

Monounsaturated fats Fatty acids found in nuts; avocados; popcorn; whole-grain wheat products; oatmeal; and olive, canola, peanut, safflower, flaxseed, and sunflower oils. Lowers low density lipoproteins (the 'bad' lipids) and possibly raises the high density lipoproteins (the 'good' lipids). Protective against heart disease.

Myocardial infarction (MI) Death of muscle tissue in the heart due to the loss of blood flow from either a blood clot or progressive narrowing of the coronary arteries. The patient feels nausea; sweating; midsternal chest pain, which may radiate to the arms and neck; weakness; and possible loss of consciousness.

MyPyramid An educational tool that translates the principles of the 2005 Dietary Guidelines for Americans and other nutritional standards to help consumers in making healthier food and physical activity choices.

Neurofibrillary tangles and plaques Tangles are protein aggregates found in the neurons in Alzheimer's disease. Beta amyloid plaques are proteins found around the neurons in Alzheimer's disease. Together, they destroy neurons in the brain.

Nitrogen balance Nitrogen intake minus the sum of all sources of nitrogen excretion.

Nonsteroidal antiinflammatory drugs (NSAIDS) Drugs used to treat pain, inflammation, and fever (antipyretic). They are not opiates nor steroids. Aspirin, ibuprofen, and naproxen are commonly used NSAIDs.

Nonviscous fiber Dietary fibers that are insoluble in water; include cellulose, lignins, resistant starches, and many hemicelluloses.

Nutrient deficiency A shortfall of any nutrient that may result in suboptimal health.

Nutrition assessment Defines nutritional status by using medical, nutritional, and medication histories; physical examination; anthropometric measurements; and laboratory data.

Nutrition screening The process of identifying factors known to be associated with nutritional problems.

Nutrition Screening Initiative's DETERMINE Checklist A 10-question tool to evaluate the nutrition risk of older adults.

Nutritional status The state of a person's overall health and body as influenced by levels of nutrients and diet.

Obesity BMI at or above 30 kg/m^2.

Old age Often defined as ages nearing the average human lifespan. Although organizations providing services to older adults define their own age criteria, most people still think of old age as those adults ages 65 and older. Some organizations' minimum age requirements are:
- The Older Americans Act (OAA): 60 years
- USDA programs: 60 years
- DRIs: 51 to 70 years and 70+ years.
- Medicare: 65 years
- Social Security: 67 years
- AARP: 51 years

Older Americans Act Nutrition Program (OAANP) The law that established the Administration on Aging; insures that all Americans age 60 and over receive necessary services to maintain health, independence, and dignity.

Olfaction Sense of smell.

Olfactory Sense of smell; one of the chemosensory functions that often declines with aging. Also negatively affected by smoking, sinusitis, respiratory disorders, dental infections, and poor oral hygiene.

Omega-3 fatty acids Any polyunsaturated fatty acid in which the first double bond starting from the methyl (CH_3) end of the molecule lies between the third and fourth carbon atoms.

Oral nutrition support The provision of supplemental nutrition products to treat or prevent malnutrition in patients who can swallow safely and have a well-functioning gastrointestinal tract with the goal of ensuring that total nutrient intake meets individual needs.

Osteoporosis Bone disease characterized by a decrease in bone mineral density and the appearance of small holes in bones due to loss of minerals.

Oxidative stress Condition caused by an imbalance between the body's level of prooxidants (free radicals, reactive oxygen, and reactive nitrogen species) and its antioxidant capabilities, resulting in tissue damage, accelerated aging, impaired immune function, and degenerative diseases. Increased oxidative stress has many causes, including factors related to nutrition, illness, and the environment.

Palliative care Care given not to cure, but rather to help the patient live better with the disease while dying.

Papillae Small bumps on the tongue. Some contain taste buds.

Parageusia Unpleasant, abnormal taste of a food; often a metallic taste; may be caused by some medications.

Parathyroid glands Two to six glands located behind the thyroid gland that produce parathyroid hormone (PTH), which regulates calcium. PTH acts directly on bone and kidneys. If greatly stimulated (by low magnesium levels or phosphate), it causes breakdown and resorption of bone. If chronic stimulation occurs, bone remodeling occurs in which bone is broken down and re-formed.

Parenteral nutrition Provision of nutrients by intravenous infusion.

Parkinson's disease A common neurological disorder characterized by bradykinesia, rigidity, resting tremor, and impaired righting reflex.

Parosmia Distorted sense of smell; the person smells something unpleasant rather than the normal smell.

Pathological aging The etiologies, mechanisms, and manifestations of disease as they influence the aging process.

Peptic ulcer disease (PUD) A duodenal or stomach ulceration or erosion often caused by the bacterium *Helicobacter pylori*, which lives in an acid environment. It is treatable with antibiotics.

Periodontitis A group of disorders affecting the gums and teeth in the mouth. The gums become reddened and painful and often bleed and recede from the teeth, exposing the root of the tooth. Part of the problem is the accumulation of plaque on the lower part of the tooth at the gum line, which changes into tartar when there is poor oral hygiene for a prolonged period of time.

Peristalsis The rhythmic, coordinated contractions by which material is moved through the gastrointestinal tract.

Pharmacodynamics The study of the effect of drugs over time.

Pharmacokinetics The study of how drug levels are affected by absorption, distribution, metabolism, and elimination.

Pituitary (anterior and posterior) The anterior part of the pituitary gland produces and secretes peptide hormones that regulate stress, growth, and reproduction. The posterior pituitary secretes antidiuretic hormone (ADH), also known as vasopressin, and oxytocin. Oxytocin causes contractions in childbirth. ADH controls blood plasma osmolality. It acts to increase the permeability of renal collecting ducts. ADH secretion is increased by changes in intravascular volume.

Platelets Tiny disk-shaped components of blood that are essential for blood clotting.

Polyunsaturated fat Fatty acids found in sunflower, corn, soybean, and cottonseed oils. A healthy fat found in grains and seafood, such as herring, mackerel, salmon, and halibut. Protects against heart disease and insulin resistance.

Postmenopausal After the female menopause, after cessation of menses.

Prehypertension A systolic blood pressure equal to or greater than 120 mm Hg and a diastolic blood pressure equal to or greater than 80 mm Hg. It is a new category of risk indicating a greater risk for hypertension.

Progressive resistance training A method of strength training based on the principle of overload, which states that a greater-than-normal load on the body requires the body to adapt. Once the adaptation takes place, the stress is gradually increased. In strength training, this involves the continuous attempt to increase weight or resistance designed to maximize gains in muscle growth and strength.

Protein-energy malnutrition (PEM) A condition resulting from long-term inadequate intakes of energy and protein that can lead to wasting of body tissues and increased susceptibility to infection.

Provitamin Inactive forms of vitamins that the body can convert into active usable forms. Also referred to as vitamin precursors.

Pruritus Itchy skin.

Pyridoxine Also known as *vitamin B6*. Promotes red blood cell production and helps balance sodium and potassium. Diminished B6 causes seizures, nerve damage (numbness in hands and feet), anemia, skin problems, and mouth sores. It can be administered orally as a pill.

Quality of life An individual's perception of well-being regarding his or her physical and mental health as well as his or her satisfaction with life as a whole.

Red blood cells *See* Erythrocytes

Renal disease Disease of the kidneys.

Sarcopenia Age-associated loss of muscle mass, associated with muscle weakness, functional limitations, and disability, as well as impairments in cardiovascular capacity and metabolic health.

Saturated fats Fatty acids found in animal products, palm oil, coconut oil, and cocoa butter. It is recommended that not more than 10% of calories come from saturated fats every day (per the 2005 Dietary Guidelines for Americans). The American Heart Association recommends less than 7% of energy per day from saturated fats.

Seborrheic keratoses Benign proliferation of basal cells producing smooth or warty lesions. Very common in older adults, who usually have multiple lesions on the chest, back, and face. Lesions are brown, tan, waxy, or flesh colored. They may be very small (mm) to large (several cm).

Sedentariness A state of low level of energy expenditure in voluntary physical activity; an overall lifestyle characterized by a habitual low level of movement in daily activities and occupational or recreational pursuits.

Selective serotonin reuptake inhibitors (SSRIs) A class of antidepressants used to treat depression and anxiety disorders.

Selenium A member of the family of antioxidant enzymes. Prevents membrane damage. Also involved in the metabolism of iodine and thyroid hormone.

Senescence The process of growing older and displaying the effects of increased age.

Sensorineural hearing loss Unknown cause of hearing loss; however, it is related to nerve damage. More common in older adults.

Sicca Condition of having dry eyes and/or dry mouth.

Sideroblastic anemia (SA) Blood disorder in which there is sufficient iron but it is not used appropriately and does not function properly.

Steatorrhea Production of stools containing an abnormally high amount of fat.

Stem cell A formative cell whose daughter cells may differentiate into other cell types.

Stroma Connective tissue cells that are associated with the bone marrow and the rest of the hematopoietic system. They make up the support structure of cells.

Telangiectasias Fine, irregular red lines on the skin that are produced by capillary dilatation. Often seen on the cheeks and nose of older adults with rosacea.

Thresholds Reduced sensitivity for taste that occurs in older adults.

Thyroid gland Composed of two lobes that lie on either side of the trachea behind the thyroid cartilage, it is not visible but is palpated on swallowing. Thyroid cells secrete polypeptides such as calcitonin and somatostatin. Thyroid hormone secretion (TH) occurs in a feedback loop with other endocrine glands, principally the anterior pituitary and hypothalamus. Thyroid-stimulating hormone (TSH) increases iodide uptake and increases synthesis and release of prostaglandins. It helps regulate somatostatin, dopamine, and catecholamines, nutritional state, the body's response to extreme cold, and steroid levels. It regulates protein, fat, and carbohydrate catabolism in all cells. It regulates the metabolic rate of all cells. It regulates body heat production, acts as an insulin antagonist, and maintains growth hormone secretion, to name just a few of its activities.

Title III of the Older Americans Act Includes congregate and home delivered meals.

Tocopherols Chemical name for vitamin E. There are four tocopherols: alpha, beta, gamma, and delta. Only alpha-tocopherol is active in the body.

Trace minerals Minerals present in the body and required in the diet in relatively small amounts compared with major minerals. Also known as microminerals.

Triglycerides Fats composed of three fatty acid chains linked to a glycerol molecule.

Trophic hormones Hormones secreted to provide for survival of various cells.

Undernutrition Poor health resulting from the depletion of nutrients due to inadequate nutrient intake over time. It is most often associated with poverty, alcoholism, and certain eating disorders.

Viscous fiber Dietary fibers that are fermentable and are soluble in water to form a gel-like consistency; include gums and mucilages, pectins, psyllium, and some hemicelluloses.

Vitamin B12 Essential for blood formation and the maintenance of the brain and nervous system. It is involved in the metabolism of every cell in the body as well as synthesis of DNA and fatty acids. A synthetic form, cyanocobalamin, can be given for deficiency.

Wellness A state of well-being achieved by a combination of emotional, environmental, mental, physical, social, and spiritual health, especially when maintained by proper diet, exercise, and habits.

Xerostomia Dry mouth due to inadequate saliva.

Index

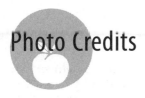

Photo Credits

Chapter 1

Page 1 Courtesy of Bill Branson/National Cancer Institute; **page 10** ©Monkey Business Images/ShutterStock, Inc.; **page 17** ©Corbis Collection/Alamy Images

Chapter 2

Page 22 ©LiquidLibrary; **page 32** ©Medical Body Scans/Photo Researchers, Inc.; **page 33** ©Photos.com; **page 36** ©Marie C. Fields/ShutterStock, Inc.; **page 38** ©Digital Stock; **page 39** ©Golf Money/ShutterStock, Inc.

Chapter 3

Page 44 ©Corbis; **page 47** ©Diana Lundin/Dreamstime.com; **page 49** ©Kathy Wynn/Dreamstime.com; **page 52** ©Glenda M. Powers/ShutterStock, Inc.

Chapter 4

Page 58 ©Photodisc; **page 60** ©Photodisc/Getty Images; **page 67** ©Geotrac/Dreamstime.com

Chapter 5

Page 72 ©Monkey Business Images/ShutterStock, Inc.; **page 73** ©Monkey Business Images/Dreamstime.com; **page 74** ©Eugene Feygin/Dreamstime.com; **page 76** ©Anthony Berenyi/Dreamstime.com; **page 79** Reproduced from *Introduction to Human Disease: Pathology and Pathophysiology Correlations, Seventh edition.* Photo courtesy of Leonard V. Crowley, M.D., Century College; **page 84** ©Simone Van Den Berg/Dreamstime.com

Chapter 7

Page 113 Reproduced from *An Introduction to Human Disease, Seventh edition.* Photo courtesy of Leonard V. Crowley, M.D., Century College.

Chapter 8

Page 127 ©Rmarmion/Dreamstime.com; **page 128** ©Ryan McVay/Photodisc/Getty Images; **page 131** ©Gualberto Becerra/ShutterStock, Inc.

Chapter 10

Page 165 Reproduced from *An Introduction to Human Disease, Seventh edition.* Photos courtesy of Leonard V. Crowley, M.D., Century College; **page 167** ©Jim Varney/Photo Researchers, Inc.; **page 176** ©Digital Vision

Chapter 11

Page 182 ©NATIVESTOCK/PhotoEdit, Inc.; **page 187** ©Rebeka Burgess/Dreamstime.com; **page 189** ©Feverpitch/ShutterStock, Inc.; **page 192** ©Monkey Business Images/Dreamstime.com; **page 196** Reproduced from *An Introduction to Human Disease, Seventh edition.* Photo courtesy of Leonard V. Crowley, M.D., Century College; **page 200 (left)** ©Bill Aron/PhotoEdit ; **page 200 (right)** ©Dr. Michael Klein/Peter Arnold, Inc.; **page 204 (top, bottom left, bottom right)** Reproduced from *An Introduction to Human Disease, Seventh edition.* Photo courtesy of Leonard V. Crowley, M.D., Century College.

Chapter 12

Page 210 (top left) ©LockStockBob/ShutterStock, Inc.; **page 210 (top right)** ©Photodisc; **page 210 (middle)** ©IRA/ShutterStock, Inc.; **page 210 (bottom)** ©Tobik/ShutterStock, Inc.; **page 211** ©Photodisc; **page 215** ©Martha Cooper/Peter Arnold

Chapter 13

Page 237 (left and right) Courtesy of the Alzheimer's Disease Education and Referral Center, a service of the National Institute on Aging; **page 243** From *An Introduction to Human Disease, Seventh edition.* Photo courtesy of Leonard V. Crowley, M.D., Century College.

Chapter 16

Page 287 ©Bilderbuch/age fotostock; **page 291 (left)** ©Robin Sachs/PhotoEdit, Inc.; **page 291 (right)** ©Monkey Business Images/Dreamstime.com; **page 295** ©Monkey Business Images/ShutterStock, Inc.

Chapter 17

Page 308 ©Pinkcandy/ShutterStock, Inc.; **page 310** ©Photos.com; **page 314** ©Alexander Raths/ShutterStock, Inc.; **page 318** Courtesy of MEIMSS.

Chapter 18

Page 323 ©Ron Chapple Studios/ShutterStock, Inc.; **page 333** ©Monkey Business Images/Dreamstime.com

Chapter 19

Page 338 ©Carme Balcells/ShutterStock, Inc.; **page 341 (top and bottom)** Courtesy of Professor Maria A. Fiatarone Singh; **page 343** ©LiquidLibrary; **pages 345, 348 (top and**